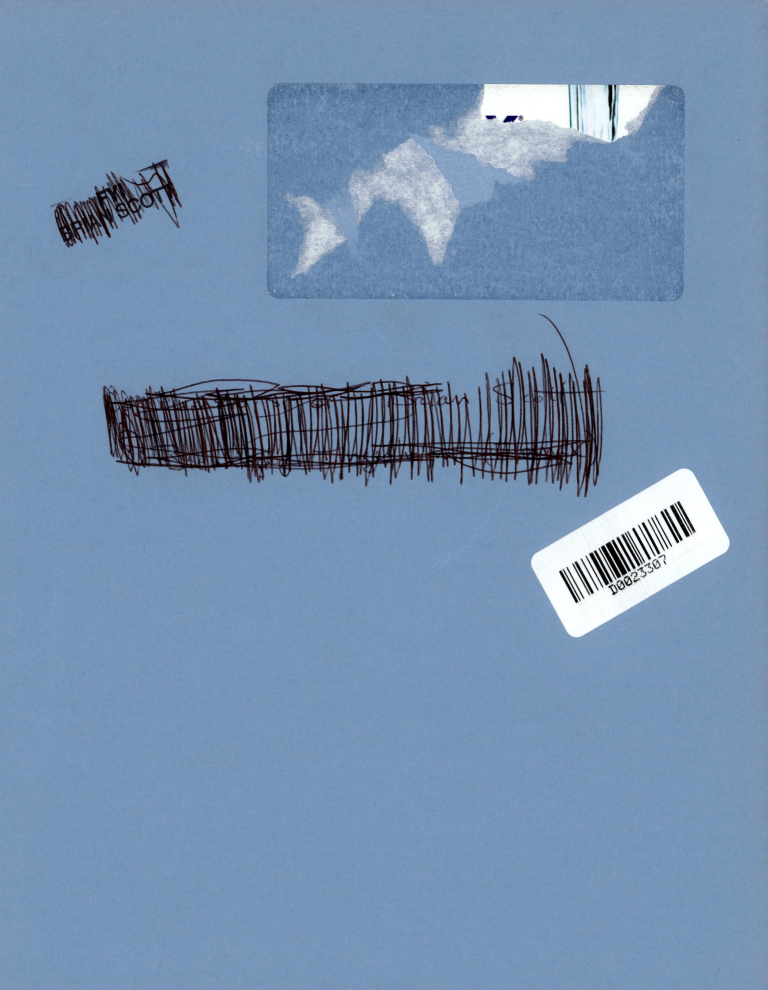

BRIAN SCOTT

TEXTBOOK OF BENIGN PROSTATIC HYPERPLASIA

Edited by

Roger Kirby MA MD FRCS (Urol) FEBU
Consultant Urologist, St. George's Hospital, London, UK

John McConnell MD
Professor and Chairman of Urology,
University of Texas Southwestern Medical Center
Dallas, Texas, USA

John Fitzpatrick MCh FRCSI FEBU
Professor of Surgery, University College, Dublin, Ireland
and Mater Misericordiae Hospital, Dublin, Ireland

Claus Roehrborn MD
Assistant Professor of Urology,
University of Texas Southwestern Medical Center,
Dallas, Texas, USA

Peter Boyle PhD
Director, Division of Epidemiology and Biostatistics,
European Institute of Oncology, Milan, Italy

Illustrated by Dee McLean and Creative Associates

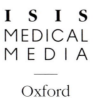

I S I S
MEDICAL
MEDIA

Oxford

© 1996 Isis Medical Media Ltd
58 St. Aldates
Oxford OX1 1ST, UK

First published 1996
Reprinted 1996, 1997, 1998

British Library Cataloguing in Publication Data
A catalogue record for this title is available from the British Library

ISBN   1 899066 24 1

Kirby R.S. (Roger)
Textbook of Benign Prostatic Hyperplasia/
Roger Kirby, John McConnell, John Fitzpatrick, Claus Roehrborn, Peter Boyle

Always refer to the manufacturer's Prescribing Information
before prescribing drugs cited in this book.

Typeset by
Creative Associates, Oxford, UK

Printed by
Jarrold Book Printing Ltd., Thetford, UK

Distributed in the USA by
Mosby-Year Book Inc.,
11830 Westline Industrial Drive
St. Louis MO 63146, USA

Distributed by
Oxford University Press
Saxon Way West
Corby, Northamptonshire NN18 9ES, UK

Contents

IV MEDICAL TREATMENT

V SURGICAL/INTERVENTIONAL OPTIONS

VI FUTURE DIRECTIONS

Preface

Ignored for decades by academia and industry alike, benign prostatic hyperplasia (BPH) has finally come of age as a subject worthy of sustained scrutiny.

Although seldom fatal, the disease is the cause of severe impairment of quality of life for many millions of men. Perhaps as a result of the "greying" of society, the 1990's have seen an exponential rise in interest in BPH — so much so that hardly a week goes by without some media focus on the problem.

In view of this we felt there was a need for a comprehensive text covering the disease itself, the methods of diagnosis and the myriad new therapies which have been developed over the past few years.

In this *Textbook of Benign Prostatic Hyperplasia* we have asked the world's leading experts in this disease to distill their knowledge and present a state-of-the-art overview of their own particular areas of interest. We hope the result will be of service to the very many urologists and physicians who daily face the challenge of diagnosing and managing this most prevalent disorder.

Roger Kirby
John McConnell
John Fitzpatrick
Claus Roehrborn
Peter Boyle

Contributors

Mohammed Al–Sudani MB FRCS
Urology Research Fellow, Department of Urology, The Lister Hospital, Corey's Mill Lane, Stevenage, Herts SG1 4AB, UK

Edwin P. Arnold MB ChB PhD FRCS FRACS
Associate Professor, Department of Urology, Christchurch Hospital, Private Bag 4710, Christchurch, New Zealand

Michael J. Barry MD
Director, Health Services Research Program, Medical Practices Evaluation Center, Massachusetts General Hospital, 50 Staniford Street, 9th Floor, Boston, MA 02114, USA

Michael L. Blute MD
Department of Urology, Mayo Clinic, 200 First Street Southwest, Rochester, MN 55905, USA

David G. Bostwick MD
Professor of Pathology, Department of Pathology, Mayo Clinic, 200 First Street Southwest, Rochester, MN 55905, USA

Peter Boyle PhD
Director, Divison of Epidemiology and Biostatistics, European Institute of Oncology, via Ripamonti 435, 20141 Milan, Italy

Reginald C. Bruskewitz MD
Professor of Surgery, Department of Surgery, Division of Urology, Clinical Science Center, 600 Highland Avenue, Madison, WI 53792, USA

Christopher R. Chapple BSc MD FRCS (Urol) FEBU
Consultant Urological Surgeon, Department of Urology, Royal Hallamshire Hospital, Glossop Road, Sheffield S10 2JF, UK

Timothy J. Christmas MD FRCS (Urol) FEBU
Consultant Urological Surgeon, Department of Urology, Charing Cross Hospital, Fulham Palace Road, London W6 8RF, UK

Leland W.K. Chung PhD
Professor of Urology, Biochemistry and Molecular Biology, The University of Texas, M.D. Anderson Cancer Center, 1515 Holcombe Boulevard, Houston, Texas 77030, USA

Louis J. Denis MD FACS
Professor of Urology, Vrije Universiteit Brussels; Chief, Department of Urology, A.Z. Middelheim, Antwerp 2020 , Belgium

Marian A. Devonec MD PhD
Service d'Urologie, Hôpital de l'Antiquaille, 1 rue de l'Antiquaille, Lyon, 69321, France

John S. Dixon BSc PhD
Senior Lecturer, Department of Anatomy, The Chinese University of Hong Kong, Shatin, New Territories, Hong Kong

Mark R. Feneley MD FRCS
Urology Research Registrar, Department of Urology, St Bartholomew's Hospital, West Smithfield, London EC1A 7BE, UK

Andrew Fitzpatrick MB BCh MRCGP DCH DObst (RCPI)
Peel View Medical Centre, Kirkintilloch, Glasgow, UK

John M. Fitzpatrick MCh FRCSI FEBU
Consultant Urologist and Professor of Surgery, Mater Misericordiae Hospital and University College, Dublin, Ireland

Clare J. Fowler MB BS MSc FRCP
Consultant in Uro-Neurology. The National Hospital for Neurology and Neurosurgery, Queen Square, London WC1N 3BG, UK

Michael R. Freeman PhD
Assistant Professor, Surgery, Children's Hospital, Boston; Harvard Medical School, Enders Research Laboratories, Rm. 1151, 300 Longwood Avenue, Boston MA 02115, USA

Martin Gleave MD FRCSC
Assistant Professor of Surgery, University of Columbia, Division of Urology, Vancouver Hospital and Health Sciences Center, D-9, 2733 Heather Street, D-8, Vancouver BC V5Z 3J5, Canada

John A. Gosling MB ChB MD FRCS (Edin)
Professor, Department of Anatomy, The Chinese University of Hong Kong, Shatin, New Territories, Hong Kong

Keith Griffiths BSc PhD DSc
Professor, Tenovus Cancer Research Centre, Tenovus Building, University of Wales, College of Medicine, Heath Park, Cardiff CF4 4XX, Wales, UK

Harry A. Guess MD
Department of Epidemiology, School of Public Health, University of North Carolina, Chapel Hill, NC 27599-7400, USA

H. Logan Holtgrewe MD FACS
Department of Urology, Johns Hopkins University School of Medicine, Baltimore, Maryland, USA

Alain Jardin MD
Professor and Chairman, Department of Urology, Hospital de Bicêtre, Universite Paris-Sud, 78 Rue General Leclerc, 94275 Kremlin-Bicêntre ,Cedex, France

Steven A. Kaplan MD
Herbert Irving Associate Professor of Urology, J. Bentley Squier Urological Clinic, College of Physicians and Surgeons, Columbia University, Columbia Presbyterian Medical Center, 622 West 168th Street, New York, NY, USA

Barry A. Kenny BSc PhD
Department of Discovery Biology, Central Research, Pfizer Limited, Sandwich, Kent CT13 9NJ, UK

Michael G. Kirby MB BS LRCP MRCS MRCP
The Surgery, Nevells Road, Letchworth, UK

Roger S. Kirby MA MD FRCS(Urol) FEBU
Consultant Urologist, St George's Hospital, Blackshaw Road, London SW17, UK

R. Karl Knight
Vice President and Director, ITRO Medical and Scientific Affairs, SmithKline Beecham Pharmaceuticals, 1250 Collegeville Road, PO Box 5089, Collegeville, PA 19426, USA

Yvonne J. Lamb
Medical Division, Smithkline Beecham Pharmaceuticals, Mundells, Welwyn Garden City, Hertfordshire, UK

Cheryl T. Lee MD
The Michigan Prostate Institute, The University of Michigan,1500 East Medical Center Drive, Ann Arbor, MI 48109-0330, USA

Herbert Lepor MD
Professor and Chairman, Department of Urology, NYU Medical Center, 550 First Avenue, New York, NY 10016, USA

Mark A. Levy PhD
Assistant Director, Department of Medicinal Chemistry, Smithkline Beecham Pharmaceuticals, 709 Swedeland Road, King of Prussia, PA 19406, USA

Ronald L. Lewis MD
Medical College of Georgia, Section of Urology, Room BA-8408, 1120 15th Street, Augusta, GA 30912-4050, USA

Thomas H. Lynch MCh FRCSI
Senior Registrar in Urology, Mater Misericordiae Hospital, Dublin, Ireland

John D. McConnell MD
Professor and Chairman, Southwestern Medical Center, 5323 Harry Hines Boulevard, Dallas, Texas, 75235-9110, USA

Tom A. McNicholas FRCS
Consultant Urological Surgeon, Department of Renal Medicine and Urological Surgery, Lister Hospital, North Hertfordshire Trust, Corey's Mill Lane, Stevenage, Herts SG1 4AB, UK.

Stephan Madersbacher MD
Department of Urology, University of Vienna, Währinger Gurtel, 18-20, A-1090 Vienna, Austria

Finn A. Madsen MD
Research Fellow, Division of Urology, G5/340 Clinical Science Center, 600 Highland Avenue, Madison WI 53792, USA

Patrick Maisonneuve PhD
Divison of Epidemiology and Biostatistics, European Institute of Oncology, via Ripamonti 435, 20141 Milan, Italy

Michael Marberger MD
Professor of Urology, Chairman, Department of Urology, University of Vienna, AKH, Wahringer Gurtel 18-20, A-1090 Vienna, Austria

James B. Meigs MD MPH
General Internal Medicine Unit,Unit S50-9, Massachusetts General Hospital, Boston, MA 02114, USA

Brian J. Miles MD
Associate Professor of Urology, Scott Department of Urology, Baylor College of Medicine, 6561 Fannin, Suite 1004, Houston, TX 77030, USA

Pavel Napalkov MD MSc
Divison of Epidemiology and Biostatistics, European Institute of Oncology, via Ripamonti 435, 20141 Milan, Italy

Alasdair M. Naylor BSc PhD
Department of Discovery Biology, Central Research, Pfizer Limited, Sandwich, Kent CT13 9NJ, UK

Jørgen Nordling MD
Chief Urologist, Department of Urology, Herlev Ringvej 75, DK-2730, Denmark

Joseph E. Oesterling MD
Professor and Chairman of Urology, The Michigan Prostate Institute, The University of Michigan, 1500 East Medical Center Drive, Ann Arbor, MI 48109, USA

Michael P. O'Leary MD MPH
Assistant Professor, Division of Urology, Brigham and Women's Hospital, 45 Francis Street, Boston, MA 02115, USA

M. Connie Parkinson
Institute of Urology and Nephrology, University College London Hospital Trust, Rockefeller Building, University Street, London WC1E 6JJ, UK

David Rickards MRCS FFRDSA FRCR
Consultant Uroradiologist, Department of Radiology, University College Hospital London, London W1N 8AA, UK

Claus G. Roehrborn MD
Assistant Professor of Urology, Southwestern Medical Center, 5323 Harry Hines Boulevard, Dallas, Texas, 75235-9110, USA

Jack A. Schalken MD
Research Director, Department of Urology, University Hospital Nijmegen, Geert Grooteplein 16, P.O. Box 9101, 6500 HB Nijmegen, The Netherlands

Claude C. Schulman MD
Professor of Urology, University Clinic of Brussels, Erasme Hospital, 808 route de Lennik, B-1070, Brussels, Belgium

Ellen Shapiro MD
Department of Urology, New York University School of Medicine, 550 First Avenue, New York, NY 10016, USA

Larry Sirls MD
Senior Staff Urologist, Co-Director, Urodynamics Laboratory, Urology K-9 Henry Ford Hospital, 2799 West Grand Boulevard, Detroit, MI 48202, USA

Barry S. Stein MD
Professor and Chief, Division of Urology, Brown University School of Medicine, 2 Dudley Street, Suite 175-185, Providence RI 02905, USA

Mitchell S. Steiner MD
Department of Urology, The University of Tennessee College of Medicine, Memphis, Tennessee, USA

Alexis E. Te MD
Assistant Professor of Urology, J. Bentley Squier Urological Clinic, College of Physicians and Surgeons, Columbia University, Columbia Presbyterian Medical Center, 622 West 168th Street, New York, NY, USA

Justin A. Vale MS FRCS (Urol)
Consultant Urological Surgeon, St Mary's Hospital, Praed Street, London W2, UK

Maureen C.W. Völler MD
Urology Research Laboratory, University Hospital Nijmegen, PO Box 9101, 6500 HB Nijmegen, The Netherlands

Michael G. Wyllie BSc PhD
Pfizer Inc, 235 East 42nd Street, New York, NY, 10017-5755, U S A

Alexandre R. Zlotta MD
Department of Urology, University Clinics of Brussels, Erasme Hospital, 808 route de Lennik, B-1070 Brussels, Belgium

Basic Science

I

Macro-anatomy of the prostate

J. S. Dixon J. A. Gosling

Introduction

The prostate is shaped like an inverted pyramid and lies between the urinary bladder and the pelvic floor (Fig. 1.1). It is a fibromuscular glandular organ that surrounds the prostatic urethra.

The prostate has a base and an apex, and anterior, posterior and inferolateral surfaces. The base is the upper surface adjacent to the bladder neck while the blunt apex is the lowest part. The anterior surface limits the retropubic space posteriorly and is connected inferiorly to the pubic bones by the puboprostatic ligaments. The inferolateral surfaces are clasped by the levator prostatae parts of the levator ani muscle, while the posterior surface lies in front of the lower rectum and is separated from it by the rectovesical fascia. The ejaculatory ducts pierce the posterior surface just below

the bladder and pass obliquely through the gland for about 2 cm to open separately into the prostatic urethra about half way along its length on the verumontanum.

A thin layer of connective tissue at the periphery of the prostate forms a 'true' capsule, outside which is a condensation of pelvic fascia forming the so-called 'false' capsule. A plexus of veins lies between these two capsules.

Blood supply and lymphatic drainage

The main arterial supply to the prostate is from the prostatic branch of the inferior vesical artery, with some small branches from the middle rectal and internal pudendal vessels passing to the lower part. Occasionally, the middle rectal artery provides the major supply. The veins from the prostate form the prostatic venous plexus

(a)   (b)

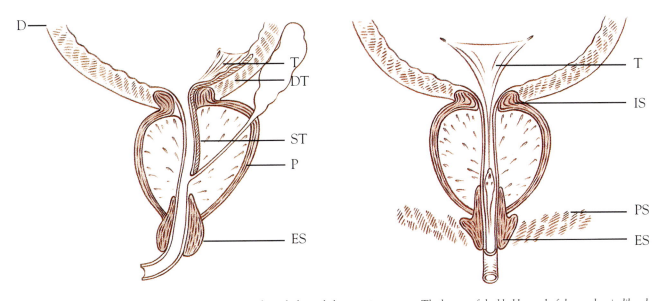

Figure 1.1. (a) Schematic diagram of a midline section through the male lower urinary tract. The lumen of the bladder and of the urethra is dilated and the right half of the trigone (T) is shown as a surface feature. The detrusor muscle (D) is in direct continuity with the deep trigone (DT). The superficial trigone (ST) extends inferiorly as far as the verumontanum. IS, internal sphincter; the external striated urethral sphincter (ES) surrounds the membranous urethra. (b) Viewed from in front, the trigone (T) is represented as a surface feature on the luminal aspect of the trigonal detrusor thickening. ES, distal or external striated urethral sphincter; IS, internal sphincter; PS, periurethral striated muscle.

situated between the true capsule of the prostate and the outer fibrous sheath.

The lymph vessels from the prostate drain into the internal iliac nodes.

The prostatic urethra

The prostatic urethra is the widest and most dilatable part of the entire male urethra. It is about 3 cm long and extends through the prostate from base to apex. The prostatic urethra is divided into proximal and distal segments of approximately equal length by an abrupt anterior angulation of its posterior wall at the midpoint between the prostate apex and bladder neck.[1] The angle of deviation is approximately 35 degrees, but can be quite variable and tends to be greater in men with nodular hyperplasia.[2] The prostatic urethra lies nearer the anterior than the posterior surface of the prostate. It is widest in the middle and narrowest below, adjoining the membranous part. In cross-section it appears crescentic in outline with the convex side facing ventrally (Fig. 1.2).

The characteristic crescentic shape is due to the presence on the posterior wall of a narrow median longitudinal ridge formed by an elevation of the mucous membrane and its subjacent tissue, called the urethral crest. On each side of the crest lies a shallow depression termed the prostatic sinus, the floor of which is pierced by the openings of the prostatic ducts. About the middle of the length of the urethral crest, the colliculus

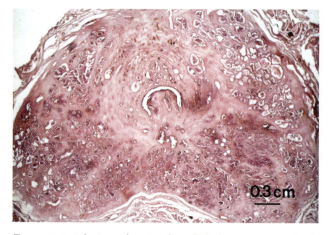

Figure 1.2. *A horizontal section through the human prostate gland. The prostatic urethra appears crescentic in outline. (H & E).*

seminalis (or verumontanum) forms an elevation on which the slit-like orifice of the prostatic utricle is situated. On each side of, or just within, this orifice are the openings of the two ejaculatory ducts. The prostatic utricle is a blind-ending diverticulum about 6 mm long which extends upwards and backwards within the substance of the prostate. It develops from the paramesonephric ducts or urogenital sinus and, as a consequence, is a remnant of the system that forms the reproductive tract in the female.

The proximal urethral segment is surrounded by a sleeve of smooth muscle fibres, forming the preprostatic sphincter. Tiny ducts and abortive acinar systems are scattered along the length of the proximal urethral segment and arborize exclusively inside the confines of the preprostatic sphincter, forming the periurethral gland region. The preprostatic sphincter is thought to function during ejaculation to prevent retrograde flow of seminal fluid from the distal urethral segment. It may also have resting tone, which maintains closure of the proximal urethral segment, thereby aiding urinary continence. The preprostatic sphincter is compact on the posterior aspect of the urethra, but anteriorly its fibres do not form complete rings but terminate within the tissue of the anterior fibromuscular stroma.

Slender bundles of smooth muscle cells also occur in the proximal part of the urethral crest, extending as far as the prostatic utricle where they become continuous with the muscle coat of the ejaculatory ducts. Proximally, these muscle bundles are continuous with those extending from the superficial trigone along the posterior wall of the preprostatic urethra.

Below the openings of the ejaculatory ducts the distal prostatic urethra possesses a thin coat of smooth muscle, consisting of both circularly and longitudinally orientated muscle bundles that are themselves continuous with the strands of smooth muscle pervading the prostate gland. The distal urethral segment is also surrounded by a sphincter formed of small-diameter, striated muscle fibres separated by connective tissue (Fig. 1.3), which represent a proximal extension of the external sphincter located distal to the prostate apex. The sphincter within the prostate gland is incomplete posterolaterally where the semicircular fibres anchor into the prostatic stroma.

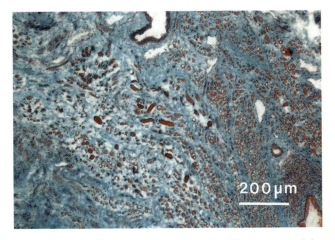

Figure 1.3. *Small-diameter striated muscle fibres, separated by connective tissue, surround the distal prostatic urethra. (Masson's trichrome stain).*

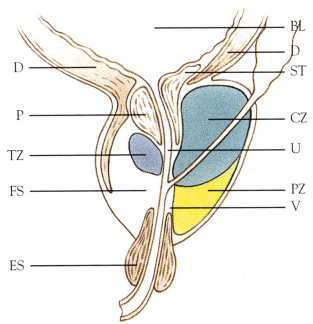

Histological structure of the prostate

In 1912 Lowsley[3] presented a detailed description of the anatomy of the human prostate, based on embryonic and foetal studies. However, his scheme of median and lateral prostatic lobes was found to be inadequate as a model for the anatomy of the adult human prostate. This early concept of prostatic structure was modified by the work of Franks[4] and by the more recent studies of McNeal[2,5–7] and Tissell and co-workers.[8,9] Although these latter authors used entirely different examination techniques, the results of their studies generally seem to coincide with those of McNeal.

McNeal studied prostates obtained at autopsy from adults and infants and from which large sections were taken in different planes. From his observations McNeal has described four distinct regions, each of which arises from a different segment of the prostatic urethra (Fig. 1.4). The largest part is the anterior or ventral fibromuscular and non-glandular region, which forms the ventral surface of the gland and which constitutes about one-third of the entire prostate.

The glandular prostate can then be subdivided into three zones, as follows:

1. A peripheral zone represents about 70% of the glandular part of the prostate. This zone forms the lateral and posterior or dorsal part of the organ. It may be regarded as a funnel that distally constitutes the apex of the prostate and cranially opens to

Figure 1.4. *Diagram of a sagittal section of prostate to show anatomical subdivisions: CZ, central zone; PZ, peripheral zone; TZ, transitional zone; V, verumontanum; FS, fibromuscular stroma; D, detrusor; P, preprostatic sphincter; ES, external sphincter; ST, superficial trigone; BL, bladder lumen; U, urethral lumen.*

receive the distal part of the wedge-shaped central zone. The ducts of the peripheral zone open into the distal prostatic urethra. They extend mainly laterally in the coronal plane, with major branches that curve anteriorly and minor branches that curve posteriorly.

2. A central zone comprises about 25% of the glandular prostate. This zone is wedge-shaped and surrounds the ejaculatory ducts with its apex at the verumontanum and its base against the bladder neck. Thus, the central zone is, at least in its distal part, surrounded by the peripheral zone and its ducts open into the prostatic urethra, in close proximity to the ejaculatory ducts.

The central zone, like the peripheral zone, has a funnel shape to accommodate the proximal segment of the urethra. Both funnels are incomplete ventrally, where their borders are held together by the fibromuscular stroma.

3. The smallest glandular part comprises only about 5–10% of the prostate and has been called a transitional zone. This zone consists of two independent small lobes whose ducts leave the

posterolateral recesses of the urethral wall at a single point, just proximal to the point of urethral angulation and at the lower border of the preprostatic sphincter. The main ducts of the transitional zone extend laterally around the distal border of the sphincter and curve sharply anteriorly, arborizing towards the bladder neck immediately external to the preprostatic sphincter and fanning out laterally. The most medial ducts and acini of the transitional zone curve medially to penetrate into the sphincter.

McNeal's concept of prostate anatomy was later confirmed by Blacklock and Bouskill,[10] although the presence of a transitional zone could not be confirmed by other workers.[11]

McNeal described distinct histological differences between the central and peripheral glandular zones that might indicate a difference in their functions.[6] In the peripheral zone and transitional zone, ducts and acini are usually 0.15–0.3 mm in diameter and have simple rounded contours that are not perfectly circular because of prominent undulations of the epithelial border. The undulations reflect the presence of corrugations of the wall that presumably provide for expansion of the lumina as secretory reservoirs. Central zone ducts and acini are distinctively larger than those of the peripheral zone and transition zone — up to 0.6 mm in diameter or larger. They become progressively larger and more elaborate as the duct territories expand toward the prostate base. Acini are clustered into lobules around a central subsidiary duct while both ducts and acini are polygonal in contour. The corrugations within the walls are very prominent and frequently form into intraluminal ridges that partially subdivide acini.

Glandular lobules in the central zone are separated by bundles of compact smooth muscle cells, but the ratio of epithelium to stroma is higher than in the peripheral and transitional zones. The more abundant peripheral zone stroma is loosely woven with randomly arranged smooth muscle bundles (Fig. 1.5). There is an abrupt contrast in stomal morphology, which delineates the boundary between the central zone and peripheral zone. However, the contrast between the peripheral and transitional zones is less obvious or consistent. The stroma of the transitional zone is composed of

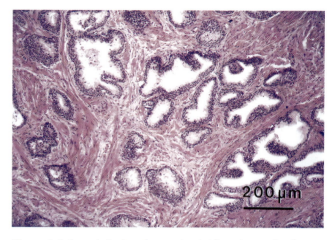

Figure 1.5. *Irregularly shaped prostatic acini from the peripheral zone. Randomly arranged smooth muscle bundles lie in the prostatic stroma. (H & E).*

interlacing bundles of compact smooth muscle cells that blend with the adjacent stroma of the preprostatic sphincter and anterior fibromuscular stroma. According to McNeal,[12] stomal distinctions are less evident in older prostates and may be obliterated by disease.

Tissell and Salander,[8,9] using a microdissection technique, were able to distinguish two dorsal, two lateral and two median lobes of the human prostate. The lobes are arranged in an onion pattern, with the median lobes lying centrally around the ejaculatory ducts and the lateral and dorsal lobes forming the outer layers. Each of these pairs of lobes was found to have its own histological characteristics,[13] which were subsequently confirmed by others.[14] Compared with the histological pattern of McNeal's central and peripheral zones,[5] the description of the histology of the median lobe given by Salander et al.[13] has obvious similarities to the central zone; similarly, the dorsal–lateral lobes correspond to the peripheral zone. Thus the two descriptions in general coincide, especially as McNeal has acknowledged that the peripheral zone might be subdivided into two zones.

The establishment of distinct anatomical and histological lobes or zones in the human prostate has led to studies of the relationship between prostatic disease and different parts of the gland, and also of the hormonal dependence of individual lobes and zones. Benign prostatic hyperplasia (BPH) largely arises in the preprostatic glandular tissue and the preprostatic urethra, and McNeal often found small nodules in this part of the organ. Furthermore, in almost half of the prostates studied by McNeal, small carcinomas — less than 0.1 cm^3 in volume — were detected, most of which originated in the peripheral zone and only a few in the central zone. Inflammatory changes were also most often seen in the peripheral zone.

The epithelium of the glandular prostate

Within each zone of the prostate, the entire duct–acinar system, with the exception of the main ducts near the urethra, is lined by columnar secretory cells, whose appearance is identical between ducts and acini. The secretory cells are separated from the basement membrane and prostatic stroma by a layer of basal cells. These cells are generally flattened and lie parallel to the basement membrane, with small dark-staining nuclei and little cytoplasm. These basal cells are often quite inconspicuous and may appear to be absent from some of the ducts and acini. They are considered to form the proliferative compartment of the prostate epithelium and divide to give rise to mature secretory cells.[15]

The secretory cells of the prostate contribute a wide variety of products to the seminal plasma, including citric acid, acid phosphatase and fibrinolysin that functions in the liquefaction of semen. Prostate-specific antigen (PSA) and prostatic acid phosphatase (PAP) are produced by the secretory cells of the ducts and acini of all zones, whereas pepsinogen II[16] and tissue plasminogen activator are normally produced only in the ducts and acini of the central zone.[17] Furthermore, it has been shown that significant differences exist between the peripheral and central zones with regard to lectin staining for cell membrane carbohydrates.[18]

Compared with other regions of the prostate, the secretory cells of the central zone have a darker, more prominently granular cytoplasm and each cell possesses a relatively large nucleus. The luminal epithelial border tends to be uneven with individual cells protruding into the lumen. The secretory cells of the peripheral zone, the transitional zone and the periurethral glands have smaller nuclei, uniformly situated towards the base. The cytoplasm is pale-staining and the cells present a relatively smooth luminal border.[12]

In all zones of the prostate, the epithelium contains a small population of randomly scattered endocrine–paracrine cells[19,20] that are rich is serotonin-containing granules and contain neuron-specific enolase.[19] Subpopulations of these cells also contain a variety of peptide hormones such as somatostatin,[20] calcitonin[21] and bombesin.[21] These cells normally occur in the basal cell layer and often possess laterally spreading dendritic processes (Fig. 1.6). However, they do not often appear to extend as far as the luminal surface. Their precise function remains unknown, although they are assumed to have a paracrine function, possibly in response to neural stimulation, thereby regulating the secretory processes of the mature gland. They may also have a significant role during prostatic growth and differentiation.

Spherical bodies called prostatic concretions (or corpora amylacea) normally occur in some of the prostatic acini. They vary greatly in size and may become calcified and exceed 1 mm in diameter. In sections they appear as concentric lamellated bodies that are believed to be condensations of prostatic secretory products.

The transitional epithelium, which lines the prostatic urethra and extends for a variable distance into the main prostatic ducts, differs histologically from that which lines the urinary bladder, and also differs from the lining of the female urethra. The transitional epithelial cells of the prostatic urethra and main ducts have

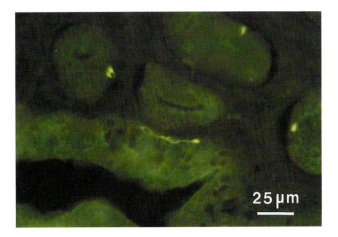

Figure 1.6. *Endocrine–paracrine cells with dendritic processes (bombesin immunocytochemistry) frequently occur in prostatic epithelium.*

relatively sparse cytoplasm with no evidence of maturation into luminal umbrella cells. Instead, the luminal surface is lined by a single layer of columnar secretory cells that appear identical to the secretory epithelium of the peripheral zone.

Innervation

The human prostate gland receives a dual autonomic innervation from both parasympathetic (cholinergic) and sympathetic (noradrenergic) nerves[11,22–26] via the prostatic nerve plexus, i.e. that part of the pelvic autonomic plexus that lies adjacent to the prostate gland. The pelvic plexus (and hence the prostatic plexus) receives parasympathetic input from the sacral segments of the spinal cord (S2–S4) and sympathetic fibres from the hypogastric (presacral) nerves (T10–L2).[27] These nerves ramify within the prostatic plexus, which contains both cholinergic and noradrenergic nerve cell bodies. The autonomic nerves that supply the prostate (and also the seminal vesicles, urethra and corpora cavernosae) arise from the pelvic plexus and travel together with the vascular supply. These neurovascular bundles approach the base of the prostate on its posterior aspect and generally lie in the same coronal plane as its rectal surface.[28] Most of the nerve branches to the prostate leave the neurovascular bundles at a level just above the prostate base and extend medially within a layer of fatty tissue. The nerve branches in these superior pedicles fan out over the prostatic capsule, which contains many autonomic ganglia embedded in a layer of fat. Some nerve branches continue medially over the prostate base to supply the central zone, while others fan out distally and penetrate the capsule at a very oblique angle. A few nerve branches leave the neurovascular bundles at the apex of the prostate via two small inferior pedicles and penetrate the capsule directly. Within the prostatic parenchyma, small nerve branches lie immediately adjacent to the walls of the ducts and acini while other nerves form branching plexuses among the smooth muscle bundles of the stroma.

According to Gosling,[25] both cholinergic (Fig. 1.7) and noradrenergic (Fig. 1.8) nerves innervate the smooth muscle bundles of the prostatic stroma, while cholinergic nerves also innervate the smooth muscle of

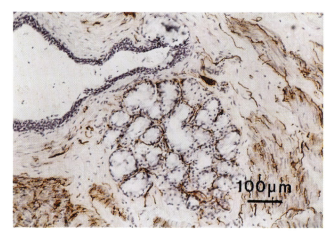

Figure 1.7. *Acetylcholinesterase-positive nerve fibres lie at the base of the prostatic acini and also occur in association with the smooth muscle bundles of the prostatic stroma.*

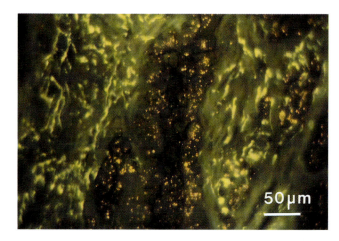

Figure 1.8. *Formaldehyde-induced fluorescence preparation showing a profusion of branching noradrenergic nerves in association with the prostatic smooth muscle bundles. The orange-coloured granules within the prostatic epithelial cells are autofluorescent lysosomes.*

the capsule. In addition, at least some of the glandular acini within the prostate receive a cholinergic secretomotor innervation. It is well known that parasympathetic stimulation increases the rate of secretion[29] and, under sympathetic stimulation (such as occurs during ejaculation), prostatic fluid is expelled into the urethra.[30] The importance of sympathetic nerves in the motor control of prostatic musculature has been demonstrated by in vivo,[31,32] in vitro and clinical studies[33–35] and forms the basis of the therapeutic use of alpha-blockade in the medical management of BPH. Although initial studies (in vitro) of prostatic capsule showed it to have a cholinergic component with an atropine-sensitive contractile response to nerve stimulation,[33] subsequent reports have failed to provide evidence that muscarinic cholinoceptor stimulation has a significant motor role within the prostate.[29,36] A decrease in the density of adrenergic and acetylcholinesterase-positive nerves has been reported in hyperplastic tissue in man.[37]

The human prostate gland is also supplied by nerves containing a variety of neuropeptides,[11,38–41] such as vasoactive intestinal polypeptide (VIP), neuropeptide Y (NPY) (Fig. 1.9), substance P (SP), calcitonin gene-related peptide (CGRP), somatostatin (SOM) and met- and leu-enkephalin (m-ENK and l-ENK). As in other organs, it seems likely that at least some of these peptides coexist within the classic cholinergic and noradrenergic nerve fibres and serve as neuromodulators, neurotransmitters or trophic factors. Both VIP and NPY are known to have motor functions elsewhere in the lower urinary and intestinal tracts. In the human urinary bladder, VIP produces a dose-related prolonged relaxation effect and is also a powerful vasodilator, whereas NPY is known as a pre- and postsynaptic modulator of adrenergic transmission. However, NPY is present not only in sympathetic nerves but also can occur in non-noradrenergic nerves. SOM, l-ENK and m-ENK have all been demonstrated in different minor populations of sympathetic nerves.

In contrast, CGRP and SP are principally co-localized in sensory nerve fibres. SP is also known to produce contraction of detrusor and intestinal smooth

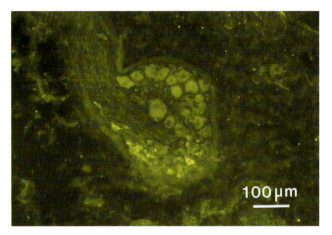

Figure 1.10. *An autonomic ganglion from the prostatic capsule containing both small dopamine-beta-hydroxylase (DBH)-positive (presumptive noradrenergic) and larger DBH-negative (presumptive cholinergic) nerve cell bodies.*

muscle. CGRP is a potent inhibitor of SP degradation and also a potent vasodilator. It seems likely that SP and CGRP fulfil a primarily sensory neurotransmitter role within the prostate during 'axon reflex' activity.[37]

The presence of intrinsic autonomic ganglion cells has also recently been reported in the human prostate[41] with a widespread distribution, occurring not only in the capsule but throughout the substance of the gland (Fig. 1.10). These ganglia contain both presumptive noradrenergic and cholinergic nerve cell bodies and, by analogy with intrinsic ganglia in other organs, it is likely that these nerve cells have an integrative and/or modulatory role in prostatic activity rather than acting as simple relay stations.[41]

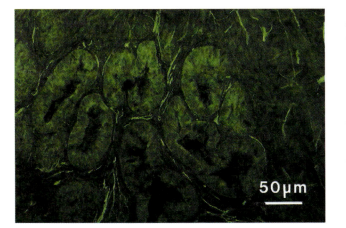

Figure 1.9. *Numerous NPY-immunoreactive nerve fibres lie at the base of these prostatic acini.*

References

1. Glenister T W. The development of the utricle and of the so-called 'middle' or 'median' lobe of the human prostate. J Anat 1962; 96: 443–455
2. McNeal J E. The prostate and prostatic urethra: a morphologic synthesis. J Urol 1972; 107: 1008–1016
3. Lowsley O S. The development of the human prostate gland with reference to the development of other structures at the next of the urinary bladder. Am J Anat 1912; 13: 299–349
4. Franks L M. Benign nodular hyperplasia of the prostate. A review. Ann R Coll Surg Engl 1954; 14: 92–106
5. McNeal J E. Regional morphology and pathology of the prostate. Am J Clin Pathol 1968; 49: 347–357
6. McNeal J E. Origin and evolution of benign prostatic enlargement. Invest Urol 1978; 15: 340–345
7. McNeal J E. Anatomy of the prostate: an historical survey of divergent views. Prostate 1980; 1: 3–13

8. Tissell L E and Salander H. The lobes of the human prostate. Scand J Nephrol 1975; 9: 185–191

9. Tissell L E, Salander H. Anatomy of the human prostate and its three paired lobes. In: Kimball F A, Buhl A E and Carter D B (eds) New approaches to the study of benign prostatic hyperplasia. New York: Alan R Liss, 1984: 55–65

10. Blacklock N J, Bouskill K. The zonal anatomy of the prostate in man and in the rhesus monkey. Urol Res 1977; 5: 163–167

11. Higgins J R A, Gosling J A. Studies on the structure and intrinsic innervation of the normal human prostate. Prostate 1989; (suppl 2): 5–16

12. McNeal J E. Prostate. In: Steinberg S S (ed) History for pathologists. New York: Raven Press, 1992: 749–763

13. Salander H, Johansson S, Tissell L G. The histology of the dorsal and medial prostatic lobes in man. Invest Urol 1981; 15: 479–484

14. Stegmayr B, Busch C, Fritjofsson A, Ronquist G. Biochemical and morphologic studies of the prostate gland in men subjected to radical cystectomy. Ups J Med Sci 1985; 90: 139–143

15. Dermer G B. Basal cell proliferation in benign prostatic hyperplasia. Cancer 1978; 41: 1857–1862

16. Reese J H, McNeal J E, Redwine E A et al. Differential distribution of pepsinogen II between the zones of the human prostate and the seminal vesicle. J Urol 1986; 136: 1148–1152

17. Reese J H, McNeal J E, Redwine E A et al. Tissue type plasminogen activator as a marker for functional zones within the human prostate gland. Prostate 1988; 12: 47–53

18. McNeal J E, Leav I, Alroy J, Skutelsky E. Differential lectin staining of central and peripheral zones of the prostate and alterations in dysplasia. Am J Clin Pathol 1988; 89: 41–48

19. Di Sant' Agnese P A, de Mesy Jensen K L, Churukian J. Human prostate endocrine–paracrine (APUD) cells: distributional analysis with a comparison of serotonin and neuron-specific enolase immunoreactivity and silver stains. Arch Pathol Lab Med 1985; 109: 607–612

20. Di Sant' Agnese P A, de Mesy Jensen K L. Somatostatin and/or somatostatin like immunoreactive endocrine–paracrine cells in the human prostate gland. Arch Pathol Lab Med 1984; 108: 693–696

21. Di Sant' Agnese P A. Calcitonin-like immunoreactive and bombesin-like immunoreactive endocrine–paracrine cells of the human prostate. Arch Path Lab Med 1986; 110: 412–415

22. Baumgarten H G, Falck B, Holstein A F et al. Adrenergic innervation of the human testis, epididymis, ductus deferens and prostate. A fluorescence microscopic and fluorimetric study. Z Zellforsch 1968; 90: 81–95

23. Gosling J A, Thompson S A. A neurohistochemical and histological study of peripheral autonomic neurons of the human bladder neck and prostate. Urol Int 1977; 32: 269–276

24. Vaalasti A, Hervonen A. Autonomic innervation of the human prostate. Invest Urol 1980; 17: 293–297

25. Gosling J A. Autonomic innervation of the prostate. In: Hinman F (ed) Benign prostatic hypertrophy. New York: Springer-Verlag, 1983: 349–360

26. Vaalasti A, Hervonen A. Nerve endings in the human prostate. Am J Anat 1980; 157: 41–47

27. Langley J N, Anderson H K. The innervation of the pelvic and adjoining viscera. VI Anatomical observations. J Physiol (Lond) 1896; 20: 372–406

28. Lepor H, Gregerman M, Crosby R et al. Precise localization of the autonomic nerves from the pelvic plexus to the corpora cavernosa: a detailed anatomical study of the adult male prostate. J Urol 1985; 133: 207–212

29. Smith E R, Lebeaux M T. The mediation of the canine prostatic secretion provoked by hypogastric nerve stimulation. Invest Urol 1970; 7: 313–318

30. Brushini H, Schmidt R A, Tanagho E A. Neurologic control of prostatic secretion in the dog. Invest Urol 1978; 15: 288–291

31. Donker P J, Ivanovici F, Noach E L. Analyses of the urethral pressure profile by means of electromyography and the administration of drugs. Br J Urol 1972; 44: 180

32. Furuya S, Kumamoto Y, Yokoyama E et al. Alpha-adrenergic activity and urethral pressure profilometry in prostatic zone in benign prostatic hypertrophy. J Urol 1982; 128: 836

33. Caine M, Raz S, Zeighler M. Adrenergic and cholinergic receptors in the human prostate, prostatic capsule and bladder neck. Br J Urol 1975; 47: 193

34. Caine M. Clinical experience with α-adrenoceptor antagonists in benign prostatic hypertrophy. Fed Proc 1986; 45: 2604

35. Caine M. The present role of α-adrenergic blockers in the treatment of benign prostatic hypertrophy. J Urol 1986; 136: 1

36. Hedlund H, Anderson K E, Larsson B. Alpha-adrenoceptors and muscarinic receptors in the isolated human prostate. J Urol 1985; 134: 1291

37. Chapple C R, Crowe R, Gilpin S A et al. The innervation of the human prostate gland — the changes associated with benign enlargement. J Urol 1991; 146: 1637–1644

38. Vaalasti A, Linnoila I, Hervonen A. Immunohistochemical demonstration of VIP, [Met^5]- and [Leu^5]-enkephalin immunoreactive nerve fibres in the human prostate and seminal vesicles. Histochemistry 1980; 66: 89–98

39. Gu J, Polak J M, Probert L et al. Peptidergic innervation of the human male genital tract. J Urol 1983; 130: 386–391

40. Adrian T E, Gu J, Allen J M et al. Neuropeptide Y in the human male genital tract. Life Sci 1984; 35: 2643–2648

41. Crowe R, Chapple C R, Burnstock G. The human prostate gland: a histochemical and immunohistochemical study of neuropeptides, serotonin, dopamine-β-hydroxylase and acetylcholinesterase in autonomic nerves and ganglia. Br J Urol 1991; 68: 53–61

2

Embryology and development of the prostate
E. Shapiro M. S. Steiner

Embryology of the prostate

The terminal end of the hindgut is termed the 'cloaca', which is the Latin word for sewer. Septation of the cloaca by the urorectal septum begins at about 28 days of gestation.[1] The rectum and primitive urogenital sinus (UGS) are evident by the 44th day of development. The primitive UGS proximal to the mesonephric duct becomes the vesicourethral canal, whereas the region distal of the mesonephric duct develops into the definitive UGS. The UGS adjacent to the bladder (the pelvic urethra) is narrow and develops into the lower portion of the prostatic and membranous urethra.[2] Embryologically, the cranial half of the pelvic urethra is derived from the endodermal UGS. Posteriorly, a component of mesonephric mesoderm originating from the bladder becomes incorporated into the pelvic urethra (superficial layer of the trigone). Later in development, this mesenchyme becomes smooth muscle that is continuous with the bladder (trigone). The caudal half of the pelvic urethra originates entirely from the UGS.[3,4]

At about the tenth week of gestation, the ductal network within the prostate originates from solid epithelial outgrowths, or prostatic buds. These prostatic buds emerge from the endodermal UGS immediately below the bladder and penetrate into the müllerian mesoderm which develops into the utricle and the mesonephric mesoderm which develops into the ejaculatory ducts.[5–9] The prostatic ducts rapidly lengthen, arborize and canalize. By 13 weeks, 70 primary ducts are present and exhibit secretory cytodifferentiation.[6,9] Prostate growth and development are dependent on androgen production by the foetal testes, which begins at about the eighth week of gestation.[10–14] Unlike development of the wolffian duct derivatives, which are dependent solely on testosterone, the differentiation of the UGS is dependent on the 5 alpha reduced form of testosterone, dihydrotestosterone (DHT). DHT is essential for the mediation of growth and development of the prostate from the pelvic portion of the UGS.[12,15,16]

Prostate morphology

Much of our understanding of prostatic ductal development has been derived from the detailed anatomical descriptions by Lowsley[9] in 1912. Lowsley serially sectioned the human foetal prostate and noted that, by 12 weeks, the branching ductal system consisted of five distinct groups. These lobes were termed the posterior, lateral (two), anterior and middle lobes. The ducts of the posterior lobes originate from the floor of the prostatic urethra distal to the openings of the ejaculatory ducts and grow posteriorly. The epithelial buds of the two lateral lobes branch lateral to the verumontanum. The ducts of the middle lobe originate on the posterior urethra proximal to the openings to the ejaculatory ducts. The anterior lobe buds branch anterior to the verumontanum. The anterior lobe is prominent until the 16th week and then involutes to become an insignificant structure by 22 weeks.

Although Lowsley's work in the foetus was meticulous and precise, it cannot be extrapolated to explain the morphology of the adult prostate gland. The distinct boundaries between the five prostate lobes that Lowsley defined cannot be identified 2.5 months postnatally, nor do the five distinct lobes exist in the prepubertal and normal young adult prostate.[5,17,18] None the less, the terms posterior, lateral, middle and anterior continue to be used to describe the lobes of the prostate, even though the middle and lateral lobes exist only in the ageing male. Although Lowsley's study emphasized the structural changes in the foetal prostate gland, Zondek and Zondek[19] examined the continuous influence of maternal placental and foetal hormones on prostatic growth. The investigators noted periodic acid–Schiff (PAS)-positive staining in the prostate as early as 14 weeks of gestation, which correlates with secretion and growth activity in the foetus. The incidence and degree of PAS-positive reactions increase as foetal development progresses.

Squamous metaplasia is found in the prostatic tubular epithelium at 22 weeks' gestation and increases as the foetus matures. The squamous metaplasia resolves by acantholysis and exfoliation, resulting in the disappearance of most foci by birth. The process appears to depend upon a delicate balance of oestrogen and testosterone. In congenital anomalies such as anencephaly, the foetus is exposed to excessive levels of circulating oestrogen in the face of abnormally low testosterone production due to the absence of gonadotropin stimulation. The prostates of foetuses with this anomaly contain extensive squamous metaplasia and cyst formation.

Zondek and Zondek[19] also examined tubular proliferation in the foetus. The foetal prostate is composed of only a few tubules widely separated by stroma. By term, glandular epithelium proliferates and interspersed stromal elements decline. More recently Xia et al.[20] qualitatively examined prostate growth, histogenesis and secretory activity in 107 specimens from normal foetuses ranging in age from 20 weeks' gestation to 1 month (postnatal). No sharply delineated 'lobules' were recognized, but two zones were apparent: these zones were identified as the inner submucosal zone (IZ) and the peripheral zone (PZ). The IZ was characterized by a concentric mass of fibromuscular connective tissue, which contained ducts at various stages of development. The PZ contained less concentrically organized fibromuscular connective tissue with secondary ducts, gland buds and groups of acinar glands. The PZ was further divided into anterior, posterior and two lateral regions.

These investigators[20] also recognized three states of development. During the bud state (20–30 weeks), the buds at the ends of the ducts were simple, solid and cellular, and contained no lumen. Columnar cells were seen basally, and spindle-shaped cells were found near the bud centre. The bud-tubule state (31–36 weeks) was characterized by small collections of cellular buds and acini in both the PZ and IZ. The histomorphogenesis of the foetal prostate further develops into the acinotubular state (37–42 weeks), in which distinct acinotubular gland clusters arise from the tubules with distinct lumina. Other investigators have noted that progression of ductal formation occurs, except in the periurethral zone. There, primitive rounded glands persist.

Xia et al.[20] also observed the presence of a glandular pattern in 25% of the foetal prostates, which resembled 'budding' atypical hyperplasia with 'back-to-back' glands, as described in the adult prostate. This pattern was seen as early as 24 weeks but occurred more frequently in glands of gestational age 37–42 weeks. PAS staining intensity was directly related to gestational age, with the region of greatest staining activity in the lateral lobes of the PZ. Prostate-specific antigen (PSA) was identified in only 20% of the specimens. When it was identified, it was usually seen in the older foetal or newborn gland. Squamous metaplasia was also noted and was always seen in association with the utricle and posterior wall of the urethra. Regions of involvement of the ducts with squamous metaplasia were variable. As the foetus progressed in gestational age, the areas of squamous metaplasia became less prominent. To date, this study is the most comprehensive examination of the embryological development of the foetal prostate.

Our understanding of prostate development has evolved from Lowsley and Venero's concept of five lobes and the organized progression of ductal budding to zonal histogenesis (IZ and PZ). These studies focus primarily on the ductal development of the gland. Popek et al.[21] examined not only development of the epithelium but also the qualitative morphological changes that occur in the mesenchyme or stroma during development. They observed that the primitive mesenchyme is initially very loose, with the epithelium budding into the stroma. As the ductal network progresses, the loose peripheral primitive mesenchyme is replaced by concentrically organized smooth muscle bundles around acini. The stroma maintains its primitive appearance in the periurethral region and does not undergo a change to smooth muscle. Two distinct smooth muscle bands are also noted: one is in association with the anterior fibromuscular stoma and one surrounds the utricle and ejaculatory ducts and is continuous with the smooth muscle of the seminal vesicles. Skeletal muscle is also seen peripherally in association with the prostatic capsule. Muscle-specific actin staining was noted as early as week 16, but mesenchymal expression was more notable by week 22. Prostate-specific acid phosphatase staining was seen in the larger ducts and cannulated acini by 17 weeks. PSA was generally absent in ductal and acinar cellular cytoplasm but was detected in areas of squamous metaplasia by 32 weeks.

Shapiro et al.[22] reported the application of computer image analysis that adapts Weibel's multipurpose test grid and line intersect stereological analysis to quantify the relative amounts of stroma and epithelium in prostate tissue. The original grey-density computer image analysis discriminated the epithelial and stromal elements of prostatic tissue sections stained with haematoxylin and eosin (H & E).

Shapiro et al.[23] recently developed a new technique for quantifying the cellular elements of the prostate. The technique involves double immunoenzymatic staining and computer-assisted colour image analysis. The epithelium and smooth muscle were labelled with rabbit anti-desmin and a mouse anti-human prostatic acid phosphatase (PSAP), respectively. A rabbit peroxidase–anti-peroxidase complex was linked to the rabbit anti-desmin by a secondary antibody to rabbit antibody. The peroxidase–anti-peroxidase complex was stained brown using the chromogen 3,3¹-diaminobenzidine tetrahydrochloride (DAB). A mouse alkaline phosphatase–anti-alkaline phosphatase (APAAP) complex was linked to the mouse anti-PSAP by a secondary antibody to mouse antibody. The APAAP complex was labelled using the chromogen fast red. The epithelium, glandular lumen, smooth muscle and connective tissue stained red, colourless, dark brown and light brown, respectively, using the double immunoenzymatic-staining technique. The thresholds for the computer-assisted colour image analysis were set to discriminate the different staining properties of the prostatic cellular elements.

Literature examining the morphometry of the prepubertal prostate is scarce.[24] The only comprehensive study of prostatic morphometry in the prepubertal male has recently been reported by Shapiro et al.[25] Quantitative morphometric studies were performed on paediatric prostates obtained from autopsy examinations. Double immunoenzymatic staining using anti-actin and anti-PSAP, as described previously,[23] was used to label the tissue components. Colour image analysis was performed to discriminate the staining properties of the epithelium, smooth muscle, connective tissue and lumen. This study demonstrated age-related changes in the density of smooth muscle that appear to parallel the postnatal testosterone surge (age 30–60 days) and the rise in testosterone at the onset of puberty.[12–14] The density of prostate smooth muscle was significantly increased in the first year of life. A progressive decrease in smooth muscle was observed throughout childhood and puberty, with a subsequent increase in the density of smooth muscle following puberty. Throughout age 1–20 years, the size of the stromal compartment remains stable. Therefore, as the age-dependent smooth muscle increases, the connective tissue component changes in an inverse fashion. No significant changes were seen in the epithelium or glandular lumen during these periods. These studies demonstrate that the paediatric prostate is a dynamic gland, and the relationship between changes in cellular content and hormone milieu may be important to our understanding of benign prostatic hyperplasia (BPH).

In addition to these observed dynamic changes in morphometry, the early testosterone surge in the young infant may be a critically important 'imprinting' event that may have an impact on the gland's propensity for future abnormal prostatic growth and disease. Hormonal imprinting has been studied in the rat.[26] Naslund and Coffey[27] showed that early hormonal surges are requisite for normal adult prostate growth in the rat and that an alteration in the normal endocrine events that occur shortly after birth can have significant and permanent effects on the androgen sensitivity and growth of the adult prostate. These hormonal surges are thought to affect prostatic growth by altering the properties of the prostatic stem cells. The absolute number of these stem cells is important because it ultimately determines the size of the gland. Hormonal events occurring before puberty can therefore imprint or programme the prostatic size, androgen sensitivity and function and maintenance of the stem cells.

In order to elucidate further the growth and development of the foetal prostate, Shapiro et al.[28] step-sectioned foetal prostates of 9.5–40 weeks' gestation to determine the macroscopic growth rate and quantitative morphometry using colour image analysis. Three-dimensional reconstruction of the foetal prostate gland has been performed to define the structural changes throughout the gland in the smooth muscle, connective tissue and urethral lumen, as well as to define ductal budding and morphogenesis.[28] Preliminary observations indicate that the mean cross-sectional area (csa) of the foetal prostate increases significantly in early gestation:[28] at gestation age 9.5, 11.5, 13.0 and 16.5 weeks, the csa is 0.42, 1.20, 1.96 and 4.95 mm^2, respectively.

The histological composition of these prostates has been determined using double immunoenzymatic staining and colour-assisted computer image analysis.[23] The authors have shown that the connective tissue comprises a significant component (approximately 65%) of the foetal gland (gestational age 9.5–16.5 weeks), whereas the smooth muscle component during these early weeks of prostatic development comprises only 25%. The epithelium and lumen together represent about 5–10% of the gland. Although the morphometry of the older foetus has yet to be determined, the stromal compartment of the gland of the neonate/infant (age 0–1 year) is known to be slightly smaller (80%), and is composed of almost 50% smooth muscle and 30% connective tissue. This again denotes dynamic changes in the stromal compartment during foetal development.

Timms et al.[29] have also investigated ductal budding and branching patterns in the developing prostate using three-dimensional computer-assisted serial section reconstruction. They studied foetal mice and rats and also examined two human foetuses (crown–rump length 70 and 100 mm). Timms and colleagues showed that ventral, lateral and dorsal lines of epithelial buds follow a ventro-dorsal and cranial–caudal axis. Their findings suggest that prostate ductal budding exhibits patterns compatible with the current concept of zonal anatomy.[30–33]

Over the past decade, McNeal[30–33] has expanded our understanding of adult prostate morphology. He described the zonal anatomy of the prostate based on examination of the gland in different planes of section. The urethra represents the primary anatomical reference point, dividing the prostate into an anterior fibromuscular and posterior glandular portion. The urethra angulates sharply (35 degrees). The point of angulation divides the urethra into proximal and distal segments of about equal length. The two principle regions of the glandular prostate are defined as the PZ

(approximately 75% of the total glandular volume) and the central zone (CZ) (approximately 25% of the total volume). The two regions have unique morphometric properties. The CZ and its ductal orifices are in close association with the ejaculatory ducts and their orifices near the verumontanum in the distal urethral segment that extends from the prostatic apex to the verumontanum. The PZ ducts enter the urethra separately from those of the CZ and are in association primarily with the distal urethral segment.

The acinar morphology of the CZ and PZ is also unique.[32,33] The CZ is composed of ducts that branch into large, irregularly contoured acini, whereas the PZ ducts branch into small, round, regular acini. The epithelial cells in the CZ have granular cytoplasm and enlarged nuclei located at various levels from the basement membrane, whereas the epithelial cells of the PZ have clear cytoplasm and small, dark nuclei located uniformly along the basal aspect of the basement membrane. Finally, the stroma of the CZ is long and compact and closely associated with the acini, whereas that of the PZ is random, with loose interconnections. These morphological histological differences between the PZ and CZ may be explained by the different embryonic origins. The ejaculatory ducts traverse the centre of the CZ, and the epithelium of the CZ is similar to that of the seminal vesicle, suggesting a wolffian duct origin. The PZ presumably is derived from the UGS.

The anatomical area of the prostate represented by the transitional zone (TZ) accounts for less than 5–10% of the glandular volume and is intimately related to the proximal urethral segment.[32,33] The cylinder of striated muscle surrounding the proximal urethral segment is termed the 'preprostatic sphincter'. Its function is to prevent the retrograde flow of semen by contracting during ejaculation. Just lateral to this sphincter are two small lobes that histologically are similar to the PZ. The stroma in the TZ is dense and compact. The TZ is adherent to the external aspect of the periprostatic sphincter, and its glands penetrate the sphincter, whereas the peripheral fibres of the sphincter penetrate the TZ stroma.

The periurethral region of the prostate comprises less than 1% of the total glandular volume.[32,33] This region contains tiny ducts arising from the proximal urethral segment that are embedded in the periurethral smooth muscle. The periurethral glands are histologically similar to those of the PZ and TZ. This is not unexpected, since the TZ and periurethral gland region have a common embryonic UGS origin. It is these two areas that are the exclusive sites of origin of BPH. Hyperplastic nodules develop in these areas as early as the fourth decade. Periurethral nodules are stromal and resemble embryonic mesenchyme, whereas TZ nodules are glandular. Nodule genesis is focal and occurs randomly within areas of susceptibility. The initial abnormality in nodule genesis may be spontaneous reversion of a clone of stromal cells to the embryonic state. Growth potential can then be mediated through coordinated stromal–epithelial interactions. This postulation is supported by qualitative observations of ductal development that is tangential to nodule borders. These ducts may show epithelial hyperplasia and budding of new branches on only the duct wall facing the centre of the nodule. These eccentric effects suggest that an induction or interaction is occurring on only one side of the duct. The hallmark of embryonic development is the formation of new architecture. It seems logical that the development of BPH nodules, which is repressed until the fourth or fifth decade of life, may be a 'reawakening of embryonic capabilities' in the adult.

Stromal–epithelial interactions in prostate development

The formation of new ductal acinar architecture of BPH deviates from that in the normal development of most organs.[32] First, the acinar development of the prostate should be completed during puberty. The prostate is the only organ that demonstrates new growth as part of the ageing process. Furthermore, formation of the ductal system in BPH differs from that of the embryonic prostate. The ducts of the embryonic prostate branch parallel and away from each other rather than towards each other, as seen in BPH nodules.

Although the specific biochemical factors initiating new growth of the prostate are unknown, there is increasing evidence that stromal cells are intimately involved. The inductive role of the stromal cells in the adult prostate, resulting in new nodule formation, is, as mentioned above, thought of as an 'embryonic reawakening'. These investigations by Cunha[15,34–44]

have examined the interaction between epithelium and mesenchyme, as well as the androgenic mediation of the events that result in prostatic growth and development.

Fundamental to an understanding of the stromal and epithelial interactions is the fact that the development of the prostate, as well as of the male internal ductal system, is androgen dependent.[45] Chemical or surgical castration of the foetus during the critical periods of sexual development results in the inhibition of development of the prostate and other male accessory sex glands.[46–53] During the postnatal period, androgen remains important for prostate growth, as castration at this time will inhibit growth and development.[45,54,55] Although the foetal testis elaborates testosterone, it is DHT that is the active intracellular androgen responsible for prostatic morphogenesis. The enzyme 5 alpha-reductase has been found in the UGS and external genitalia of humans.[12,16,39] Inhibition of this enzyme in the male rat results in feminization of the external genitalia and urethra and the partial inhibition of prostatic development.[56] Although DHT is important for prostatic growth, the developing prostate may be responsive to exceedingly low levels of DHT or other androgens.[56] Furthermore, some aspects of postnatal growth may be independent of androgen, as castration in the rat during this period does not completely inhibit prostate development.[45,54,55] This suggests that other non-androgen growth factors such as peptide growth factors are capable of mediating arborization and growth of prostatic ducts.

A human model to study the sexual differentiation of males who lack DHT is provided by those individuals with 5 alpha-reductase deficiency.[57,58] This syndrome is a form of autosomal recessive male pseudo-hermaphroditism characterized by severe penoscrotal hypospadias, a blind vaginal pouch and normal testes with normal epididymides, vasa deferentia and seminal vesicles. The ejaculatory ducts terminate in the blind-ending vagina, and the prostate is small or undetectable. Overall, the phenotypic appearance is female without breast development. Because the defect in virilization during embryogenesis is limited to the UGS and the anlage of the external genitalia, the selective effects of testosterone and DHT can be understood.

Testicular feminization syndrome (Tfm) is another disorder resulting in complete failure of the prostate to develop.[59] Androgen receptors (ARs) are defective or absent in this syndrome. The wolffian ducts undergo degeneration. Although the testes elaborate normal amounts of testosterone, the external genitalia are feminized. Testicular feminization and 5 alpha-reductase deficiency syndromes provide a clinical basis for understanding the profound effect of DHT on prostate morphogenesis.

In addition to human models that delineate the importance of androgen for prostatic development, analysis of tissue recombinant experiments utilizing Tfm mice have demonstrated the role of stromal–epithelial interactions.[60] These mice have defective ARs and fail to develop prostates. When tissue recombinants constructed of wild-type mesenchyme and Tfm epithelium are exposed to physiological androgen levels as a result of grafting of the recombinants into intact male hosts, normal prostatic morphogenesis ensues.[37,43,61] Prostates do not form when the Tfm mesenchyme is used with either the Tfm or the wild-type epithelium. These findings show that the mesenchyme is the actual target and elaborates other local growth factors that mediate androgen effects on the epithelium. The importance of DHT in prostate development is further supported by the presence of DHT-receptor-binding sites in wild-type UGS.[62–65] Such binding sites are absent in the Tfm urogenital mesenchyme.[43]

Our current understanding of the pre- and postnatal development of the prostate has evolved from investigations using the rat and mouse model.[42,66,67] These studies have delineated the lobar and ductal development, hormonal receptor status and sex steroid requirements for growth. In the rodent, prostatic morphogenesis continues from late foetal life until sexual maturity.[42] In these rodent species the prostatic ducts are organized and encapsulated into individual lobes that emerge centrally from the urethra and extend peripherally before branching. Microdissections of these glands have shown a compound ductal system lacking true acini.[66] Each of the four paired lobes has a distinct ductal branching pattern. The ducts are lined with pseudostratified columnar secretory epithelium and each duct is surrounded by a layer of smooth muscle.[68–72] Along the basement membrane are non-secretory basal epithelial cells that may function as reserve or stem cells

capable of differentiation. The epithelial morphology varies along the proximal–distal axis of the ducts, accompanied by differences in the function of the cells. For example, plasma membrane proteins,[42] secretory proteins[73] and proteins governing cell death and degeneration[73–75] are differentially expressed in specific regions along the duct. Therefore, growth, secretion and cell death occur heterogeneously throughout the gland, due to their regionalization. The stoma consists of fibroblasts, smooth muscle cells, blood vessels, connective tissue, nerve terminals and lymphatics with an extracellular matrix of collagen.[76] The stroma is subdivided into periacinar and interacinar stroma.[77] The periacinar stroma constitutes several layer of smooth muscle separated from the ductal epithelium by the basal lamina.[69,78]

Endocrinology of prostatic development

Development of the prostate prenatally as well as postnatally is androgen dependent.[11,12,14,42] DHT is the active intracellular androgen. Castration of neonatal mice inhibits continued growth and development, although some aspects of neonatal growth may be androgen independent.[42,55,79] In rodents, ARs are expressed prenatally in the mesenchyme but not in the epithelium.[62–65] These epithelial ARs appear at the end of the first postnatal week when duct canalization starts to occur.[62]

The timetable and distribution of AR expression have been further studied by Cooke et al.[80] They showed that functional foetal mouse ARs (capable of ligand binding) are present on gestational days 13–14 in the UGS and wolffian duct (WD) mesenchyme, but not in the epithelium. At this early time, only AR mRNA is present in the epithelium. When functional epithelial ARs appear, they do so in a cranial–caudal direction in the WD and UGS over the late foetal/early neonatal periods.

Since differentiation, growth and early morphogenesis of the UGS and WD structures are androgen dependent, early androgen effects must be mediated through the ARs of the mesenchyme of these structures.[80] This is supported by the elegant tissue recombinant experiments by Cunha,[42,43] in which prostate developed from normal UGS mesenchyme

(UGM) and Tfm UGS epithelium grafted into a male host. These experiments demonstrate the critical paracrine relationship between the mesenchyme and epithelium during androgen-dependent morphogenesis.

Regional differences in androgen sensitivity have been demonstrated along the ductal axis.[66,73,75] The proximal duct is relatively androgen independent, whereas the distal duct tips are highly androgen dependent. Prins et al.[81] have shown no differences in functional AR levels and 5 alpha-reductase levels along the ducts in the 15-, 30- or 100-day-old rat.

Recent investigations by Prins and Birch,[82] using antibodies to rat ARs, have shown that in the rat the basal epithelium expresses ARs as early as day 1. These ARs may act as direct targets of androgen effects of the epithelium during prostate development, even though initial epithelial AR induction may be an androgen-dependent process mediated by AR+ mesenchyme during late foetal life. Luminal epithelium does not appear until days 5–10; when present, it stains intensely for ARs. In addition, periductal mesenchyme shows differentiation into smooth muscle by days 3–5. These smooth muscle cells are also strongly AR+, whereas interductal fibroblasts have fewer AR+ cells. These smooth muscle cells may be important targets for androgen-mediated morphogenesis.

Prins' study[82,83] also examined the effects of neonatal oestrogen exposure on the development of the ARs. Oestrogen receptors (ERs) have been shown to be strongly expressed in the mouse prostate mesenchyme.[84] Whereas the stroma is strongly ER+, the prostate smooth muscle is weakly to negatively staining after differentiating from mesenchyme. Fibroblasts remain strongly ER+. The epithelium of the prostate never expresses ER. Brief exposure to neonatal oestrogen will downregulate ARs and permanently alter its expression, as well as retarding ductal development.[82,83] Smooth muscle development proceeds without significant delay, as does the development of basal cells. Oestrogenization does not block epithelial cell differentiation (determined by the appearance of luminal cell cytokeratins) completely, indicating that initiation of cytodifferentiation precedes elevated AR expression, rather than increasing ARs triggering cytodifferentiation. These experiments do suggest that functional differentiation is dependent on AR expression in

epithelial cells. The ventral prostate epithelial cells express prostate-binding protein only after cytodifferentiation of distal duct tips occurs where AR immunostaining was seen.

These studies support previous observations by Donjacour and Cunha,[85] using tissue recombinant techniques. Although UGM from normal mice instructively induced prostate morphology in WT, as well as the Tfm urinary tract epithelium, tissue recombinants of UGM and Tfm bladder or urethral epithelium cannot produce complete prostate cytodifferentiation or secretory proteins. Epithelial ARs are, therefore, important to the final states of morphogenesis and the initiation of prostate secretory activity.

Tissue recombinant experiments have also been used to examine the role of epithelial–mesenchymal interactions on the differentiation and organization of prostatic smooth muscle.[86] Experiments combined adult prostatic epithelium with UGM or seminal vesicle mesenchyme (SVM) or bladder epithelium with UGM or SVM. Prostatic ducts developed in all tissue recombinants when UGM was used with either epithelium. Smooth muscle cells also organized into sheets resembling prostate. When SVM was combined with either epithelium, the prostatic ducts were surrounded by thick smooth muscle cells resembling seminal vesicle. The smooth muscle was unorganized in grafts of SVM or UGM. These experiments suggest that male urogenital gland mesenchyme dictates spatial organization, but smooth muscle differentiation is induced by epithelium. Urothelium may also direct the organization in, for example, the bladder. This may occur as urothelium is probably a potent inducer of smooth muscle differentiation. Cunha[42] has in fact shown that the proximal segments of prostatic ducts near the urethra express urothelial membrane antigen and have associated thick layers of smooth muscle cells surrounding them.

Role of growth factors in prostatic development

Peptide growth factors may be direct mediators of androgen action and may be responsible for mediating the epithelial–mesenchymal microenvironment through either autocrine or paracrine pathways.[87–90] These growth factors have been shown to be regulated by androgens, suggesting that androgens may only indirectly influence growth. These growth factors are part of a large family of proliferating and differentiating regulatory factors. There is strong experimental evidence that peptide growth factors may be important in prostate growth. Almost a decade ago, Norman et al.[91] combined mouse UGM with an adult prostate epithelial duct tip. The mesenchyme induced ductal proliferation and arborization of adult epithelium, which demonstrated that the adult prostate has the potential for new growth by 'reawakening' of early prostatic embryonic mesenchymal–epithelial interactions.[29–33,42] These findings — that adult prostates treated with androgens do not grow but that embryonic mesenchyme is effective in inducing growth of the adult prostate — suggest that the mesenchyme may elaborate other local factors that stimulate adult prostatic growth.

For the following reasons, peptide growth factors appear to be those local factors directly responsible for mediating the mesenchymal and epithelial interactions that are important for prostate development:

1. Peptide growth factors are expressed in either mesenchymal or epithelial components of developing prostate.[42,44,92]

2. Isolated prostatic, epithelial and stromal cells respond to peptide growth factors in vitro.[44,93]

3. Prostatic mesenchymal and epithelial cells express specific membrane receptors for peptide growth factors.[94–96]

4. Neutralizing antibodies for a peptide growth factor or its receptor inhibit biological effects.[97–100]

5. Overexpression of peptide growth factors in transgenic mice perturbs prostatic growth and development.[101–103]

6. Androgens directly influence the expression of peptide growth factors by prostate cells.[100,104,105]

7. Androgen production is modulated by peptide growth factors.[106,107]

Epidermal growth factor (EGF), fibroblast growth factor (FGF), insulin-like growth factor (IGF) and transforming growth factor-beta (TGFβ) family members have been detected in normal prostate.[108–110] The interplay between the stimulatory growth factors [EGF, transforming growth factor-alpha (TGFα), IGF, and FGF] and inhibitory growth factors (TGFβ-1–3) regulate the epithelial and mesenchymal interactions responsible for prostatic development.[111] Although TGFα and EGF utilize the same EGF receptor to enhance prostate cell proliferation, TGFα is preferentially expressed during periods of prenatal and postnatal prostate epithelial development.[112] TGFα appears to stimulate prostatic ductal proliferation during development, since overproduction of TGFα in prostates from TGFα transgenic mice resulted in prostatic ductal hyperplasia.[103] Interestingly, FGF family members are mitogenic for both prostatic epithelial and mesenchymal cells.[97,113,114] Perhaps the strongest evidence for their role in the embryonic reawakening of mesenchymal and epithelial interactions leading to prostate growth is based on transgenic mice that overproduce int-2, which is FGF-like growth factor.[101,102] These int-2 transgenic mice exhibit exuberant prostatic hyperplasia with prostates up to 20-fold larger than those of control animals. The prostatic hyperplasia observed is similar to human BPH in many respects.[101,102] Another FGF family member, keratinocyte growth factor, is unique as it is produced by stromal cells but stimulates only epithelial growth.[115] Similarly, IGF appears to stimulate prostatic epithelial proliferation selectively.[116] This suggests that peptide growth factors can specifically influence either epithelial or mesenchymal cells during prostatic development.

TGFβ family members have multifunctional biological properties. TGFβ inhibits normal prostatic epithelial growth, but stimulates prostatic mesenchymal cells.[111] Steiner[117] has performed preliminary studies focusing on defining the important factors for prostate development. He has utilized TGFβ-1 transgenic mice, which overexpress TGFβ-1.[118,119] Overexpression of TGFβ-1 appears to alter prostate development by decreasing prostate ductal branching and increasing smooth muscle surrounding the acinar ducts.[101–103,117] Moreover, the anterior prostate had evidence of only primary ductal branching — the involuted or 'aborted' ductal branching — as seen in the development of distal ductal tips in androgen-deprived animals.[117]

The effects of androgens on growth factors have generally been investigated in adult rats when glandular growth is minimal.[44] This is the case with studies on TGFβ that have shown that, following castration, there is a cascade of events, one of which is a marked increase in the level of TGFβ-1 mRNA expression and TGFβ-1 receptor binding sites in the rat ventral prostate.[100,105,120] TGFβ-1 has also been shown to inhibit normal proliferation of prostatic epithelial cells in culture. Foster and Cunha (unpublished data) have recently investigated the role of TGFβ-1 during prostate development.[90] Rat anterior prostate is grown in vitro in a serum-free culture. The newborn rat anterior prostate consists of mesenchyme and unbranched epithelial buds. When testosterone is added for 6 days, ductal branching morphogenesis occurs. The trophic effect of testosterone and DHT can be inhibited by adding TGFβ-1 to the culture medium. This blocking effect occurs in a dose-dependent fashion. Thus, TGFβ has a role in limiting ductal proliferation and arborization as well as stimulating mesenchymal cell growth (smooth muscle).

Peptide growth factors appear to be the direct mediators of androgen action. Following androgen withdrawal, the production of stimulatory peptide growth factors EGF, IGF and FGF by prostate cells decreases whereas there is an increase in the expression of the inhibitory peptide growth factor TGFβ-1 and TGFβ-2 receptors.[104,109,121,122] The net effect of these peptide growth factor alterations is prostatic involution. Androgen replacement re-establishes normal EGF, IGF and FGF levels and suppresses TGFβ-1, and the prostate regrows towards its original size.[111]

Peptide growth factors may be the embryonic inducers that initiate adult prostatic growth. FGF and TGFβ family members have been implicated in the development of BPH.[111] Mori et al.[123] have reported that basic FGF (bFGF) and TGFβ-2 mRNA are elevated in human BPH. Moreover, extracts of human BPH contain bFGF-like activity that enhances growth of human prostate epithelial cells and prostate-derived fibroblasts in culture.[97] TGFβ is known to stimulate production of bFGF mRNA and protein in prostate-derived stromal cells.[124] Thus, a stromal BPH nodule may be formed when bFGF and TGFβ-2 both stimulate stromal proliferation. The degree of interplay between TGFβ-2 and bFGF will have differential effects on prostatic epithelial–stromal interactions, resulting in varying amounts of stromal and glandular hyperplasia.

Although the exact role of peptide growth factors in prostate development remains to be elucidated, peptide growth factors will almost certainly be a critical component. A greater understanding of peptide growth factors using transgenic mice and other models will help to define the precise contribution of these growth factors to normal and abnormal prostatic growth.

References

1. Stephens F D. Congenital malformations of the urinary tract. New York: Praeger, 1993
2. Hamilton W J, Mossman H W. The urogenital system. In: Human embryology: prenatal development of form and function, 4th ed. New York: Macmillan, 1976: 201
3. McNeal J E. The prostate and prostatic urethra: a morphologic synthesis. J Urol 1972; 107: 1008
4. McNeal J E. Developmental and comparative anatomy of the prostate. In: Grayhack J T, Wilson J D, Scherbenske M J (eds) Benign prostatic hyperplasia. NIAMDD Workshop Proceedings, 20–21 Feb 1975. DHEW. Publication No. NIH 76-1113. Washington: US Government Printing Office, 1976; 1–9
5. Johnson F P. The later development of the urethra in the male. J Urol 1920; 4: 447
6. Kellokumpu-Lehtinen P. The histochemical localization of acid phosphatase in human fetal urethral and prostatic epithelium. Invest Urol 1980; 17: 435–440
7. Kellokumpu-Lehtinen P. Development of sexual dimorphism in human urogenital sinus complex. Biol Neonate 1985; 48: 157
8. Kellokumpu-Lehtinen P, Santti R, Pelliniemi L J. Correlation of early cytodifferentiation of the human fetal prostate and leydig cells. Anat Rec 1980; 196: 263–273
9. Lowsley O S. The development of the human prostate gland with reference to the development of other structures at the neck of the urinary bladder. Am J Anat 1912; 13: 299–346
10. Pointis G, Latreille M T, Cedard L. Gonado-pituitary relationships in the fetal mouse at various times during sexual differentiation. J Endocrinol 1980; 86: 48
11. Resko J A. Androgen secretion by the fetal and neonatal Rhesus monkey. Endocrinology 1978; 87: 680
12. Siiteri P K, Wilson J D. Testosterone formation and metabolism during male sexual differentiation in the human embryo. J Clin Endocrinol Metab 1974; 38: 113
13. Weniger J P, Zeis A. Sur la sécrétion précoce de testosterone par le testicule embryonnaire de souris. C R Acad Sci 1972; 275: 1431
14. Winder J S D, Faiman C, Reyes F. Sexual endocrinology of fetal and perinatal life. In: Austin C R, Edward R G (eds) Mechanisms of sex differentiation in animal and man. New York: Academic Press, 1981; 205
15. Cunha G R. Epithelio-mesenchymal interactions in primordial gland structures which become responsive to androgenic stimulation. Anat Rec 1972; 172: 179
16. Wilson J D, Griffin J E, Leshin M et al. Role of gonadal hormones in development of the sexual phenotypes. Hum Genet 1981; 58: 78

17. Franks L M. Benign nodular hyperplasia of the prostate. A review. Ann R Coll Surg Engl 1954; 14: 92–106

18. Franks L M. Benign prostatic hyperplasia. Gross and microscopic anatomy. In: Grayhack J T, Wilson J D, Scherbenske M J (eds) Benign prostatic hyperplasia. NIAMDD Workshop Proceedings, 20–21 Feb 1975. DHEW Publication No (NIH) 76-1113. Washington: US Government Printing Office, 1976: 63–89

19. Zondek T, Zondek L H. The fetal and neonatal prostate. In: Goland M (ed) Normal and abnormal growth of the prostate. Springfield: C.C. Thomas, 1975: 5–28

20. Xia B T, Blackburn X T, Gardner W A. Fetal prostate growth and development. Pediatr Pathology. 1990; 10: 527–537

21. Popek E J, Tyson R W, Miller G J, Caldwell S A. Prostate development in prune belly syndrome and posterior urethral valves: etiology of PBS — lower urinary tract obstruction or primary mesenchymal defect? Pediatr Pathol 1991; 11: 1–29

22. Shapiro E, Hartanto V, Becich M J, Lepor H. The relative proportion of stromal and epithelial hyperplasia is related to the development of symptomatic BPH. J Urol 1992; 147: 1293

23. Shapiro E, Hartanto V, Lepor H. Quantifying the smooth muscle content of the prostate using double-immunoenzymatic staining and colour assisted image analysis. J Urol 1992; 147: 1167–1170

24. Andrews G S. The histology of the human fetal and prepubertal prostates. J Anat 1951; 85: 44–54

25. Shapiro E, Hartanto V, Perlman E, Lepor H. Morphogenesis of the prostate. Abstract 93. New Orleans: American Academy of Pediatrics Section of Urology, 1991

26. Rajfer J, Coffey D S. Sex steroid imprinting of the immature prostate: long-term effects. Invest Urol 1978; 16: 186–190

27. Naslund M J, Coffey D S. The differential effects of neonatal androgen, oestrogen and progesterone on adult rat prostate growth. J Urol 1986; 136: 1136–1140

28. Shapiro E. Unpublished data

29. Timms B G, Mohs T J, Didio L J A. Ductal budding and branching patterns in the developing prostate. J Urol 151; 1427–1432

30. McNeal J E. The zonal anatomy of the prostate. Prostate 1981; 2(1): 35–49

31. McNeal J E. The prostate gland: morphology and pathology. Monogr Urol 1983; 4: 3

32. McNeal J E. The prostate gland: morphology and pathobiology. Monogr Urol 1988; 9: 3

33. McNeal J E. Normal histology of the prostate. Am J Surg Pathol 1988; 12: 619

34. Cunha G R. The role of androgens in the epithelio-mesenchymal interactions involved in prostatic morphogenesis in embryonic mice. Anat Rec 1972; 175: 87

35. Cunha G R. Support of normal salivary gland morphogenesis by mesenchyme derived from accessory sexual glands of embryonic mice. Anat Rec 1972; 173: 205

36. Cunha G R. Epithelial–stromal interactions in development of the urogenital tract. Int Rev Cytol 1976; 47: 137–194

37. Cunha G R, Lung B. The possible influences of temporal factors in androgenic responsiveness of urogenital tissue recombinants from wild-type and androgen-insensitive (Tfm) mice. J Exp Zool 1978; 205: 343

38. Cunha G R, Chung L W K, Shannon J M, Reese B A. Stromal–epithelial interactions in sex differentiation. Biol Reprod 1980; 22: 19–43

39. Cunha G R, Chung L W K. Stromal–epithelial interactions: induction of prostatic phenotype in urothelium of testicular feminized (Tfm/y) mice. J Steroid Biochem 1981; 14: 1317

40. Cunha G R, Chung L W K, Shannon J M et al. Hormone-induced morphogenesis and growth: role of mesenchymal–epithelial interaction. Recent Prog Horm Res 1983; 39: 599–598

41. Cunha G R, Donjacour A A. Stromal–epithelial interactions in normal and abnormal prostatic development. Prog Clin Biol Res 1987; 239: 251–272

42. Cunha G R, Donjacour A A, Cooke P S et al. The endocrinology and developmental biology of the prostate. Endocr Rev 1987; 8: 388

43. Cunha G R, Donjacour A A. Mesenchymal–epithelial interaction in the growth and development of the prostate. In: Lepor H, Ratliff T L (eds) Urologic oncology. Boston: Kluwer Academic, 1989: 159

44. Cunha G R, Alarid E T, Turner T et al. Normal and abnormal development of the male urogenital tract: role of androgens, mesenchymal–epithelial interactions, and growth factors. J Androl 1992; 13: 465

45. Donjacour A A, Cunha G R. The effect of androgen deprivation on branching morphogenesis in the mouse prostate. Dev Biol 1988; 128: 1

46. Burns R K. Role of hormones in the differentiation of sex. In: Young W C (ed) Sex and internal secretions. Baltimore: Williams and Wilkins, 1961: 76

47. Elger W, Graf K J, Steinbeck H et al. Hormonal control of sexual development. Adv Biosci 1974; 13: 41

48. Greene R. Hormonal factors in sex inversion. The effects of sex hormones in embryonic sexual structures of the rat. Biol Symp 1940; 9: 105

49. Greene R R, Burrill M W, Ivy A C. The effects of estrogens on the antenatal sexual development of the rat. Am J Anat 1939; 67: 305

50. Jost A. Problems of fetal endocrinology: the gonadal and hypophyseal hormones. Recent Prog Horm Res 1953; 8: 379–418

51. Neumann F, Elger W, Steinbeck H. Antiandrogens and reproductive development. Phil Trans R Soc Lond (Biol) 1970; 25: 179

52. Neumann F, Graf K J, Elger W. Hormone-induced disturbances in sexual differentiation. Adv Biosci 1974; 13: 71

53. Raynaud A, Frilley M. Destruction de cerveau des embryos de souris au treizieme jour de la gestation, par irradiation au moyen des rayon X. C R Soc Biol 1947; 141: 658

54. Lung B, Cunha G R. Development of seminal vesicles and coagulating glands in neonatal mice 1: The morphogenetic effects of various hormonal conditions. Anat Rec 1981; 199: 73

55. Price D. Normal development of the prostate and seminal vesicles of the rat with a study of experimental postnatal modifications. Am J Anat 1936; 60: 79

56. Imperato-McGinley J, Binienda Z, Arthur A et al. The development of a male pseudohermaphroditic rat using an inhibitor of the enzyme 5α reductase. Endocrinology 1985; 116: 807

57. Imperato-McGinley J, Guerrero L, Gautieer T et al. Steroid 5α-reductase deficiency in man. An inherited form of pseudohermaphroditism. Science 1974; 186: 1213

58. Walsh P C, Madden J D, Harrod M J et al. Familial incomplete male pseudohermaphroditism type 2: decreased dihydrotestosterone formation in pseudovaginal perineoscrotal hypospadias. N Engl J Med 1974; 291: 944

59. Griffin J E, Wilson J D. Disorder of sexual differentiation. In: Walsh P C, Gittes R F, Perlmutter A D, Stamey T A (eds) Campbell's Urology, 5th ed. Philadelphia: Saunders, 1986: 1819

60. Ohio S. Major sex determining genes. New York: Springer-Verlag, 1979: 1–140

61. Lasnitzki I, Mizuno T. Prostatic induction and interaction of epithelium and mesenchyme from normal wild-type and androgen-insensitive mice with testicular feminization. J Endocrinol 1980; 85: 423

62. Shannon J M, Cunha G R. Autoradiographic localization of androgen binding in the developing mouse prostate. Prostate 1983; 4: 367–373

63. Shannon J M, Cunha G R, Vanderslice K D. Autoradiographic localization of androgen receptors in the developing urogenital tract and mammary gland. Anat Rec 1981; 199: 232

64. Takeda H, Mizuno T, Lasnitzki I. Autoradiographic studies of androgen-binding sites in the rat urogenital sinus and postnatal prostate. J Endocrinol 1985; 104: 87–92

65. Wasner G, Hennermann I, Kratochwil K. Ontogeny of mesenchymal androgen receptors in the embryonic mouse mammary gland. Endocrinology 1983; 113: 1771

66. Sugimura Y, Cunha G R, Donjacour A A. Morphogenesis and histologic study of castration-induced degeneration and androgen-induced regeneration in the mouse prostate. Biol Reprod 1980; 22: 19–43

67. Hayashi N, Sugimura Y, Kawamura J et al. Morphological and functional heterogeneity in the rat prostate gland. Biol Reprod 1991; 45: 308–321

68. Bazer G T. Basal cell proliferation and differentiation in regeneration of the rat ventral prostate. Invest Urol 1979; 17: 470

69. Ichihara I, Pelliniemi L J. Ultrastructure of the basal cell and the acinar capsule of rat ventral prostate. Anat Anz 1975; 138: 355

70. Dahl E, Kjaerheim A, Tveter K. The ultrastructure of the accessory sex organs of the male rat. 1. Normal structure. Z Zellforsch 1973; 137: 345

71. Timms B G, Chandler J A, Sinowatz F. The ultrastructure of basal cells of rat and dog prostate. Cell Tissue Res 1976; 173: 542

72. Rowlatt C, Franks L M. Myoepithelium in mouse prostate. Nature 1964; 202: 707

73. Lee C, Sensibar J, Dudek S et al. Prostatic ductal system in rats: regional variation in morphological and functional activities. Biol Reprod 1990; 43: 1079–1086

74. Sensibar J, Griswold M, Sylvester S et al. Prostatic ductal system in rats: regional variation in localization of an androgen-repressed gene product, sulfated glycoprotein-2. Endocrinology 1991; 128: 2091–2102

75. Rouleau M, Legert J, Tenniswood M. Ductal heterogeneity of cytokeratins, gene expression, and cell death in the rat ventral prostate. Mol Endocrinol 1990; 4: 2003–2013

76. Aumuller G. Morphologic and endocrine aspects of prostatic function. Prostate 1983; 4: 195

77. English H F, Drago J R, Santen R J. Cellular response to androgen depletion and repletion in the rat ventral prostate; autoradiography and morphometric analysis. Prostate 1985; 7: 41

78. Brandes D. Fine structure and cytochemistry of male accessory organs. In: Brandes D (ed) Male accessory sex organs: structure and function. New York: Academic Press, 1974: 18

79. Berry S, Isaacs J T. Comparative aspects of prostatic growth and androgen metabolism with aging in the rat versus the dog. Endocrinology 1984; 114: 511

80. Cooke P S, Young P, Cunha G R. Androgen receptor expression in developing male reproductive organs. Endocrinology 1991; 128: 2867

81. Prins G, Cooke P, Birch L et al. Androgen receptor expression and 5α reductase activity along the proximal–distal axis of the rat prostatic duct. Endocrinology 1992; 130: 3066–3073

82. Prins G S, Birch L. The developmental pattern of androgen receptor expression in rat prostate lobes is altered after neonatal exposure to oestrogen. Endocrinology 1995; 136: 1303–1314

83. Prins G. Neonatal Oestrogen exposure induces lobe-specific alterations in adult rat prostate and androgen receptor expression. Endocrinology 1992; 130: 3703–3714

84. Cooke P S, Young P, Hess R A, Cunha G R. Estrogen receptor expression in developing epididymis, efferent ductules, and other male reproductive organs. Endocrinology 1991; 128: 2874–2879

85. Donjacour A A, Cunha G R. Assessment of prostatic protein secretion in tissue recombinants made of urogenital sinus mesenchyme and urothelium from normal or androgen-insensitive mice. Endocrinology 1993; 132: 2342–2350

86. Cunha G R, Battle E, Young P et al. Role of epithelial–mesenchymal interaction in the differentiation and spatial organization of visceral smooth muscle. Epith Cell Biol 1992; 1: 76–83

87. Aaronson S A, Bottaro D P, Miki T et al. Keratinocyte growth factor: a fibroblast growth factor family member with unusual target cell specificity. Ann NY Acad Sci 1991; 638: 62–77

88. Nilsen-Hamilton M. Transforming growth factor-β and its actions on cellular growth and differentiation. Curr Top Dev Biol 1990; 24: 95–136

89. Partanen A M. Epidermal growth factor and transforming growth factor-α in the development of epithelial–mesenchymal organs of the mouse. Curr Top Dev Biol 1990; 24: 31–55

90. Cunha G R. Role of mesenchymal–epithelial interactions in normal and abnormal development of the mammary gland and prostate. Cancer 1994; 74: 1030–1043

91. Norman J T, Cunha G R, Sugimura Y. The induction of new ductal growth in adult prostatic epithelium in response to an embryonic prostatic inductor. Prostate 1986; 8: 209–220

92. Steiner M S, Barrack E R. Transforming growth factor-β1 overproduction in prostate cancer: effects on growth in vivo and in vitro. Mol Endocrinol 1992; 6: 15

93. Mansson P E, Adams P, Kan M, McKeehan W L. Heparin-binding growth factor gene expression and receptor characteristics in normal rat prostate and two transplantable rat prostate tumors. Cancer Res 1989; 49: 2485

94. Connolly J M, Rose D P. Production of epidermal growth factor and transforming growth factor-α by the androgen-responsive LNCaP human prostate cancer cell line. Prostate 1990; 16: 209

95. Story M T, Livingston B, Baeten L et al. Cultured human prostate-derived fibroblasts produce a factor that stimulates their growth with properties indistinguishable from basic fibroblast growth factor. Prostate 1989; 15: 355

96. Wilding G, Zugmeier G, Knabbe C et al. Differential effects of transforming growth factor beta on human prostate cancer cells in vitro. Mol Cell Endocrinol 1989; 62: 79

97. McKeehan W L, Adams P S. Heparin-binding growth factor/prostatropin attenuates inhibition of rat prostate tumor epithelial cell growth by transforming growth factor type beta. In Vitro Cell Dev Biol 1988; 24: 243

98. Wilding G, Valverius E, Knabbe C, Gelmann E P. Role of transforming growth factor-α in human prostate cancer cell growth. Prostate 1989; 15: 1

99. Shain S A, Lin A L, Koger J D, Karaganis A G. Rat prostate cancer cells contain functional receptors for transforming growth factor-beta. Endocrinol 1990; 126: 818

100. Kyprianou N, Isaacs J T. Identification of a cellular receptor for transforming growth factor-beta in rat ventral prostate and its negative regulation by androgens. Endocrinol 1988: 123: 2124

101. Muller W J, Lee F S, Dickson C et al. The int-2 gene product acts as an epithelial growth factor in transgenic mice. EMBO J 1990; 9: 907

102. Tutrone R F, Ball, R A, Ornitz D M et al. Benign prostatic hyperplasia in a transgenic mouse: a new hormonally sensitive investigatory model. J Urol 1993; 149: 633

103. Sandgren E P, Luetteke N C, Palmiter R D et al. Overexpression of TGFα in transgenic mice: induction of epithelial hyperplasia, pancreatic metaplasia and carcinoma of the breast. Cell 1990; 61: 1121

104. Katz A E, Benson M C, Wise G J et al. Gene activity during the early phase of androgen-stimulated rat prostate regrowth. Cancer Res 1989; 49: 5889

105. Kyprianou N, Isaacs J T. Expression of transforming growth factor-beta in the rat ventral prostate during castration-induced programmed cell death. Mol Endocrinol 1989; 3: 1515

106. Avallet O, Vigier M, Perrard-Saporj M H, Saez J M. Transforming growth factor beta inhibits Leydig cell functions. Biochem Biophys Res Commun 1987; 146: 575

107. Lin T, Blaisdell J, Haskell J F. Transforming growth factor-beta inhibits Leydig cell steroidogenesis in primary culture. Biochem Biophys Res Commun 1987; 146: 387

108. Steiner M S. The role of peptide growth factors in the prostate. A review. Urology 1993; 42: 99

109. Fiorelli G, DeBellis A, Longo A et al. Insulin-like growth factor-I receptors in human hyperplastic prostate tissue: characterization, tissue localization and their modulation by chronic treatment with a gonadotropin-releasing hormone analog. J Clin Endocrinol Metab 1991; 72: 740

110. Kimura G, Kasuya J, Giannini S et al. Inhibition of IGF-II-stimulated growth of prostate cancer cells by IGF-I receptor-specific monoclonal antibody and antisense oligonucleotide of IGF-II messenger RNA. J Urol 1994; 151: 367A (abstr)

111. Steiner M S. Review of peptide growth factors in benign prostatic hyperplasia and urologic malignancy. J Urol 1995; 153: 1085

112. Taylor T B, Ramsdell J S. Transforming growth factor-α and its receptor are expressed in the epithelium of the rat prostate gland. Endocrinology 1993; 133: 1306

113. McKeehan W L, Adams P S, Fast D. Different hormonal requirements for androgen-independent growth of normal and tumor epithelial cells from rat prostate. In Vitro Cell Dev Biol 1987; 23: 147

114. Smith E P, Russell W E, French F S, Wilson E M. A form of basic fibroblast growth factor is secreted into the adluminal fluid of the rat coagulating gland. Prostate 1989; 14: 353

115. Marchese C, Rubin J, Ron D et al. Human keratinocyte growth factor activity on proliferation and differentiation of human keratinocytes: differentiation response distinguishes KGF from EGF family. J Cell Physiol 1990; 144: 326

116. Iwamura M, Sluss P M, Casamento J B, Cockett A T K. Insulin-like growth factor I: action and receptor characterization in human prostate cancer cell lines. Prostate 1993; 22: 243

117. Steiner M S. Unpublished data

118. Matsui Y, Halter S A, Holt J T et al. Development of mammary hyperplasia and neoplasia in MMTV-TGF alpha transgenic mice. Cell 1990; 61: 1147

119. Halter S A, Dempsey P, Matsui Y et al. Distinctive patterns of hyperplasia in MMTV-TGFα transgenic mice. Characterization of mammary gland and skin proliferations. Am J Pathol 1992; 140: 1131

120. Martikainen P, Kyprianou N, Isaacs J T. Effect of transforming growth factor-beta 1 on proliferation and death of rat prostatic cells. Endocrinology 1990; 127: 2963–2968

121. Hiramatsu M, Kashimata M, Minami N et al. Androgenic regulation of epidermal growth factor in the mouse ventral prostate. Biochem Int 1988; 17: 311

122. McKeehan W L, Adams P S, Rosser M P. Direct mitogenic effects of insulin, epidermal growth factor, glucocorticoid, cholera toxin, unknown pituitary factors and possibly prolactin, but not androgen, on normal rat prostate epithelial cells in serum-free, primary cell culture. Cancer Res 1984; 44: 1998

123. Mori H, Maki M, Oishi K et al. Increased expression of genes for basic fibroblast growth factor and transforming growth factor type beta 2 in human benign prostatic hyperplasia. Prostate 1990; 16: 71

124. Story M T, Hopp K A, Meier D A et al. Influence of transforming growth factor β1 and other growth factors on basic fibroblast growth factor level and proliferation of cultured human prostate-derived fibroblasts. Prostate 1993; 22: 183

3

Molecular control of prostate growth
K. Griffiths

Introduction

It is well accepted that the clinical manifestations of symptomatic benign prostatic hyperplasia (BPH) are generally recognized in men over the age of 50 years. Indeed, the ageing factor is considered a risk factor relating to the disease. Also now accepted is the evidence[1,2] that a large proportion of men in their later years will have some degree of prostate enlargement, often causing bladder outlet obstruction that requires surgical intervention. Moreover, as life expectancy is extended around the world, it would be expected that the proportion of men requiring a transurethral prostatectomy will consequently increase, and it is currently predicted[3] that in the USA, for example, a man of 40 years of age now has a 30% chance of undergoing such surgical treatment in his lifetime. Twenty-five years ago, approximately 10% could be expected to have surgery.[4]

Prostatectomy remains the second most common operation performed on males, but new initiatives directed to the medical management of BPH are now being created. One is centred on the use of 5 alpha-reductase inhibitors, which suppress the conversion of testosterone to 5-alpha-dihydrotestosterone (DHT), the principal 'active androgen' within the prostate gland. Concurrently, intense research activity attempts to understand better the molecular process through which DHT influences prostatic growth and function.[5,6]

It is noteworthy that clinical BPH occurs during a period when testicular function is declining and the concentrations of testosterone in plasma (Fig. 3.1), and also in saliva (Fig. 3.2), are falling with increasing age.[7,8] Despite this, most of the related evidence tends to indicate that androgens are implicated in the pathogenesis of the disease. Early castration, or hypopituitarism, appear to prevent the development of BPH. Furthermore, the enlarged prostate regresses following castration or after the administration of luteinizing hormone (LH)-releasing hormone (LHRH) treatment, or after treatment with anti-androgens.[9]

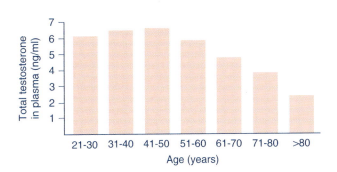

Figure 3.1. *Decline in the concentration of testosterone in plasma with increasing age. (Data from ref. 8.)*

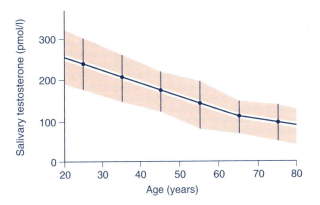

Figure 3.2. *Range of salivary testosterone determinations in a large population of males of different ages. The salivary steroid concentration represents the plasma levels of the free, non-protein-bound metabolically available steroid moiety. The concentrations decline significantly with age.*

Plasma hormones, the prostate and ageing

Although the prostate grows and functions within a multihormonal environment, responding to a range of regulatory factors, the functional activity of the human gland is primarily dependent on the maintenance of normal concentrations of plasma testosterone. Approximately 90–95% of the 6–7 mg testosterone that is produced daily and that appears in the plasma is synthesized by the Leydig cells of the testis[10,11] under the control of LH. The remainder originates in the adrenal gland, either by direct synthesis and secretion or from its production by the peripheral metabolism of the adrenal androgens, the C19-steroids dehydroepiandrosterone (DHA), DHA sulfate or androstenedione, by muscle and adipose tissue (Fig. 3.3).

The concentration of testosterone in the spermatic vein is approximately 75 times higher than that in the peripheral venous plasma. LH secretion by the pituitary gland is controlled by LHRH, a decapeptide released by the hypothalamus in a pulsatile manner, thereby promoting a similar, corresponding pulsatile secretion of LH. Both the androgens and oestrogens are involved in negative feedback control processes in order to regulate LH synthesis and secretion.[12]

In man, approximately 30% of the plasma oestrogens are synthesized and secreted by the testis,[13,14] with the major proportion, however, being produced[15] by the peripheral aromatization of androstenedione and testosterone (Fig. 3.4). The secretion of the adrenal androgens is controlled by adrenocorticotrophic hormone (ACTH), although prolactin may exercise a synergistic influence with ACTH.

Testosterone would be considered the most important plasma androgen, but it is the free, non-protein-bound form (Fig. 3.5) that is generally accepted as the biologically active moiety that enters the prostate target cells. The free testosterone level normally provides a reasonable indicator of the androgenic status of the male. In the plasma of the younger man,[16–19] approximately 57% of the testosterone is specifically and avidly bound to sex hormone-binding globulin (SHBG), with about 40% less well bound to albumin. A smaller amount, 1%, is bound to corticosteroid-binding globulin (CBG) and approximately 2% constitutes the free' fraction (Fig. 3.5). The oestrogens are similarly bound to SHBG with, again, approximately 2% in the free fraction.

SHBG is synthesized and secreted by the liver by processes regulated to some extent by oestrogens, with the thyroid hormones and insulin also implicated.[20–22] The decline in testicular function with age would generally be considered of primary testicular origin.[8] Although plasma levels of LH rise in the elderly man, there is also an impaired testicular response to LH and, moreover, a decreasing number of Leydig cells with increasing age with a consequent fall in plasma testosterone concentrations (Fig. 3.1). Ageing generally increases SHBG levels, giving rise to a corresponding reciprocal decrease in the free testosterone concentration. Therefore, although the total plasma testosterone level of an 80-year-old man is approximately 30–40% of that of a 25-year-old, the free concentration represents only 15–20% of that of the younger man (Fig. 3.5).

The 'active' androgenic steroid hormone within the prostate gland is DHT,[23,24] synthesized from testosterone by the 5 alpha-reductase enzyme system located on the nuclear membrane of prostatic cells (Fig. 3.6). It is interesting that testosterone and DHT are also synthesized[25,26] from the adrenal androgens within prostatic tissue (Fig. 3.7) and this particular source of DHT has been implicated by some[27,28] in the

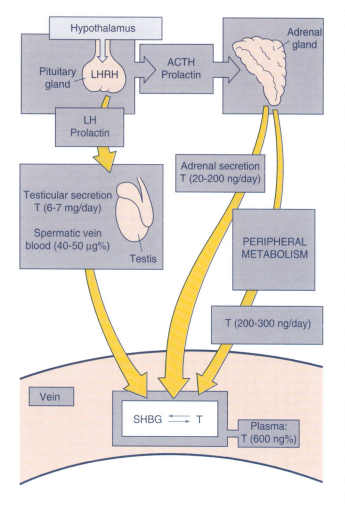

Figure 3.3. *Testosterone (T) production by the human male.*

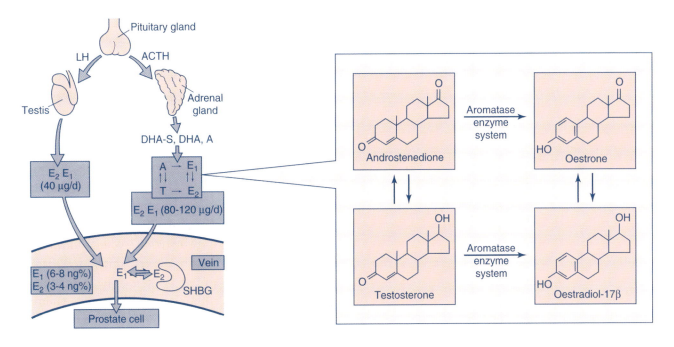

Figure 3.4. *Production of oestrogens by the human male: E_1, oestrone; E_2, oestradiol-17-beta; T, testosterone.*

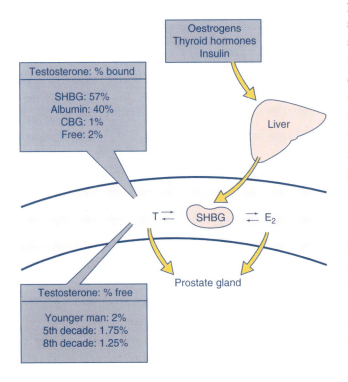

Figure 3.5. *Factors concerned with the levels of free, non-protein-bound steroid hormone in plasma that is considered to be the biologically active moiety that enters the target cell. E_2, oestradiol; T, testosterone.*

progression of disseminated prostatic cancer after primary endocrine therapy such as castration, or the administration of LHRH analogues.[29] Studies in animals[30] certainly suggest that the adrenal steroids can influence prostatic growth and function, but they cannot restore the size nor maintain the morphology of the prostate of the castrated rat. The significance of the role of the adrenal androgens in the normal prostate has yet to be clarified; at present, there are few, if any, data from man to indicate that they are involved in the pathogenesis of BPH. Of interest and rarely considered, is that certain of the metabolites of DHT, the 5-alpha-androstanediols, and androst-5-ene-3-beta,17-beta-diol, a metabolite of DHA, elicit weak oestrogenic effects[31] by binding to the oestrogen receptor (ER) protein and promoting certain biological responses similar to, but weaker than, those effected by oestradiol (Fig. 3.7).

There is some controversy as to the precise changes in the endocrine status of the male as he ages.[5,6,32,33] It is reported that, as testicular function declines with increasing age, there is a corresponding increase in the rate of peripheral aromatization[34,35] such that the levels of oestradiol in plasma rise relative to those of testosterone. The SHBG-binding capacity is stated[17,36] to increase in the elderly (Fig. 3.8), possibly in response

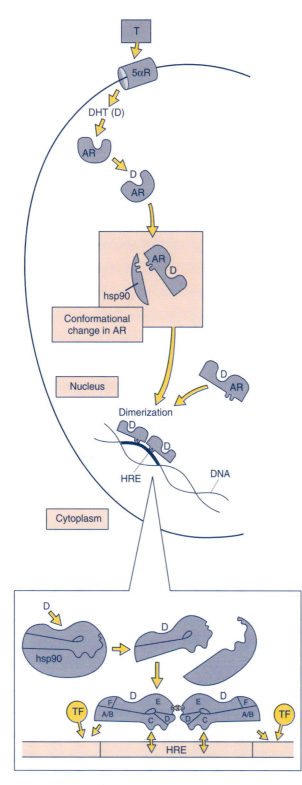

Figure 3.6. *A simple representation of the intracellular processes relating to the binding of DHT (D) to the androgen receptor (AR) and to the dimerization of the DHT–AR complex when binding to the hormone response elements (HRE), the nucleotide recognition sequences on the genome. T, testosterone; TF, the transcription factors binding to the DNA adjacent to the DHT–AR complexes.*

to the elevated oestrogenic status in the older man, the consequent effect being seen as an increased ratio of the plasma free oestradiol to free testosterone. The ageing prostate is therefore subjected to a changing oestrogen/androgen balance that would be expected to influence the amounts of steroid hormones that are transferred into the prostate cell.

It is generally accepted that the free steroid is transferred into the prostate cell by a process of passive diffusion, although there is still much to understand about these biological mechanisms, with reports[37] that the testosterone–SHBG complex specifically binds to receptors on the cell membrane (Fig. 3.9) to activate signal transduction systems.

Androgens, androgen receptors and gene transcription

As already stated, DHT is formed from testosterone within the prostate cells. DHT can then be further metabolized[33] to the 5-alpha-androstanediols (Fig. 3.7) by a reaction regulated by the enzyme 3-alpha(beta)-hydroxysteriod oxidoreductase [$3\alpha(\beta)$OHSOR]. It is DHT, however, that is the active androgen. It specifically binds to the androgen receptor (AR) with a binding affinity fivefold greater than that for testosterone and elicits the androgenic effects within the prostate cells.[23,24] In muscle cells, however, which do not have a 5 alpha-reductase enzyme, testosterone is the principal androgen.

Of interest in relation to this is an inherited clinical disorder, recognized in the Dominican Republic and referred to as male pseudohermaphroditism, in which patients are 5 alpha-reductase deficient.[38] At puberty, males with this condition show an adequately developed musculature, manifest relatively normal genitalia, libido and erections, presumable promoted by testosterone, but have only a vestigial prostate gland because of the lack of the 5 alpha-reductase enzyme and, consequently, a lack of DHT.

The androgenic action of DHT within the prostate depends on the specific binding of the steroid ligand to the nuclear AR protein. The androgenic signal is then transmitted through the DHT–AR complex to the genome (Fig. 3.6) by the consequent association of the complex with the nucleotide recognition sequences of

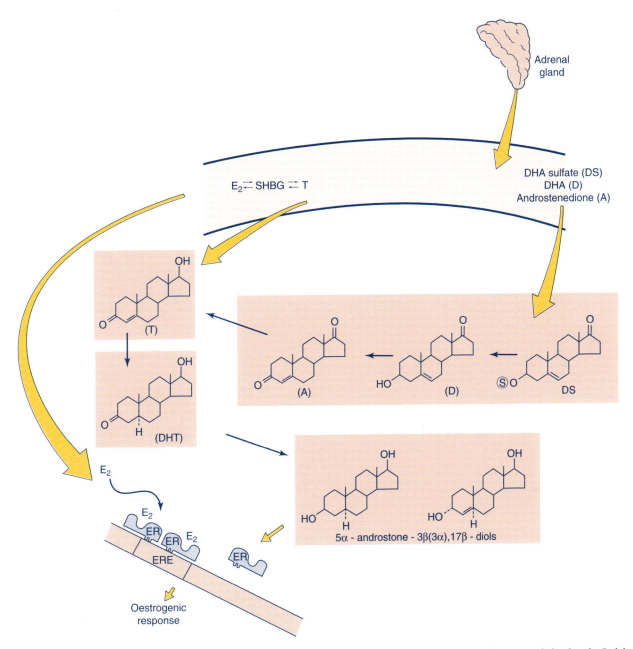

Figure 3.7. *Metabolism of the adrenal androgens by the human prostate gland to produce DHT. The DHT is further metabolized to the 5 alpha-androstanediols, which can elicit weak oestrogenic effects by association with the ER. E_2, oestradiol; T, testosterone.*

the DNA referred to as hormone response elements (AREs). The AR is, essentially, an intracellular gene-regulatory protein, one of a large family of such chromatin-binding proteins.[39]

The DHT–AR complexes have a high affinity for the HREs and bind as homodimers (Fig. 3.6), a process facilitated by the particular symmetry of the nucleotide recognition sequences. Thus, the DHT–AR complexes associate with the response element related to the

appropriate androgen-responsive genes (Fig. 3.10). This interaction allows the DHT–AR complex to modulate, or initiate, the transcription of such genes, although it must be remembered that the complexes may also suppress gene transcription.

The steroid receptor complexes therefore modulate gene transcription depending on the particular functions of the cell. In the prostate gland, the DHT–AR complexes will modulate genes that encode,

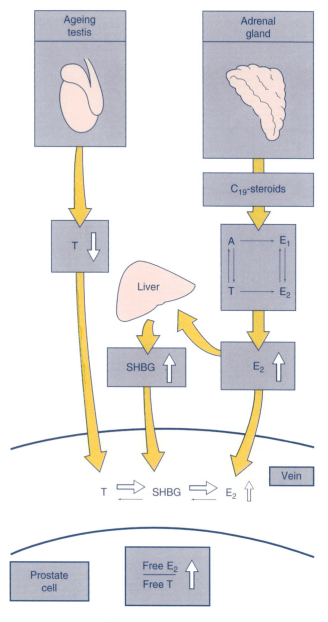

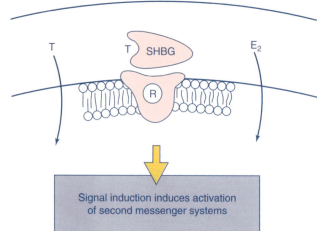

Figure 3.9. *Simple representation of the reported cell membrane receptor that is activated by the testosterone (t)–SHBG complex to promote intracellular cyclic adenosine monophosphate (cAMP) production. E_2, oestradiol.*

In order to understand better certain aspects of androgen action at the molecular level, some revision of DNA biology, simply portrayed, may be of value at this stage. The sequences of nucleotides on the 5′ end of the gene (Figs 3.10, 3.11), stated to be '*upstream*', are called the '*promoter region*'. These sequences are concerned with the regulation of transcription. The '*core promotor*' sequences, nearer the gene, are involved in the *initiation* of the transcription process, whereas those further upstream influence the *rate* of gene transcription. These promoter regions would therefore be recognized by the *RNA polymerase*, the enzyme that is involved in the transcription process (Fig. 3.12).

At a point 10 base pairs (bp) upstream of the gene, the DNA strands separate, a process referred to as '*melting*' and a prerequisite to the process, since only one DNA strand is transcribed (Fig. 3.12). The particular sequence of the nucleotides making up the gene is therefore copied as a strand of RNA, called a *messenger RNA (mRNA) transcript*.

On many genes, an upstream *TATA box* (Fig. 3.10) in which the bases thymine (T) and adenine (A) predominate, directs the RNA polymerase to the initiation site. Sequences of nucleotides that can influence the adjacent neighbouring gene are said to be *enhancers*, and *cis-acting modulators* of transcription. The different proteins such as DHT–AR and the various growth regulatory transcription factors such as the Fos,

Figure 3.8. *Diagram illustrating changes that have been recognized in the endocrine status of the middle-aged man. Declining testicular function and decreasing testosterone (T) output are associated with increased peripheral aromatization of adrenal androgens. The elevated oestradiol (E_2) levels have been implicated in the increased SHBG-binding capacity and the resultant changes in the free-E_2/free-T ratio in plasma, the overall effect giving rise to an enhanced oestrogenic influence on the prostate gland.*

for example, secretory proteins such as prostate-specific antigen (PSA) or structural proteins, but also the growth regulatory peptides such as the Fos and Jun proteins intimately concerned in the control of cellular growth processes and with the maintenance of homoeostasis.

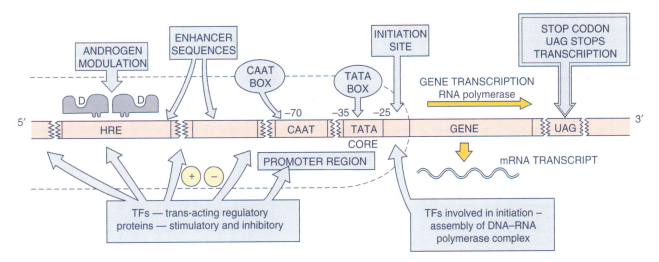

Figure 3.10. *Diagrammatical representation of the influence of various factors on the promoter region of an androgen-responsive gene. The figure shows the DHT–AR homodimers and the possible stimulatory or inhibitory influence of growth-regulatory factors that could influence gene transcription.*

Jun and myc proteins that bind to DNA, are considered to be *trans-acting modulators*.

The genetic message transcribed from the nucleotide sequence of the gene and carried by the mRNA transcript is then *translated* into the corresponding chain of amino acids that make up the protein encoded by that gene. Genes are therefore '*switched on*' or activated by the various growth-regulatory mechanisms. It is important to understand, however, that the mRNA is not a faithful transcript of the gene and certain sequences of a gene are not copied, but loop out of the process (Fig. 3.13). Those regions that loop out are called *introns*; they are interspersed between *exons*, which are encoded, copied and processed to form the mature mRNA transcript. The process whereby specific enzymes remove the introns is referred to as *splicing out*.

Steroid hormone receptor structure

Analysis of the nucleotide sequences of the DNA that encode steroid-receptor proteins clearly illustrates how they represent a family of receptor genes.[39] The receptors are ligand- or steroid-activated modulators of gene transcription, in which various domains have been identified[39] for particular functions (Fig. 3.14). Of the six domains of the oestrogen receptor, for example, two — the C and E regions — show a very marked homology to similar regions of other receptors. The E-domain is the region to which the steroid binds and the C-domain is the region of the protein that is involved in associating with the hormone response elements of the DNA. A similar relationship is illustrated for one of the series of receptors for retinoic acid (RA), also members of this receptor family. Again, the RA binds to the E-domain of the 462 amino acid alpha-retinoic acid receptor (αRAR) protein, encoded by the corresponding gene localized on chromosome 17q.

The 919 amino acid AR was one of the later steroid receptors to be sequenced and characterized,[40] with studies indicating that the F-domain could be further divided into three regions (Fig. 3.14). The AR protein is encoded by a gene situated on the X-chromosome. A genetic male without a functional AR receptor develops female external genitalia, a condition referred to as androgen insensitivity syndrome, sometimes as testicular feminization, clinical disorders relating to the X-chromosome.

Various gene deletions have been identified[41,42] in patients with the syndrome (Fig. 3.14). From the knowledge of the nucleotide sequences of the AR gene, oligonucleotide primers were made in order to amplify, by polymerase chain reaction (PCR) technology, DNA fragments containing the AR gene-coding exons, thereby allowing the identification of various gene mutations. These mutants included deletions of exons

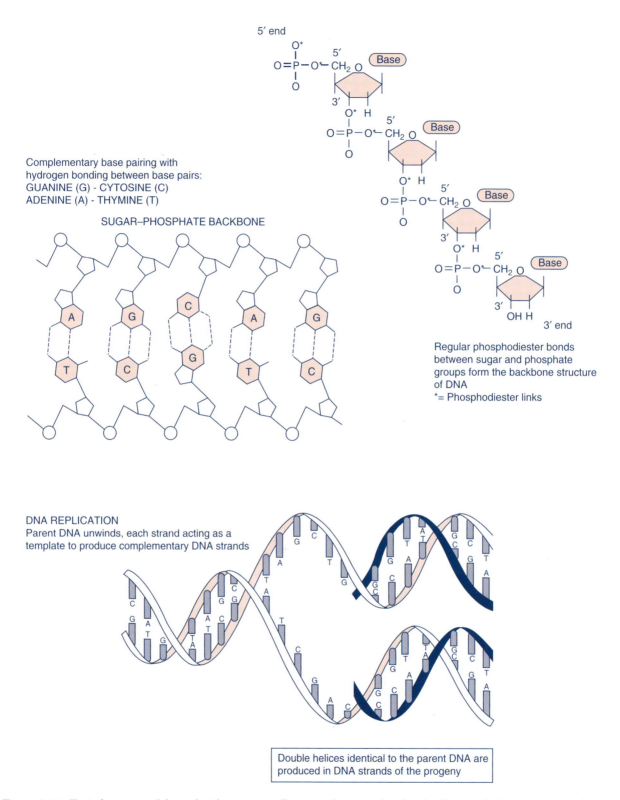

Figure 3.11. *Typical structure of the nucleotide sequences, illustrating the sugar–phosphate backbone with the complementary base-pairing through hydrogen bonding. The unwinding of the DNA provides the template on which to produce the complementary strands during replication of the DNA.*

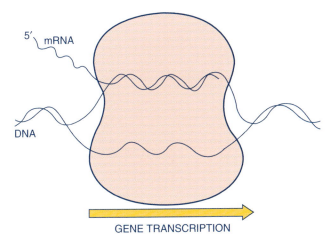

Figure 3.12. *Unwinding, or melting, of DNA in association with the RNA polymerase enzyme that controls gene transcription, thereby providing a single-strand template for the production of the complementary mRNA transcript.*

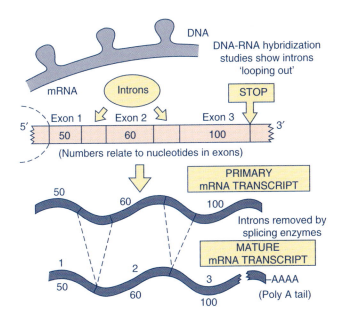

Figure 3.13. *Simple illustration of the processing of the mRNA transcript and the looping out of the introns.*

encoding the steroid-binding domain, complete gene deletion and also point mutations in the E-domain, for example, the 866 amino acid codon GTG changing to ATG, resulting in a methionine rather than valine being built into the E-domain of the AR.

In passing, it is worth noting that there is a possibility that such AR mutants could be implicated in the processes by which a prostatic cancer could lose androgen sensitivity as it progresses and de-differentiates, although studies from the Tenovus Cancer Research Centre[43] suggest that such mutant AR proteins are not common. A mutant AR could well influence growth-regulatory processes by an uncontrolled constitutive activation of androgen-responsive genes in association with other growth-stimulatory transcription factors.

Association of DHT–AR with DNA

The association of DHT with the steroid-binding region of the AR (Fig. 3.6) triggers a conformational change in the protein to reveal the DNA-binding domain, thus allowing DHT–AR to interact with the ARE adjacent to the androgen-responsive gene. Evidence[44] suggests that the unmasking of the DNA-binding domain is associated with the release from the complex of a protein referred to as the heat-shock protein 90 (hsp90). These conformational changes would also appear to be a prerequisite to the dimerization of the complexes,[45] a process that seems necessary for the androgenic regulatory action on the genome. The E-domain is also important for the *trans*-acting modulating function of the receptor, activating the transcription process.

It is the C-domain of the DHT–AR complex that, however, specifies the target gene. If a '*chimaeric receptor*' is prepared in which the DNA-binding domain of the glucocorticoid receptor (GR) is inserted in the place of the C-region of the ER — a process called '*finger swapping*' — the resultant chimaeric receptor will activate genes responsive to the GR,[46] when oestradiol is bound to the steroid-binding E-domain of the protein (Fig. 3.15).

The AR, like other steroid-receptor proteins and various transcription factors, contains within the C-domain a highly conserved core of amino acids, a sequence rich in cysteine residues, which, by coordinate binding of zinc, form two DNA-binding '*zinc fingers*',[47] illustrated diagrammatically in Figure 3.16. These zinc fingers are unmasked by the conformational changes

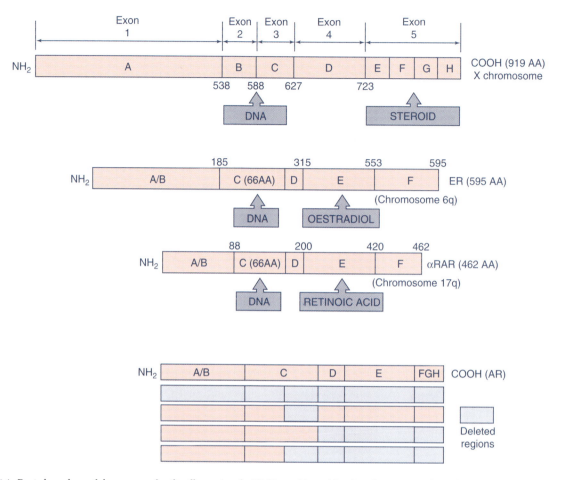

Figure 3.14. *Basic homology of the receptor family, illustrating the DNA- and ligand-binding domains. In the androgen insensitivity syndrome, androgen receptors with deleted regions (   ) have been identified.*

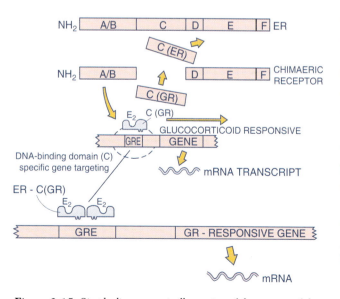

Figure 3.15. *Simple diagrammatic illustration of the concept of the chimaeric receptor. E_2, oestradiol; GRE, glucocorticoid response element.*

induced by the association of steroid with the receptor, and they subsequently facilitate the binding of the steroid-receptor complex to the response elements, looping into the major DNA grooves. The particular dyad symmetry of the response element relates effectively to the binding of DHT–AR as dimers, an association that confers stability (Fig. 3.17) to the transcription complex formed between the RNA polymerase, DNA and the various transcription factors involved in the process.

The CI zinc finger motif, containing four cysteine residues, appears to be responsible for determining target gene specificity through its association with the hormone response element (HRE), whereas the CII motif, with five cysteines, would appear to stabilize the receptor–response element association and the dimerization process by less specific binding. This dimerization function of the C-domain is, however,

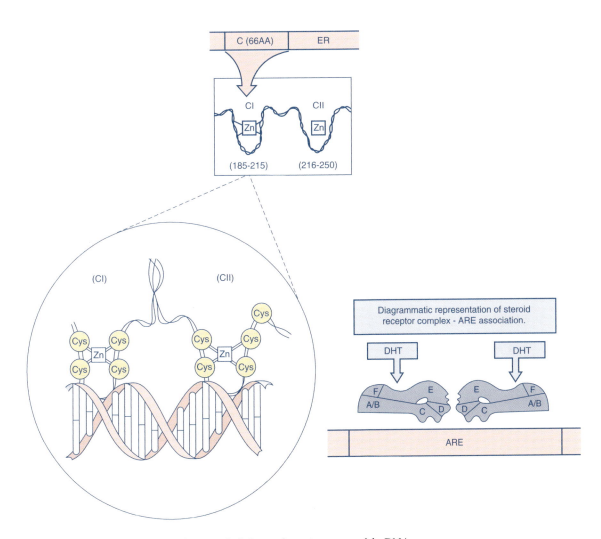

Figure 3.16. *Zinc fingers of the DNA-binding domain, which fit into the major grooves of the DNA.*

constitutive and, moreover, is a weaker function than that of the steroid-binding E-domain (Fig. 3.17), which is steroid ligand inducible. In the process of unmasking the DNA-binding domain, the conformational change resulting from the association with the steroid may also unmask an E-domain-located dimerization region.

Although understanding of many of these molecular processes is only slowly being achieved,[44] it would seem that the binding of the receptor protein to the response element may modify the spatial orientation of the DNA strands in such a way that it facilitates an easier access to the other transcription factors that are implicated in the regulation of these transcriptional processes. If the steroid-binding E-domain is removed from the receptor protein, the steroid-inducible transcriptional activation effect is also lost. However, such a protein can bind to

DNA and, through the A/B domain, can still constitutively promote transcription at the level of up to 10% of that induced by the binding with a steroid. This is possibly due to the interaction of the A/B domain with adjacent transcription factors associated with the DNA (Fig. 3.17).

Androgens and the regulation of prostate growth

Androgens are, therefore, the principal determinants of prostatic growth during adult life and their removal by castration results in dramatic prostatic atrophy. It is well accepted, from an accumulation of evidence derived from both human and animal studies, that, despite the fact that the prostate gland grows within a

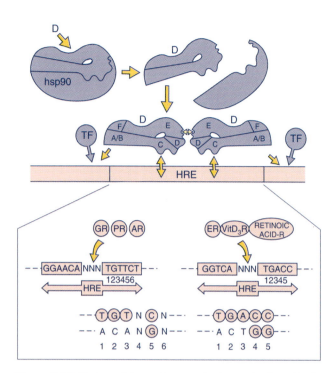

Figure 3.17. *Regions of the receptor protein that are implicated in the dimerization process and in the maintenance of the stability of the homodimer complex in association with the HRE. A transcription activation function relating to the N-terminal region is illustrated. The putative nucleotide sequences of the HREs that recognize particular receptor complexes are depicted, with the important bases of the DNA strands that have a role in the association of the ligand–receptor complexes to the DNA, making contact with the receptor amino acids.*

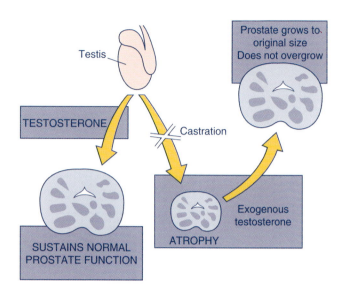

Figure 3.18. *Testosterone will not cause prostate overgrowth.*

multihormonal environment, the development, growth, function and maintenance of the gland are primarily androgen dependent.[48] The human embryonic prostate differentiates in response to androgens secreted by the foetal testis after week 8 of gestation. Exogenous administration of testosterone accelerates the growth of an immature prostate, but only to the normal maximal adult size and the gland does not overgrow. Prostate weight increases dramatically after puberty. Castration prior to puberty prevents prostatic development. Moreover, the administration of exogenous testosterone to the castrated adult causes the gland to grow to the normal adult size, but the prostate does not normally enlarge in response to exogenous androgen (Fig. 3.18).

It is now clear that testosterone, by way of its conversion to DHT, modulates these growth processes through a balance between the influence of the androgenic hormone on cellular proliferation and also

by way of certain antagonistic effects of DHT on the processes involved in apoptosis, or programmed cell death.[49] This balance is diagrammatically illustrated in Figure 3.19. DHT, therefore, tends to restrain apoptosis and maintain cell number. Depletion of DHT, and thereby a lowering of intracellular AR, instigates involution of the gland, whereas subsequent reaccumulation of androgen within the gland and the resynthesis of new AR initiate active cellular proliferation,[50] both being active biological processes with associated selective gene expression.

With little evidence for a direct positive stimulation of DNA synthesis by androgenic hormones, it would appear that DHT essentially 'switches on' the growth processes,[50] after which a series of 'functional intermediaries' are then expressed between the point in time when AR levels increase within the prostate of a castrated rat in response to androgen, and the period of DNA replication and cell division (Fig. 3.20). Many of these intermediaries are directly implicated in cell proliferation,[51–54] and considerable research activity is currently being directed to the identification of these growth-regulatory factors and a greater understanding of their role, not only in the maintenance of normal cellular homoeostasis, but also in abnormal growth processes in relation to the pathogenesis of prostatic disease.

Androgens are, therefore, essential but not primarily responsible for the initiation of cell proliferation. The

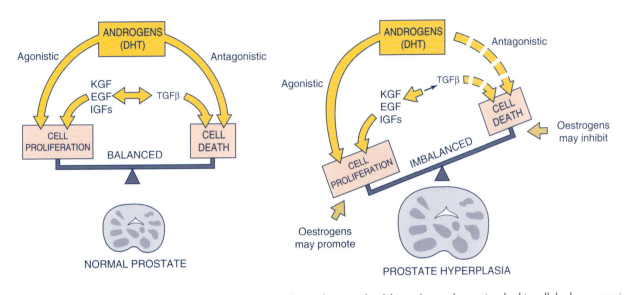

Figure 3.19. *Schematic representation of the balance between growth-stimulatory and -inhibitory factors that are involved in cellular homoeostasis in the prostate gland. Imbalance results in abnormal growth and BPH.*

androgenic effects are mediated by the intercession of growth-regulatory factors. As DHT switches on cell proliferation, it induces the synthesis of mitogenic peptides such as the growth-stimulatory epidermal growth factor (EGF), keratinocyte growth factor (KGF) and the insulin-like growth factors (IGFs) I and II. It would also appear mandatory that, if a steady state is to be maintained, a 'stop-mechanism' would also have to be encoded in order to restrain growth. In this regard, the growth-inhibitory factor transforming growth factor-beta (TGFβ) has been seen as having a major inhibitory role in balancing the effect of the growth-stimulatory peptides (Fig. 3.21). An early response of androgen-responsive prostatic cells to EGF, for example, results in the early expression (Fig. 3.20) of the proto-oncogenes, c-fos and c-jun. The products encoded by c-fos and c-jun, the Fos and Jun proteins, are implicated in growth-regulatory processes and act as transcription factors (Fig. 3.22) in influencing the activity of other genes concerned with growth, and also autoregulate the expression of their own genes. The effect of EGF on the expression of c-jun gene is illustrated in Figure 3.23. The immediate stimulatory response[55] probably relates to the dephosphorylation and release of Jun protein from the phosphorylated 'stored product', prior to the activation of c-jun, a process that provides an immediate induction of activity of related growth genes (Fig. 3.24).

Growth-regulatory factors

Growth factors, therefore, may stimulate or restrain cell proliferation[54,56] and are involved in normal cellular growth control mechanisms. Clearly, homoeostasis requires an equilibrium between the biological effects of stimulatory and inhibitory factors and it is not unreasonable to suspect that an imbalance of these factors could cause abnormal growth as seen in BPH. Moreover, if the genes encoding these proteins are overactive or mutated, such that processes that regulate their activity are usurped, then uncontrolled growth, characteristic of cancer, would follow.

Classically, an endocrine effect is when hormones are synthesized by a gland and are then transported to the target cell by way of the circulation. Growth-regulatory factors act through paracrine, autocrine or possibly intracrine effects (Fig. 3.25). With the former, growth factors produced by one cell diffuse to a neighbouring cell to promote their biological effects, whereas, with an autocrine response, a cell produces a growth factor that is used by the cell itself. With intracrine effects, the factors remain internal. Various growth-regulatory factors that act in this manner have been isolated from the prostate gland:[33,54] some are also secreted by prostatic cells and specific cell membrane-associated receptors have been identified for some of them.

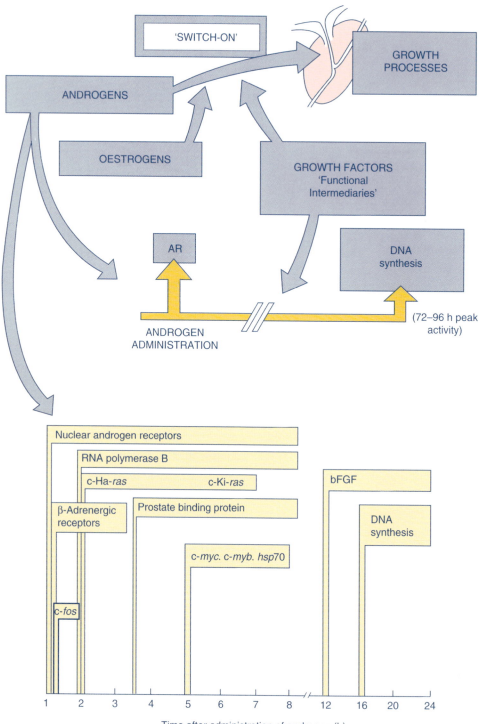

Figure 3.20. *Castration causes involution of the prostate, with a decline in cell number and in the DNA content of the gland to a level approximately 10% of normal by 10 days after castration. The surviving cells are presumed to be stem cells. Androgen administration promotes proliferation and restores cell number. There is, however, a significant interval between androgen stimulation and a rise in the rate of DNA synthesis. The figure depicts that androgens are essential, but not responsible, for inducing proliferation and that the intercession of other 'intermediary factors' is necessary for the growth processes.*

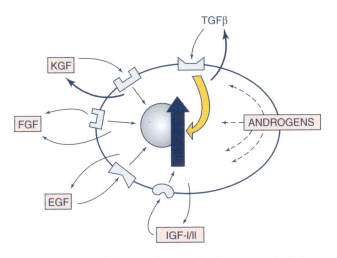

EGF, rather than DHT, is known to stimulate the proliferation of prostate epithelial cells in culture (Fig. 3.26), with possibly a more specific action localized to the basal cells of the gland. TGFβ is produced by many cells and is generally regarded as an inhibitor of epithelial cell growth.[56] Other factors, such as IGF-I and IGF-II, TGFα and platelet-derived growth factor (PDGF), may also influence prostate growth, but, in recent years, good evidence has been made available by McKeehan and his colleagues[57–60] to suggest most compellingly that KGF may have a particularly important role in this regard. This is discussed later in the text.

Figure 3.21. *Modulating influence of androgens on the balance between growth-stimulatory and growth-inhibitory factors.*

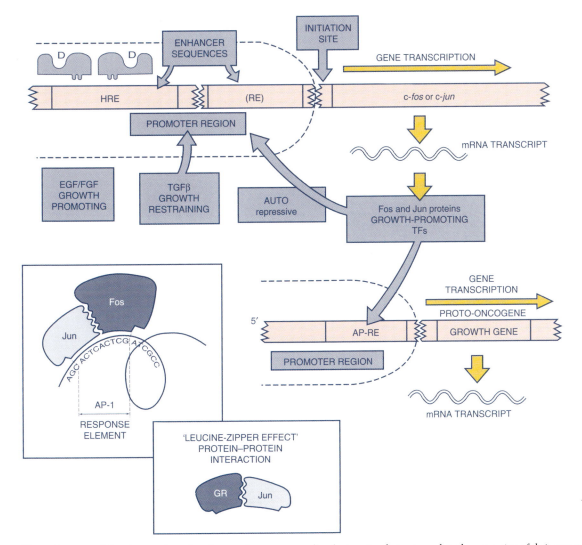

Figure 3.22. *The androgen-modulated expression of a c-fos or c-jun gene, encoding for proteins that autoregulate the expression of their own gene and influence the transcriptional activity of other genes concerned with growth regulation. The concept of protein–protein or leucine-zipper interactions, and the implication of Fos–Jun heterodimers associating with the AP-1 recognition site on the genome, are diagrammatically portrayed.*

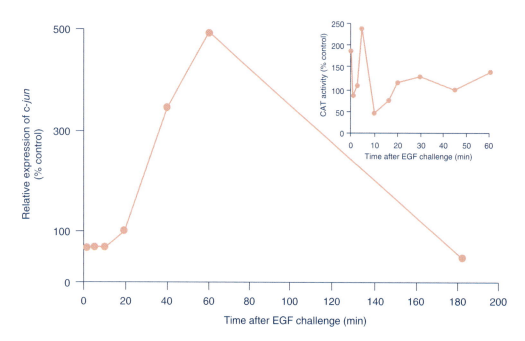

Figure 3.23. *Induction of c-jun mRNA expression (main diagram) and the activity of a transfected reporter gene construct TPA responsive element–chloramphenicolacetyl transferase (TRE-CAT) which was designed to be potentially modulated by Fos/Jun product when experimentally introduced into living cells. Normal canine epithelial cells (CAPE cell line) were challenged with EGF in culture. Upregulation of c-jun transcript was observed 40–60 min after treatment. However, an increase in the activity of the potential Fos/Jun protein product was observed, as determined by reporter gene activity, 5 min after treatment, suggesting that significant levels of the Fos/Jun product existed in the cells prior to challenge, that are rapidly activated by the EGF stimulus. Subsequent transcription of at least one Fos/Jun family member, the c-Jun gene, is enhanced, presumably to replenish intracellular stored levels of c-Jun protein.*

Cell membrane-associated receptors for many of the growth factors have been recognized in prostate tissue and, through intracellular signal transduction pathways, growth-regulatory factors activate various proto-oncogenes, increasing the expression of their protein products which then become involved in growth processes (Fig. 3.27). The stimulatory action of the growth factor therefore induces proto-oncogene transcription, with androgens appearing to modulate these effects, thereby influencing cell proliferation processes in a permissive, rather than direct, manner.

Epithelial–stromal interaction

As our understanding of the growth-regulatory processes of the prostate increases, so does the realization that the system is, indeed, complex. The human prostate gland is a branched glandular structure, with 40–50 ductal systems, each duct lined with epithelial cells and embedded in a matrix of stromal components.[61,62]

Although suspected a number of years ago,[63] it is becoming increasingly more apparent that there is an important interactive relationship between stroma and epithelium, with the stromal elements of the gland playing a major part in regulating the functional activity of the epithelial cells. Conversely, it would also appear that the epithelial tissue could well influence the behaviour of the stromal compartment.[64]

The elegant embryological studies of Cunha and his colleagues[65,66] strongly support this concept of a close interrelationship between stroma and epithelial elements, with inductive signalling between the compartments, controlled by growth-regulatory factors, influencing growth, differentiation and, possibly, function. Imbalance of this complex interaction between the two compartments could be concerned in the pathogenesis of BPH, if not cancer.

With regard to this interrelationship (Fig. 3.28), it is important to recognize that both the epithelial and stromal tissues contain 5 alpha-reductase[25,67] and

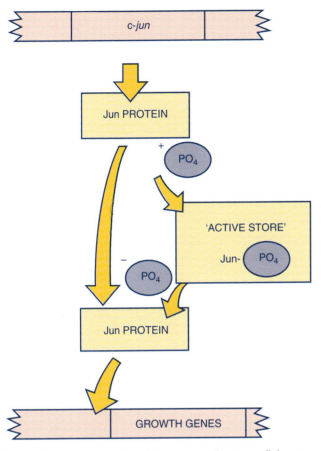

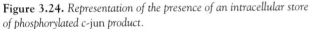

Figure 3.24. *Representation of the presence of an intracellular store of phosphorylated c-jun product.*

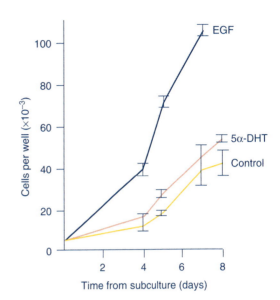

Figure 3.26. *Various growth factors stimulate proliferation of prostate epithelial cells. Illustrated is the effect of EGF on a normal canine epithelial cell line (CAPE) in culture; DHT had little, if any, effect.*

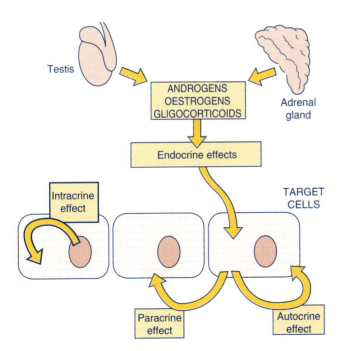

Figure 3.25. *Diagrammatic illustration of intracrine, paracrine and autocrine effects.*

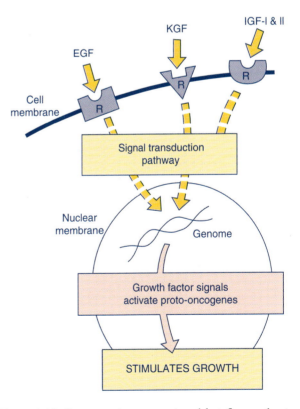

Figure 3.27. *Diagrammatic representation of the influence of various growth-stimulatory factors on the activity of growth-related proto-oncogenes. The influence of the growth factors on signal transduction pathways within the cell is effected through the cell membrane-localized specific receptors.*

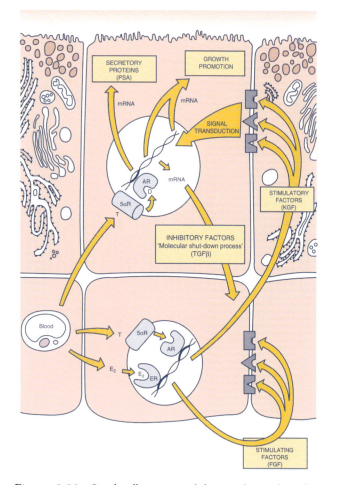

Figure 3.28. *Simple illustration of how androgen-dependent 'mediators' of stromal origin influence epithelial proliferation and prostate growth. It is presumed that, to establish and maintain homoeostasis, the system encodes for a growth-restraining mechanism to be induced once normal gland size is attained. Receptors for oestrogens are shown, localized in the stromal elements, whereas the AR is found in both compartments. E_2, oestradiol; PSA, prostate-specific antigen; T, testosterone.*

AR.[68,69] Although ERs can be located in both compartments,[54] studies on human prostatic tissues[70,71] indicate that ER levels are higher in the stroma.

The current belief, therefore, is that many of the biological processes of epithelial tissue are indirectly controlled by androgens through androgen-dependent mediators of stromal origin (Fig. 3.28). Presumably, growth-stimulatory factors produced by the stromal elements through the action of the DHT–AR complex elicit these mitogenic effects on the epithelium. It is interesting to consider how this interaction between stomal tissue and the epithelium is probably involved in

the development of the adult, mature prostate gland and, furthermore, in the pathogenesis of BPH.

At birth, the prostate is approximately the size of a pea and grows little until adolescence. After puberty, there is a rapid increase in size (Fig. 3.29) until the gland attains its normal, maximal adult size during the early part of the third decade.[72,73] The mature weight of the prostate, between 20 and 25 g, normally remains constant until the age of 50 or more when, in many men, the gland enlarges, often associated with 'bothersomeness', an effect on the quality of life but, in many men, related to the clinical symptoms of bladder outlet obstruction. Noteworthy, however, and illustrated in Figure 3.29, is the increasing prevalence with increasing age of microscopic BPH — epithelial hyperplasia — identified as early as the third decade. It develops into microscopic nodular hyperplasia,[74] with the number of micronodules localized in the transition zone[75] and periurethral tissue (Fig. 3.30) increasing with age. Also of particular interest is the similar prevalence of microscopic BPH in the prostates of men of all races, worldwide.[72,73]

It would appear that the early growth and differentiation of the prostate and the postpubertal growth of the gland are indirectly promoted by androgens through the androgen-dependent production of growth-stimulatory factors of stromal origin. It would be assumed that, once the adult size is attained, a growth-restraining molecular shut-down procedure would become effective under the influence of growth-restraining factors such as TGFβ (Fig. 3.28). Homoeostasis would normally prevail with a balance between growth-stimulatory and -inhibitory factors.

The precise mechanisms by which cells escape from normal growth-regulatory control remain to be identified, but presumably either a limited but sustained growth promotion or, alternatively, ineffective restraint of cell proliferation, produces an imbalance (Fig. 3.19), with a consequent development of epithelial hyperplasia and nodular growth. Essentially, overstimulation, or a decreased capacity of the prostatic cells to respond to TGFβ could play a role in the pathogenesis of BPH. The permissive or promotional role of androgens is accepted, but the earlier reports[76–79] that the intraprostatic concentration of DHT is elevated in patients with BPH, which led to the proposal that DHT was the central causal agent,[80] have been refuted.[81]

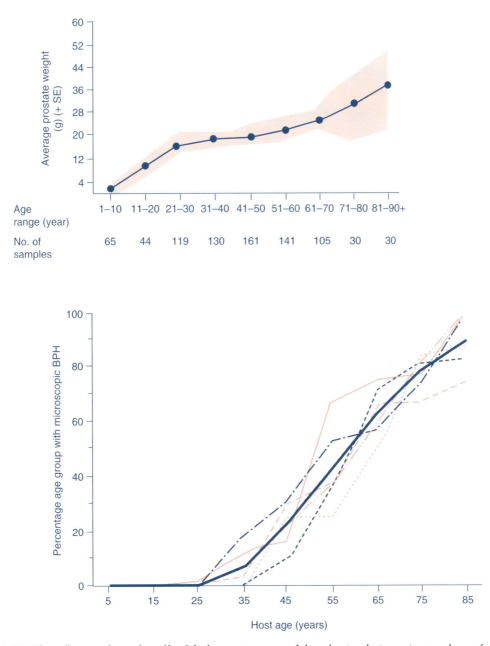

Figure 3.29. *The well-accepted growth profile of the human prostate, and data showing the increasing prevalence of microscopic BPH, epithelial hyperplasia, that is recognized in men as they age from the mid-20s to later life:* ——, *USA;* ----, *England;* ......, *Denmark;* – – –, *Austria;* —·—, *India;* —··—, *Japan;* ——, *composite (average).*

McNeal[75,82] indicates that the majority of the nodules that can be identified at an early age are glandular and are located in the transition zone, the site of origin of clinical obstructive BPH. Nodular formation begins with a cluster of new, glandular epithelial branches, budding eccentrically from the wall of a duct, with the stroma implicated as the source of growth factors. The random focal development of the nodules suggests that this is a locally regulated process, most probably promoted by androgens.

Epithelial–stromal interaction: regional duct heterogeneity

Noteworthy, in relation to the establishment of prostatic homoeostasis after the postpubertal growth

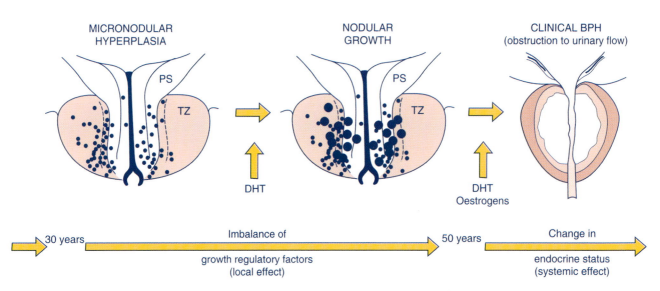

Figure 3.30. *Diagrammatic illustration of the natural history of clinical BPH that causes bladder outlet obstruction. TZ, transitional zone.*

phase, are the elegant studies of Chung Lee.[83,84] He describes regions of the rat ductal system (Fig. 3.31) as proximal, intermediate or distal segments relative to their distance from the urethra. Distinct regional variation in the functional activity of epithelial cells was identified. Cells in the distal region were actively proliferating; the differentiated intermediate section — the major component — secreted protein, and the proximal segment was associated with programmed cell death. The latter segment exclusively expressed sulfated glycoprotein-2, and androgen-suppressed gene product similar to the castration-induced protein referred to as testosterone-repressed prostatic message-2.[85]

This regional variation in morphology and function, occurring in the presence of normal circulating levels of testosterone, suggests a corresponding regional variability in the response to DHT, or to the stromally derived growth regulators. Moreover, the data could also suggest that there is a migration of cells from the distal segment along the duct, to the proximal region where programmed cell death, or apoptosis, prevails. It is equally of interest to recognize the proliferative distal segment of the rat prostate as a region that could be considered related to the peripheral zone in the human gland (Fig. 3.32), the area in which cancer primarily originates.[86]

This more sophisticated concept of cellular homoeostasis, with regional variability in response to androgens, would suggest that epithelial hyperplasia could then be a consequence of an imbalance in the equilibrium between the biological effects of the growth-stimulatory and -inhibitory factors, dysfunctional cell migration, or ineffective programmed cell-death processes.

Oestrogens and the prostate gland

Earlier, it was suggested that androgens played a major part in promoting the development of microscopic BPH and nodular hyperplasia, conditions in which epithelial cell proliferation was prominent. Through the years, however, oestrogens have consistently been implicated in the pathogenesis of BPH, not only in man, but also in the dog.[5] Since ageing is a factor relating to BPH in man, it is interesting that benign enlargement of the prostate is also a universal disorder of the elderly dog, and it is reasonable to search for a factor, common to both species, that might predispose to this condition.

Glandular BPH can be induced in young castrated dogs by administration of oestradiol together with either DHT or the 5-alpha-androstanediol, 5-alpha-androstane-3-alpha,17-beta-diol,[87–91] with at least part of the effect due to an oestrogen-mediated increase in AR and ER levels in the prostate. Neither treatment with either of these C19-steroids alone, nor with testosterone, promoted the development of glandular BPH. Elevated levels of nuclear AR have also been reported[92] in prostatic tissue of the spontaneous BPH that develops in the elderly dog.

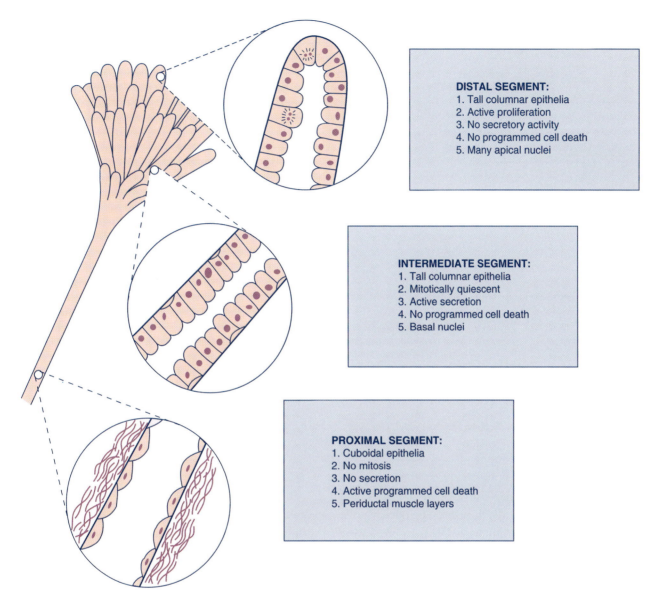

DISTAL SEGMENT:
1. Tall columnar epithelia
2. Active proliferation
3. No secretory activity
4. No programmed cell death
5. Many apical nuclei

INTERMEDIATE SEGMENT:
1. Tall columnar epithelia
2. Mitotically quiescent
3. Active secretion
4. No programmed cell death
5. Basal nuclei

PROXIMAL SEGMENT:
1. Cuboidal epithelia
2. No mitosis
3. No secretion
4. Active programmed cell death
5. Periductal muscle layers

Figure 3.31. *Concept of regional duct heterogeneity.*

Stromal hyperplasia can be induced in the prostates of the monkey and dog by administration of androstenedione, the adrenal androgen, which can be metabolized peripherally (Fig. 3.4) to produce oestrogens. Treatment with an aromatase inhibitor[93–95] prevents this effect, an action compatible with the localization of ERs in stromal tissue. It has also been suggested[96] that oestradiol might be essential to support the androgen-mediated stimulation of prostatic epithelial proliferation, with oestrogen administration to dogs not only increasing the intraprostatic concentration of DHT but also inhibiting the rate of programmed death (Fig. 3.19).

Immunocytochemical studies on the canine prostate[97] indicate that the ER is localized in both stromal and ductal epithelium of the periurethral region, the site of origin of BPH and the region in the prostate of the castrated *Cynomolgus* monkey that is reported to be most responsive to the administration of oestrogen.

The increased 'oestrogenic status' of the human male as he moves into his 50s, relating to an elevated plasma free-oestradiol/free-testosterone ratio, discussed earlier in the text, could be the primary factor responsible for the stromal hyperplasia associated with the development of the prostatic adenoma and bladder outflow obstruction. In most cases, most of the

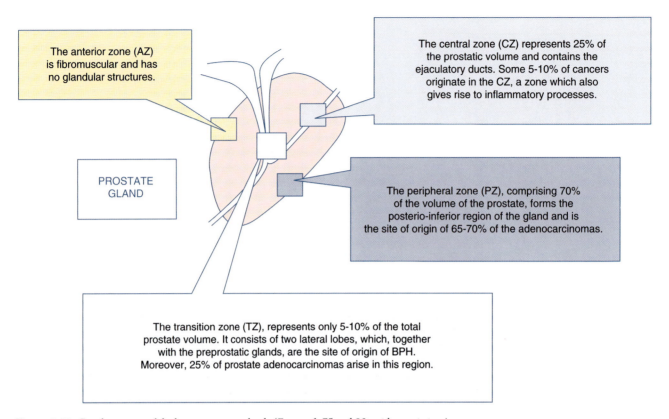

The anterior zone (AZ) is fibromuscular and has no glandular structures.

The central zone (CZ) represents 25% of the prostatic volume and contains the ejaculatory ducts. Some 5-10% of cancers originate in the CZ, a zone which also gives rise to inflammatory processes.

PROSTATE GLAND

The peripheral zone (PZ), comprising 70% of the volume of the prostate, forms the posterio-inferior region of the gland and is the site of origin of 65-70% of the adenocarcinomas.

The transition zone (TZ), represents only 5-10% of the total prostate volume. It consists of two lateral lobes, which, together with the preprostatic glands, are the site of origin of BPH. Moreover, 25% of prostate adenocarcinomas arise in this region.

Figure 3.32. *Zonal anatomy of the human prostate gland. (From refs 75 and 82, with permission.)*

adenomas principally comprise stromal elements, and Figure 3.28 diagrammatically illustrates the putative role of oestradiol, synergistically with DHT, in promoting stromal hyperplasia through the possible mediation and autocrine action of a growth-stimulatory factor, probably basic fibroblast growth factor (bFGF: FGF-2).

It must be stated that the factors that control the growth and differentiation of the stromal cell population are not well understood. Conditioned medium from fibroblasts in culture certainly contains factors that promote fibroblast growth (Fig. 3.33). DHT alone has no effect on the proliferation of prostatic fibroblasts in culture,[98] although it has in association with bFGF. Moreover, both ERs and ARs have been identified[99–100] in fibroblasts and smooth muscle cells, with androgen inhibiting and oestrogen stimulating smooth muscle growth.[101,102] In relation to this, it has been shown[103] that cardiac fibroblasts differentiate into smooth muscle cells after the addition of TGFβ in culture. Fibroblasts co-cultured with epithelial cells undergo a similar change.[104,105]

A locally manifest and variable cell–cell interaction between epithelial and stromal components in the different segments of the ductal system[83,84] could, to some degree, explain the regional heterogeneity in androgen responsiveness of prostatic epithelial cells. The influence of androgens and oestrogens on the promotion of smooth muscle hyperplasia[106] and on the production of growth-stimulatory factors by stromal tissue would seem particularly relevant to abnormal growth. The midlife change in the oestrogenic status of men could impinge on a prevailing imbalance of growth-regulatory mechanisms (Fig. 3.30) when stromal hyperplasia then results from systemic, rather than local, endocrine effects in an individual.

Diet and prostatic disease

It is interesting that the prevalence of microscopic epithelial hyperplasia is similar for men in the East as in the West (Fig. 3.29), yet the incidence of clinical BPH would appear[107] to be much lower in the Oriental male

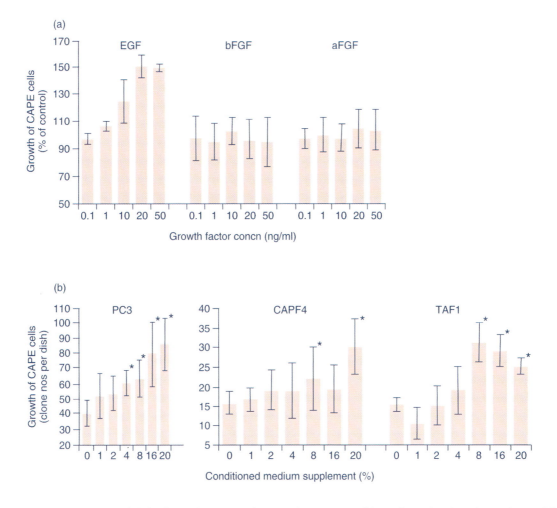

Figure 3.33. *(a) Normal prostatic epithelial cells in culture respond to EGF but not FGF. (b) Conditioned medium from cultures of the PC3 cancer cell line also promotes growth, as does medium from fibroblasts in culture (CAPF4 and TAF1). CAPE, canine epithelial cell line.*

than in his counterpart in the West. It is equally interesting that the incidence of latent prostatic cancer is the same in all men of different races,[108,109] yet there is a greater incidence of the malignant disseminating disease[110] in the West (Fig. 3.34). Evidence is accumulating[111,112] to suggest that dietary components, which are essentially weak oestrogens, could well be implicated in restraining both the development of the clinical adenoma of BPH and also the progression of latent carcinoma into the aggressive malignant disease (Fig. 3.35).

The Asian diet is essentially one of low fat, high fibre. Grain and fibre-rich food, vegetables and legumes, are sources of lignans such as enterolactone and enterodiol, which are weak oestrogens. Soya protein, a major constituent of the Japanese diet, is a source of particular isoflavonoids such as genistein and diadzein, again weak oestrogens and referred to as phyto-oestrogens (Fig. 3.36). The action of the microflora of the gut converts various precursors in certain foodstuffs into the dietary oestrogens, which are absorbed and appear in various body fluids, including prostatic fluid secreted by the prostate gland.[113] There is good evidence that these weak oestrogens could act as a 'natural form of tamoxifen' in restraining breast cancer development in the East by acting, like tamoxifen, as an anti-oestrogen. Furthermore, in their (albeit weak) capacity as 5 alpha-reductase and aromatase inhibitors,[114–116] and possibly as tyrosine kinase and angiogenesis inhibitors, these compounds could well have an important role in restraining the progression of prostatic disease. Some fundamental and exciting work

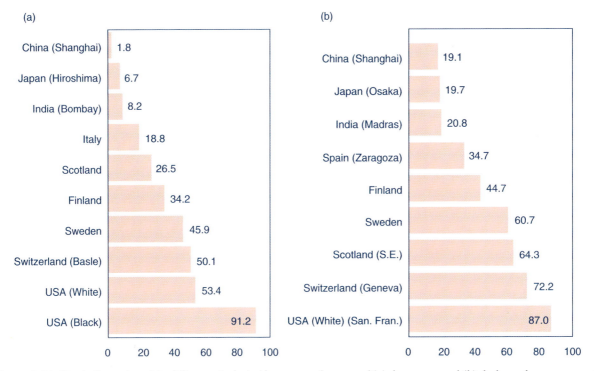

Figure 3.34. *Simple illustration of the differences in the incidence rates of cancers of (a) the prostate and (b) the breast between countries in the East and the West. (Data from ref. 110.)*

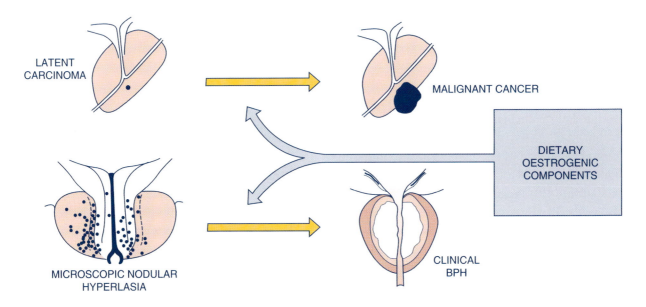

Figure 3.35. *Possible restraining influence of dietary or environmental factors on the development of clinical BPH and possibly on the progression of a latent carcinoma to the aggressive malignant phenotype.*

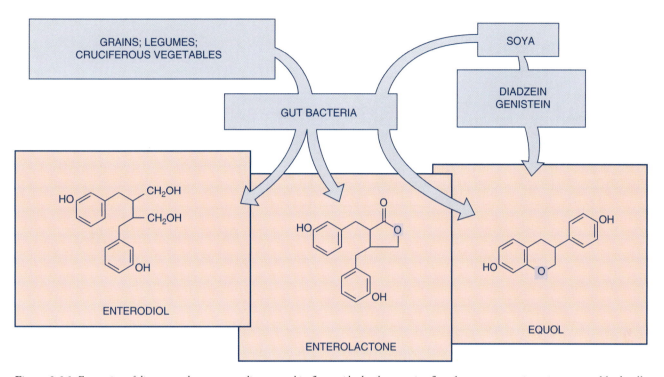

Figure 3.36. *Formation of dietary weak oestrogens, lignans and isoflavonoids, by the gut microflora from precursors in various types of foodstuffs.*

is required in this field to identify the role of such dietary components in disease processes.

Transition zone cancer

It was originally believed that the major proportion of prostatic cancer originated in the peripheral zone of the gland (Fig. 3.32), with the transition zone accepted as the site of origin of BPH. The general consensus has been that prostatic cancer and BPH represented independent disorders, with distinct aetiologies. Recent reports[117] indicate that, although 70% of cancers do originate in the peripheral zone, approximately 25% develop in the centrally located transition zone and are identified as 'incidental carcinoma' in transurethrally resected tissue removed at prostatectomy (TURP) for BPH. Transition zone cancer and BPH show an increasing incidence with ageing, have related natural histories and are androgen-associated conditions that respond to androgen-withdrawal therapy. Cancer is found incidentally in approximately 10% of TURP specimens, with an incidence that is age dependent, and neither BPH nor cancer develop in men castrated early in life. Resected tissue also contains lesions resembling

low-grade acinar carcinoma, referred to as atypical adenomatous hyperplasia (AAH),[118] which could be analogous to prostatic intraepithelial neoplasia (PIN), considered a premalignant lesion in the peripheral zone.[119,120] Both AAH and PIN represent early stages in the escape of epithelial cell proliferation from growth regulation.

AAH may well represent an intermediate phase between microscopic BPH, epithelial hyperplasia in which genetic aberrations can occur, and stage T1 prostate cancer (Fig. 3.37), which does not always have a low metastatic propensity.[121,122] AAH would at least be seen as a dysfunctional imbalance in normal growth-regulatory processes in the prostate, and information is needed on the molecular events that are involved in the initiation of AAH and PIN, their progression to focal cancer, and the development of the clinically asymptomatic slowly growing latent carcinoma into the aggressive malignant phenotype.

Growth-regulatory imbalance

Previous discussion in the text related to the mitogenic activity of KGF, IGF-I and -II and EGF in cultures of

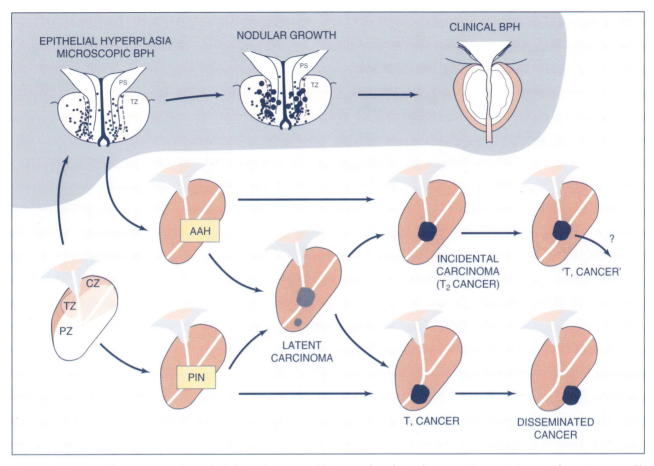

Figure 3.37. *Atypical adenomatous hyperplasia (AAH) — a possible intermediary lesion between microscopic BPH and transition zone T1 cancer. CZ, central zone; PZ, peripheral zone; TZ, transitional zone.*

normal prostatic epithelial cells. The capacity of TGFβ to inhibit epithelial cell proliferation is also well recognized,[56,123,124] the androgen-orchestrated homoeostasis (Fig. 3.21) being the balance between growth-stimulatory and -inhibitory factors. Imbalance results in the development of BPH. Information is accumulating on the roles of these various regulatory peptides in the complex inter- and intracellular signalling processes of the prostate, particularly as they impinge on prostatic disease.

Interesting, too, are reports that using transgenic mice, overexpression of the *int-2* gene encoding for a member of the FGF family — FGF-3 — resulted in epithelial hyperplasia of the prostate.[125] Conditioned media derived from the culture of fibroblasts (Fig. 3.33) are also mitogenic in isolated epithelial cells in culture,[126] but epithelial cells respond neither to acidic FGF (aFGF: FGF-1) nor to bFGF (FGF-2). FGF-1 and FGF-2 are mitogenic for prostatic stromal cells[127,128] and

FGFs have been shown to be mitogenic in certain prostatic tumour cell populations.[129]

Recent investigations have focused on KGF, which is also a member of the FGF family, referred to as FGF-7. KGF, in contrast to aFGF and bFGF, is mitogenic in cultures of normal prostatic epithelial cells, but does not promote stromal proliferation.[130] KGF is produced by prostatic fibroblasts in culture, where its expression is regulated by androgens. Moreover, the growth-stimulatory effects of KGF are inhibited by TGFβ.

Particularly interesting in relation to the FGF family of growth factors and their corresponding receptors is the marked complexity of the mechanisms by which some of the FGF-R genes are regulated and expressed. Four FGF-R genes, FGF-R1 to FGF-R4, have been recognized (Fig. 3.38). The FGF-R1 (*flg*) gene encodes a receptor protein that is normally recognized in stromal cells.[57,131] The prostate epithelial cells express a 'splice variant' of the FGF-R2 (*bek*) gene, a receptor (referred

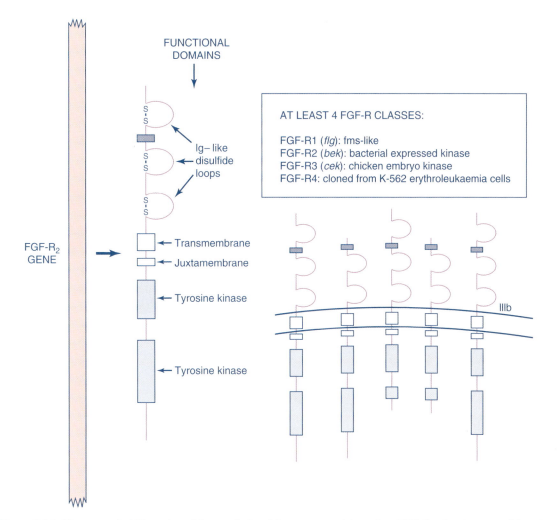

Figure 3.38. *Diagrammatical illustration of the complexity of the structures of the various FGF-Rs, showing external domains that bind FGF and heparin, the trans- and juxtamembrane domains and the intracellular tyrosine kinase. The different splice variants would display different ligand specificities. Ig, immunoglobulin.*

to as FGF-R2-exonIIIb) that specifically recognizes KGF.[132] The splicing enzymes (Fig. 3.13) structure the primary mRNA to produce the mature mRNA transcript. Splicing variants are produced by varying the length of the exons that are built into the mature mRNA, with corresponding synthesis of receptors with structural heterogeneity in both the extracellular FGF-binding domain of the protein and in the intracellular signal transduction domain.[59,133]

Studies on liver cells[58,60] indicate that such differing receptor phenotypes can elicit a stimulatory or inhibitory signal in response to different FGFs.

In the prostate gland, the KGF-specific FGF-R2-exonIIIb receptor is expressed in the slowly growing,

non-metastatic and well-differentiated Dunning R-3327 prostatic acid phosphatase (PAP) prostate tumours (Fig. 3.39). This receptor is not present in the rapidly growing, undifferentiated cancer, although FGF-R2-exonIIIc was recognized in the cancer, a receptor with a high binding avidity for bFGF (FGF-2), as well as the FGF-R1 (*flg*) gene, which encodes the receptor normally localized in the stromal cells.[57,131]

Natural history of prostatic disease

On the basis of the foregoing discussion, it is not unreasonable to consider that the steps outlined in Figure 3.37 represent the various growth phases in the

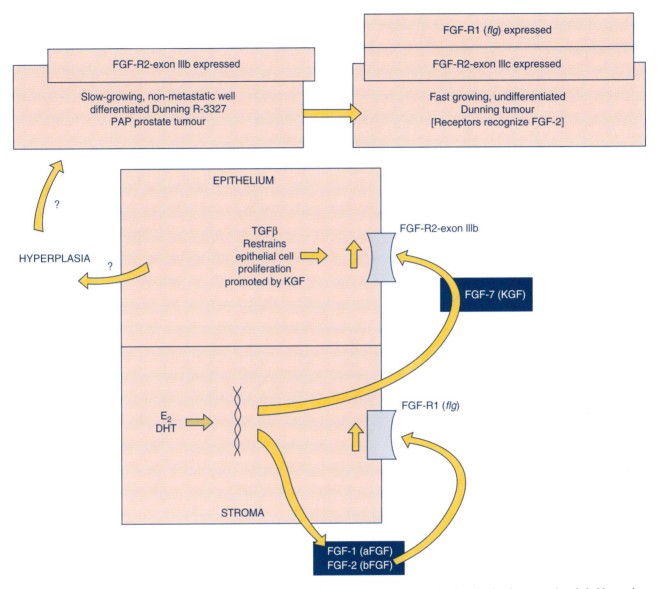

Figure 3.39. *Illustrated scheme to portray the changes in the FGF-R expression that may be related to the development of epithelial hyperplasia and early cancer, with progression to the malignant disease. E_2, oestradiol. (Data from refs 57 and 131.)*

natural history associated with the pathogenesis of BPH and prostate cancer. The complex mechanisms by which the expression of genes can lead to structural variation and ligand specificity for various members of the FGF family, as a result of differential splicing of RNA transcripts, provide concepts as to the possible changes that could occur as disease progresses. It is interesting to speculate on the biological effects of these multiple autocrine and intracrine loops, which influence the family of FGF-receptor proteins. Such alterations in the specificity of an FGF-R that make it unable to recognize KGF, but avidly bind to FGF-2, may underlie the early

imbalance of growth-regulatory processes within the prostate that leads to epithelial hyperplasia and, ultimately, to malignancy.

Earlier investigations such as those from the author's laboratory,[134] relating to the increased specific receptor-binding capacity of tissue preparations from grade II and III prostate cancers for radiolabelled IGF-I, relative to those found for tissue from grade I and from BPH samples, suggest that the imbalance of growth control probably involves many components.[5,6] The complexity and sophistication of these steroid hormone-modulated gene-regulatory processes is now well recognized.[44,135–137]

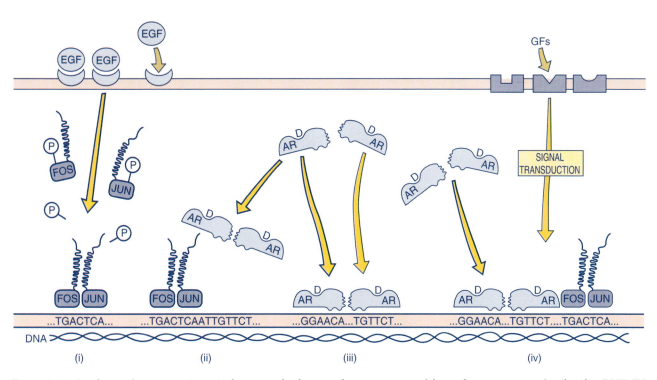

Figure 3.40. *Regulation of gene transcription in the prostate by the particular arrangements of the regulatory sequences of nucleotides. DHT (D) binds to AR, which then associates with the HRE to influence gene expression (iii). Signal transduction pathways are activated by various growth factors (GFs) such as KGF, EGF and the IGFs to enhance the activity of certain growth-related genes such as the c-fos and c-jun. They encode proteins which, as heterodimers, bind to the AP-1 recognition sites (i) involving the nucleotide sequence TGACTCA. The relative positioning of these regulatory sequences can result in competition for the site (ii) or, as in (iv), cooperation. An inhibitory growth factor can introduce a regulatory agent that prevents the association of a transcription factor to DNA.*

Clearly, the androgenic influence on the prostate is dependent on the association between the DHT–AR complex and the AREs of the genome. Equally important are the closely related cell-specific transcription factors, together with the optimal spatial orientation of chromatin in the sequences of nucleotides associated with the gene promoter regions that 'read' the response signals. The intercession and binding of the other growth-regulatory transcription factors in juxtaposition flanking the AREs would seem mandatory to the growth-regulatory processes (Fig. 3.40).

The integrated response of cells to signalling language, reading sense from the messages induced by the various growth factors and hormones, is clearly a finely tuned system. The 'crosstalk' between the steroid receptor-controlled pathways and those activated by growth factors would appear to be at the very fulcrum of these regulatory processes. Essentially, they malfunction as cellular proliferation overrides growth-restraining influences, causing epithelial hyperplasia. As cells escape from growth-regulatory control, carcinogenesis prevails.

References

1. Garraway W M, Collins G N, Lee R J. High prevalence of benign prostatic hypertrophy in the community. Lancet 1991; 338: 469–471
2. Barry M J, Beckley S, Boyle P et al. Importance of understanding the epidemiology and natural history of BPH. In: Cockett A T K, Aso Y, Chatelain C et al. (eds) The first international consultation on benign prostatic hyperplasia (BPH). Paris: SCI Press, 1991: 13–21
3. Glynne R J, Campion E W, Bouchard G R, Silbert J E. The development of benign prostatic hyperplasia among volunteers in the normative aging study. Am J Epidemiol 1985; 121: 78–90
4. Lytton B, Emery J M, Harvard B M. The incidence of benign prostatic obstruction. J Urol 1968; 99: 639–645
5. Griffiths K, Akaza H, Eaton C L et al. Hormones, growth factors and benign prostatic hyperplasia (BPH). In: Cockett A T K, Aso Y, Chatelain C et al. (eds) The first international consultation on benign prostatic hyperplasia (BPH). Paris: SCI Press, 1991: 25–49

6. Griffiths K, Akaza H, Eaton C L et al. Regulation of prostatic growth. In: Cockett A T K, Khoury S, Aso Y et al. (eds) The second international consultation on benign prostatic hyperplasia (BPH). Paris: SCI Press, 1993: 49–75

7. Riad-Fahmy D, Read G F, Walker R F, Griffiths K. Steroids in saliva for assessing endocrine function. Endocr Rev 1982; 3: 367–395

8. Vermeulen A, Deslypere J P, Meirleir K. A new look at the andropause: altered function of the gonadotrophs. J Steroid Biochem 1989; 32: 163–165

9. Schroeder F H, Westerhof M, Bosch R J L H, Kurth K H. Benign prostatic hyperplasia treated by castration or the LH-RH analogue buserelin: a report on six cases. Eur Urol 1986; 12: 318–321

10. Baird D T, Uno A, Melby J C. Adrenal secretion of androgens and oestrogens. J Endocrinol 1969; 45: 135–136

11. Lipsett M B. Steroid secretion by the human testis. In: Rosemberg E, Paulsen C A (eds) The human testis. New York: Plenum Press, 1970: 407–421

12. Santen R J, Bardin C W. Episodic luteinizing hormone secretion in man. Pulse analysis, clinical interpretation, physiological mechanisms. J Clin Invest 1973; 52: 2617–2628

13. Longcope C, Widrich W, Sawin C T. The secretion of estrone and estradiol-17β by human testis. Steroids 1972; 20: 439–448

14. Baird D T, Galbraith A, Fraser I S, Newsam J E. The concentration of oestrone and oestradiol-17β in spermatic venous blood in man. J Endocrinol 1973; 57: 285–288

15. McDonald P C. Origin of oestrogen in man. In: Grayhack J T, Wilson J D, Scherbenske M J (eds) Benign prostatic hyperplasia. NIAMDD Workshop Proc. NIH Publ. No. (NIH) 76-1113. Bethesda: DHEW, 1976: 191–193

16. Vermeulen A, Rubens R, Verdonck L. Testosterone secretion and metabolism in male senescence. J Clin Endocrinol Metab 1972; 34: 730–735

17. Vermeulen A, Van Camp A, Mattelaer J, De Sy W. Hormonal factors relating to abnormal growth of the prostate. In: Coffey D S, Isaacs J T (eds) Prostate cancer. UICC Tech Rep Ser Vol 48. Geneva: UICC, 1979: 81–92

18. Vermeulen A. Testicular hormone secretion and aging in males. In: Grayhack J T, Wilson J D, Scherbenske M J (eds) Benign prostatic hyperplasia. NIAMDD Workshop Proc. NIH Publ. No. (NIH) 76-1113. Bethesda: DHEW, 1976: 177–182

19. Rubens R, Dhont M, Vermeulen A. Further studies on Leydig cell function in old age. J Clin Endocrinol Metab 1974; 39: 40–45

20. Rosner W. The functions of corticosteroid-binding globulin and sex hormone-binding globulin: recent advances. Endocr Rev 1990; 11: 80–91

21. Loukovaara M, Carson M, Adlercreutz H. Regulation of production and secretion of sex hormone-binding globulin in HepG2 cell cultures by hormones and growth factors. J Clin Endocrinol Metab 1995; 80: 160–164

22. Mousavi Y, Adlercreutz H. Genistein is an effective stimulator of sex hormone-binding globulin production in hepatocarcinoma human liver cancer cells in culture. Steroids 1993; 58: 301–304

23. Bruchovsky N, Wilson J D. The intranuclear binding of testosterone and 5α-androstan-17β-ol-3-one by rat prostate. J Biol Chem 1968; 243: 5953–5960

24. Bruchovsky N, Wilson J D. The conversion of testosterone to 5α-androstan-17β-ol-3-one by rat prostate in vivo and in vitro. J Biol Chem 1968; 243: 2012–2021

25. Harper M E, Pike A, Peeling W B, Griffiths K. Steroids of adrenal origin metabolized by human prostatic tissue both in vivo and in vitro. J Endocrinol 1974; 60: 117–125

26. Harper M E, Peeling W B, Griffiths K. Adrenal androgens and the prostate. In: Motta M, Serio M (eds) Hormonal therapy of prostatic disease: basic and clinical aspects. Amsterdam: Medicom Europe, 1988: 81–94

27. Labrie F, Dupont A, Belanger A et al. New approach in the treatment of prostatic cancer: complete instead of partial withdrawal of androgens. Prostate 1983; 4: 579–594

28. Labrie F, Dupont A, Belanger A. Spectacular response to combined antihormonal treatment in advanced prostate cancer. In: Labrie F, Prouix L (eds) Endocrinology, International Congress Series. Amsterdam: Excerpta Medica, 1984: 450–453

29. Denis L J. Controversies in the management of localised and metastatic prostatic cancer. Eur J Cancer 1991; 27: 333–341

30. Muntzing J. The androgenic action of adrenal implants in the ventral prostate of adult, castrated and oestrogen-treated rats. Acta Pharmacol Toxicol 1971; 30: 203–207

31. Nicholson R I, Davies P, Griffiths K. Interaction of androgens with oestradiol-17β receptor proteins in DMBA-induced mammary tumours — a possible oncolytic mechanism. Eur J Cancer 1978; 14: 439–445

32. Griffiths K, Davies P, Harper M E et al. The etiology and endocrinology of prostatic cancer. In: Rose D (ed) Endocrinology of cancer, Vol 2. Boca Raton: CRC Press, 1979: 1–55

33. Griffiths K, Davies P, Eaton C L et al. Cancer of the prostate: endocrine factors. In: Clarke J R (ed) Oxford Reviews of Reproductive Biology, Vol 9. Oxford: Oxford University Press, 1987; 192–259

34. MacDonald P C, Grodin J M, Siiteri P K. Dynamics of androgen and oestrogen secretion. In: Baird D T, Strong J A (eds) Control of gonadal steroid secretion. Baltimore: Williams and Wilkins, 1972: 157–167

35. Kley H K, Nieschlag E, Bidlingmaier F, Kruskemper H L. Possible age-dependent influence of estrogens on the binding of testosterone in plasma of adult men. Horm Metab Res 1974; 6: 213–221

36. Baker H W G, Burger H G, De Kretser D M et al. Changes in the pituitary–testicular system with age. Clin Endocrinol 1976; 5: 349

37. Hryb D J, Kahn M S, Romas N A, Rosner W. Solubilization and partial characterization of the sex hormone-building globulin receptor from human prostate. J Biol Chem 1989; 264: 5378–5383

38. Imperato-McGinley J, Guerrero L, Gautier T, Peterson R E. Steroid 5α-reductase deficiency in men: an inherited form of male pseudohermaphroditism. Science 1974; 186: 1213–1215

39. Green S, Chambon P. Nuclear receptors enhance our understanding of transcription regulation. Trends Genet 1988; 4: 309–314

40. McPhaul M J, Marcelli M, Zoppi S et al. The spectrum of mutations in the androgen receptor gene that causes androgen resistance. J Clin Endocrinol Metab 1993; 76: 17–23

41. Pinsky L, Kaufman M. Genetics of steroid receptors and their disorders. In: Harris H, Hirschhorn K (eds) Advances in human genetics. New York: Plenum Press, 1987: 299–472

42. Brown T R, Lubahn D B, Wilson E M et al. Functional characterization of naturally occurring mutant androgen receptors from subjects with complete androgen insensitivity. Mol Endocrinol 1990; 4: 1759–1772

43. Evans B A J, Harper M E, Daniells C E et al. Low incidence of androgen receptor gene mutations in human prostatic tumors using single strand conformation polymorphism analysis. Prostate 1996; in press

44. Truss M, Beato M. Steroid hormone receptors: interaction with deoxyribonucleic acid and transcription factors. Endocr Rev 1993; 14: 459–479

45. Kumar V, Chambon P. The oestrogen receptor binds tightly to its responsive element as a ligand-induced homodimer. Cell 1988; 55: 145–156

46. Green S, Chambon P. Oestradiol induction of a glucocorticoid-responsive gene by a chimaeric receptor. Nature 1987; 325: 75–78

47. Evans R M, Hollenberg S M. Zinc fingers: gilt by association. Cell 1988; 52: 1–3

48. Coffey D S. The structure and function of the prostate gland and the sex accessory tissues in prostate cancer. In: Khoury S, Chatelain C, Murphy G, Denis L (eds) Physiologie de la Proside. Paris: FIIS, 1990: 70–103

49. Isaacs J T. Antagonistic effect of androgen on prostatic cell death. Prostate 1984; 5: 545–557

50. Bruchovsky N, Lesser B, Van Doorn E, Craven S. Hormonal effects of cell proliferation in rat prostate. Vitam Horm 1975; 33: 61–102

51. Katz A E, Benson M C, Wise G J et al. Gene activity during the early phase of androgen-stimulated rat prostate regrowth. Cancer Res 1989; 49: 5889–5894

52. Quarmby V E, Beckman W C Jr, Wilson E M, French F S. Androgen regulation of a c-myc messenger ribonucleic acid levels in rat ventral prostate. Mol Endocrinol 1987; 1: 865–874

53. Buttyan R, Zakeri S, Lockshin R, Wolgemuth D. Cascade induction of c-fos, c-myc, and heat shock 70K transcriptions during regression of the rat ventral prostate gland. Mol Endocrinol 1988; 2: 650–657

54. Griffiths K, Davies P, Eaton C L et al. Endocrine factors in the initiation, diagnosis, and treatment of prostatic cancer. In: Voigt K D, Knabbe C (eds) Endocrine dependent tumours. New York: Raven Press, 1991: 83–130

55. Jones H E, Eaton C L, Barrow D et al. Growth response of normal and neoplastic prostatic cell lines to retinoic acid: influence on the expression of retinoic acid receptor. Prostate 1996; in press

56. Sporn M B, Roberts A B. TGF-β: problems and prospects. Cell Regul 1990; 1: 875–882

57. Xu J, Nakahara M, Crabb J W et al. Expression and immunocytochemical analysis of rat and human fibroblast growth factor (flg) isoforms. J Biol Chem 1992; 267: 17792–17803

58. Kan M, Huang J, Mansson P E et al. Heparin-binding growth factor type I (acidic fibroblast growth factor): a potential biphasic autocrine and paracrine regulation of hepatocyte regeneration. Proc Natl Acad Sci USA 1989; 86: 7432–7436

59. Hou J, Kan M, McKeehan K et al. Fibroblast growth factor receptors from liver vary in three structural domains. Science 1991; 251: 665–668

60. Kan M, DiSorbo D, Hou J et al. High and low affinity binding of heparin-binding growth factor to a 130-kDa receptor correlates with stimulation and inhibition of growth of a differentiated human hepatoma cell. J Biol Chem 1988; 263: 11306–11313

61. Rohr H P, Bartsch G. Human benign prostatic hyperplasia: a stromal disease? New perspectives by quantitative morphology. Urology 1980; 16: 625–633

62. McNeal J E. Normal histology of the prostate. Am J Surg Pathol 1988; 12: 629–633

63. Franks L M, Riddle P M, Carbonell A W, Gey G O. A comparative study of the ultrastructure and lack of growth capacity of adult human prostate epithelium mechanically separated from its stroma. J Pathol 1970; 100: 113–119

64. Tenniswood M. Role of epithelial–stromal interactions in the control of gene expression in the prostate: an hypothesis. Prostate 1986; 9: 375–385

65. Cunha G R, Chung L W K, Shannon J M et al. Hormone-induced morphogenesis and growth: role of mesenchymal–epithelial interactions. Recent Prog Horm Res 1983; 39: 559–595

66. Cunha G R, Donjacour A A, Cooke P S et al. The endocrinology and development biology of the prostate. Endocr Rev 1987; 8: 338–362

67. Schweikert H U, Totzauer P, Rohr H P, Bartschi G. Correlated biochemical and stereological studies on testosterone metabolism in the stromal and epithelial compartment of human benign prostatic hyperplasia. J Urol 1985; 134: 403–407

68. Krieg M. Biochemical endocrinology of human prostatic tumours. Prog Cancer Res Ther 1984; 31: 425–440

69. Kyprianou N, Davies P. Association state of androgen receptors in nuclei of human benign hypertrophic prostate. Prostate 1986; 8: 363–380

70. Krieg M, Bartsch W, Thomsen M, Voigt K D. Androgens and estrogens: their interaction with stroma and epithelium of human benign prostatic hyperplasia and normal prostate. J Steroid Biochem 1983; 19: 155–161

71. Tunn S, Krieg M Z. Androgen metabolism in human prostate: influence of aging. In: Aumuller G, Krieg M, Senge T (eds) New aspects in the regulation of prostatic function. Munich: W Zuckshwerdt Verlag, 1989: 134–142

72. Isaacs J T, Coffey D S. Etiology and disease process of benign prostatic hyperplasia. Prostate 1989; (suppl 2): 33–50

73. Berry S J, Coffey D S, Walsh P C, Ewing L L. The development of human benign prostate hyperplasia with age. J Urol 1984; 132: 474–479

74. Walsh P C. In: Walsh P C, Gittes R E, Perlmutter A D, Stamey T A (eds) Campbell's urology, Vol 2 5th ed. Philadelphia: Saunders, 1986: 1248–1265

75. McNeal J E. Anatomy of the prostate and morphogenesis of BPH. In: Kimball F A, Buhl A E, Carter D B (eds) New approaches to the study of benign prostatic hyperplasia. New York: Alan R. Liss, 1984: 27–53

76. Siiteri P K, Wilson J D. Dihydrotestosterone in prostatic hypertrophy. The formation and content of dihydrotestosterone in the hypertrophied prostate of man. J Clin Invest 1970; 49: 1737–1745

77. Geller J, Albert J, Lopez D et al. Comparison of androgen metabolites in benign prostatic hypertrophy (BPH) and normal prostate. J Clin Endocrinol Metab 1976; 43: 686–688

78. Habib F K, Lee I R, Stitch S R, Smith P H. Androgen levels in the plasma and prostatic tissues of patients with benign hypertrophy and carcinoma of the prostate. J Endocrinol 1976; 71: 99–107

79. Meikle A W, Stringham J D, Olsen D C. Subnormal tissue 3α-androstanediol and androsterone in prostatic hyperplasia. J Clin Endocrinol Metab 1978; 47: 909–913

80. Geller J. Pathogenesis and medical treatment of benign prostatic hyperplasia. Prostate 1989; (suppl 2): 95–104

81. Walsh P C, Hutchins G M, Ewing L L. Tissue content of dihydrotestosterone in human prostatic hyperplasia is not supranormal. J Clin Invest 1983; 72: 1772–1777

82. McNeal J E. Origin and evolution of benign prostatic enlargement. Invest Urol 1978; 15: 340–345

83. Lee C, Sensibar J A, Dudek S M et al. Prostatic ductal system in rats: regional variation in morphological and functional activities. Biol Reprod. 1990; 43: 1079–1086

84. Sensibar J A, Griswold M D, Sylvester S R et al. Prostatic ductal system in rats: regional variation in localization of an androgen-repressed gene product, sulfated glycoprotein-2. Endocrinology 1991; 128: 2091–2102

85. Wong P, Pineault J, Lakins J N et al. Genomic organisation and expression of the rat TRPM-2 (clusterin) gene, a gene implicated in apoptosis. J Biol Chem 1993; 268: 5021–5031

86. McNeal J E. Age related changes in prostatic epithelium associated with carcinoma. In: Griffiths K, Pierrepoint C G (eds) Some aspects of the aetiology and biochemistry of prostatic cancer. Proc Third Tenovus Workshop. Cardiff: Alpha Omega, 1970: 23–32

87. Walsh P C, Wilson J D. The induction of prostatic hypertrophy in the dog with androstanediol. J Clin Invest 1976; 57: 1093–1097

88. DeKlerk D P, Coffey D S, Ewing L L et al. Comparison of spontaneous and experimentally induced canine prostatic hyperplasia. J Clin Invest 1979; 64: 842–849

89. Moore R J, Gazak J M, Quebbeman J F, Wilson J D. Concentration of dihydrotestosterone and 3α-androstanediol in naturally occurring and androgen-induced prostatic hyperplasia in the dog. J Clin Invest 1979; 64: 1003–1010

90. Tunn U, Senge T, Schenck B, Neumann F. Biochemical and histological studies on prostates in castrated dogs after treatment with androstanediol, oestradiol and cyproterone acetate. Acta Endocrinol 1979; 91: 373–384

91. Tunn U, Senge T, Schenck B, Neumann F. Effects of cyproterone acetate on experimentally induced canine prostatic hyperplasia: a morphological and histochemical study. Urol Int 1980; 35: 125–140

92. Trachtenberg J, Hicks L L, Walsh P C. Androgen and estrogen receptor content in spontaneous and experimentally induced canine hyperplasia. J Clin Invest 1980; 65: 1051–1059

93. El Etreby M F, Habenicht U-F. Experimental induction of stromal hyperplasia in prostate of castrated dogs treated with 4-androstene-3,17-dione. Effect of the aromatase inhibitor 4-hydroxyandrostene-3,17-dione. In: Rodgers C H, Coffey D S, Cunha G R et al (eds) Benign prostatic hyperplasia, Vol II. NIH Publ. No. 87-2881, Dept Health, Human Serv, NIH. Bethesda: DHEW, 1987; 303–310

94. Habenicht U-F, El Etreby M F. Synergic inhibitory effects of the aromatase inhibitor 1-methyl-androsta-1,4-diene-3,17-dione and the antiandrogen cyproterone acetate on androstenedione-induced hyperplastic effects on the prostates of castrated dogs. Prostate 1987; 11: 133–143

95. Habenicht U-F, Schwartz K, Neumann F, El Etreby M L. Induction of estrogen-related hyperplastic changes in the prostate of the *Cynomolgus* monkey (*Macaca fascicularis*) by androstenedione and its antagonization by the aromatase inhibitor 1-methyl-androsta-1,4-diene-3,17-dione. Prostate 1987; 11: 313–326

96. Coffey D S, Berry S J, Ewing L L. An overview of current concepts in the study of benign prostatic hyperplasia. In: Rodgers C H, Coffey D S, Cunha G R (eds) Benign prostatic hyperplasia, Vol II. NIH Publ. No. 87-2881, Dept Health, Human Serv. Bethesda: DHEW, 1987; 1–13

97. Schulze H, Barrack E R. Immunocytochemical localization of oestrogen receptors in spontaneous and experimentally induced canine benign prostatic hyperplasia. Prostate 1987; 11: 145–162

98. Sherwood E R, Fong C J, Lee C, Kozlowski J M. Basic fibroblast growth factor: a potential mediator of stromal growth in the human prostate. Endocrinology 1992; 130: 2955–2963

99. Cooke P S, Young P, Cunha G R. Androgen receptor expression in developing male reproductive organs. Endocrinology 1991; 128: 2867–2873

100. Cooke P S, Young P, Hess R A, Cunha G R. Estrogen receptor expression in developing epididymis, efferent ductules, and other male reproductive tissues. Endocrinology 1991; 128: 2874–2879

101. Toney T W, Danzo B J. Developmental changes in and hormonal regulation of estrogen and androgen receptors present in the rabbit epididymis. Biol Reprod 1988; 39: 818–828

102. Toney T W, Danzo B J. Androgen and estrogen effects on protein synthesis by the adult rabbit epididymis. Endocrinology 1989; 125: 243–249

103. Eghbali M, Tomek R, Woods C, Bhambi B. Cardiac fibroblasts are predisposed to convert into myocyte phenotype: specific effect of transforming growth factors. Proc Natl Acad Sci USA 1991; 88: 795–799

104. Cunha G R, Battle E, Young P et al. Role of epithelial–mesenchymal interactions in the differentiation and spacial organization of visceral smooth muscle. Epith Cell Biol 1992; 1: 76–83

105. Kedinger M, Simon-Assmann P, Bouziges F et al. Smooth muscle actin expression during rat gut development and induction in fetal skin fibroblastic cells associated with intestinal embryonic epithelium. Differentiation 1990; 40: 87–97

106. Bruengger A, Mariotti A, Rohr H P et al. Androgen and estrogen effect on guinea pig seminal vesicle muscle: a combined stereological and biochemical study. Prostate 1986; 9: 303–310

107. Ekman P. BPH epidemiology and risk factors. Prostate 1989; (suppl 2): 23–31

108. Breslow N E, Chan C W, Dhom G et al. Latent carcinoma of prostate at autopsy in seven areas. Int J Cancer 1977; 20: 680–688

109. Yatani R, Chigusa I, Akazaki K et al. Geographic pathology of latent prostatic cancer. Int J Cancer 1982; 29: 611–616

110. Dhom G. Epidemiology of hormone-depending tumours. In: Voight K D, Knabbe C (eds) Endocrine dependent tumours. New York: Raven Press, 1991; 1–42

111. Griffiths K, Adlercreutz H, Boyle P et al. Nutrition and cancer. Isis Medical Media, Oxford: 1995; 77–98

112. Adlercreutz H. Western diet and western diseases: some hormonal and biochemical mechanisms and associations. Scand J Clin Invest 1990; 50 (suppl): 3–23

113. Finlay E M H, Wilson D W, Adlercreutz H, Griffiths K. The identification and measurement of 'phyto-oestrogens' in human saliva, plasma, breast aspirate or cyst fluid, and prostatic fluid using gas chromatography–mass spectrometry. J Endocrinol 1991; 129 (suppl): 49

114. Evans B A J, Griffiths K, Morton M S. Inhibition of 5-α-reductase in genital skin fibroblasts by dietary lignans and isoflavonoids. J Endocrinol 1995; 147: 296–302

115. Adlercreutz H, Bannwart C, Wahala K et al. Inhibition of human aromatase by mammalian lignans and isoflavonoid phytoestrogens. J Steroid Biochem Molec Biol 1993; 44: 147–153

116. Campbell D R, Kurzer M S. Flavonoid inhibition of aromatase enzyme activity in human preadipocytes. J Steroid Biochem Molec Biol 1993; 46: 381–388

117. Bostwick D G, Barcells F S, Cooner W H et al. Benign prostatic hyperplasia (BPH) and cancer of the prostate. In: Cockett A T K, Aso Y, Chatelain C et al. (eds) The first international consultation on benign prostatic hyperplasia (BPH). Paris: SCI Press, 1991; 139–159

118. Kovi J, Mostofi F K. Atypical hyperplasia of the prostate. Urology 1987; 34 (suppl): 23–27

119. McNeal J E, Bostwick D G, Kindrachuk R A et al. Patterns of progression of prostatic cancer. Lancet 1986; i: 60–63

120. Bostwick D G, Brawer M K. Prostatic intra-epithelial neoplasia and early invasion in prostatic cancer. Cancer 1987; 59: 788–794

121. Epstein J I, Paull G, Eggleston J C, Walsh P C. Prognosis of untreated stage A1 prostatic carcinoma: a study of 94 cases with extended follow-up. J Urol 1986; 136: 837–839

122. Whitmore W F. Stage A prostatic cancer — Editorial. J Urol 1986; 136: 883

123. Wilding G, Valverius E, Knabbe C, O'Elmann E P. Role of transforming growth factor-α in human prostate cancer cell growth. Prostate 15: 1989; 1–12

124. Sporn M B, Roberts A B. Interactions of retinoids and transforming growth factor-β in regulation of cell differentiation and proliferation. Mol Endocrinol 1991; 5: 3–7

125. Muller W J, Lee F S, Dickson C et al. The int-2 gene product acts as an epithelial growth factor in transgenic mice. EMBO J 1990; 9: 907–913

126. Kabalin J N, Peehl D M, Stamey T A. Clonal growth of human prostatic epithelial cells is stimulated by fibroblasts. Prostate 1989; 14: 251–263

127. Mansson P E, Adams P, Kan M, McKeehan W L. Heparin-binding growth factor gene expression and receptor characteristics in normal rat prostate and two transplantable rat prostate tumours. Cancer Res 1989; 49: 2485–2494

128. Story M T, Livingstone B, Baeten L et al. Cultured human prostate-derived fibroblasts produce a factor that stimulates their growth with properties indistinguishable from basic fibroblast growth factor. Prostate 1989; 15: 355–365

129. Chaproniere D M, McKeehan W L. Serial culture of single adult human prostatic epithelial cells in serum-free medium containing

low calcium and a new growth factor from bovine brain. Cancer Res 1986; 46: 819–824

130. Yan G, Fukabori Y, Nikolaropoulos S et al. Heparin-binding keratinocyte growth factor is a candidate stromal to epithelial cell andromedin. Mol Endocrinol 1992; 6: 2123–2128

131. Yan G, Wang F, Fukabori Y et al. Expression and transforming activity of a variant of the heparin-binding fibroblast growth factor receptor (flg) gene resulting from splicing of the alpha exon at an alternate 3'-acceptor site. Biochem Biophys Res Commun 1992; 183: 423–430

132. Miki T, Bottaro D P, Fleming T P et al. Determination of ligand-binding specificity by alternate splicing: two distinct growth factor receptors encoded by a single gene. Proc Natl Acad Sci USA 1992; 89: 246–250

133. Jaye M, Schlessinger J, Dionne C A. Fibroblast growth factor receptor tyrosine kinases: molecular analysis and signal transduction. Biochem Biophys Acta 1992; 1135: 185–199

134. Davies P, Eaton C L, France T D, Phillips M E A. Growth factor receptors and oncogene expression in prostate cells. Am J Clin Oncol 1988; 11 (suppl 2): S1–S7

135. Beato M. Gene regulation by steroid hormones. Cell 1989; 56: 335–344

136. Yamamoto K R. Steroid receptor regulated transcription of specific genes and gene networks. Ann Rev Genet 1985; 19: 209–252

137. Gronemeyer H. Transcription activation by estrogen and progesterone receptors. Ann Rev Genet 1991; 25: 89–123

4

Stromal–epithelial interactions: molecular aspects and relevance to benign prostatic hyperplasia

M. R. Freeman   M. E. Gleave   L. W. K. Chung

Introduction

Despite research on benign prostatic hyperplasia (BPH) undertaken by a large number of laboratories and spanning nearly a century,[1,2] the molecular mechanisms underlying the age-related enlargement of the prostate in humans are still obscure. In the last decade, however, there has been an explosive growth of new knowledge on molecular aspects of cellular growth control, the function of secreted and cell-surface proteins, the regulatory role of the extracellular matrix (ECM), pathways of transmission of external signals to the cell interior and to the cell nucleus, and the mechanics of cell cycle regulation. Although much of this research has been carried out in other organ systems or in experimental models, the new findings provide important clues about potential mechanisms of prostatic neoplasia. There is now strong evidence that biochemical mediators sequestered or originating from within the prostatic connective tissue have a crucial role in the functional state and the growth potential of the mature gland. In the prostate and in other organ systems, both diffusible (soluble) and solid-state (insoluble) mediators are involved in tissue interactions responsible for differentiative change, as well as changes in patterns of cell growth. The identification of some of these regulatory molecules, and in some cases the discovery of their specific functional roles, suggest the possibility that BPH occurs as a result of aberrant cellular interactions resulting from alteration in expression, localization and function of cytokines and growth factors as well as insoluble regulatory molecules comprising the connective tissue matrix. This chapter provides an overview of the concept of stromal (mesenchymal)–epithelial interaction as it pertains to development and growth of the prostate, and attempts to integrate findings from more classic studies of tissue and cell recombination with recent results from molecular investigations of cell regulation by soluble regulatory factors and the ECM. The objective of this treatment is to provide a framework for the development of testable hypotheses of the molecular processes underlying the clinical dilemma of BPH, with the ultimate goal of devising novel and effective therapies for this common neoplasm.

Stromal–epithelial interactions in prostatic functional differentiation and growth

The prostate gland is composed of two histologically distinct tissue compartments — a branching acinar–ductal epithelium and fibromuscular stroma. Morphometric analyses have demonstrated that each compartment (when luminal spaces are considered part of the epithelial compartment) make up about one-half of the glandular volume of the human prostate.[3] Each of these tissue elements is further composed of a variety of cell types, including secretory and basal epithelial cells, smooth muscle cells, undifferentiated fibroblasts, nerve bundles and inflammatory cell infiltrates. Each of these specialized cells can be further grouped by histological criteria into distinct subcompartments, such as simple columnar versus pseudostratified epithelium, and vascular and connective smooth muscle. However, a precise categorization of all of the specialized cells in the prostate awaits the identification of more informative molecular markers than are available at present. None of the specialized cell types found within the human prostate has yet been thoroughly characterized in molecular terms.

The prostatic stroma provides a supporting matrix for the ductal epithelial cells, which synthesize, concentrate and secrete the components of the prostatic fluid into the ductal lumina. In addition, the connective smooth muscle compartment mediates contractions required to expel the prostatic secretions from the gland. There is strong evidence from experimental models that the stromal and epithelial compartments communicate with each other, and that prostatic growth and functional differentiation, both during development and in the adult, are dependent on regulatory signalling between them.

The development of the prostate occurs in response to inductive signals originating from the endodermal urogenital sinus mesenchyme. In tissue recombination experiments in which mouse foetal urogenital sinus (UGS) is microdissected into epithelial (UGE) and mesenchymal (UGM) components, prostatic growth, morphogenesis and functional differentiation occur when homotypic (prostatic) or certain types of heterotypic epithelia are recombined with UGM and implanted under the kidney capsule of a syngeneic or athymic host.[4–10] Under these conditions, reconstituted prostatic tissue is formed, with histological and immunological evidence of normal glandular architecture and secretory functions. Prostatic morphogenesis does not occur in the absence of UGM, or in the presence of non-inductive heterotypic mesenchymes, indicating a high degree of tissue or developmental specificity underlying the morphological outcome of these experiments.[11] These tissue-specific inductive mechanisms are highly conserved in evolution, as demonstrated by the capability of human foetal bladder epithelium to differentiate into ductal structures lined by columnar epithelium in response to heterotypic recombination with mouse UGM.[7] It is now well established that foetal prostatic development and morphogenesis is absolutely dependent on inductive signals originating from the mesenchymal compartment. This is consistent with similar findings in other organ systems.[8,12] Remarkably, however, the ability of adult epithelia to respond functionally to these inductive signals has also been demonstrated for *adult* prostatic, seminal vesicle, adult ureter and bladder epithelium.[4,5,9,10,13,14] These investigators have demonstrated directly that adult urogenital epithelia maintain the capability to respond to stromal mediators of growth and differentiation. This information is consistent with the hypothesis, first proposed by McNeal,[15] that benign prostatic growth occurring later in life in humans is the result of a 'reawakening' of the inductive potential of the prostatic stroma.

There is general agreement that BPH is mediated in part by gonadal androgens. Boys castrated prepubertally do not develop BPH.[16] The prostate is an androgen-dependent organ and circulating androgens are required for maintenance of prostatic function in adulthood and for embryonic and foetal prostatic development.[17] The rat prostate, which is primarily a parenchymal organ with an epithelial:stromal ratio of 5:1 loses approximately 80% of its cellular content after castration.[18] On the basis of a variety of studies of prostatic dependence and response to androgens, the epithelial compartment appears to be more sensitive to the effects of androgen withdrawal than is the stromal compartment. This correlates with the observation that high-affinity androgen receptors are more abundant in the adult prostatic epithelium than in the neonatal prostatic stroma or in the stromal compartment of the adult.[19,20] However, during foetal prostatic development, androgen receptors are expressed exclusively in the mesenchyme,[20,21] indicating that androgen-mediated effects on development prostatic epithelial ductal growth and morphogenesis are proximally regulated by androgen receptor-mediated mechanisms confined initially to the mesenchymal compartment. This was demonstrated most convincingly by recombination experiments in which androgen receptor-deficient bladder epithelium (Tfm/y) was recombined heterotypically with androgen receptor-positive UGM, resulting in dramatic growth and prostatic functional differentiation in the epithelium.[9,22–24] These results demonstrate that mesenchyme-mediated regulation of epithelium is not only permissive — in which epithelial glandular morphogenesis occurs in cells previously committed to expressing a prostatic phenotype — but also can be instructive — in which epithelium previously directed to a distinct, non-secretory, non-glandular lineage is nevertheless capable of expressing a heterotypic, secretory phenotype specified by the adjacent mesenchyme. Studies on androgen receptor localization in these reconstituted prostatic tissues have confirmed the absence of androgen receptors in the epithelial compartment, and the presence of androgen receptors (identified by binding analyses revealing the presence of functional, high-affinity androgen-binding sites) in the mesenchyme.[23,24]

A critical role for the mesenchyme in prostatic development parallels that revealed by studies on the mechanisms of hormonally induced regression of the mammary gland, in which steroid hormone-mediated degenerative responses in the parenchyma are mediated by the mesenchyme.[12,25,26] Similarities between the prostate and mammary gland in cellular and molecular mechanisms of organ function are of interest in the study of prostatic disease because of the functional, structural and endocrinological similarities between these two organs.[11] The tissue specificity of inductive mesenchymal–epithelial interactions was demonstrated by tissue recombination experiments in which mammary gland and preputial gland mesenchyme were each capable of eliciting dramatic growth and cytodifferentiation of mammary epithelium in vivo, whereas other mesenchymes (vaginal, uterine, UGS, genital tubercle) were either incapable of inducing growth, or induced an aberrant histomorphological architecture.[8]

There is also experimental evidence that the epithelial tissue compartment is capable of directing events in neighbouring mesenchyme. Tissue recombination experiments similar to those described above have recently provided evidence that spatial organization of urogenital smooth muscle involves critical, tissue-specific paracrine mediation from the neighbouring epithelium.[27]

The potential for stromal mediation of neoplastic growth has also been demonstrated with experimental models. Chung and collaborators have presented results of a series of studies using cell recombination techniques, which show that the presence of stromal cells greatly enhances neoplastic growth of immortalized epithelial cells or adenocarcinoma cells in vivo.[28–34] In these experiments, carcinomas or carcinosarcomas are created experimentally in syngeneic or athymic rodent hosts by in vivo injection of epithelial cells in a co-inoculum with homotypic or heterotypic fibroblasts cultured in vitro. Tumorigenic potential and tumour growth rate are subsequently measured directly. Initially, Chung et al.[28] demonstrated the potential for tumorigenic rat prostate fibroblasts to evoke neoplastic growth in vivo of non-tumorigenic rat prostate-derived epithelial cells. Subsequent studies demonstrated the potential for heterotypic fibroblasts to accelerate the growth of human prostate, breast, bladder and kidney carcinoma cells when co-inoculated subcutaneously in athymic hosts.[29] Using the androgen receptor-positive LNCaP cell line, which expresses the androgen-regulated prostate-specific proteinase, prostate-specific antigen (PSA), Gleave et al.[31] demonstrated the

capability of prostate and bone fibroblasts, but not lung and kidney fibroblasts, to induce PSA-secreting tumours in vivo. In this study, LNCaP tumours grew preferentially in male hosts, suggesting a role for androgens in fibroblast-mediated acceleration of epithelial tumour growth. An inductive role for the organ-specific microenvironment in prostate tumour growth was also shown in studies in which LNCaP tumours were generated within prostatic tissue by orthotopic inoculation into mouse dorsal prostate.[32] In these studies, PSA-secreting tumours did not form when LNCaP cells were injected under the renal capsule or under the skin, even when higher numbers of tumour cells were injected at these ectopic sites. The capability for mouse prostate to serve as a preferred site for growth of human prostate tumour cells also suggests that inductive stromal influences on prostate tumour growth are evolutionarily conserved. Intraprostatic implantation of human prostate tumour cells has also been demonstrated to result in enhanced rates of tumour metastasis to distant sites,[35] consistent with the idea that the intraprostatic environment contains regulatory factors that can enhance tumour development and progression to the metastatic state.

In contrast to the above studies, which demonstrate the capability of stromal cells to promote normal and neoplastic growth of prostatic epithelial cells, mesenchyme has also been shown to induce differentiation of transplantable rat prostatic tumours carried in animals for decades. UGM was able to induce glandular, secretory and biochemical differentiation of androgen-sensitive, well-differentiated Dunning prostatic tumours but not the poorly differentiated, androgen-independent Dunning and Noble prostatic tumours.[36,37] This induction of histomorphological and functional differentiation in a tumour of nearly historical origin (the Dunning tumour has been passaged in animals continuously for over 30 years) is likely to be tissue specific, based on the failure of neonatal bladder mesenchyme to induce differentiation of tumour in Dunning tumour–bladder mesenchyme chimaeras.[37] These studies are consistent with reports from other laboratories demonstrating the capability of embryonic tissues to induce the differentiation of a variety of neoplasms, including embryonal carcinoma,[38] colon carcinoma,[39] neuroblastoma[40] and mammary carcinoma.[41] These studies provide an intriguing contrast to the growth-promoting role of fibroblasts in carcinomas created by in vivo injections of single-cell suspensions. These differences illustrate the limitations of model systems in extrapolating directly to clinical conditions; however, they also provide clear demonstrations of the potential for in vivo growth of tumours to be altered in drastic ways by the stromal microenvironment.

Role of soluble growth factors

The results presented above are consistent with the hypothesis that mesenchyme-derived paracrine factors direct growth, branching morphogenesis and secretory function of prostatic epithelium during critical phases of prenatal and adult life. A common assumption is that enlargement of tissues occurs as a result of the paracrine activity of one or more growth factors — soluble polypeptides belonging to a spectrum of gene families that stimulate proliferation of cells in culture. Although this is partly correct, nevertheless it is a highly oversimplified assumption. Most of the molecules identified as growth factors by functional criteria using in vitro systems actually show a wide range of biological activities in cell culture, depending on the experimental conditions or on the cell types used for analysis. Further, for many of these factors, evidence from in vivo systems indicates that their roles in development, tissue homoeostasis or wound repair may be distinctly different from (or even unrelated to) the control of cell growth per se. Basic fibroblast growth factor (bFGF, also known as FGF-2) is a pleiotropic polypeptide capable of stimulating the proliferation of a variety of cultured cells,[42] including human prostate fibroblasts.[43] bFGF/FGF-2 also induces endothelial cell growth in vitro, initiates neovascularization in vivo, and is an important tumour angiogenesis factor. Recently, however, bFGF/FGF-2 was identified as a mediator of apical ectodermal ridge development in the developing chick limb bud.[44] From the in vitro studies of bFGF/FGF-2 alone, it would have been difficult to predict this important developmental role for this molecule. The reader is directed to a recent review on growth factors in relation to prostatic and urological malignancy, for a comprehensive overview.[45]

The pleiotropic nature of most growth factors makes it difficult to construct hypotheses regarding the potential role of specific forms in BPH. Although the prostatic volume enlarges in BPH in humans, physiological changes such as remodelling of the microvasculature[46] and relative increases in the non-muscular (fibroblastic) compartment of the prostatic stroma[3] have also been reported. These and other findings in experimental systems suggest that BPH is a complex physiological process involving growth as well as remodelling of tissue architecture.[47] Individual growth factors might therefore have multiple roles, whereas other growth factors, although present, may play no functional part in BPH. Studies of growth factor localization and function in human and rodent prostatic tissues have been less common than studies with cultured cell lines. To date, few differences between growth factor levels in human BPH and normal prostatic tissue have been reported. In some reports, where investigators used mRNA expression techniques to examine growth factor or growth factor receptor levels, no differences between normal and BPH tissues were found.[48,49]

Perhaps the best-studied example of a single factor that is capable of mediating a wide range of distinct activities in vitro and in vivo is transforming growth factor-beta-1 (TGFβ-1). TGFβ-1 is a member of a family of growth and differentiation factors which includes the related but genetically distinct isoforms TGFβ-2 and TGFβ-3 in mammals, and a variety of other molecules such as müllerian-inhibiting substance (involved in masculinization during foetal development), activins, inhibins and bone morphogenetic proteins.[50] The identification of TGFβ-related molecules as mediators of cell differentiation exemplifies the role of growth factors in normal developmental processes unrelated to cell growth. TGFβ-1 is a potent mitogen for fibroblasts and other mesenchymal cell types, but may also be the most important physiological inhibitor of epithelial cell proliferation. TGFβ-1 also regulates ECM biosysnthesis and degradation, is a potent immunosuppressor, and can stimulate cells to undergo apoptosis. Carcinoma cells, including prostate tumour cells, often lose their normal pattern of growth inhibition in response to TGFβ-1.[51,52] The TGFβ-insensitivity of carcinoma cells is thought to be an important mechanism of tumour expansion during malignant progression. TGFβ-1 may also enhance the invasive potential of tumour cells,[53] thereby promoting malignant progression by a mechanism not directly related to an absence of its normal growth-inhibitory function. It is clear from studies of the diverse biological activities of TGFβ-1, and of a host of other growth factors belonging to different gene families, that the physiological activities of specific growth factors in vivo are dependent on the temporal and spatial context in which they act.

It has been proposed that alteration in the functional status of TGFβ-1 in prostatic tissue may have a role in BPH. This hypothesis is based partly on the observation that, although TGFβ-1 negatively regulates prostate stromal cell growth, it also upregulates the production of bFGF/FGF-2, an autocrine growth factor for prostate stromal cells.[43,54] Therefore, this growth factor axis, which consists of mechanisms for both positive and negative effects on stromal cell proliferation, could be altered during the natural history of BPH to favour expansion of the stromal compartment. TGFβ-1 has been found in human seminal plasma, suggesting that it is a secretory product of the normal prostate gland.[55] Elevation of TGFβ isoform accumulation has been observed in human prostate cancer[56] and in rodent prostatic tumours in several model systems.[57–59] Human and rat prostate cell lines and normal and neoplastic tissues also express TGFβ-like bone morphogenetic protein mRNAs.[60] In the developing mouse prostate, TGFβ-1, -2 and -3 isoforms were detected in UGM, with expression levels appearing higher in UGM than in UGE.[61] During development, highest levels of TGFβ-1 were found in areas of active epithelial branching morphogenesis, suggesting a role for the growth factor in morphogenesis of the ductal network and in epithelial differentiation. Expression of the TGFβ-1 isoform was retained, predominantly in the mesenchyme, in the adult. Expression patterns of the TGFβ-1–3 isoforms in development have also suggested a role for these factors in mesenchymal–epithelial interactions outside the developing urogenital tract.[62] The potential for TGFβ isoforms to regulate smooth muscle cell physiology[63] suggests the possibility that TGFβ-related factors may be physiological regulators of prostatic smooth muscle cells in vivo. An indirect role for TGFβ in tissue growth can also be inferred from studies in which TGFβ has been shown to upregulate production of angiogenic factors by vascular smooth muscle cells.[64]

Growth factors identified as belonging to the epidermal growth factor (EGF), FGF or insulin-like growth factor (IGF) families have also been identified in the human or rodent prostate. The majority of published data concern FGF- or EGF-like factors. Two major prostatic growth factor activities identified in functional tests have been identified as FGF-like and EGF-like.[65,66] bFGF/FGF-2 is detectable at significant levels in normal human and rodent prostate and in prostatic fluid.[67,68]

The EGF and FGF gene families each contain multiple, structurally similar but functionally distinct factors, which bind and activate distinct cell-surface receptors in a cell type-specific fashion. Conclusions about the functional role of specific EGF- and FGF-like factors obtained from studies carried out in the 1980s, when many fewer growth factors had been identified, will have to be revised as new EGF- and FGF-related molecules are identified in the prostate and studies are undertaken to assess their possible roles in prostatic physiology and disease. The functional roles of the known EGF and FGF family members are still not well defined, a problem that grows more complex because a variety of new FGF- and EGF-related factors and FGF- and EGF-receptor-related receptors have been discovered in recent years. Nine members of the FGF family have been found at the time of writing, but only two of these — acidic FGF (aFGF/FGF-1) and bFGF/FGF-2 — have been studied extensively.[42] aFGF/FGF-1 and bFGF/FGF-2 represent a distinct subclass of FGF family members because these polypeptides, unlike the other known FGFs, lack a secretion signal at their amino termini. The FGF-3–FGF-9 isoforms are secreted into the extracellular space by a conventional protein-secretory pathway. However, aFGF/FGF-1 and bFGF/FGF-2 bind to high-affinity receptors displayed on the outside cell surface. Therefore, the physiological context and the regulatory signals mediating the secretion of these two factors remain unclear. Wounding and cell death, which cause damage to cell membranes, may result in the release of the normally intracellular aFGF/FGF-1 and bFGF/FGF-2 into the extracellular space, thereby making these factors available to their cognate receptors.[69,70] These observations provide a logical bridge between studies designed to define the circumstances in which apoptotic cell death occurs in the prostate and mechanisms of growth factor action and intercellular communication.

Keratinocyte growth factor (KGF/FGF-7), an FGF-family member, was recently identified as a product of prostatic stromal cells.[71] This factor is of special significance in terms of identifying mechanisms of stromal–epithelial interaction because, unlike all other members of the FGF family, cell-surface receptors for stromal-derived KGF/FGF-7 are expressed exclusively by epithelial calls. Consequently, KGF/FGF-7 may be involved in stromal-mediated hormonal regulation of prostatic epithelium. Such soluble factors have long been predicted to exist, on the basis of results of tissue recombination experiments described above. Neutralizing anti-KGF/FGF-7 antibodies inhibited androgen-dependent seminal vesicle (SV) growth and ductal branching morphogenesis in organ culture, and exogenously applied KGF/FGF-7 was able to substitute in part for androgens in SV maturation in this system.[72] These results provide direct evidence for a role for stromal-derived KGF-FGF-7 in hormone-dependent growth and epithelial differentiation in an organ known to require mesenchymal–epithelial interactions for normal development. In order to define further the physiological significance of KGF/FGF-7 in androgen-dependent epithelial maturation, it will be necessary to demonstrate that the expression of this growth factor is androgen regulated and associated temporally with androgen induction and patterns of developmental morphogenesis of the male accessory glands.

In the Dunning prostate tumour model, foetal UGM, when recombined with poorly differentiated Dunning tumour pieces, induced the differentiation of the adenocarcinoma cells consistent with a reversion of the malignant phenotype.[36,37] These observations suggest that neoplastic growth of the Dunning tumour cells can be controlled by their connective tissue environment. McKeehan and co-workers have determined that, in the Dunning model, a transition from a stromal-dependent, non-malignant form of tumour growth, to a stromal-independent, malignant form is accompanied by a switch in FGF receptor isoforms.[71,73,74] This switch is the result of an alternative mRNA splicing event in

which the FGF-receptor-2 (FGF-R2) isoform containing the IIIb region of the third immunoglobulin-like loop domain (a segment of the extracellular FGF-binding region) is replaced by the alternative IIIc region. This confers a change in FGF ligand receptor responsitivity by the cells, resulting in an inability to respond to KGF/FGF-7 (a ligand for the IIIb form of the FGF-R2 receptor). Because this switch in receptor expression is also accompanied by an upregulation of the bFGF/FGF-2 gene, as well as genes for several other FGF receptors,[74] these data suggest that loss of regulation by stromal-derived KGF/FGF-7, possibly accompanied by acquisition of cellular responsiveness to other FGF-like factors, may accompany progression to a state of uncontrolled, stromal-independent growth in prostatic tumours.

Additional evidence indicates that FGF-like factors are involved in BPH. The most direct demonstration of the possibility for growth factors to induce hyperplastic growth in the prostate has been the creation of a transgenic mouse line expressing the int-2/FGF-3 growth factor targeted to the mammary gland and, fortuitously, to the male accessory glands. Expression of this oncoprotein in male mice results in an androgen-sensitive epithelial/glandular hyperplasia histologically similar to human and canine BPH.[75] Begun et al.[68] used a sensitive radioimmunoassay to measure levels of bFGF/FGF-2 accumulation in a significant series of normal prostatic glands and glands with BPH. The BPH glands showed two- to threefold elevation of this growth factor compared with the histologically normal glands. This is the only evidence from published studies that has implicated alteration in levels of a specific regulatory polypeptide in BPH versus normal prostatic tissues. Recent evidence suggests that bFGF/FGF-2 accumulation in human prostatic tissue may not be responsive to androgens.[76]

The identification of other stromal-derived prostatic growth factors, like KGF/FGF-7, will be of great interest. Other candidates for physiologically relevant stromal growth factors include platelet-derived growth factor (PDGF) isoforms, which are potent fibroblast and smooth muscle cell mitogens. PDGFs could conceivably drive proliferation of most of the cells in the fibromuscular prostatic stroma (e.g. non-differentiated fibroblasts and smooth muscle cells). Stromal cells derived from human prostate tissue were shown to express high-affinity receptors for the PDGF-BB isoform and demonstrated an increased proliferative response to exogenous PDGF-BB.[77] A stromal-derived nerve growth factor-like (NGF-like) protein was identified in the conditioned medium of human prostatic stromal cells and neoplastic epithelial cells and was localized immunocytochemically to the stromal component of normal and hyperplastic prostates and prostatic adenocarcinoma.[78] Interestingly, NGF receptors were localized predominantly to the epithelium, suggesting that NGF-like polypeptides may be stroma-derived mediators of epithelial cell proliferation or function in the human prostate. Several abnormalities in the IGF axis have recently been identified in cultured human stromal cells derived from BPH specimens compared with stromal cells derived from histologically normal specimens. Cohen et al.[79] found evidence for enhanced expression of IGF-2 and diminished expression of IGF-binding protein 5, a stoichiometric regulator of IGF activity. These data suggest that IGF activity might be enhanced in BPH stroma relative to normal, owing to increases in both stromal growth factor synthesis and localization, as well as release of inhibitory control over growth factor function. Human prostatic stromal cells also produce and respond to bFGF/FGF-2.[43,54]

The EGF family now contains five members known to activate the canonical EGF receptor (ErbB-1): these are EGF, transforming growth factor-alpha (TGFα), amphiregulin, heparin-binding EGF-like growth factor (HB-EGF) and betacellulin. Additional EGF-like factors bind and activate three additional EGF-receptor (EGF-R)-related tyrosine kinases (ErbB-2/Neu, ErbB-3 and ErbB-4). The soluble receptor ligands that do not activate the EGF-R are known collectively as the neu differentiation factors (NDFs) or heregulins.[80] Crosstalk between the ErbB receptor isoforms and their ligands occurs in a variety of cells and is poorly understood at present.[81] Because of the physiological importance of the EGF-R, and the well-known capability of the ErbB family of molecules to be involved in control of growth regulation, EGF-like factors and their cognate receptors are good candidates for mediators of stromal–epithelial interaction in urogenital tissues. At the time of writing, any or all of the above factors might potentially be involved in growth regulation in the prostate. EGF-like

activities have been detected in the intact prostate and in prostatic secretions.[82] TGFα has been detected in the human prostate by immunological and molecular techniques.[83–85] Amphiregulin, a third EGF-related factor and one with heparin-binding affinity, has been identified as a product of human prostatic epithelial cells and its expression in culture is regulated by androgens in the androgen-responsive LNCaP prostate cell line.[86] The ErbB-2/Neu protein has also been identified in human benign hyperplastic and carcinomatous prostatic tissue.[87,88]

A second heparin-binding EGF receptor ligand, HB-EGF, has recently been identified as a product of prostate smooth muscle cells in vivo (M. Freeman and M. Klagsbrun, unpublished data; Fig. 4.1). HB-EGF binds and activates the EGF receptor with a potency similar to EGF and TGFα; however, it has also been shown to be a potent smooth muscle cell mitogen, as potent as the canonical smooth muscle cell mitogen, PDGF.[89] HB-EGF stimulation of smooth muscle cell growth is dependent on the presence of cell-surface heparin-like molecules, most likely heparan sulfate proteoglycans. Immunohistochemical staining of human BPH and prostate adenocarcinoma tissues with an antibody raised against the cytoplasmic domain of the membrane-anchored HB-EGF precursor identified smooth muscle cells specifically; undifferentiated fibroblasts, normal epithelial cells and prostatic adenocarcinoma cells expressed low or undetectable levels of HB-EGF in these experiments. The use of an antibody that recognizes the cell-associated precursor form of HB-EGF allows cells that synthesize HB-EGF to be identified immunocytochemically. These data suggest the possibility that HB-EGF, synthesized by prostatic smooth muscle cells, may play a part in the expansion of the stromal compartment in BPH.

The cell-associated form of HB-EGF has also been detected in prostatic epithelial cells growing in culture.[90] HB-EGF and amphiregulin are distinct members of the EGF family, in that they possess an intrinsic affinity for heparin-like molecules, unlike EGF or TGFα. This heparin-binding affinity is likely to be a general requirement for activation of EGF receptors by amphiregulin and HB-EGF.[89,91] The identification of the HB-EGF transmembrane precursor as a major product of prostatic cells suggests the possibility that HB-EGF

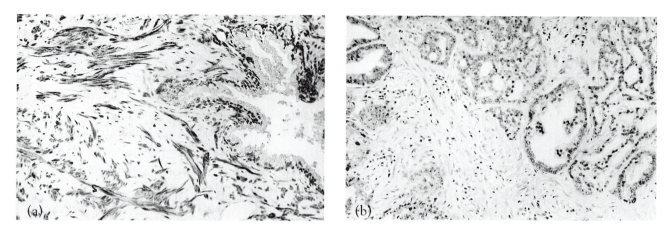

Figure 4.1. *Localization of the sites of synthesis of heparin-binding epidermal growth factor-like growth factor (HB-EGF) in human prostate carcinoma as determined by immunohistochemistry. A monospecific anti-HB-EGF polyclonal antibody, which specifically recognizes the transmembrane, cell-associated HB-EGF precursor, was used in this experiment. This type of antibody allows cells that synthesize HB-EGF to be identified. (a) HB-EGF staining is evident in prostatic smooth muscle cells (elongated, spindle-shaped cells in the stroma). (b) Negative control using pre-immune serum, showing an absence of staining in the stroma. Slides in (a) and (b) were counterstained with haematoxylin to show cell and tissue structure. (From M. Freeman and M. Klagsbrun with permission.)*

binding to cell-surface receptors, and to ancillary molecules such as heparan sulfate proteoglycans, might occur at the cell membrane as part of a so-called 'juxtracrine' regulatory mechanism. Growth factors that can exist in a membrane-anchored form, including HB-EGF, amphiregulin, TGFα, colony stimulating factor-1 (CSF-1) and tumour necrosis factor-alpha (TNFα), might bind to and activate cell-surface receptors on adjacent cells without a requirement for proteolytic processing from the cell surface. This capability for juxtracrine activity has been demonstrated for some of the above factors in experimental models.[92–94] The possibility that juxtracrine cell signalling mediates aspects of intercellular communication in the prostate has not yet been explored.

A potentially important component of the prostatic stroma that has not been studied extensively is represented by inflammatory cell infiltrates, including lymphocytes and monocyte-derived macrophages. Extensive infiltration of human BPH tissues by chronically activated T cells has been reported to be common.[95] The absence of granulocytes in these infiltrates suggests that mononuclear cell accumulation in the prostate is unlikely to be the result of infection (reaction to foreign antigens). Peripheral blood T cells, in the absence of a requirement for a T-cell-receptor-mediated stimulus, have recently been shown to produce and secrete three heparin-binding growth factors: these

are HB-EGF and bFGF/FGF-2,[96] as well as vascular endothelial growth factor (VEGF), a potent angiogenic factor and endothelial cell mitogen.[97] (bFGF/FGF-2 is also an endothelial cell mitogen and angiogenic factor, as stated previously.) VEGF synthesis was also recently identified as a product of T cells infiltrating human prostate and bladder cancers.[97] Human tumour-derived lymphocytes were shown to produce bioactive HB-EGF and bFGF/FGF-2 capable of stimulating the growth of breast and ovarian tumour cells, as well as smooth muscle cells and fibroblasts.[98] These results suggest that T cells have the capability to secrete potent epithelial, vascular and stromal mitogens into the interstitial tissues in a fashion that is not dependent on active immunoregulatory (T-cell-receptor-dependent) signals. Within the context of BPH, this could mean that T-cell infiltrates, not functioning as part of a sustained immunological reaction but present in significant numbers, might contribute directly to stromal as well as glandular hyperplasia.

Role of the extracellular matrix

The potential role of the ECM in the promotion of neoplastic growth in vivo has been demonstrated in model systems in which isolated matrix, such as the basement membrane-like matrix from the EHS sarcoma, promotes growth initiated by injection of a variety of tumour cells, including human prostatic carcinoma cells, into athymic hosts.[99–101] These studies may be analogous to the previously mentioned experiments in which carcinomatous growth can be promoted by co-inoculating epithelial tumour cells with heterotypic or homotypic fibroblasts, a source of ECM.[33] In prostate tumour models, stroma or ECM have been found to have a promotional[28,29,31,32,99,101,102] or suppressive[36,37,74] effect on the malignant phenotype of carcinoma cells, indicating the dramatic potential for the connective tissue environment to direct or alter the natural course of epithelial tumours. Freeman et al.[102] demonstrated that long-term cell contact with basement membrane ECM increased cell motility and invasive properties and resulted in stably altered patterns of gene expression in a poorly differentiated prostatic tumour line. These data suggest that cell association with specific matrices has the potential to induce hyperplastic — and even malignant — growth of epithelial cells in vivo. What is occurring at the molecular level that can explain how seemingly simple contextual cues can dramatically regulate cell growth and malignant phenotype?

The ECM is capable of sequestering soluble regulatory molecules such as growth factors, and releasing them during degradative or inflammatory conditions, where they become available to cognate cell-surface receptors. Heparin-binding growth factors, such as bFGF/FGF-2, can accumulate at significant levels in ECM, particularly in basement membranes.[103] Some matrix components, such as heparan sulfate proteoglycans (HSPGs), appear to be specialized to bind and store heparin-binding growth factors in extracellular sites.[104] Certain membrane-bound HSPGs also appear to be required on cell surfaces for the presentation of bound growth factors to receptors, thereby acting as co-receptors for cell activation by growth factors.[89,91,105] This may be a general mechanism for cell activation by growth factors with a high affinity for heparin, where intimate, specialized contacts between growth factor ligand, cell-surface receptor and HSPGs activate the receptor. Evidence for this mechanism includes the identification of discrete heparin-binding domains on growth factor receptors. For example, the FGF-receptor type 1 (FGF-R1/*flg*), a receptor for aFGF/FGF-1 and bFGF/FGF-2, contains a low-affinity heparin-binding site necessary for high-affinity FGF ligand binding.[106]

Heparin-binding growth factor interaction with HSPGs is also likely to be highly specific, with some interactions resulting in significant biological responses in target cells, while others do not. The isoform of the cell-surface CD44 proteoglycan (the hyaluronic acid receptor) containing the so-called V3 region is modified with heparan sulfate and binds two heparin-binding growth factors, bFGF/FGF-2 and HB-EGF, but does not bind the heparin-binding growth factor amphiregulin.[107] This is an interesting and unexpected observation because amphiregulin and HB-EGF have nearly identical affinity for heparin, as determined by heparin-affinity chromatography. It has been demonstrated that heparin-like molecules are likely to be co-receptors for EGF-receptor activation by amphiregulin,[91] as is the case for other heparin-binding growth factors. The CD44 family of proteoglycans has been implicated in regulation of inflammation and malignant progression. The V3-containing CD44 isoform is expressed on keratinocytes, monocytes and dendritic cells in inflamed skin tissue, but is not detectable immunocytochemically on endothelial cells, which are known to be activated by heparin-binding growth factors, in the same specimens.[107] These observations indicate that heparan sulfate-containing proteoglycans are likely to be highly specialized for presentation of particular growth factor subsets to high-affinity cell-surface receptors. Further, this mechanism of growth factor regulation probably occurs in a context-dependent or tissue-specific manner.

The above data indicate that HSPG components of the ECM are critical regulators of cellular interaction, in that they coordinate growth factor localization and presentation to cell-surface receptors. Interestingly, in epithelial–mesenchymal culture models of cell differentiation, formation of HSPGs at the basement membrane interface has been found to be dependent on the presence of both epithelial and stromal cells.[108] Formation of HSPG-containing matrices can be controlled directly by heterologous matrix–cell interaction.[109] These observations suggest the importance of heterotypic cell–cell interactions in the establishment of connective tissue networks that regulate tissue differentiation and function.

Remodelling of the ECM during tumorigenesis or inflammation may alter the normal homoeostasis of these growth factor–ECM interactions, resulting in the alteration of the proliferative state of cells. Matrix remodelling occurs by release of matrix-degrading enzymes, such as serine/threonine proteases, cysteine proteases and metalloproteinases from parenchymal, interstitial and inflammatory cells. Alteration of the normal balance between matrix synthesis and degradation occurs in response to proliferative signals and may be mediated by matrix-associated growth factors such as TGFβ-1, which control synthesis of ECM components, as well as specific ECM-degradative mechanisms involving proteases and protease inhibitors.[110] Matrix has also been proposed to be a storage site for growth factors involved in the sustained elevation of local proteolysis.[111] Metastatic tumour cells appear to stimulate their own growth and movement through matrix by releasing HSPG-degrading enzymes (heparinases), an activity that also presumably releases pleiotropic HSPG-resident growth factors, such as bFGF/FGF-2.[112]

Are growth factors likely to be the major growth-promoting elements of the ECM? The matrix was once considered to be an inert scaffold of insoluble material serving to anchor cells to each other and to connective tissues. It is now clear, however, that the ECM is a dynamic structure linking a complex network of extracellular sites to cytoplasmic and nuclear locations within cells. The large ECM proteins, such as collagens I, III and IV, fibronectin and laminin, consist of arrays of distinct multidomain structures with diverse functions. These molecules bind specifically to each other, either directly or by mutual interaction with other glycoproteins and glycosaminoglycans. The complexity of the ECM in most tissues is formidable: as an example, the abundant interstitial collagens I and III represent only two of a family of structurally related collagen molecules with at least 19 members.[113]

Cells make contact with specific matrices using cell-surface receptors known as integrins.[114] Integrins belong to a large family of multifunctional heterodimeric transmembrane proteins that bind specific matrix sites on their extracellular face and components of the cytoskeleton in the cell interior. Extracellular ligands that bind integrins include ECM glycoproteins, cellular

adhesion molecules, thrombolytic proteins and components of the complement cascade. Integrins provide a functional link between the outside and the inside of the cell by serving as mechanical connectors between the ramifying ECM scaffolds and their associated molecules, the intracellular cytoskeletal systems and the cell nucleus. Regulatory signals are transmitted to the cell interior through this network. Cytoplasmic proteins involved in intracellular cell-signalling events are recruited to protein complexes containing integrins following integrin binding to extracellular ligands. Subsequent to binding ligand, integrins typically cluster on the cell surface, resulting in amplification and transmission of mechanochemical information to the cell interior. Extracellular signals for a variety of cellular activities, such as growth, migration and differentiation, have been found to be dependent on specific integrins.[115,116] The complexity of these signals is made plain by the fact that most integrins can be demonstrated by biochemical techniques specifically to bind multiple ligands, in some cases seven or more. Integrins, therefore, appear to be unusually permissive regulatory proteins with respect to ligand binding and activation resulting from protein–protein interaction. A variety of integrins bind the large ECM glycoproteins, such as fibronectin (bound by αsβ1, α3β1 and α4β1 integrins) and laminin (bound by α1β1, α2β1, α3β1, α6β1, α7β1 and α6β4 integrins). Signal transduction through ECM receptors, resulting in changes in cellular physiology reminiscent of signals through membrane-bound growth factor receptors, have been demonstrated for a number of specific integrins.[117–119] Integrins are thus capable of 'outside-in' signalling, in addition to their role as structural connecting sites. Non-integrin matrix receptors capable of cell regulation have also been identified.[120]

Because many of the ligands for the more than 30 known integrins have been identified and many are, in fact, matrix molecules rather than growth factors or cytokines, it is clear that important cellular events are mediated directly by cell contact with matrix. This would include cell-adhesion molecules connected to the matrix and soluble molecules sequestered within the matrix. It is also clear that cellular interactions with purified matrices can transmit signals to the cell nucleus and regulate the expression of specific genes.[121,122]

Alterations of integrin expression on the surface of tumour cells have been shown to result in some of the abnormal cell behaviour associated with malignant transformation. The ECM itself, therefore, is an important regulator of cellular physiology and the notion that connective tissue and basement membrane elements are mere support structures is not valid. Basement membrane matrices are particularly potent at eliciting dramatic behavioural changes within cells, at least in cell culture.[102,123–125] Morphogenesis and differentiation of isolated lactogenic mammary epithelial cells into secretory acini occurs in culture on basement membrane gels.[121,125] These multicellular structures resemble milk-producing acini in vivo. There is now extensive evidence that this differentiation event is mediated in large part by cell interaction with basement membrane ECM.[12]

How does the ECM control cell growth? The mechanisms appear to be diverse and complex. For over 15 years it has been known that transformed, growth-factor-independent cells frequently lose the ability to contact components of the ECM,[126] suggesting that adhesive interactions with extracellular sites may be required for normal growth control. This possibility has been confirmed with the recent identification of adhesion-dependent intracellular regulators of cell cycle progression.[127,128] Growth control by the ECM can be negative or positive. Consistent with observations showing a loss of cell-surface ECM, particularly fibronectin, correlating with an increase in malignant properties,[129–131] overexpression of the fibronectin receptor — $\alpha 5\beta 1$ integrin — can suppress the tumorigenic phenotype and partly suppress growth of cells in culture.[132] A dramatic and potentially clinically significant example of negative growth regulation by integrins is the finding that synthetic or immunological antagonists to the $\alpha v\beta 3$ integrin, expressed on microvascular endothelial cells undergoing angiogenesis, induce endothelial cell apoptosis and a resultant loss of blood vessels.[133] This regression of the microvasculature can culminate in tumour regression.

Positive growth regulation by integrins appears to involve temporal coordination between integrin signalling mechanisms and growth factor receptor interactions. An in vitro system in which this interplay between ECM and growth factors has been studied in some detail is the formation of capillary tubes from pure endothelial cell cultures, a process that may mimic angiogenesis in vivo. This complex morphogenetic process, which involves intricate cell movements and interactions as well as differentiative change, is dependent on both soluble and insoluble extracellular signals.[134] Tumour growth is dependent on angiogenesis, and remodelling of the microvasculature is a common feature of growing solid tumours. Evidence of microvascular remodelling in human BPH has recently been reported.[46]

Growth-factor-mediated signalling systems regulating cell proliferation can be dependent on appropriate matrix-dependent cues from the extracellular environment. In mammary epithelial cells, the TGFβ-1 gene, in contrast to the gene for the related isoform TGFβ-2, responds to cell contact with basement membrane ECM, by downregulation.[122] This suggests that growth factor synthesis by cells is dependent on, and controlled by, cell–ECM contact. These findings also imply that disruption of the basement membrane ECM as a consequence of malignant growth may result in the upregulation of TGFβ-1, a potent pleiotropic factor capable of stromal remodelling, immunosuppression and induction of angiogenesis. As described above, TGFβ isoforms have been implicated by several laboratories in human prostatic disease. Because of the likelihood that TGFβ regulates the connective tissue environment directly in prostate as well as in other organ systems,[50] aberrant stromal localization of TGFβ-1 in experimental and human prostate carcinoma suggests that remodelling of the prostatic stroma occurs as a consequence of neoplastic prostatic growth.[56]

A generalizable mechanism for cell regulation by growth factors and ECM, which probably applies to growth control as well as cell differentiation, is that chemomechanical signals provided by the ECM act in concert with soluble signalling molecules to regulate cell physiology and behaviour. That is, ECM and growth factors may each be obligatory components of many regulatory pathways and act cooperatively to initiate, maintain and redirect regulated cellular responses to extracellular cues.

Purified matrices, proteolytic fragments of matrix molecules and synthetic peptides corresponding to discrete domains of matrix molecules can initiate a variety of cellular responses in model systems in cell culture.[124,135–137] These effects have been shown to be highly dependent on the molecular structure of individual matrix molecules and therefore the result of highly specific cell–matrix interactions. Culture of human breast carcinoma cells in collagen I gels results in activation of the latent form of matrix metalloproteinase 2 (MMP-2), a matrix-degrading enzyme whose expression pattern in human mammary tumours correlates well with prognosis and tumour grade.[138] This appears to be a specific property of intact polymeric collagen I and not of laminin, fibronectin, collagen IV or gelatin. This observation suggests an important role for interstitial collagen, frequently considered to be primarily a support structure in tissues, in the growth of solid tumours. Signals transmitted to cells through matrix are frequently found to be dependent on mechanical information presented to the cell by the three-dimensional matrix structure.[139]

Roles for specific cell–ECM interactions in human BPH remain speculative at present. A variety of specific integrins have been identified in human prostatic tissue.[140–142] Some of these molecules, such as the hemidesmosome-associated $\alpha6\beta4$ integrin, which is localized to prostatic basal epithelia, are likely to perform similar matrix-adhesion functions in the prostate as in other organs. The $\alpha6\beta1$ and $\alpha2\beta1$ integrins, localized to acinar basement membranes in normal and hyperplastic prostatic tissue, appear to be present in distinct patterns and expressed abnormally in organ-confined and metastatic carcinoma.[140] This information suggests a role for altered expression of integrins in prostatic disease; however, the functional involvement of integrins in prostatic pathophysiology awaits further study.

Given the general dependence of prostatic growth on circulating androgens, a fertile area of investigation is the potential for synthesis and deposition of stroma-derived matrices to be regulated by dihydrotestosterone, the primary prostatic androgen. Tenascin, a mesenchyme-derived matrix glycoprotein, has been shown to appear in prostatic stroma in response to androgen deprivation.[143] This hormonal-dependent expression of tenascin in the prostate may be associated with a low-degree epithelial differentiation. In human prostates, tenascin was detected in normal and hyperplastic tissue and prostatic carcinoma.[144] Studies with the androgen-responsive human prostate cell line LNCaP indicate that effects of androgens on differentiated properties of prostatic cells can be mediated in part by cell–ECM contact in concert with soluble stromal-derived factors.[145] Tumorigenic growth of LNCaP cells in vivo is enhanced by ECM and bFGF/FGF-2.[32,99] It is likely that differentiated functions of the adult prostate are dependent on regulatory networks maintained by epithelial–mesenchymal interactions using solid-state and soluble mediators. Although the best evidence for this hypothesis derives from studies of mammary epithelia in culture, limited numbers of co-culture systems employing urogenital cells, especially testicular Sertoli cells and mesenchymal peritubular cells,[146] support this view.

Future directions

The current experimental evidence suggests an important role for stromal-derived paracrine factors in prostatic development, maintenance of prostatic function, and benign and malignant prostatic growth. At present, however, there is still a limited understanding of the precise mechanistic nature of age-related benign prostatic growth. Experimental models suggest that soluble molecules produced by stromal cells, in concert with ECM-associated cell-signalling mechanisms (which may include mechanochemical signalling as well as biochemical mediation), may have a role. A stage has been reached, however, where likely candidate BPH mediators are still being identified, on the basis of experiments using prostatic cells and tissues, experiments in other organ systems, and models that involve specific molecules but that do not necessarily possess definable physiological correlates or contexts. Hypotheses involving these candidate molecules have to be developed and experiments to test these hypotheses designed. The authors believe, however, that further studies designed to identify new soluble as well as insoluble stromal cell products will complement existing studies and provide additional insights. The ability to transfect genes specifically into the prostate and into distinct prostatic compartments in rodents has now become a reality;[57,147–149] this new technology should enhance the power of traditional rodent experimental models. New methods of scanning the expressed genome for proteins synthesized differentially among normal and pathological tissues, and rapid cloning of their respective genes,[150] should allow the pace of discovery to increase markedly. The identification of genes regulated by androgens, and therefore potentially involved in androgen-induced growth of the prostate, should benefit considerably from this new technology.

The potential for molecular and cellular biology to affect human health problems has never been greater than it is today. It will be the obligation of the basic scientist and the clinician, working together, to apply this new technology in creative ways to discover the fundamental mechanisms, and to devise simple and effective treatments for human BPH and other urological diseases.

References

1. Albarran J, Halle N. Hypertrophie et neoplasies epitheliades de la prostate. Ann Mal Org Genito-Urin (Paris) 1900; 17: 113

2. Reischauer F. Die Entstehung der sogenannten Prostatahypertrophie. Virchows Arch [B] 1925; 256: 357–389

3. Deering R E, Bigler S A, King J et al. Morphometric quantitation of stroma in human benign prostatic hyperplasia. Urology 1994; 44: 64–70

4. Chung L W K, Cunha G R. Stromal–epithelial interactions II. Regulation of prostatic growth by embryonic urogenital sinus mesenchyme. Prostate 1983; 4: 503–511

5. Chung L W K, Matsura J, Runner M N. Tissue interaction and prostatic growth. I. Induction of adult mouse prostatic hyperplasia by renal urogenital sinus implants. Biol Reprod 1984; 31: 155–163

6. Neubauer B L, Chung L W K, McCormick K A et al. Epithelial–mesenchymal interactions in prostatic development II. Biochemical observations of prostatic induction by urogenital sinus mesenchyme in epithelium of the adult rodent urinary bladder. J Cell Biol 1983; 96: 1671–1676

7. Cunha G R, Sekkingstad M, Meloy B A. Heterospecific induction of prostatic development in tissue recombinants prepared with mouse, rat, rabbit and human tissues. Differentiation 1983; 24: 174–180

8. Cunha G R, Young P, Hamamoto S et al. Developmental response of adult mammary epithelial cells to various fetal and neonatal mesenchymes. Epithelial Cell Biol 1992; 1: 105–118

9. Donjacour A A, Cunha G R. Assessment of prostatic protein secretion in tissue recombinants made of urogenital sinus mesenchyme and urothelium from normal or androgen-insensitive mice. Endocrinology 1993; 132: 2342–2350

10. Hayashi N, Cunha G R, Parker M. Permissive and instructive induction of adult rodent prostatic epithelium by heterotypic urogenital sinus mesenchyme. Epithelial Cell Biol 1993; 2: 66–78

11. Cunha G R. Role of mesenchymal–epithelial interactions in normal and abnormal development of the mammary gland and prostate. Cancer 1994; 74: 1030–1044

12. Howlett A R, Bissell M J. The influence of tissue microenvironment (stroma and extracellular matrix) on the development and function of mammary epithelium. Epithelial Cell Biol 1993; 2: 79–89

13. Higgins S J, Young P, Brody J R, Cunha G R. Induction of functional cytodifferentiation in the epithelium of tissue recombinants. I. Homotypic seminal vesicle recombinants. Development 1989; 106: 219–234

14. Norman J T, Cunha G R, Sugimura Y. The induction of new ductal growth in adult prostatic epithelium in response to an embryonic prostatic inductor. Prostate 1986; 8: 209–220

15. McNeal J E. Origin and evolution of benign prostatic enlargement. Invest Urol 1978; 15: 340–345

16. Wu C P, Gu F L. The prostate in eunuchs. In: EORTC Genitourinary Group Monograph 10. Urologic oncology: reconstructive surgery, organ preservation, and restoration of function. New York: Wiley-Liss, 1992: 249–255

17. Cunha G R, Donjacour A, Cooke P S et al. The endocrinology and development biology of the prostate. Endocrine Rev 1987; 8: 338–362

18. Lee C. Physiology of castration-induced regression in rat prostate. In: Karr J P, Sandberg A A, Murphy G P (eds) The prostate cell: structure and function, Part A. New York: Alan R Liss, 1981

19. Schleicher G, Stumpf W E, Drews U et al. Differential distribution of ^{3}H dihydrotestosterone and ^{3}H estradiol nuclear binding sites in mouse male accessory sex organs: an autoradiographic study. Histochemistry 1985; 82: 453–461

20. Takeda H, Mizuno T, Lasnitzki I. Autoradiographic studies of androgen-binding sites in the rat urogenital sinus and postnatal prostate. J Endocrinol 1985; 104: 87–92

21. Shannon J M, Cunha G R. Autoradiographic localization of androgen binding in the developing mouse prostate. Prostate 1983; 4: 367–373

22. Cunha G R, Chung L W K. Stromal–epithelial interactions: I. Induction of prostatic phenotype in urothelium of testicular feminized (Tfm/y) mice. J Steroid Biochem 1981; 14: 1317–1321

23. Thompson T C, Cunha G R, Shannon J M, Chung L W K. Androgen-induced biochemical response in epithelium lacking androgen receptors: characterization of androgen receptors in the mesenchymal derivative of the urogenital sinus. J Steroid Biochem 1986; 25(5A): 627–634

24. Sugimura Y, Cunha G R, Bigsby R M. Androgenic induction of DNA synthesis in prostatic glands induced in the urothelium of testicular feminized (Tfm/y) mice. Prostate 1986; 9: 217–225

25. Drews U. Regression of mouse mammary gland anlagen in recombinations of Tfm and wild-type tissues: testosterone acts via the mesenchyme. Cell 1977; 10: 401–404

26. Kratochwil K, Schwartz P. Tissue interaction in androgen response of embryonic mammary rudiment of mouse: identification of target for testosterone. Proc Natl Acad Sci USA 1976; 73: 4041–4044

27. Cunha G R, Battle E, Young P et al. Role of epithelial–mesenchymal interactions in the differentiation and spatial organization of visceral smooth muscle. Epithelial Cell Biol 1992; 1: 76–83

28. Chung L W K, Chang S M, Bell C et al. Co-inoculation of tumorigenic rat prostate mesenchymal cells with nontumorigenic epithelial cells results in the development of carcinosarcoma in syngeneic and athymic animals. Int J Cancer 1989; 43: 1179–1187

29. Camps J L, Chang S M, Hsu T C et al. Fibroblast-mediated acceleration of human epithelial tumor growth in vivo. Proc Natl Acad Sci USA 1990; 87: 75–79

30. Chung L W K. Fibroblasts are critical determinants in prostate cancer growth and dissemination. Cancer Metastasis Rev 1991; 263–274

31. Gleave M E, Hsieh J T, Gao C A et al. Acceleration of human prostate cancer growth in vivo by factors produced by prostate and bone fibroblasts. Cancer Res 1991; 51: 3753

32. Gleave M E, Hsieh J T, von Eschenbach A C, Chung L W K. Prostate and bone fibroblasts induce human prostate cancer growth in vivo: implications for bidirectional tumor–stromal cell interaction in prostatic carcinoma growth and metastasis. J Urol 1992; 147: 1151–1159

33. Chung L W, Li W, Gleave M E et al. Human prostate cancer model: roles of growth factors and extracellular matrices. J Cell Biochem 1992; (suppl 16H): 99–105

34. Zhau H-Y E, Hong S J, Chung L W K. A fetal urogenital sinus mesenchymal cell line (rUGM): accelerated growth and conferral of androgen-induced growth reponsiveness upon a human bladder cancer epithelial cell line in vivo. Int J Cancer 1994; 56: 706–714

35. Stephenson R A, Dinney C P, Gohji K et al. Metastatic model for human prostate cancer using orthotopic implantation in nude mice. J Natl Cancer Inst 1992; 84: 951–957

36. Chung L W K, Zhau H, Ro J. Morphologic and biochemical alterations in rat prostatic tumors induced by fetal urogenital sinus mesenchyme. Prostate 1990; 17: 165–174

37. Hayashi N, Cunha G R, Wong Y C. Influence of male genital tract mesenchymes on differentiation of Dunning prostatic adenocarcinoma. Cancer Res 1990; 50: 4747–4754

38. Pierce G B, Aguilar D, Hood G, Wells R S. Trophectoderm in control of murine embryonal carcinoma. Cancer Res 1984; 44: 3978–3996

39. Fukamachi H, Mizuno T, Kim Y S. Morphogenesis of human colon cancer cells with fetal rat mesenchymes in organ culture. Experientia 1986; 42: 312

40. Podesta A H, Mullins J, Pierce G B, Wells R S. The neurula stage mouse embryo in control of neuroblastoma. Proc Natl Acad Sci USA 1984; 81: 7608–7611

41. DeCrosse, Gossens C L, Kuzma J F. Breast cancer: induction of differentiation by embryonic tissue. Science 1973; 181: 1057

42. Klagsbrun M. The fibroblast growth factor family: structural and biological properties. Prog Growth Factor Res 1990; 1: 207–235

43. Story M T, Livingston B, Baeten L et al. Cultured human prostate-derived fibroblasts produce a factor that stimulates their growth with properties indistinguishable from basic fibroblast growth factor. Prostate 1989; 15: 355–365

44. Fallon J F, Lopez A, Ros M A et al. FGF-2: apical ectodermal ridge growth signal for check limb development. Science 1994; 264: 104–107

45. Steiner M S. Review of peptide growth factors in benign prostatic hyperplasia and urological malignancy. J Urol 1995; 153: 1085–1096

46. Deering R E, Bigler S A, Brown S A, Brawer M K. Microvascularity in benign prostatic hyperplasia. Prostate 1995; 26: 111–115

47. Coffey D S, Walsh P C. Clinical and experimental studies of benign prostatic hyperplasia. Urol Clin North Am 1990; 17: 461–475

48. Glynne-Jones E, Harper M E, Goddard L et al. Transforming growth factor beta 1 expression in benign and malignant prostatic tumors. Prostate 1994; 25: 210–218

49. Bonnet P, Reiter E, Bruyninx M et al. Benign prostatic hyperplasia and normal prostate aging: differences in types I and II 5-alpha-reductase and steroid hormone receptor messenger ribonucleic acid (mRNA) levels, but not in insulin-like growth factor mRNA levels. J Clin Endocrinol Metab 1983; 77: 1203–1208

50. Roberts A B, Sporn M B. Physiological actions and clinical applications of transforming growth factor-beta (TGF-beta). Growth Factors 1993; 8: 1–9

51. McKeehan W L, Adams P S. Heparin binding growth factor/prostatropin attenuates inhibition of rat prostate tumor epithelial cell growth by transforming growth factor type beta. In Vitro Cell Dev Biol 1988; 24: 243

52. Wright J A, Turley E A, Greenberg A H. Transforming growth factor beta and fibroblast growth factor as promoters of tumor progression to malignancy. Crit Rev Oncog 1993; 4: 473–492

53. Mooradian D L, McCarthy J B, Komanduri K V, Furcht L T. Effects of transforming growth factor-beta 1 on human pulmonary adenocarcinoma cell adhesion, motility and invasion in vitro. J Natl Cancer Inst 1992; 84: 523–527

54. Story M T, Hopp K A, Meier D A et al. Influence of transforming growth factor beta 1 and other growth factors on basic fibroblast growth factor level and proliferation of cultured human prostate-derived fibroblasts. Prostate 1993; 22: 183–197

55. Lokeshwar B L, Block N L. Isolation of a prostate carcinoma cell proliferation-inhibiting factor from seminal plasma and its similarity to transforming growth factor beta. Cancer Res 1992; 52: 5821–5825

56. Truong L D, Kadmon D, McCune B K et al. Association of transforming growth factor-beta 1 with prostate cancer: an immunohistochemical study. Hum Pathol 1993; 24: 4–9

57. Merz V W, Miller G J, Krebs T et al. Elevated transforming growth factor β1 and β3 mRNA levels are associated with ras+myc-induced carcinoma in reconstituted mouse prostate: evidence for a paracrine role during progression. Mol Endocrinol 1991; 5: 503–513

58. Steiner M S, Barrack E R. Transforming growth factor-beta 1 overproduction in prostate cancer: effects on growth in vivo and in vitro. Mol Endocrinol 1992; 6: 15–25

59. Thompson T C, Timme T L, Kadmon D et al. Genetic predisposition and mesenchymal–epithelial interactions in ras+myc-induced carcinogenesis in reconstituted mouse prostate. Mol Carcinog 1993; 7: 165-179

60. Harris S E, Harris M A, Mahy P et al. Expression of bone morphogenetic protein messenger RNAs by normal rat and human prostate and prostate cancer cells. Prostate 1994; 24: 204–211

61. Timme T L, Truong L D, Merz V W et al. Mesenchymal–epithelial interactions and transforming growth factor-beta expression during mouse prostate morphogenesis. Endocrinology 1994; 134: 1039–1045

62. Millan F A, Denhez F, Kondaiah P, Akhurst R J. Embryonic gene expression patterns of TGF beta 1, beta 2 and beta 3 suggest different development functions in vivo. Development 1991; 111: 131–143

63. Orlandi A, Ropraz P, Gabbiani G. Proliferative activity and alpha-smooth muscle actin expression in cultured rat aortic smooth muscle cells are differently modulated by transforming growth factor beta-1 and heparin. Exp Cell Res 1994; 214: 528–536

64. Brogli E, Wu T, Namiki A, Isner J M. Indirect angiogenic cytokines upregulate VEGF and bFGF gene expression in vascular smooth muscle cells, whereas hypoxia upregulates VEGF expression only. Circulation 1994; 90: 649–652

65. Jacobs S C, Story M T, Sasse J, Lawson R K. Characterization of growth factors derived from the rat ventral prostate. J Urol 1988; 139: 1106–1110

66. Mydlo J H, Bulbul M A, Richon V M et al. Heparin-binding growth factor isolated from human prostatic extracts. Prostate 1988; 12: 343–355

67. Smith E P, Russell W E, French F S, Wilson E M. A form of basic fibroblast growth factor is secreted into the adluminal fluid of the rat coagulating gland. Prostate 1989; 14: 353

68. Begun F P, Story M T, Hopp K A et al. Regional concentration of basic fibroblast growth factor in normal and benign hyperplastic human prostates. J Urol 1995; 153: 839–843

69. Muthukrihnan L, Warder E, McNeil P. Basic fibroblast growth factor is efficiently released from a cytosolic storage site through plasma membrane disruptions of endothelial cells. J Cell Physiol 1991; 148: 1–16

70. Ku P-T, D'Amore P. Regulation of basic fibroblast growth factor (bFGF) gene and protein expression following its release from sublethally injured endothelial cells. J Cell Biochem 1995; 58: 328–343

71. Yan G, Fukabori Y, Nikolaropoulos S et al. Heparin-binding keratinocyte growth factor is a candidate stromal-to-epithelial cell andromedin. Mol Endocrinol 1992; 6: 2123–2128

72. Alarid E T, Rubin J S, Young P et al. Keratinocyte growth factor functions in epithelial induction during seminal vesicle development. Proc Natl Acad Sci USA 1994; 91: 1074–1078

73. McKeehan W L, Hou J, Adams P et al. Heparin-binding fibroblast growth factors and prostate cancer. Adv Exp Med Biol 1993; 330: 203–221

74. Yan G, Fukabori Y, McBride G et al. Exon switching and activation of stromal and embryonic fibroblast growth factor (FGF)-FGF receptor genes in prostate epithelial cells accompany stromal independence and malignancy. Mol Cell Biol 1993; 13: 4513–4522

75. Tutrone R F, Ball R A, Ornitz D M et al. Benign prostatic hyperplasia in a transgenic mouse: a new hormonally sensitive investigatory model. J Urol 1993; 149: 633–639

76. Geller J, Sionit L R, Baird A et al. In vivo and in vitro effects of androgen on fibroblast growth factor-2 concentrations in the human prostate. Prostate 1994; 25: 206–209

77. Vlahos C J, Kriauciunas T D, Gleason P E et al. Platelet-derived growth factor induces proliferation of hyperplastic human prostatic stromal cells. J Cell Biochem 1993; 52: 404–413

78. Graham C W, Lynch J H, Djakiew D. Distribution of nerve growth factor-like protein and nerve growth factor receptor in human prostatic hyperplasia and prostatic adenocarcinoma. J Urol 1992; 147: 1444–1447

79. Cohen P, Peehl D M, Baker B et al. Insulin-like growth factor axis abnormalities in prostatic stromal cells from patients with benign prostatic hyperplasia. J Clin Endocrinol Metab 1994; 79: 1410–1415

80. Tzahar E, Levkowitz G, Karunagaran D et al. ErbB-3 and ErbB-4 function as the low and high affinity receptors of all Neu differentiation factor/heregulin isoforms. J Biol Chem 1994; 269: 25226–25233

81. Karunagaran D, Tzahar E, Liu N et al. Neu differentiation factor inhibits EGF binding. A model for trans-regulation within the ErbB family of receptor tyrosine kinases. J Biol Chem 1995; 270: 9982–9990

82. Gregory H, Willshire I R, Kavanagh J P et al. Urogastrone–epidermal growth factor concentrations in prostatic fluid of normal individuals and patients with benign prostatic hypertrophy. Clin Sci 1986; 70: 359–363

83. Ching K Z, Ramsey E, Pettigrew N et al. Expression of mRNA for epidermal growth factor, transforming growth factor-alpha and their receptor in human prostate tissues and cell lines. Mol Cell Biochem 1993; 126: 151–158

84. Yang Y, Chisholm G D, Habib F K. Epidermal growth factor and transforming growth factor alpha concentrations in BPH and cancer of the prostate: their relationships with tissue androgen levels. Br J Cancer 1993; 67: 152–155

85. Robertson C N, Robertson K M, Herzberg A J et al. Differential immunoreactivity of transforming growth factor alpha in benign, dysplastic and malignant prostatic tissues. Surg Oncol 1994; 3: 237–242

86. Sehgal I, Bailey J, Hitzemann K et al. Epidermal growth factor receptor-dependent stimulation of amphiregulin expression in androgen-stimulated human prostate cancer cells. Mol Biol Cell 1994; 5: 339–347

87. Zhau H-Y E, Wan D S, Zhou J et al. Expression of c-erbB2/neu proto-oncogene in human prostatic cancer tissues and cell lines. Mol Carcinog 1992; 5: 320–327

88. Giri D K, Wadhwa S N, Upadhaya S N, Talwar G P. Expression of NEU/HER-2 oncoprotein (p185neu) in prostate tumors: an immunohistochemical study. Prostate 1993; 23: 329–336

89. Higashiyama S, Abraham J A, Klagsbrun M. Heparin-binding EGF-like growth factor stimulation of smooth muscle cell migration: dependence on interactions with cell surface heparan sulfate. J Cell Biol 1993; 122: 933–940

90. Freeman M R, Uchida T, Soker S et al. HB-EGF expression is decreased and VEGF is increased in the progression of normal to transformed prostate epithelia. J Cell Biochem 1994; (suppl 18D): 221

91. Johnson G R, Wong L. Heparan sulfate is essential to amphiregulin-induced mitogenic signalling by the epidermal growth factor receptor. J Biol Chem 1994; 269: 27149–27154

92. Wong S T, Winchell L F, McCune B K et al. The TGFα precursor expressed on the cell surface binds to the EGF receptor on adjacent cells leading to signal transduction 1989; 56: 495–506

93. Stein J, Borzillo G V, Rettenmier C W. Direct stimulation of cells expressing receptors for macrophage colony stimulating factor (CSF-1) by a plasma membrane-bound precursor of human CSF-1. Blood 1990; 76: 1308–1314

94. Higashiyama S, Iwamoto R, Goishi K et al. The membrane protein CD9/DRAP 27 potentiates the juxtacrine growth factor activity of the membrane-anchored heparin-binding EGF-like growth factor. J Cell Biol 1995; 128: 929–938

95. Theyer G, Kramer G, Assman I et al. Phenotypic characterization of infiltrating leukocytes in benign prostatic hyperplasia. Lab Invest 1992; 66: 96–107

96. Blotnick S, Peoples G E, Freeman M R et al. T lymphocytes synthesize and export heparin-binding epidermal growth factor-like growth factor and basic fibroblast growth factor, mitogens for vascular cells and fibroblasts: differential production and release by CD4+ and CD8+ T cells. Proc Natl Acad Sci USA 1994; 91: 2890–2894

97. Freeman M R, Schneck F X, Gagnon M et al. Peripheral blood T lymphocytes and T cells infiltrating human cancers express vascular endothelial growth factor: a potential role for T cells in angiogenesis. Cancer Res 1995; 55: 4140–4145

98. Peoples G E, Blotnick S, Takahashi K et al. T lymphocytes that infiltrate tumors and atherosclerotic plaques produce HB-EGF and bFGF: a pathologic role. Proc Natl Acad Sci USA 1995; 92: 6547–6551

99. Passanti A, Isaacs J T, Haney J A et al. Stimulation of human prostatic carcinoma tumor growth in athymic mice and control of migration in culture by extracellular matrix. Int J Cancer 1992; 51: 318–324

100. Fridman R, Kibbey M C, Royce L S et al. Enhanced tumor growth of both primary and established human and murine tumor cells in athymic mice after coinjection with Matrigel. J Natl Cancer Inst 1991; 83: 769–774

101. Pretlow T G, Delmoro C M, Dilley G G et al. Transplantation of human prostatic carcinoma into nude mice in Matrigel. Cancer Res 1991; 51: 3814–3817

102. Freeman M R, Bagli D J, Lamb C C et al. Culture of a prostatic cell line in basement membrane gels results in an enhancement of malignant properties and constitutive alterations in gene expression. J Cell Physiol 1994; 158: 325–336

103. Folkman J, Klagsbrun M, Sasse J et al. Heparin-binding angiogenic protein — basic fibroblast growth factor — is stored within basement membrane. Am J Pathol 1988; 130: 393–400

104. Bernfield M, Sanderson R D. Syndecan, a developmentally regulated cell surface proteoglycan that binds extracellular matrix and growth factors. Phil Trans R Soc Lond B 1990; 327: 171–186

105. Yayon A, Klagsbrun M, Esko J D et al. Cell surface, heparin-like molecules are required for binding of basic fibroblast growth factor to its high affinity receptor. Cell 1991; 64: 841–848

106. Kan M, Wang F, Xu J et al. An essential heparin-binding domain in the fibroblast growth factor receptor kinase. Science 1993; 259: 1918-1921

107. Bennett K L, Jackson D G, Simon J C et al. CD44 isoforms containing exon V3 are responsible for the presentation of heparin-binding growth factor. J Cell Biol 1995; 128: 687–695

108. Vachon P H, Durand J, Beaulieu J F. Basement membrane formation and re-distribution of the beta1 integrins in a human intestinal co-culture system. Anat Rec 1993; 235: 567–576

109. Austria M R, Couchman J R. Enhanced assembly of basement membrane matrix by endodermal cells in response to fibronectin substrata. J Cell Sci 1991; 99: 443–451

110. Presta M, Maier J A, Rusnati M et al. Modulation of plasminogen activator activity in human endometrial adenocarcinoma cells by basic fibroblast growth factor and transforming growth factor beta. Cancer Res 1989; 48: 68–74

111. Flaumenhaft R, Moscatelli D, Saksela O, Rifkin D B. Role of extracellular matrix in the action of basic fibroblast growth factor: matrix as a source of growth factor for long-term stimulation of plasminogen activator production and DNA synthesis. J Cell Physiol 1989; 140: 75–81

112. Vlodavsky I, Korner G, Ishai-Michaeli R et al. Extracellular matrix-resident growth factors and enzymes: possible involvement in tumor metastasis and angiogenesis. Cancer Metastasis Rev 1990; 9: 203–226

113. Fukai N, Apte S S, Olsen B R. Methods Enzymol 1994; 245: 3

114. Hynes R O. Integrins: versatility, modulation and signalling in cell adhesion. Cell 1992; 69: 11–25

115. Sorokin L, Sonnenberg A, Aumailley M et al. Recognition of the laminin E8 cell-binding site by an integrin possessing the α6 subunit is essential for epithelial polarization in developing kidney tubules. J Cell Biol 1990; 111: 1265–1273

116. Juliano R L, Haskill S. Signal transduction from the extracellular matrix. J Cell Biol 1993; 120: 577–585

117. Werb Z, Tremble P M, Behrendtsen O et al. Signal transduction through the fibronectin receptor induces collagenase and stromolysin gene expression. J Cell Biol 1989; 109: 877–889

118. Kornberg L J, Earp H S, Turner C E et al. Signal transduction by integrins: increased protein phosphorylation caused by clustering of β1 integrins. Proc Natl Acad Sci USA 1991; 88: 8392–8395

119. Pelletier A J, Bodary S C, Levinson A D. Signal transduction by the platelet integrin αIIbβ3: induction of calcium oscillations required for protein–tyrosine phosphorylation and ligand-induced spreading of stably transfected cells. Mol Biol Cell 1992; 3: 989–998

120. Mecham R P, Hinek A, Entwistle R et al. Elastin binds to a multifunctional 67kD peripheral membrane protein. Biochemistry 1989; 28: 3716–3722

121. Schmiddhauser C, Bissell M J, Myers C A, Casperson G F. Extracellular matrix and hormones transcriptionally regulate bovine β-casein in stably transfected mouse mammary cells. Proc Natl Acad Sci USA 1990; 87: 9118–9122

122. Streuli C H, Schmidhauser C, Kobrin M et al. Extracellular matrix regulates expression of the TGF-beta 1 gene. J Cell Biol 1993; 120: 253–260

123. Kleinman H K, McGarvey M L, Hassell J R et al. Basement membrane complexes with biological activity. Biochemistry 1986; 25: 312–318

124. Vukicevic S, Luyten F P, Kleinman H K, Reddi A H. Differentiation of canalicular cell processes in bone cells by basement membrane matrix components: regulation by discrete domains of laminin. Cell 1990; 63: 437–445

125. Streuli C H, Bailey N, Bissell M J. Control of mammary epithelial differentiation: basement membrane induces tissue-specific gene expression in the absence of cell–cell interaction and morphological polarity. J Cell Biol 1991; 115: 1383–1395

126. Wagner D, Ivatt R, Destree A, Hynes R. Similarities and differences between fibronectins of normal and transformed hamster cells. J Biol Chem 1981; 256: 11708–11715

127. Guadagno T M, Ohtsubo M, Roberts J M, Assoian R K. A link between cyclin A expression and adhesion-dependent cell cycle proliferation. Science 1993; 262: 1572–1575

128. Symington B E. Fibronectin receptor modulates cyclin-dependent kinase activity. J Biol Chem 1993; 267: 25744–25747

129. Vaheri A, Ruoslahti E. Fibroblast surface antigen produced but not retained by virus-transformed human cells. J Exp Med 1975; 142: 530–535

130. Schreiner C, Fisher M, Hussein S, Juliano R L. Increased tumorigenicity of fibronectin receptor deficient Chinese hamster ovary cell variants. Cancer Res 1991; 51: 1738–1740

131. Freeman M R, Song Y, Carson D D et al. Extracellular matrix and androgen receptor expression associated with spontaneous transformation of rat prostate fibroblasts. Cancer Res 1991; 51: 1910–1916

132. Giancotti F G, Ruoslahti E. Elevated levels of the α5β1 integrin suppresses the transformed phenotype of Chinese hamster ovary cells. Cell 1990; 60: 849–859

133. Brooks P C, Montogomery A M P, Rosenfed M et al. Integrin αVβ3 antagonists promote tumor regression by inducing apoptosis of angiogenic blood vessels. Cell 1994; 79: 1157–1164

134. Ingber D E, Folkman J. How does extracellular matrix control capillary morphogenesis? Cell 1989; 58: 803–805

135. Turpeenniemi-Hujanen T, Thorgeirsson U P, Rao C N, Liotta L A. Laminin increases the release of type IV collagenase from malignant cells. J Biol Chem 1986; 261: 1883–1889

136. Graf J, Iwamoto Y, Sasaki M et al. Identification of an amino acid sequence in laminin mediating cell attachment, chemotaxis and receptor binding. Cell 1987; 48: 989–996

137. Sephel G C, Tashiro K-I, Sasaki M et al. Laminin A chain synthetic peptide which supports neurite outgrowth. Biochem Biophys Res Commun 1989; 162: 821–829

138. Thompson E W, Yu M, Bueno J et al. Collagen induced MMP-2 activation in human breast cancer. Breast Cancer Res Treat 1994; 31: 357–370

139. Hohn H P, Parker C R, Boots L R et al. Modulation of differentiation markers in human choriocarcinoma cells by extracellular matrix: on the role of a three-dimensional matrix structure. Differentiation 1992; 51: 61–70

140. Bonkoff H, Stein U, Remberger K. Differential expression of alpha 6 and alpha 2 very late antigen integrins in the normal, hyperplastic and neoplastic prostate: simultaneous demonstration of cell surface receptors and their extracellular ligands. Hum Pathol 1993; 24: 243–248

141. Knox J D, Cress A E, Clark V et al. Differential expression of extracellular matrix molecules and the alpha 6-integrins in the normal and neoplastic prostate. Am J Pathol 1994; 145: 167–174

142. Nagle R B, Knox J D, Wolf C et al. Adhesion molecules, extracellular matrix, and proteases in prostate carcinoma. J Cell Biochem 1994; 19: 232–237

143. Vollmer G, Michna H, Ebert K, Knuppen R. Androgen ablation induces tenascin expression in the rat prostate. Prostate 1994; 25: 81–90

144. Ibrahim S N, Lightner V A, Ventimiglia J B et al. Tenascin expression in prostatic hyperplasia, intraepithelial neoplasia, and carcinoma. Hum Pathol 1993; 24: 982–989

145. Fong C J, Sherwood E R, Braun E J et al. Regulation of prostatic carcinoma cell proliferation and secretory activity by extracellular matrix and stromal secretions. Prostate 1992; 21: 121–131

146. Verhoeven G, Swinnen K, Cailleau J et al. The role of cell–cell interactions in androgen action. J Steroid Biochem Mol Biol 1992; 41: 487–494

147. Thompson T C, Southgate J, Kitchner G, Land H. Multistage carcinogenesis induced by ras and myc oncogenes in a reconstituted organ. Cell 1989; 56: 917–930

148. Greenburg N M, DeMayo F, Sheppard P C et al. The rat probasin promoter directs hormonally and developmentally regulated expression of a heterologous gene specifically to the prostate in transgenic mice. Mol Endocrinol 1994; 8: 230–239

149. Greenburg N M, DeMayo F, Finegold M et al. Prostate cancer in a transgenic mouse. Proc Natl Acad Sci USA 1995; 92: 3439–3443

150. Liang P, Pardee A. Differential display of eukaryotic messenger RNA by means of the polymerase chain reaction. Science 1992; 257: 967–970

5

Prostatic adrenoceptors

B. A. Kenny A. M. Naylor M. G. Wyllie

Historical aspects

The treatment of benign prostatic hyperplasia (BPH) with alpha-1-adrenoceptor antagonists stemmed from the pioneering studies of Marco Caine. This work has contributed greatly to our understanding of the autonomic innervation of the prostate. Although the prostate, like most organs, receives a dual adrenergic/cholinergic innervation (Fig. 5.1), the former is of particular interest to the urologist and is the prime determinant of fibromuscular prostate smooth muscle tone. Bladder outlet obstruction in BPH is thought to consist of two components — a static component related to prostatic tissue mass and a dynamic component related to prostatic tone. Since

approximately one-third of the tissue within the prostate is fibromuscular and related to the bladder both anatomically and functionally,[1] a reduction in tone might be postulated to reduce prostatic urethral pressure and improve obstructive symptoms. In this context, Caine demonstrated in the mid-1970s that the contractile response of the prostatic capsule adenoma, derived from patients undergoing retropubic prostatectomy, was mediated primarily by alpha-1- rather than beta-adrenoreceptors.[2,3]

On the basis of these data and several animal studies, Caine postulated that specific blockade of prostate alpha-1-adrenoceptors would reduce urethral resistance, thereby increasing flow and improving symptoms. Shortly thereafter, he reported the first clinical data

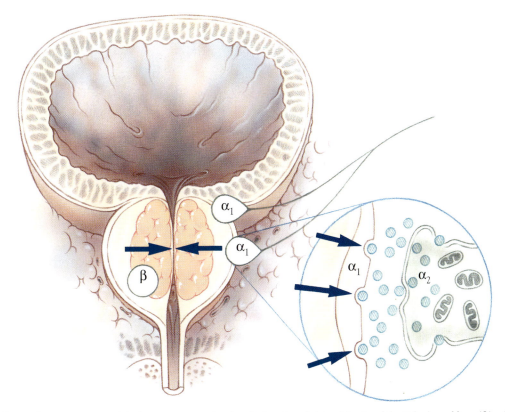

Figure 5.1. *Sympathetic innervation of the human prostate showing the location of alpha-1 (α_1)-, alpha-2 (α_2)- and beta (β)-adrenoceptors.*

with the adrenoceptor antagonist phenoxybenzamine.[3] Although this antagonist was effective, the study would no longer be considered to represent unequivocal evidence of a predominant role of alpha-1-adrenoceptors, as phenoxybenzamine also has high affinity for alpha-2-adrenoceptors, which are also found in the prostatic neuroeffector synapse (Fig. 5.1). Subsequently, however, several studies with more selective alpha-1-adrenoceptor antagonists have demonstrated a key role for alpha-1-adrenoceptors in the control of prostatic tone. In particular, although the densities of alpha-1- and alpha-2-receptors in the prostate are similar, Lepor and Shapiro have demonstrated that alpha-1-adrenoceptors are the prime determinant of tone.[4,5]

These, and other studies, provided the rationale for the use of more selective alpha-1-adrenoceptor antagonists. Although phenoxybenzamine was clinically effective, the incidence and severity of side effects, arising from interactions at sites other than the alpha-1-adrenoceptor, limited its use. Considerable advances with respect to tolerance have been made with the advent of the more selective alpha-1-adrenoceptor antagonists such as prazosin, terazosin, doxazosin and tamsulosin, which are effective treatments of BPH. However, as none of these agents was designed specifically to target the prostate, signs of cardiovascular activity, such as dizziness and light-headedness, may be apparent at high doses. Current understanding of the heterogeneity of alpha-1-adrenoceptors offers an opportunity to target the prostatic alpha-1-adrenoceptor selectively while minimizing activity at other sites.

Heterogeneity of alpha-1-adrenoceptors

Over the last few years, considerable evidence for the existence of multiple alpha-1-adrenoceptor subtypes has emerged. Since the development of the original concept of alpha-1-adrenoceptor heterogeneity there has been much debate regarding classification and terminology, which has only recently been resolved. It is important to recognize the impact of the emerging nomenclature when interpretating historical data, as previous conclusions have been reached on the basis of different classification criteria. On this basis, therefore, it is not surprising that characterization of the alpha-1-adrenoceptor subtype mediating contraction of human prostate has been, apparently, highly dependent on the group undertaking the study.

A major difficulty in interpretation has arisen because of the differences in classifying adrenoceptors in native tissues in relation to those identified using molecular cloning. Current nomenclature now allows for the alignment of cloned and native alpha-1-adrenoceptors (Table 5.1). This consensus in alpha-1-adrenoceptor terminology should help to facilitate the unambiguous identification of the prostatic alpha-1-adrenoceptor subtype involved in the contractile response in man.

Evidence for multiple alpha-1-adrenoceptors

Heterogeneity of alpha-1-adrenoceptors was originally suggested on the basis of radioligand-binding studies to native rat tissues.[6,7] Thereafter, a number of findings using both receptor-binding and functional approaches have clearly demonstrated the existence of multiple alpha-1-adrenoceptor subtypes. Two types of pharmacologically defined alpha-1-adrenoceptors have consistently been detected in native tissues. One of these subtypes displays high affinity for the agonists methoxamine and oxymetazoline as well as the antagonists WB 4101, phentolamine, 5-methylurapidil (5-MU) and (+)-niguldipine, but is resistant to alkylation by chloroethylclonidine (CEC) (Table 5.1): this subtype has been named the alpha-1A-adrenoceptor. Another subtype displays considerably lower affinity for the above competitive agonists and antagonists but is sensitive to alkylation and inactivation by CEC (Table 5.1): this subtype has been named the alpha-1B-adrenoceptor.

Receptor cloning studies have revealed the existence of at least three subtypes of alpha-1-adrenoceptors, encoded by distinct genes and located on different human chromosomes. In an attempt to align cloned and pharmacologically defined subtypes, apart from affinities for competitively acting drugs and CEC sensitivities, tissue distribution of mRNA has been used as a criterion for subtype identification. A receptor cDNA that was originally cloned from hamster smooth muscle cells, and

Table 5.1. *Molecular and pharmacological properties of alpha-1-adrenoceptor subtypes*

Property	Pharmacological designation (and clone subtype)		
	1A (alpha-1c)	1B (alpha-1b)	1D (alpha-1a/d)
Structure	466 aa, 7TM human, bovine, rat	515 aa, 7TM human, hamster, rat	560 aa, 7TM human, rat
Human chromosomal localization	C8	C5	C20
Distribution of mRNA	Liver, heart, cerebral cortex, lung, prostate (human); vas deferens, cerebral cortex, heart, submaxillary gland (rat)	Aorta, spleen, lung (human); cerebral cortex, kidney, liver, heart (rat)	Aorta, cerebral cortex, prostate (human); hippocampus, cerebral cortex, vas deferens (rat)
Tissues expressing homogeneous populations (radiological binding)	Rat submaxillary gland, rabbit liver, human liver	Rat liver, rat spleen	?
Functional preparations	Rat kidney vasoconstriction, rat vas deferens contraction; **human prostate contraction**?	Rat spleen contraction	Rat aorta contraction
Selective antagonists	(+)-Niguldipine, 5-methylurapidil, RS 17053	Spiperone	BMY 7378

subsequently from rat and human sources, encodes for a protein that has low affinity for all known alpha-1A-adrenoceptor-selective drugs and is readily alkylated by CEC; hence it was named the alpha-1b subtype (note the initially used designation of cloned receptors in lower case). Several studies have now demonstrated that this cDNA encodes a receptor protein equivalent to the tissue alpha-1B-adrenoceptor based on its pharmacological and tissue expression profile.[8,9] Two other cloned alpha-1-adrenoceptor subtypes have been isolated from bovine and rat sources and were initially termed alpha-1c and alpha-1a/d; the latter designation has arisen since two groups independently cloned an apparently identical cDNA and initially referred to it as alpha-1a[10] and alpha-1d.[11] Since the properties of the cloned alpha-1a/d subtype differ from the native alpha-1A subtype (see below), referral to this cloned receptor as an alpha-1D subtype is clearly more appropriate.

Whereas it is clear that the identity of the alpha-1b-cDNA is consistent with the pharmacologically defined alpha-1B-adrenoceptor, the situation with regard to

cloned alpha-1d and alpha-1c subtypes and pharmacologically defined native alpha-1-adrenoceptors has, until recently, remained controversial. Recently, a number of [³H]prazosin-binding studies have shown that the profile of a range of subtype selective compounds at cloned alpha-1c-adrenoceptors is very similar to the profile obtained using rat submaxillary gland membranes, a model tissue of the pharmacologically characterized alpha-1A-adrenoceptor.[12] In addition, Clarke and colleagues[12] have obtained similar functional affinities using vasoconstriction in the perfused rat kidney as a model of alpha-1A-adrenoceptors. Taken together with mRNA distribution studies, all these findings suggest that the cloned alpha-1c-adrenoceptor is the molecular correlate of the native alpha-1A subtype. Native correlates for the cloned alpha-1d-adrenoceptor are less well defined. The presence of this receptor has been suggested in some tissues containing heterogeneous populations of alpha-1-adrenoceptors and it has been suggested that it is the predominant receptor mediating the contractile response of rat aorta to noradrenalin.[13] However, a homogeneous population of receptors has yet to be identified.

Thus, the current alpha-1-adrenoceptor classification recognizes three native and cloned subtypes, which have been designated alpha-1A, alpha-1B and alpha-1D (corresponding to previous cloned subtypes alpha-1c, alpha-1b and alpha-1a/d, respectively) Since the properties of both recombinant and native receptor subtypes are similar when appropriately defined (Table 5.1), the use of lower and upper-case letters is now recommended for both cloned and tissue-defined alpha-1-adrenoceptors respectively.[14] It must be emphasized that this classification scheme accounts only for those alpha-1-adrenoceptor subtypes identified by molecular cloning, together with their endogenous correlates. The pharmacological profile exhibited by compounds on a number of tissue preparations is inconsistent with this classification. In particular, the relatively low affinity exhibited by prazosin and other compounds in some function studies (particularly from the dog and rabbit) suggests the existence of an additional population of alpha-1-adrenoceptors, which have been termed alpha-1L.[15] The relationship between these receptors and those accounted for by current classification, if any, remains to be confirmed.

Contractile responses of prostatic tissue in vitro

The application of quantitative pharmacological analysis of the interaction of agonists and antagonists is often used to facilitate the characterization and classification of receptors mediating contractile responses of smooth muscle in vitro. Activation of muscarinic receptors does not elicit a contractile response of human prostatic tissue in vitro, and it is well established that noradrenaline and phenylephrine mediate contractile responses almost exclusively through an interaction with alpha-1-adrenoceptors, as the selective alpha-2-agonists UK 14304 and clonidine are relatively ineffective.[16–19] In this respect, it is interesting to note that smooth muscle strips taken from hyperplastic prostatic tissues have been found to be more responsive to the alpha-1-agonist phenylephrine than is normal tissue.[16] This finding may relate to

observations made by Shapiro and colleagues, in which a direct relationship was found between the extent of urinary flow improvement with alpha-1-adrenoceptor antagonists and the density of prostatic smooth muscle mass.[20] This finding suggests a direct action of these drugs that reduce the dynamic tone associated with bladder outlet obstruction.

Antagonism of alpha-1-receptor-mediated responses has been determined for a range of antagonists (Table 5.2, Fig. 5.2), unequivocally demonstrating the contractile role of alpha-1-adrenoceptors. A number of studies have attempted to elucidate the alpha-1-adrenoceptor subtype mediating the functional response of human prostatic tissue in vitro. However, across the literature a number of differing conclusions have been reached, mainly as a reflection of the limited pharmacological tools previously available and the various criteria applied to classify the functional response.[21–25] Most of these studies have used competitive alpha-1-adrenoceptor antagonists, together with the alkylating agent CEC.

The availability of compounds that have different selectivity profiles for the various alpha-1-adrenoceptor subtypes outlined above have been important in elucidating the predominant subtype mediating contractile responses of prostatic smooth muscle in vitro. Estimates of antagonist affinity for a range of competitive alpha-1-antagonists suggest that alpha-1A-adrenoceptors mediate functional responses (Fig. 5.2). A clear correlation exists between the affinity of compounds for cloned human alpha-1A-adrenoceptors and their corresponding estimates against alpha-1-mediated contractions of human prostatic smooth muscle in vitro. Particularly noteworthy are compounds with differing degrees of selectivity for the cloned alpha-1A subtype, such as 5-MU, WB 4101, indoramin and SNAP 1069, reported by Forray et al.[24] and Kenny et al.[13] (Table 5.2), which exhibit functional affinity estimates consistent with their alpha-1A-binding affinities.

However, this conclusion is not uniformly accepted because of conflicting data generated with other compounds. The relatively low affinity exhibited by prazosin against alpha-1-mediated contractile responses (pA_2 affinity estimates <9.0) in contrast to the affinity for cloned alpha-1A-receptors (pK_i > 9.5) has been

Table 5.2. *Binding affinities (pK_i) for compounds at cloned human alpha-1-adrenoceptors*

Compound	pK_i		
	Human alpha-1A	Human alpha-1B	Human alpha-1D
BMY 7378	6.2 ± 0.10	6.7 ± 0.11	8.2 ± 0.10
Prazosin	9.7 ± 0.20	9.6 ± 0.14	9.5 ± 0.10
Doxazosin	8.5 ± 0.20	9.0 ± 0.20	8.4 ± 0.12
WB 4101	9.3 ± 0.10	8.2 ± 0.16	9.2 ± 0.06
5-Methylurapidil	8.5 ± 0.09	6.8 ± 0.13	7.8 ± 0.09
Benoxathian	8.9 ± 0.23	7.8 ± 0.14	8.6 ± 0.12
Phentolamine	8.1 ± 0.09	7.1 ± 0.15	7.8 ± 0.03
SNAP 1069	7.8 ± 0.19	7.6 ± 0.18	6.8 ± 0.20
Indoramin	8.3 ± 0.03	8.0 ± 0.12	7.3 ± 0.15
Alfuzosin	8.0 ± 0.20	8.0 ± 0.13	8.5 ± 0.07
Spiperone	7.6 ± 0.12	8.8 ± 0.16	8.1 ± 0.03

Affinities were determined by displacement of 0.2 nM [3H]prazosin from rat-1 fibroblasts stably expressing cloned alpha-1-adrenoceptor subtypes by 12 concentrations of competing drug. Values represent mean ± SEM for three to five separate determinations. Hill slopes for displacement curves were not significantly different from unity. (Data from ref. 13 with permission.)

suggested to be indicative of a different functional receptor.[26] The affinity of 5-MU against noradrenaline-mediated contractions of human prostate has been suggested to be intermediate between its affinity for alpha-1A- and alpha-1B-adrenoceptors in several studies, which might suggest the existence of a non-alpha-1A, alpha-1B-adrenoceptor.[27] More recently, other compounds such as the highly selective and potent alpha-1A-antagonist RS 17053 (alpha-1A-binding affinity=9.5) have been shown to be relatively weak antagonists on human prostate (pA_2=6.9).[28] Taken together, these data suggest that the cloned alpha-1A-adrenoceptor and the alpha-1-subtype mediating contractile responses of human prostate in vitro may not be identical. In support of this conclusion, the ability of CEC to attenuate the contractile response of human prostate[27,29] contrasts with the reported insensitivity of other alpha-1A-mediated functional responses,[7,9,14,27] suggesting a response or at least a component of the response that is non-alpha-1A-mediated. However, it must be noted that the agonist response following alkylation of receptors with CEC can depend on a number of factors, including receptor reserve for the agonist, tissue type, species and exposure time to CEC, making interpretation of comparative data difficult.

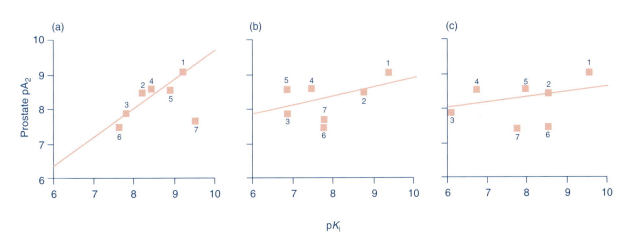

Figure 5.2. *Correlation plots of the potency of several alpha-1-adrenoceptor antagonists (1, prazosin; 2, terazosin; 3, indoramin; 4, SNAP 1069; 5, 5-methylurapidil; 6, SK & F104856; 7, RS 17053) for cloned human and animal (RS 17053) alpha-1-adrenoceptors (a, alpha-1A; b, alpha-1B; c, alpha-1D) versus their potency at inhibiting alpha-1-mediated contractions of the human prostate in vitro. These data illustrate a good correlation between functional alpha-1-adrenoceptor affinity (pA_2) on human prostate and binding affinity (pK_i) for most, but not all, alpha-1-antagonists at the cloned human alpha-1A subtype. (Adapted from refs 24 and 28.)*

If the prostatic alpha-1-adrenoceptor is not entirely consistent with its designation of a typical alpha-1A-adrenoceptor, it appears to be at least closely related. However, exhaustive attempts have thus far failed to identify additional alpha-1-adrenoceptor subtypes using homology-based molecular cloning. As genes encoding the alpha-1-adrenoceptor possess introns, splice variants of existing receptors cannot be fully excluded, which may give rise to several isoforms of the alpha-1A-receptor having different pharmacological properties. Whether such a receptor is functionally predominant on human prostate awaits confirmation.

Radioligand-binding studies

Characterization of prostatic alpha-1-adrenoceptors has been carried out with iodinated or tritiated alpha-1-adrenoceptor-antagonist radioligands, principally [3H]prazosin, [3H]tamsulosin and [125I]HEAT (iodo-4-hydroxyphenyl-ethyl-aminomethyl-tetralone), using homogenized prostatic tissue (which will consist of stromal, epithelial and vascular elements). Localization of alpha-1-adrenoceptors by receptor autoradiography using [3H]prazosin indicates that the majority (85%) of alpha-1-adrenoceptor sites are on the fibromuscular stroma, with a much lower density (15%) on glandular epithelium.[30,31] Some studies suggest that the density of binding sites in hyperplastic prostate homogenates is higher than in corresponding non-BPH tissue, although this is not found in all studies.[32,33] In addition, binding parameters (affinity K_d and density B_{max}) have been found to be similar for different regions (anterior, posterior, lateral and central) of the prostate.[34] Recent binding studies from two groups, using either [125I]HEAT[35] or [3H]prazosin,[36] indicates that these ligands label a single population of high-affinity alpha-1-adrenoceptors in human and canine prostatic homogenates. Competitive displacement of these radioligands by a wide range of competing compounds was consistent with an interaction at a single receptor that exhibited the characteristics of an alpha-1A-adrenoceptor. In the study carried out by Goetz et al.[35] the profile of more than 20 compounds was examined: binding affinities determined against [125I]HEAT in human and canine prostatic tissue homogenates were highly correlated with affinities for the same compounds

at cloned human alpha-1A-adrenoceptors, but not with alpha-1B or alpha-1D subtypes. Similar conclusions have also been reached by Testa et al.[36]

However, although the majority of studies suggest the presence of a single population of binding sites, other studies suggest that at least two alpha-1-adrenoceptor subtypes can be detected from binding studies to prostatic homogenates. Perhaps this is not surprising, given the composition of prostate-binding homogenates. However as shown in Table 5.2, prazosin displays similar affinity for all currently identified cloned receptors, yet several groups have reported that two receptors with differing affinities for prazosin (and some other compounds) can be identified on human prostate. Prostatic receptors displaying different affinities for prazosin cannot be fully reconciled with the profile of prazosin at currently cloned alpha-1-adrenoceptors. In the studies by Muramatsu and colleagues,[26] it has been shown that the detection of these putative sites is dependent on the ability of certain compounds to differentiate between them, with a component of [3H]prazosin-binding insensitive to certain agents such as phentolamine and 5-MU. Thus, only a single site can be detected for 5-MU in competition studies, in contrast to other compounds such as prazosin and WB 4101, which appear to inhibit an additional component of the total number of sites labelled by [3H]prazosin. Similarly, in several other studies using human,[25] canine[37] and bovine[38] prostatic alpha-1-adrenoceptors, displacement studies with a small number of competing compounds have been found to be biphasic, suggesting that these drugs distinguish between two different alpha-1-adrenoceptor subtypes on prostatic membranes. Similarly, in a comparative study, [3H]tamsulosin was found to label 75% of the sites in human prostate labelled by prazosin, suggesting that tamsulosin may have relatively low affinity for a subpopulation of the total sites identified by prazosin,[39] although neither of these quinazoline alpha-1-antagonists discriminates between currently identified cloned alpha-1-adrenoceptors.

A key question is how the affinity of compounds for these different sites relates to their functional affinity against noradrenaline-mediated contractile responses, especially as binding homogenates contain more than purely stromal elements. In almost all published studies for those compounds exhibiting high and low affinities for prostatic binding sites (such as prazosin, WB 4101, oxymetazoline and RS 17053), the low-affinity site has been claimed to be consistent with the identity of the functional alpha-1-adrenoceptor.[25,26,28] As the low binding and functional affinities exhibited by these compounds are not consistent with their profile at currently identified cloned alpha-1-adrenoceptors, these data suggest the existence of a distinct subtype that is functionally predominant.

In summary, an alpha-1-adrenoceptor with the characteristics of an alpha-1A subtype can be detected in human prostatic tissue. Consensus as to whether an alpha-1A-adrenoceptor, or a similar but distinct subtype, mediates the contractile response of this tissue to noradrenaline has not been reached. This situation will be resolved with the impact of more selective competitive antagonists.

Localization of prostatic alpha-1-adrenoceptors at the molecular level

All three human alpha-1-adrenoceptors have been cloned from human prostate, either by reverse transcriptase–polymerase chain reaction (RT–PCR) of cDNA fragments or from human prostate cDNA libraries. Sequencing of full-length cDNAs shows a high degree of identity to other mammalian alpha-1-adrenoceptor homologues. Using RNA extracted from human prostate, RNase protection assays have shown that the alpha-1A-adrenoceptor subtype represents more than 70% of the total alpha-1-mRNA in human prostate. In situ hybridization experiments carried out by Price et al.[40] have shown that alpha-1A-mRNA localizes to the stromal compartment, consistent with radioligand binding to prostatic tissue sections using receptor autoradiography.[21] In agreement with radioligand-binding studies, molecular techniques also identify multiple alpha-1-adrenoceptors in human prostate tissue with mRNA transcripts for all three currently cloned alpha-1-adrenoceptors having been detected.[25] Using cDNA probes, Faure et al.[25] have examined, by Northern analysis, the expression of different alpha-1-adrenoceptors in different prostatic regions of human prostatic adenoma, which has been found to be similar in the apex, base, lateral lobe and periurethral zones. It must be emphasized, however, that expression of high levels of mRNA for any given subtype does not necessarily correlate with high levels of receptor protein and confirms the importance of other techniques such as radioligand binding and functional analysis, especially given the possible presence of more than one subtype. Thus far, extensive efforts have failed to identify additional alpha-1-adrenoceptor subtypes at the molecular level using homology-based techniques, although, by definition, additional subtypes may not have been detected if they are sufficiently divergent in sequence.

Alpha-2- and beta-adrenoceptors

In addition to alpha-1-adrenoceptors, the presence of alpha-2- and beta-adrenoceptors have been demonstrated on human prostatic tissue. Radioligand-binding studies clearly demonstrate the presence of alpha-2-adrenoceptors, and autoradiography findings suggest an association with blood vessels and glandular epithelial cells.[31] As noted above, selective alpha-2-agonists fail to contract human prostate smooth muscle in vitro. In addition, alpha-2-antagonists such as rauwolscine inhibit noradrenaline-mediated contractions at concentrations consistent with their affinity for alpha-1- rather than alpha-2-adrenoceptors. These compounds also have no effect on field-stimulated contractions of human prostate at concentrations known to block alpha-2-mediated responses. It is now well established that several alpha-2-adrenoceptor antagonists such as [^{3}H]idazoxan label non-alpha-1, alpha-2, which relate to the imidazoline structure of such compounds and are referred to as non-adrenoceptor imidazoline-binding sites. In human prostate, these distinct imidazoline sites are present at twice the density of alpha-2-receptors, although, as with alpha-2-adrenoceptors, no functional role has been described.

The presence of beta-adrenoceptors on human prostate has been demonstrated on the basis of ligand-binding studies with [^{3}H]dihydroalprenolol by several groups.[41,42] A consistent finding has been that the number of beta-adrenoceptor-binding sites in BPH tissue is markedly lower than in corresponding controls. The functional role of beta-adrenoceptors has been studied by Tsujii and co-workers[41] in relation to these apparent differences in receptor density. Using tonically contracted prostate smooth muscle in vitro, it has been shown that the beta-adrenoceptor agonist isoprenaline caused a much larger relaxant response in control tissue than in hyperplastic prostates. These authors suggested, therefore, that a decrease in the number of beta-adrenoceptors in BPH tissue, associated with a concomitant reduction in beta-adrenoceptor-mediated relaxation might contribute to an increase in dynamic tone of the prostate enveloping the urethra in subjects with clinical BPH.

Effect of alpha-1-adrenoceptor antagonists in vivo

The clinical profile of a number of potent alpha-1-adrenoceptor antagonists clearly shows that these agents are effective in reducing the symptoms of outlet obstruction, as improvements in both urinary flow and subjective symptom scores have been described. The emerging pharmacology associated with prostatic alpha-1-adrenoceptors clearly provides an opportunity for developing drugs with potency and selectivity for prostatic alpha-1-adrenoceptors, while producing fewer of the cardiovascular effects associated with other alpha-1-adrenoceptors. On this basis, therefore, it is desirable to profile the effects of putatively selective agents in vivo, in models allowing the differentiation of prostatic and blood-pressure effects.

There have been several reports of the effects of alpha-1-adrenoceptor antagonists decreasing urethral resistance in animals.[43–47] Indeed, such animal models can be used to determine the potency and selectivity of alpha-1-adrenoceptor antagonists for the prostate over other parameters such as blood pressure. One such anaesthetized dog model for simultaneously assessing the effects of alpha-1-adrenoceptor antagonists on prostate and blood pressure has been described.[43] Phenylephrine can be used to increase both prostatic and blood pressure, and the ability of alpha-1-adrenoceptor antagonists to block each response can be determined. Compounds with greater potency and selectivity for the alpha-1-adrenoceptor subtype on the prostate (putatively alpha-1A) should selectively block phenylephrine-induced rises in prostatic pressure while being less active against phenylephrine-induced increases in blood pressure. As no prostate-selective alpha-1-adrenoceptor antagonists are currently clinically available, the profile of several non-selective alpha-1-adrenoceptor antagonists is shown in comparison with 5-MU, a compound that shows selectivity for the alpha-1A subtype (Fig. 5.3). These data clearly show that compounds that show no subtype selectivity for any of the alpha-1-adrenoceptor subtypes exhibit a balanced profile in vivo towards prostatic and blood pressure. However, compounds such as 5-MU, which show selectivity for the prostatic alpha-1A subtype, preferentially antagonize phenylephrine-induced

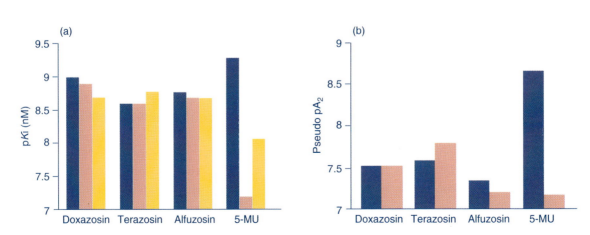

Figure 5.3. (a) Selectivity profile of doxazosin, terazosin, alfuzosin and 5-methylurapidil (5-MU) for the cloned human alpha-1-adrenoceptor subtypes (■, alpha-1A; ■, alpha-1B; ■, alpha-1D). 5-MU is the only compound that shows selectivity for the cloned human alpha-1A-adrenoceptor. (b) Selectivity profile of doxazosin, terazosin, alfuzosin and 5-MU in the anaesthetized dog. All compounds are equi-active on prostate pressure (■) and blood pressure (■), except the alpha-1A-selective compound 5-MU, which is approximately 30-fold prostate selective.

rises in prostate pressure relative to blood pressure. The advantage of this and other similar models (e.g. refs 46 and 47) is that parameters are obtained simultaneously, providing an index of selectivity in the same animal, in which non-selective alpha-1-antagonists show balanced profiles on both parameters. In other studies in which changes in urethral tone are determined in one model in comparison with haemodynamic changes in another, relative selectivity is harder to assess. An exception to this is the effect of compounds on orthostatic blood pressure, which is best determined in 'tilt' or 'lift' models which predict well for the orthostatic effects associated with alpha-1-antagonists.

Thus, it should be possible to target the prostate selectively by optimizing affinity for the prostatic subtype while minimizing affinity at the others. Understanding of alpha-1-adrenoceptors, together with the pharmacology associated with prostatic adrenoceptors, will undoubtedly lead to a new generation of prostate-selective drugs that will be highly beneficial in the medical management of BPH.

References

1. McNeal J E. The zonal anatomy of the prostate. Prostate 1981; 2: 35–49
2. Caine M, Raz S, Ziegler M. Adrenergic and cholinergic receptors in the human prostatic capsule and bladder neck. Br J Urol 1975; 47: 193–202
3. Caine M. The present role of alpha adrenergic blockers in the treatment of benign prostatic hypertrophy. J Urol 1986; 136: 1–4
4. Lepor H, Shapiro E. Characterisation of alpha$_1$ adrenergic receptors in human benign prostatic hyperplasia. J Urol 1984; 132: 1226–1229
5. Shapiro E, Lepor H. Alpha$_2$ adrenergic receptor in hyperplastic human prostate: identification and characterization using [^{3}H] rauwolscine. J Urol 1986; 135: 1038–1043
6. McGrath J C, Brown C M, Wilson V G. Alpha adrenoceptors: a critical review. Med Res Rev 1989; 9: 407–533
7. Bylund D B. Subtypes of α_1 and α_2 adrenergic receptors. FASEB J 1992; 6: 832–840
8. Cotecchia S, Schwinn D S, Randall R et al. Molecular cloning and expression of the cDNA for the hamster alpha$_1$ adrenergic receptor. Proc Natl Acad Sci USA 1988; 85: 7159–7163
9. Ruffolo R R, Nichols A J, Stadel J M, Hieble J P. Structure and function of α-adrenoceptors. Pharmacol Rev 1991; 43: 475–506
10. Lomasney J W, Cotecchia S, Lorenz W et al. Molecular cloning and expression of the cDNA for the α_{1A} adrenergic receptor. J Biol Chem 1991; 266: 6365–6369
11. Perez D M, Piascik M T, Graham R M. Solution-phase library screening for the identification of rare clones: isolation of an α_{1D} adrenergic receptor cDNA. Mol Pharmacol 1991; 40: 876–883
12. Ford A P D W, Williams T J, Blue D R, Clarke D E. α_1 Adrenoceptor classification: sharpening Occam's razor. Trends Pharmacol Sci 1994; 15: 167–170
13. Kenny B A, Chalmers D H, Philpott P C, Naylor A M. Characterization of an α_{1D} adrenoceptor mediating the contractile response of rat aorta to noradrenaline. Br J Pharmacol 1995; 115: 981–986
14. Hieble J P, Bylund D B, Clarke D E et al. Recommendation for nomenclature of α_1 adrenoceptors: consensus update. Pharmacol Rev 1995; 47: 267–270
15. Muramatsu I, Ohmura T, Kigoshi S et al. Pharmacological subclassification of α_1 adrenoceptors in vascular smooth muscle. Br J Pharmacol 1990; 99: 197–201
16. Kitada S, Kumazawa J. Pharmacological characteristics of smooth muscle in benign prostatic hyperplasia and normal prostatic tissue. J Urol 1987; 138: 158–160
17. Hieble J P, Caine M, Zalaznik E. In vitro characterization of the alpha-adrenoceptors in human prostate. Eur J Pharmacol 1985; 107: 111–117
18. Hedlund H, Andersson K E, Larsson B. Alpha adrenoceptors and muscarinic receptors in the isolated human prostate. J Urol 1985; 134: 1291–1298
19. Lepor H, Gup D I, Bavmann M, Shapiro E. Laboratory assessment of terazosin and α_1 blockade in prostatic hyperplasia. Urology 1988; 32: 21–26
20. Shapiro E, Hartanto V, Lepor H. The response to alpha blockade in benign prostatic hyperplasia is related to the percent area density of prostate smooth muscle. Prostate 1992; 21: 297–307
21. Chapple C R, Aubrey M L, James S. Characterization of human prostatic adrenoceptors using pharmacology receptor binding and localisation. Br J Urol 1989; 63: 487–496
22. Smith D J, Chapple C R, Marshall I et al. Human alpha 1C adrenoceptors: functional characterisation in the human prostate. J Urol 1993; 149: 434A
23. Lepor H, Tang R, Shapiro E. The alpha-adrenoceptor mediating the tension of human prostatic smooth muscle. Prostate 1993; 22: 301–307
24. Forray C, Bard J A, Wetzel J M et al. The α_1 adrenoceptor that mediates smooth muscle contraction in human prostate has the pharmacological properties of the cloned human α_{1c} subtype. Mol Pharmacol 1994; 45: 703–708
25. Faure C, Pimoule C, Vallancien G et al. Identification of α_1 adrenoceptor subtypes present in the human prostate. Life Sci 1994; 54: 1595–1605
26. Muramatsu I, Oshita M, Ohmura T et al. Pharmacological characterisation of α_1 adrenoceptor subtypes in the human prostate; functional and binding studies. Br J Urol 1994; 74: 572–578
27. Teng C H, Guh J H, Ko F N. Functional identification of α_1 adrenoceptor subtypes in human prostate: comparison with those in rat vas deferens and spleen. Eru J Pharmacol 1994; 265: 61–66
28. Ford A P D W, Arredondo N F, Blue D R et al. Do α_{1A} (α_{1C})-adrenoceptors (AR) mediate prostatic smooth muscle contraction in man? Studies with a novel, selective α_{1A}-AR antagonist, RS 17053. Br J Pharmacol 1995; 114: 249
29. Chapple C R, Burt R P, Andersson P O et al. Alpha 1 adrenoceptor subtypes in the human prostate. Br J Urol 1994; 74: 585–589
30. Chapple C R, Aubry M L, James S et al. Characterization of human prostatic adrenoceptors using pharmacology receptor binding and localization. Br J Urol 1982; 62: 487–496
31. Kobayashi S, Tang R, Shapiro E, Lepor H. Characterisation and localization of prostatic alpha$_1$ adrenoceptors using radioligand binding on slide-mounted tissue sections. J Urol 1993; 150: 2002–2006
32. Yamada S, Ashizawa N, Ushijima H et al. Alpha-1 adrenoceptors in human prostate: characterizations and alteration in benign prostatic hypertrophy. J Pharmacol Exp Ther 1987; 242: 326–330
33. Kitada S, Kumazawa J. Pharmacological characteristics of smooth muscle in benign prostatic hyperplasia and normal prostatic tissue. J Urol 1987; 138: 158–160

34. Lepor H, Tang R, Meretyk S, Shapiro E. Binding and functional properties of alpha$_1$ adrenoceptors in different regions of the human prostate. J Urol 1993; 150: 252–256

35. Goetz A S, Lutz M W, Rimele T J, Saussy D L. Characterization of alpha-1 adrenoceptor subtypes in human and canine prostate membranes. J Pharmacol Exp Ther 1994; 271: 1228–1233

36. Testa R, Guarneri L, Ibba M et al. Characterization of α_1 adrenoceptor subtypes in prostate and prostatic urethra of rat, rabbit, dog and man. Eur J Pharmacol 1993; 249: 307–315

37. Ohmura T, Sakamoto S, Hayashi H et al. Identification of α_1-adrenoceptor subtypes in the dog prostate. Urol Res 1993; 21: 211–215

38. Muruyama K, Tsuchihashi H, Baba S et al. α_1-Adrenoceptor subtypes in bovine prostate. J Pharm Pharmacol 1992; 44: 727–730

39. Yamada S, Tanaka C, Ohkura T et al. High affinity specific [^{3}H] tamsulosin binding to α_1 adrenoceptors in human prostates with benign prostatic hypertrophy. Urol Res 1994; 22: 272–278

40. Price D T, Schwinn D A, Lomasney J W et al. Identification, quantification and localization of mRNA for three distinct alpha$_1$ adrenergic receptor subtypes in human prostate. J Urol 1993; 149: 324A

41. Tsujii T, Azuma H, Yamaguchi T, Oshima H. A possible role of decreased relaxation mediated by β-adrenoceptors in bladder outlet obstruction by benign prostatic hyperplasia. Br J Pharmacol 1992; 107: 803–807

42. Yokoyama E, Furuya S, Kumamoto E. Quantitation of alpha$_1$ and beta adrenergic receptor densities in the normal and hypertrophied prostate. Jpn J Urol 1985; 76: 525–327

43. Kenny B A, Naylor A M, Carter A J et al. Effect of alpha$_1$ adrenoceptor antagonists on prostatic pressure and blood pressure in the anaesthetised dog. Urology 1994; 44: 52–57

44. Imigawa J, Akima M, Saki K. In vivo experiments for the evaluation of α_1 adrenoceptor antagonistic effects of SGB-1534 on canine urethra. Eur J Pharmacol 1989; 167: 167–172

45. Lefevre-Borg F, O'Connor S E, Schoemaker H et al. Alfuzosin, a selective α_1 adrenoceptor antagonist in the lower urinary tract. Br J Pharmacol 1993; 109: 1282–1289

46. Shibaski M, Sudoh K, Inagaki O et al. Effect of optical isomers of YM-12617 on increased intra-urethral pressure induced by phenylephrine in anaesthetised dogs. J Autonom Pharmacol 1992; 12: 263–268

47. Breslin D, Fields D W, Chou T C et al. Medical management of benign prostatic hyperplasia: a canine model comparing the in vivo efficacy of alpha-1 adrenergic antagonists in the prostate. J Urol 1993; 149: 395–399

6

5 Alpha-reductase in prostate disease
J. D. McConnell

Background

The initiation of benign prostatic hyperplasia (BPH) requires the presence of functional testes during foetal development, puberty and at least a portion of adulthood. Patients castrated before puberty, or who are affected by a variety of inborn errors of metabolism that impair androgen action or production, do not develop BPH. It is also known that intraprostatic levels of dihydrotestosterone (DHT), as well as the androgen receptor, remain high with ageing, despite the fact that peripheral levels of testosterone are decreasing. Moreover, recent evidence demonstrates that androgen ablation by medical or surgical castration leads to programmed death (apoptosis) of benign and malignant prostate epithelial cells.

It was assumed that DHT was only made locally in the normal and neoplastic prostatic epithelial cells by 5 alpha-reductase. Recent studies, however, suggest that intraprostatic DHT is produced exclusively in prostatic stomal and basal cells. Thus, DHT effects on the epithelial cells are likely to be paracrine rather than autocrine in nature. Moreover, presumptive evidence suggests that DHT — made in peripheral tissues, such as the skin and liver — may have a true endocrine effect on the prostate. These studies have significant implications for the role of 5 alpha-reductase inhibitors in the treatment of BPH.

5 Alpha-reductase-isozymes

DHT is synthesized from testosterone by the nuclear membrane-bound enzyme steroid 5 alpha-reductase in target tissues (Fig. 6.1).[1] Growth of the prostate at puberty, as well as benign and neoplastic proliferation of prostatic epithelial and stromal cells in elderly men, require DHT.[2] Molecular cloning studies by David Russell and colleagues have identified two genes that encode the isozymes of 5 alpha-reductase termed type 1 and type 2 (Table 6.1).[1] Mutations in the type 2 gene cause the syndrome of 5 alpha-reductase deficiency in

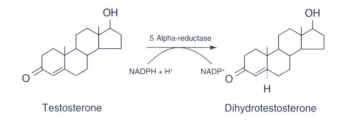

Figure 6.1. *The enzymatic reaction catalysed by steroid 5 alpha-reductase. Other substrates are 20-alpha-hydroxy-preg-4-en-3-one, 17-alpha-hydroxy-progesterone, epitestosterone, progesterone and androstenedione.*

which affected individuals fail to have development of normal external genitalia and prostates.[2] Consistent with these genetic observations, immunoblotting studies indicate that the type 2 isozyme is present in the normal foetal and adult urogenital tract.[3] This isozyme is also found in peripheral tissues, such as the liver and skin, and expression is developmentally regulated.[3] The type 1 isozyme is predominantly expressed in the skin and liver. The 5 alpha-reductase inhibitors tested clinically in patients with BPH — finasteride and episteride — effectively block type 2 isozyme activity, but have little effect on type 1 activity.

Table 6.1. *Characteristics of human 5 alpha-reductase isozymes*

| | Isozyme | |
Characteristic	Type 1	Type 2
Chromosome location	5	2
Prostate abundance	Low	High
pH optimum	Neutral–basic	Acidic
Status in 5-alpha-reductase deficiency	Normal	Mutated
Inhibition by finasteride	Insensitive $(K_i \geq 300 \text{ nM})$	Sensitive $(K_i = 5 \text{ nM})$
Prostate expression (protein)	Absent	Abundant

(From ref. 3 with permission.)

To gain further insight into the role of 5 alpha-reductase and its role in prostate disease, Russell and colleagues have investigated the cell type-specific expression of 5 alpha-reductase by immunohistochemical staining and immunoblot analysis.[4,5]

5 Alpha-reductase expression in the androgen target organs

Immunoblots in which protein extracts from various human adult tissues were incubated with affinity-purified antiserum directed against the 5 alpha-reductase type 2 isozyme demonstrate a protein of molecular weight 23 000 that is specifically detected by the antiserum in the foreskin, prostate, seminal vesicle, epididymis and liver (Fig. 6.2).[4] The recognition of the type 2 isozyme is blocked by preincubating the antiserum with the peptide used for immunization.

Normal prostate

Immunohistochemical staining of formalin-fixed sections of normal prostate demonstrate an intense reaction localized in two cell types.[4] In some specimens, staining was predominantly detected in the basal epithelial cells, while in others the type 2 antigen was detected in stromal and basal epithelial cells. In both cell types the stain was in the perinuclear region. No antigen was detected in the luminal (glandular)

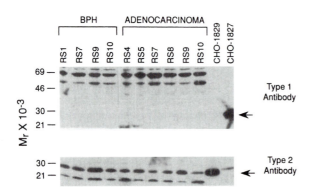

Figure 6.2. *Detection of 5 alpha-reductase type 2 in BPH and prostate cancer is illustrated in the lower panel. The lower band represents non-specific binding. The upper panel demonstrates an absence of detectable type 1 isozyme protein. CHO-1827 and CHO-1829 represent Chinese hamster ovary cells transfected with type 1 and type 2 cDNAs, respectively. (Reproduced from ref. 3 with permission.)*

epithelial cells with type 2 antibody. Kirschenbaum and colleagues have demonstrated significant basal cell staining in ducts closest to the urethra (personal communication). Moreover, using duct antibody techniques, they have suggested that the stromal cells containing 5 alpha-reductase may be fibroblasts rather than smooth muscle cells (personal communication).

Seminal vesicle

Silver et al. determined which cell types express the 5 alpha-reductase type 2 isozyme in seminal vesicles.[4] The results indicate that the isozyme is present in a perinuclear distribution in the stromal cells of this tissue. Staining appeared to be more intense in stroma adjacent to the epithelial cells.

Epididymis

In contrast to the results obtained in the seminal vesicle, immunohistochemical analysis of epididymal sections demonstrates expression of the type 2 isozyme predominantly in the epithelial cells lining the tubules. Intracellular localization is unclear, given the resolution of the images.

Benign prostatic hyperplasia

BPH specimens stained with an affinity-purified immune antiserum recognizing the 5 alpha-reductase type 2 isozyme demonstrate an intense staining pattern in the stromal cells (Fig. 6.3).[5] Positive cells are localized throughout BPH nodules. At higher power, the subcellular staining appears to be largely perinuclear and predominantly localized within the stromal cells rather than the basal epithelial cells. Within some sections, the stromal cells of adjacent normal tissue appear to exhibit less intense staining than those in BPH nodules. Once again, it remains unclear whether the stromal type 2 isozyme is in smooth muscle or fibroblasts. This is further complicated by the similarity between the biochemical phenotype of these two stromal cell populations when the muscle cells are actually proliferating.

Prostate cancer

Silver et al. examined the cell type-specific expression pattern of the type 2 isozyme in prostate intraepithelial neoplasia (PIN) and prostate cancers.[5] Staining of high-grade PIN revealed the type 2 isozyme in stromal cells

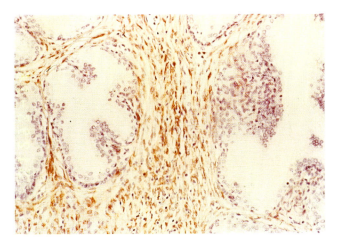

Figure 6.3. *Immunohistochemical demonstration of type 2 5 alpha-reductase in stroma adjacent to a BPH nodule.*

separating the proliferating epithelium, but no staining in the PIN epithelial cells. A stromal-specific staining pattern was also detected in prostatic cancers. No type 2 isozyme staining was detected in a lymph node containing a metastatic tumour.[5]

Androgen regulation of 5 alpha-reductase

The androgen regulation of the 5 alpha-reductase type 2 isozyme expression has been studied in the epididymis and prostate tissue from men on androgen ablation therapies.[5] Three different androgen ablation therapies (leuprolide, diethylstilboestrol and flutamide) each abolish expression of the type 2 isozyme in the epididymis. Substantially different results are obtained in the prostate. A combination androgen ablation therapy for prostate cancer, consisting of leuprolide and flutamide administration for either 10 weeks or 3 months, did not abolish expression of the type 2 isozyme.[5] Six months after orchiectomy for prostate cancer, the expression of 5 alpha-reductase persists, but at a decreased level. In men with BPH on finasteride, expression does not change relative to untreated tissue. When these same prostate samples are subjected to immunoblotting using an affinity-purified antiserum that recognizes the type 1 isozyme,[3] no expression of this isozyme is detected.[5]

To examine the cell type-specific expression pattern of the type 2 isozyme in a finasteride-treated individual with prostate cancer, immunohistochemistry was performed on a section from a prostate needle biopsy. As

in the normal prostate, the type 2 isozyme was predominantly detected in the stromal cells of the gland.[5] The type 1 isozyme could not be detected by immunohistochemical staining of this sample.

New concepts of androgen action

The stromal cell has a central role in androgen-dependent prostatic growth and suggests a new paracrine model for androgen action in the gland (Fig. 6.4). Moreover, it is likely that circulating DHT — produced in the skin and liver — may act on prostate cells in a true endocrine fashion.

Expression of 5 alpha-reductase in the prostate is detected in basal epithelial cells and stromal cells. Russell's group has, at the time of writing, not been able to demonstrate expression of the type 1 protein or enzyme activity in the human prostate.[3–5] Thus, it would appear that a majority of intraprostatic DHT synthesis is accomplished by the type 2 isozyme in these two cell types of the human prostate (Fig. 6.4). Once synthesized, the hormone acts in a paracrine fashion on the androgen-dependent luminal epithelium, where the androgen receptor is present in the nuclei of luminal epithelial cells.[6,7] This enzymatic step in the prostate is presumably interrupted by treatment with 5 alpha-reductase inhibitors, such as finasteride.[8] In addition, DHT produced in the skin and liver (type 1 and type 2 5 alpha-reductase-derived) could act in a true endocrine fashion on prostatic cells (Fig. 6.4).

It seems likely that the cell type-specific expression pattern varies within the gland, possibly reflecting the growth rate of different regions or a more specialized anatomical hierarchy (for example differential expression in the peripheral versus transition zone). The asymmetric nodular hyperplasia noted in the prostates of many patients may be explained by such local variation in 5 alpha-reductase expression. The basal cell type 2 isozyme expression is interesting, given the close association between this population of cells and neuroendocrine cells.

In contrast to the situation in the human prostate, both 5 alpha-reductase isozymes are expressed in the rat ventral prostate.[9] In the rat gland, basal epithelial cells express the type 1 isozyme and stromal cells express the type 2 isozyme.[10] Human prostate sections do not stain

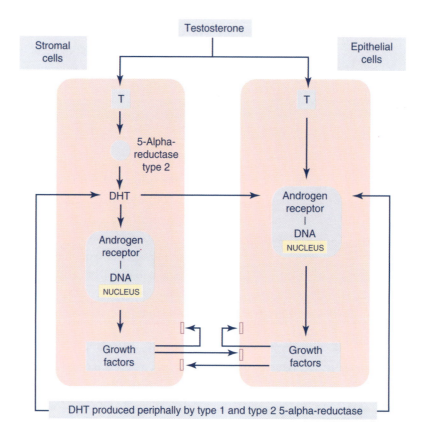

Figure 6.4. *Androgen action in the prostate gland. Testosterone (T) diffuses into the prostate epithelial and stromal cells. T can interact directly with the androgen (steroid) receptors bound to the promoter region of androgen-regulated genes. In the stromal cells a majority of T is converted into dihydrotestosterone (DHT) — a much more potent androgen —that can act in an autocrine fashion in the stromal cells, or in a paracrine fashion by diffusing into epithelial cells in close proximity. DHT produced peripherally, primarily in the skin and liver, can diffuse into the prostate from the circulation and act in a true endocrine fashion. In some cases, the basal cells in the prostate may serve as a DHT production site, similar to the stromal cells. Autocrine and paracrine growth factors may also be involved in androgen-dependent processes within the prostate.*

positively when probed with a type 1-specific antibody. Thus, expression of the type 2 isozyme in human basal epithelial cells may serve the same physiological function in these cells as the type 1 isozyme of the prostate.

Stromal cells of the seminal vesicle have been found to express the 5 alpha-reductase type 2 isozyme. However, expression in the epididymis was in the epithelial cells. This suggests that the cell type-specific expression patterns of the type 2 isozyme are independent of the embryonic origin of the tissue, since the prostate and seminal vesicle/epididymis arise from different anlagen (urogenital sinus and wolffian ducts, respectively).[3] In the embryo, 5 alpha-reductase enzyme activity is detected in the urogenital sinus several weeks

before that in the wolffian duct deviates,[2] suggesting that expression in the two structures is regulated by different mechanisms. Given this temporal pattern of expression and the findings reported regarding the role of androgens in expression of 5 alpha-reductase in the epididymis,[5] it is possible that the synthesis of DHT by the urogenital sinus brings about the expression of 5 alpha-reductase in tissues derived from the wolffian duct.

Silver et al. demonstrated that the stromal cells of the prostate express the type 2 isozyme of 5 alpha-reductase in BPH and prostate cancer specimens.[5] In some sections, the number of cells expressing the isozyme appears to increase in BPH to the point that almost every stromal cell in a nodule stains positively for the isozyme (Fig. 6.3). Androgen ablation leads to a dramatic decrease in 5 alpha-reductase type 2 expression in the epididymis, but has little effect on expression in the prostate. Short-term finasteride treatment has little effect on the steady-state levels of isozyme in the prostate, whereas long-term treatment appears to decrease expression slightly.

The development of BPH requires the action of DHT synthesized by 5 alpha-reductase.[13] Stromal cells appear to be the predominant cell type expressing the type 2 isozyme in BPH. Indeed, there may be more expression in BPH nodules than in adjacent normal tissue. These observations stem from qualitative immunohistochemical analyses of a limited number of samples and it cannot be stated with certainty whether the overall expression of 5 alpha-reductase type 2 is higher in BPH than in normal tissue. However, several studies have previously shown that 5 alpha-reductase enzyme activity is higher in BPH than in the normal prostate.[14–16] The differences in the relative staining intensity of immunohistochemically positive cells between the normal and BPH specimens may prove useful in diagnostic assays to assess the status of benign stromal cell growth in the gland, or possibly to predict response to 5 alpha-reductase inhibition therapy.

Although prostatic adenocarcinoma, like BPH, is characterized by a proliferation of epithelial cells,[17] the role of 5 alpha-reductase in the process of malignant growth is uncertain. In cancer specimens, the expression of the type 2 isozyme is confined to the stromal cells of the tumour. The absence of the type 2 isozyme in the tumour epithelium is supported by the failure to detect this protein in metastatic tumour deposits.[5] The presence of the type 2 isozyme in tumoral stroma, when considered with the androgen dependence of early-stage prostate cancer,[17] suggests that inhibitors of 5 alpha-reductase may be useful as a chemopreventative for some prostate tumours. In contrast, the absence of type 2 expression in the tumoral epithelium suggests that the addition of a 5 alpha-reductase inhibitor to a total androgen ablation treatment strategy in advanced tumours is unlikely to produce benefit, as indicated in a previous study.[18]

Numerous investigators have demonstrated the expression of the androgen receptor, the recipient of the DHT signal produced by 5 alpha-reductase, in BPH and prostate cancer.[19–23] In general, androgen receptor expression predominates in the luminal epithelium; however, it is not yet clear whether this expression correlates with any clinical parameters.[19–23] The knowledge that androgen receptor expression occurs in luminal epithelial cells, and the finding that 5 alpha-reductase type 2 expression occurs predominantly in stromal cells, suggest that DHT is acting as a paracrine hormone to drive cell growth in prostate disease. The endocrine contribution of circulating DHT in BPH and prostate cancer is less certain.

The addition of a 5 alpha-reductase inhibitor to a programme of luteinizing hormone-releasing hormone (LHRH) and flutamide for advanced prostate cancer — as suggested by Labrie et al.[25] —is unlikely to achieve further therapeutic benefit, since 5 alpha-reductase can not be measured in cancer cells. However, the finasteride Prostate Cancer Prevention Trial recently begun by the National Cancer Institute may have a biological rationale, given the distribution of the type 2 isozyme in stromal cells in close proximity to intraprostatic tumours and PIN. If finasteride proves of chemopreventative benefit in this trial, then current data suggest that the drug would do so by inhibiting 5 alpha-reductase enzyme activity in the stroma rather than in the tumorigenic epithelium. In this context, it is interesting to note that recent evidence suggests that DHT synthesized by the type 1 isozyme in the liver and skin can act as a true endocrine (circulating) hormone, and may thus contribute to androgen-dependent growth of the prostate.[3] Thus, a more effective 5 alpha-reductase-inhibitor therapy for BPH and prostate cancer prevention may require blockade of both intraprostatic 5 alpha-reductase type 2 and peripheral 5 alpha-reductase type 1.

References

1. Russell D W, Wilson J D. Steroid 5α-reductase: two genes/two enzymes. Rev Biochem 1994; 63: 25

2. Wilson J D, Griffin J E, Russell D W. Steroid 5α-reductase 2 deficiency. Endocr Rev 1993; 14: 577

3. Thigpen A E, Silver R I, Guileyardo J M et al. Tissue distribution and ontogeny of steroid 5α-reductase isozyme expression. J Clin Invest 1993; 92: 903

4. Silver R I, Wiley E L, Thigpen A E et al. Cell type specific expression of steroid 5α-reductase 2. J Urol 1994; 152: 438

5. Silver R I, Wiley E L, Davis D L et al. Expression and regulation of steroid 5α-reductase 2 in prostate disease. J Urol 1994; 152: 433

6. Lubahn D B, Joseph D R, Sar M et al. The human androgen receptor: complementary deoxyribonucleic acid cloning, sequence

analysis and gene expression in prostate. Mol Endocrinol 1988; 2: 1265

7. Liao S S, Kokontis J, Sai T, Hiipakka R A. Androgen receptors: structures, mutations, antibodies and cellular dynamics. J Steroid Biochem 1989; 34: 41

8. Gormley G J, Stoner E, Bruskewitz R C et al. The effect of finasteride in men with benign prostatic hyperplasia. N Engl J Med 1992; 327: 1185

9. Normington K, Russell D W. Tissue distribution and kinetic characteristics of rat steroid 5α-reductase isozymes. Evidence for distinct physiological functions. J Biol Chem 1992; 267: 19548

10. Berman D M, Russell D W. Cell type specific expression of rat steroid 5α-reductase isozymes. Proc Natl Acad Sci USA 1993; 90: 9359

11. Choudry R, Hodgins M B, van der Kwast T H et al. Localisation of androgen receptors in human skin by immunohistochemistry: implications for the hormonal regulator of hair growth sebaceous glands and sweat glands. J Endocrinol 1992; 133: 467

12. Liang T, Hoyer S, Yu R et al. Immunocytochemical localizations of androgen receptors in human skin using monoclonal antibodies against the androgen receptor. J Invest Dermatol 1993; 100: 663

13. Walsh P C. Benign prostatic hyperplasia. In: Walsh P C, Retik A B, Stamey T E, Vaughn E D Jr (eds) Campbell's Urology, 6th ed. Philadelphia: Saunders, 1992: 1009–1027

14. Bruchovsky N, Rennie P S, Batzoid F H et al. Kinetic parameters of 5α-reductase activity in stroma and epithelium of normal, hyperplastic, and carcinomatous human prostates. J Clin Endocrinol Metab 1988; 67: 806

15. Hudson R W, Wherrett D. Comparison of the nuclear 5α-reduction of testosterone and androstenedione in human prostatic carcinoma and benign prostatic hyperplasia. J Steroid Biochem 1990; 35: 231

16. Brendler C B, Follansbee A L, Isaacs J T. Discrimination between normal, hyperplastic and malignant human prostatic tissues by enzymatic profiles. J Urol 1985; 133: 495

17. Stamey T A, McNeal J E. Adenocarcinoma of the prostate. In: Walsh P C, Retik A B, Stamey T A, Vaughn E D Jr (eds) Campbell's Urology, 6th ed. Philadelphia: Saunders, 1992: 1159–1220

18. Presti J C Jr, Fair W R, Andriole G et al. Multicenter, randomized, double-blind, placebo controlled study to investigate the effect of finasteride (MK-906) on stage D prostate cancer. J Urol 1992; 148: 1201

19. Ruizeveld de Winter J A, Trapman J, Brinkmann A O et al. Androgen receptor heterogeneity in human prostatic carcinomas visualized by immunohistochemistry. J Pathol 1990; 160: 329

20. Masai M, Sumiya H, Akimoto S et al. Immunohistochemical study of androgen receptor in benign hyperplastic and cancerous human prostates. Prostate 1990; 17: 293

21. Sadi M V, Walsh P C, Barrack E R. Immunohistochemical study of androgen receptors in metastatic prostate cancer. Comparison of receptor content and response to hormonal therapy. Cancer 1991; 67: 3057

22. van der Kwast T H, Schalken J, Ruizeveld de Winter J A et al. Androgen receptors in endocrine-therapy-resistant human prostate cancer. Int J Cancer 1991; 48: 189

23. Miyamoto K K, McSherry S A, Dent G A et al. Immunohistochemistry of the androgen receptor in human benign and malignant prostate tissue. J Urol 1993; 149: 1015

24. George F W, Russell D W, Wilson J D. Fee-forward control of prostate growth: dihydrotestosterone induces expression of its own biosynthetic enzyme, steroid 5α-reductase. Proc Natl Acad Soc USA 1991; 88: 8044

25. Labrie F, Belanger A, Duport A et al. Science behind total androgen blockade: from gene to combination therapy. Clin Invest Med 1993; 16: 475–492

7

Pathology of benign prostatic hyperplasia

D. G. Bostwick

Introduction

Benign enlargement of the prostate [benign prostatic hyperplasia (BPH), nodular hyperplasia or adenofibromyomatous hyperplasia (AFH)] consists of overgrowth of the epithelium and fibromuscular tissue of the transition zone and periurethral area. Lower urinary tract symptoms are caused by interference with muscular sphincteric function and obstruction of urine flow through the prostatic urethra. There is a positive but weak correlation between the amount of hyperplastic tissue and clinical symptoms.

This chapter describes the pathological spectrum of BPH, including usual epithelial and stromal hyperplasia and the numerous variants and other benign proliferative lesions.

Usual epithelial and stromal hyperplasia in BPH

At puberty, rising serum testosterone concentration results in a rapid increase in prostatic growth; with the prostate doubling in size about every 3 years.[1] The normal adult prostate contains about 50% stroma, 30% acinar lumens and 20% epithelium, according to morphometric studies. Between the ages of 31 and 50 years, hyperplastic tissue grows exponentially, with a doubling time of 4.5 years.[2] From 55 to 70 years, the doubling time for BPH is 10 years, decreasing to more than 100 years in men older than 70 years. The proliferative rate of the epithelium and stroma of BPH is much higher than that of the normal prostate (nine and 37 times higher, respectively).[3]

Pathogenesis of BPH

The prevalence of histological BPH increases rapidly, beginning in the fourth decade of life, culminating in nearly 100% prevalence in the ninth decade. The age-specific prevalence is remarkably similar in populations throughout the world (Fig. 7.1).[4] Epidemiological studies have shown that the risk of undergoing

prostatectomy for BPH is fourfold greater in first-degree relatives of young men with BPH than in controls.[5] The concordance rate for BPH among identical (monozygotic) twins is greater than among non-identical twins (dizygotic), suggesting a hereditary influence in BPH.[6]

Development of BPH includes three pathological stages — nodule formation, diffuse enlargement of the transition zone and periurethral tissue, and enlargement of nodules.[7–9] In men under 70 years of age, diffuse enlargement predominates; in older men, epithelial proliferation and expansile growth of existing nodules predominates, probably as the result of androgenic and other hormonal stimulation.

The pathogenesis of BPH is uncertain, but multiple overlapping theories have been proposed, all of which may be operative.[10] Essential to all are advancing age and the presence of circulating androgens. Regression of BPH can be reversibly induced by luteinizing hormone-releasing hormone (LHRH) agonists, indicating that androgens have at least an important supportive role in BPH.[11]

Ageing theory of pathogenesis

As men age, there is an increase in cumulative lipid peroxidation, resulting in an increase in tissue

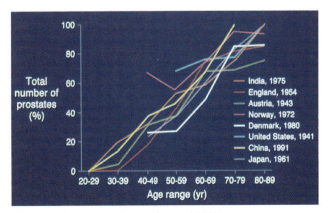

Figure 7.1. *Age-specific prevalence of BPH in autopsy specimens from human prostates according to country. (From ref. 4 with permission.)*

concentration of cofactors such as NAD and NADPH. This, in turn, increases 5 alpha-reductase concentration (sensitive to changes in NADPH) and prostatic dihydrotestosterone (DHT) concentration, ultimately inducing epithelial and stromal growth, which culminates in BPH. This theory is supported by the consistent observation of high DHT concentration in patients with BPH.[10]

Oestrogen theory of pathogenesis

The ratio of plasma oestrogen to testosterone increases with age, and this may result in stromal overgrowth because of the greater amount of hormone receptors in the stroma compared with the epithelium. This theory explains why BPH is chiefly a stromal disease. Attempts to correlate the amount of BPH with serum hormone concentrations have yielded conflicting results,[12] although testosterone and oestrogen are clearly influential.

Embryonic reawakening theory of pathogenesis

McNeal[8,9] suggested that the earliest lesion of BPH is a proliferation of epithelium, probably under the influence of DHT, with branching and budding due to 'reawakening' of the embryonic inductive potential of the prostatic stoma during adulthood. This theory accounts for the presence of the common fibroadenomatous nodules of BPH.

Oxidoreductase theory of pathogenesis

Abnormal activity of certain enzymes may cause BPH by promoting the retention of tissue DHT, resulting in higher DHT levels. Isaacs et al. found significantly lower concentrations of two enzymes that remove DHT from tissue (17-beta-hydroxysteroid and 3-alpha-hydroxysteroid reductase) in BPH patients than in controls.[1]

Inflammation/growth factor theory of pathogenesis

Inflammation and the release of growth factors such as platelet-derived growth factor (PDGF) may play a part in the development of BPH;[13] Steiner et al.[14] found that the number of T cells in BPH is greater than that in the normal prostate, and these T cells are preactivated and functionally capable of producing sufficient amounts of autocrine growth factors necessary for T-cell

proliferation. Conversely, Helpap showed that there is no significant correlation between the amount of chronic inflammation and the extent of BPH.[15]

Pathology of BPH

Grossly, BPH consists of variably sized nodules that are soft or firm, rubbery and yellow-grey, and bulge from the cut surface upon transection (Fig. 7.2). If there is prominent epithelial hyperplasia in addition to stromal hyperplasia, the abundant luminal spaces create soft and grossly spongy nodules which ooze a pale-white watery fluid. If BPH is predominantly fibromuscular, there may be diffuse enlargement or numerous trabeculations without prominent nodularity. Degenerative changes include calcification and infarction. BPH usually involves the transition zone, but occasionally nodules arise from the periurethral tissue at the bladder neck. Protrusion of bladder neck nodules into the bladder lumen is referred to as median lobe hyperplasia (Fig. 7.2). Rarely, hyperplastic nodules are present in the peripheral zone.

Microscopically, BPH is invariably nodular, composed of varying proportions of epithelium, fibrous connective tissue and smooth muscle. There are five types of nodules, including adenomyofibromatous (most common), fibromuscular, muscular (uncommon), fibroadenomatous and stromal (Fig. 7.3). In practice, pathologists do not subclassify BPH histologically because of the wide variation in composition. Common associated findings include chronic inflammation, acinar atrophy and luminal corpora amylacea and microcalculi.

The diagnosis of BPH is often used by pathologists in reporting the findings in needle biopsy specimens when only normal benign peripheral zone tissue is present. The transition zone is infrequently sampled by needle biopsy unless the urologist specifically targets this area or there is massive BPH that compresses the peripheral zone. The presence of at least part of a nodule is required for the diagnosis of BPH. Narrow 18-gauge biopsies virtually never contain the entire nodule unless it is very small and fortuitously sampled. Casual use of the term BPH for benign prostatic tissue may mislead the urologist into believing that a palpable nodule or hypoechoic focus of concern has been sampled and histologically evaluated; it is important for the

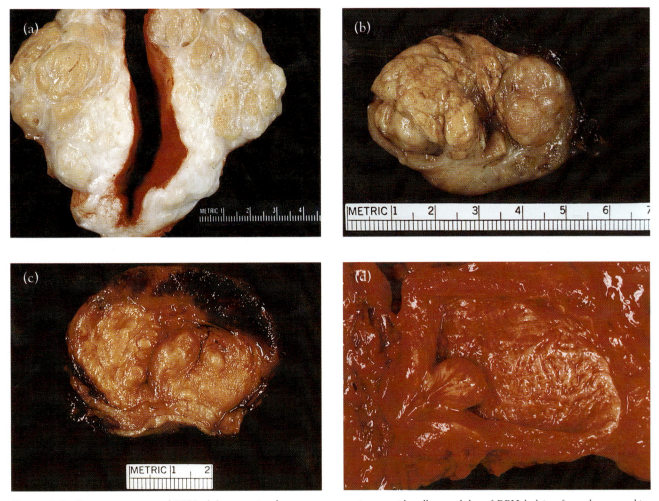

Figure 7.2. *Gross appearance of BPH: (a) prostatic adenomectomy specimen, with yellow nodules of BPH bulging from the grey-white fibromuscular stroma; (b) the rubbery nodules have replaced and expanded the transition zone, distorting and compressing the urethral lumen and adjacent prostate; the peripheral zone is compressed at the bottom, and contains foci of adenocarcinoma which are subtle and appear pale yellow; (c) BPH and a large infarct; (d) a BPH nodule protrudes into the bladder lumen, acting as a ball valve with intermittent urinary obstruction.*

pathologist to correlate the light-microscopic findings with the clinical impression, so communication with the urologist is vital.

Vascular insufficiency probably accounts for infarction of BPH nodules, seen in up to 20% of resected cases (Fig. 7.3). The centre of the nodule undergoes haemorrhagic necrosis, often with reactive changes in the residual epithelium at the periphery, including squamous metaplasia and transitional cell metaplasia.

Peripheral zone BPH

BPH sometimes protrudes from the transition zone into the peripheral zone, creating a palpable abnormality that may be clinically or radiographically mistaken for adenocarcinoma.[16–18] Rarely, fibroadenomatous nodules may originate in the peripheral zone that are spatially distinct from the transition zone.[19] These nodules are present in about 2% of radical prostatectomies with cancer, and are of unknown aetiology. Possible explanations include embryonic reawakening, similar to that proposed for transition zone BPH, parasitic nodules from the transition zone extending into the peripheral zone, and implantation of transition zone tissue in the peripheral zone during embryogenesis. There is no apparent relationship between peripheral zone BPH nodules and cancer.

Giant BPH (giant prostatic hyperplasia)

Prostatic enlargement due to BPH rarely exceeds 100 g, and does so in only 4% of men over 70 years of age[2] (Fig. 7.3). Giant BPH is arbitrarily defined as specimens over 200 g[20] or 500 g;[21] the lower threshold was suggested by Japanese authors,[20] probably because BPH is rare in their country. The largest adenoma ever removed by suprapubic prostatectomy weighed 820 g, but the patient died of haemorrhage.[22] Giant BPH tends to have the typical adenomyofibromatous pattern.

Morphometry of BPH: ratio of epithelium to stroma

Numerous techniques have been used to study the ratio of epithelium to stroma in BPH, including light microscopy,[23] computer-assisted digital image analysis,[24,25] stereological analysis[26] and texture analysis.[27] The relative proportions of epithelium and stroma are 21.6–40% and 60–78%, respectively.

The clinical importance of the ratio of epithelium and stroma is that men with symptomatic BPH have a significantly higher proportion of stroma than men with asymptomatic BPH.[24] It is likely that the predominant component of the BPH nodule determines the response to therapy: smooth muscle-predominant nodules would respond to alpha-blockers, epithelial nodules to androgen-deprivation therapy (LHRH agonists, steroid anti-androgens and 5 alpha-reductase inhibitors), and fibrous nodules to surgery.

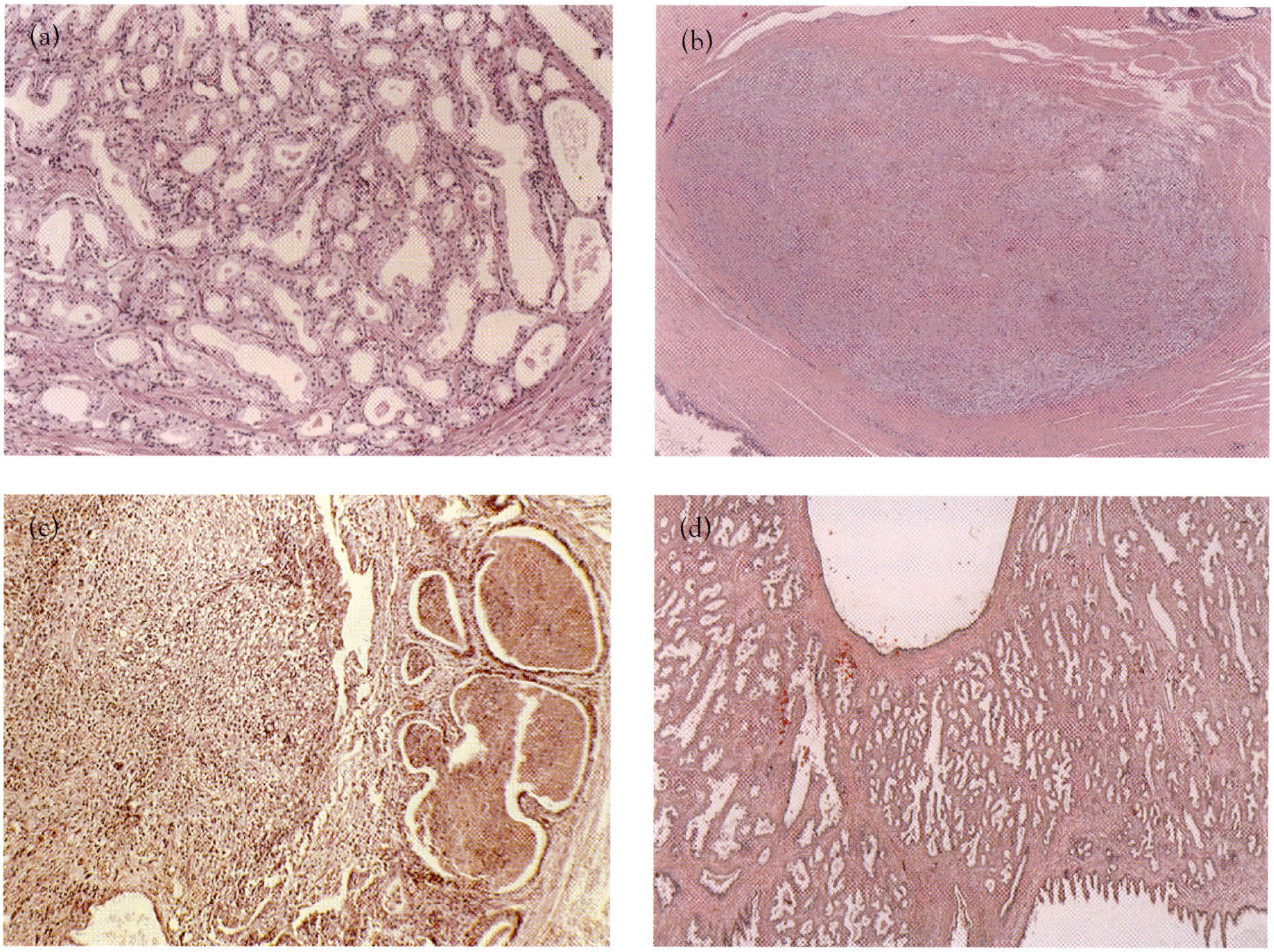

Figure 7.3. *Microscopic appearance of BPH: (a) fibroadenomatous pattern of BPH, showing a circumscribed elongate nodule of glands and fibrous stroma; (b) pure stomal nodule of BPH; (c) edge of BPH nodule with infarct; note the presence of acute inflammation (left) and dilated glands with necrotic debris (right); (d) section from giant BPH from a 16-year-old boy who underwent suprapubic prostatectomy for massive enlargement of the prostate.*

Association of BPH and prostate cancer

There are a number of similarities between BPH and cancer[4] (Table 7.1). Both display a parallel increase in prevalence with patient age, according to autopsy studies, although cancer lags by 15–20 years. Both require androgens for growth and development, and both may respond to androgen-deprivation treatment. Most cancers arise in prostates with concomitant BPH, and cancer is found incidentally in a significant number (10%) of transurethral prostatectomy specimens. BPH may be related to prostate cancer arising in the transition zone, perhaps in association with certain forms of hyperplasia, but BPH is not a premalignant lesion nor a precursor of carcinoma.

The optimal number of chips to submit for histological evaluation from a transurethral resection of the prostate (TURP) specimen remains controversial, with some authors preferring partial sampling and others advocating complete submission, even with large specimens that would require many cassettes.[28–31] The Cancer Committee of the College of American Pathologists recommends a minimum of six cassettes for the first 30 g tissue and one cassette for every 10 g thereafter.[32]

Histological variants of hyperplasia and associated benign lesions

There is a wide morphological spectrum of epithelial and stromal hyperplasia (see Figs 7.4–7.11). Awareness of these variants is important to avoid misinterpretation as adenocarcinoma (Table 7.2).

Table 7.1. *Prostatic carcinoma: comparison based on anatomical site of origin**

Characteristic	Transition zone cancer	Peripheral zone cancer
Incidence		
Stage T/a	75%	–
Stage T/b	79%	–
All stage T1	78%	–
All stages	24%	70%
Origin		
In or near BPH	Yes	No
Near apex	Yes	Yes
Detection rate by TURP	78%	–
Pathological features		
Tumour volume	Usually small	Small to large
Tumour pattern	Alveolar–medullary	Tubular–scirrhous
Tumour grade (Gleason)	Usually 1 or 2	Usually 2, 3 or 4
Clear cell pattern	Most cases	Rare
Stromal fibrosis	Uncommon	Common
Associated putative premalignant changes	AAH or PIN[†]	PIN
Aneuploidy[‡]	6%	31%
Clinical behaviour		
Extracapsular extension[‡]	11%	44%
Site of extracapsular extension	Anterolateral and apical	Lateral
Average tumour size with extracapsular extension[‡]	4.98 cm^3	3.86 cm^3
Risk of seminal vesicle invasion[‡]	0%	19%
Risk of lymph node metastases	Low	High

*Central zone cancers (5–10% of total) were excluded. [†]Atypical adenomatous hyperplaia or prostatic intraepithelial neoplasia. [‡]Data from ref. 65 for stage T1 and T2 cancers.

Table 7.2. *Histopathological variants of BPH*

Variant	Microscopic features	Usual location
Postatrophic hyperplasia	Atrophic acini with epithelial proliferative changes. Easily mistaken for adenocarcinoma owing to architectural distortion	All zones
Stromal hyperplasia with atypical giant cells	Stromal nodules in the setting of BPH with increased cellularity and nuclear atypia	Transition zone
Basal cell hyperplasia	Proliferation of basal cells, two or more cells in thickness; may have prominent nucleoli (atypical basal cell hyperplasia) or form a nodule (basal cell adenoma)	Transition zone
Cribriform hyperplasia	Acini with distinctive cribriform pattern, often with clear cytoplasm. Easily mistaken for proliferative acini of the central zone	Transition zone
Atypical adenomatous hyperplasia	Localized proliferation of small acini in association with BPH nodule which architecturally mimics adenocarcinoma but lacks cytological features of malignancy	Transition zone
Sclerosing adenosis	Circumscribed proliferation of small acini in a dense spindle-cell stroma without significant cytological atypia. Usually solitary and microscopic	Transition zone
Verumontanum mucosal gland hyperplasia	Small benign acinar proliferation involving the verumontanum	Verumontanum
Hyperplasia of mesonephric remnants	Rare benign lobular proliferation of small acini with colloid-like material in the lumens. May mimic nephrogenic metaplasia focally. Acini do not apparently express PSA or PAP	All zones (very rare)

Atrophy and postatrophic hyperplasia (postinflammatory hyperplasia; partial atrophy; post-sclerotic hyperplasia)

Atrophy is a common microscopic finding, consisting of small distorted glands with flattened epithelium, hyperchromatic nuclei and stromal fibrosis. It is usually idiopathic and the prevalence increases with advancing age. At low magnification, atrophy may be confused with adenocarcinoma owing to the prominent acinar architectural distortion. At high magnification, atrophy usually lacks nuclear and nucleolar enlargement, except in cases of postatrophic hyperplasia (PAH).

Clusters of atrophic prostatic acini that display proliferative epithelial changes are referred to as PAH.[33,34] PAH is at the extreme end of the morphological continuum of acinar atrophy that most closely mimics adenocarcinoma. This continuum varies from mild acinar irregularity with a flattened layer of attenuated cells with scant cytoplasm to that of PAH, in which the lining cells are low cuboidal with moderate cytoplasm. There is no sharp division in this continuum between atrophy and PAH, challenging the utility of PAH as a distinct entity. However, the morphological mimicry of PAH and carcinoma creates the potential for misdiagnosis, sometimes resulting in unnecessary prostatectomy.[34] To avoid this potentially tragic misinterpretation, the pathologist should have an understanding of this extreme morphological variant of atrophy. In the author's opinion, PAH is a diagnostic category for atrophic acini that most closely mimic adenocarcinoma, recognizing that this is merely a descriptive term.

PAH consists of a microscopic lobular cluster of five to 15 small acini with distorted contours reminiscent of atrophy (Fig. 7.4). One or more larger dilated acini are usually present within these small round to oval clusters, and the small acini appear to bud off the dilated acinus, imparting a lobular appearance to the lesion. The small acini are lined by a layer of cuboidal secretory cells with mildly enlarged nuclei with an increased nucleus-to-cytoplasmic ratio when compared with adjacent benign epithelial cells. The nuclei contain finely granular chromatin, and nucleoli are usually small, although mildly enlarged nucleoli are focally present in 39% of cases. The cytoplasm is often basophilic or finely granular to clear, and luminal apocrine-like blebs are present in 33% of cases. Luminal mucin is occasionally present in PAH. Corpora amylacea are present in 75% of cases of PAH but crystalloids are rarely, if ever, seen.

The basal cell layer is usually present in PAH but is often inconspicuous by routine light microscopy. Basal cell hyperplasia is rarely seen in foci of PAH. Immunohistochemical stains for high-molecular-weight keratin (antibody 34βE12) reveal a focally fragmented basal cell layer in some cases. Adjacent prostatic acini always show at least focal atrophy.

Stromal changes are always present in PAH, ranging from smooth muscle atrophy to dense sclerosis with compression of acini. In cases with sclerosis, the acinar lumens are compressed and showed marked distortion. Subtyping of PAH into the lobular and post-sclerotic subtypes is useful only to allow recognition of PAH and distinguish it from mimics such as low-grade adenocarcinoma; it is preferable not to subtype PAH. In addition, PAH is often associated with patchy chronic inflammation; infrequently, dilated acini contain luminal neutrophils.

PAH is distinguished from carcinoma by its characteristic lobular architecture, intact or fragmented basal cell layer, inconspicuous or mildly enlarged nucleoli, and adjacent acinar atrophy with stromal fibrosis or smooth muscle atrophy. Low-grade adenocarcinoma is the most important differential diagnostic consideration with PAH. PAH usually has a lobular pattern on low power, similar to Gleason pattern 2 and 3 adenocarcinoma. However, the lobular pattern is less distinct in cases with abundant stromal sclerosis, and there may be a pseudoinfiltrative growth pattern with fibrous entrapment of acini. Nucleolar changes are also useful in separating PAH and carcinoma, although some cases of low-grade carcinoma have only patchy large nucleoli or even micronucleoli. Mildly enlarged nucleoli may be present in PAH, but only focally, and the majority of cells have micronucleoli. The separation of PAH from carcinoma is most difficult in needle biopsy specimens in which only a portion of the lesion is sampled, and awareness of this entity assists in this distinction. In about half of the biopsies containing PAH, the lesion extends to the edge of the tissue core, indicating incomplete sampling.

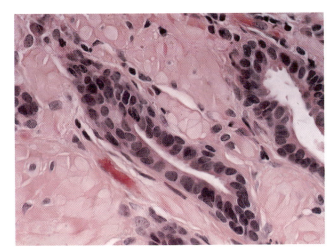

Figure 7.4. *Postatrophic hyperplasia; these distorted glands are embedded in sclerotic stroma in an area of atrophy.*

Stromal hyperplasia with atypical giant cells

Stromal hyperplasia with atypia consists of stromal nodules in the setting of BPH with increased cellularity and nuclear atypia (Fig. 7.5).[35,36] These may appear as solid stromal nodules (often referred to as atypical leiomyoma) or with atypical cells interspersed with benign glands. Stromal nuclei are large, hyperchromatic and rarely multinucleated or vacuolated, with inconspicuous nucleoli. There are no mitotic figures and

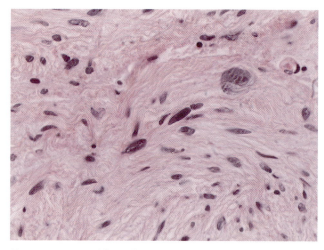

Figure 7.5. *Stromal hyperplasia with atypical giant cells.*

no necrosis. Stromal hyperplasia with atypia has no malignant potential, and the atypical cells are considered degenerative.

Basal cell hyperplasia and basal cell proliferations

There are three patterns of benign basal cell hyperplasia —typical basal cell hyperplasia (Fig. 7.6), atypical basal cell hyperplasia (Fig. 7.7) and basal cell adenoma (Fig. 7.8).[37,38]

Basal cell hyperplasia

Basal cell hyperplasia consists of a proliferation of basal cells, two or more cells in thickness, at the periphery of prostatic acini (Fig. 7.6).[37–40] It sometimes appears as small nests of cells surrounded by a few concentric layers of compressed stroma, often associated with chronic inflammation. The nests may be solid or cystically dilated, and occasionally are punctuated by irregular rounded luminal spaces, creating a cribriform pattern. Basal cell hyperplasia frequently involves only part of an acinus, and sometimes protrudes into the lumen, retaining the overlying secretory cell layer; less commonly, there is symmetrical duplication of the basal cell layer at the periphery of the acinus. The proliferation may protrude into the acinar lumen, retaining the overlying secretory luminal epithelium. Symmetrical circumferential thickening of the basal cell layer is less frequent than eccentric thickening, and these changes do not result from tangential sectioning.

The basal cells in basal cell hyperplasia are enlarged, ovoid or round, and plump (epithelioid), with large pale ovoid nuclei, finely reticular chromatin and a moderate amount of cytoplasm. Nucleoli are usually inconspicuous (less than 1 μm in diameter) except in atypical basal cell hyperplasia (see below). It is rarely associated with atypical adenomatous hyperplasia.

Atypical basal cell hyperplasia

Atypical basal cell hyperplasia is identical to basal cell hyperplasia except for the presence of large prominent nucleoli (Fig. 7.7). The nucleoli are round to oval and lightly eosinophilic. There is chronic inflammation in the majority of cases, suggesting that nucleolomegaly is a reflection of reactive atypia. A morphological

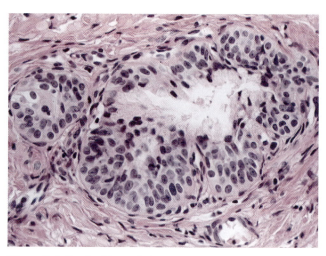

Figure 7.6. *Basal cell hyperplasia.*

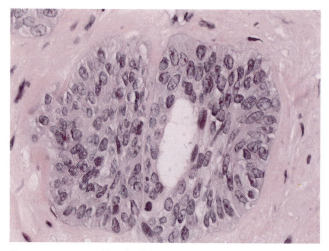

Figure 7.7. *Atypical basal cell hyperplasia.*

spectrum of nucleolar size is observed in basal cell proliferations, and only these with more than 10% of cells exhibiting prominent nucleoli are considered atypical.[37]

Basal cell adenoma

Basal cell adenoma consists of a large round, usually solitary, circumscribed nodule of acini with basal cell hyperplasia in the setting of BPH (Fig. 7.8). The nodule contains uniformly spaced aggregates of hyperplastic basal cells, which form small solid nests or cystically dilated acini. Condensed stroma is seen at the periphery of the nodule. In addition, stromal connective tissue traverses the adenomatous nodule, creating incomplete lobulation in some cases. Stroma is normal or slightly increased in density, and may be basophilic without myxoid change adjacent to cell nests.

The basal cells in basal cell adenoma are plump, with large nuclei, scant cytoplasm and usually inconspicuous nucleoli, although large prominent nucleoli are rarely observed. Many cells are cuboidal or 'epithelioid', particularly near the centre of the cell nests, and some contain clear cytoplasm. Prominent calcific debris is often present within acinar lumens.

Multiple basal cell adenomas are referred to as basal cell adenomatosis. Basal cell adenoma invariably arises in association with BPH, and appears to be a variant.

Immunohistochemical findings

Basal cell hyperplasia (typical and atypical forms) displays intense cytoplasmic immunoreactivity in virtually all of the cells with high-molecular-weight keratin 34βE12. Immunoreactivity for prostate-specific antigen (PSA), prostatic acid phosphatase (PAP), chromogranin, S-100 protein, and neuron-specific enolase is present in rare basal cells in the majority of cases.

Role of basal cells

Basal cells may act as 'reserve' cells that are capable of dividing and replenishing the prostatic epithelium, including the ability to differentiate into other cell types such as secretory cells.[41] Basal cells and secretory cells retain the ability to divide; transition forms have rarely been identified. Basal cells apparently retain the ability to undergo metaplasia, including squamous differentiation in the setting of prostatic infarction and myoepithelial differentiation in the setting of sclerosing adenosis. Epidermal growth factor receptors have been identified in basal cells but not in secretory cells, suggesting that these cells play a part in growth regulation.[42,43]

Cribriform hyperplasia

Cribriform hyperplasia, including clear-cell cribriform hyperplasia, consists of a nodule composed of glands arranged in a distinctive cribriform pattern (Fig. 7.9). The cells from such glands usually have pale to clear cytoplasm and small uniform nuclei with inconspicuous nucleoli.[44,45]

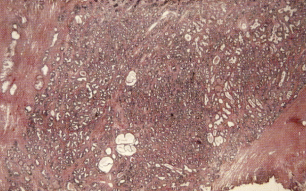

Figure 7.8. *Basal cell adenoma.*

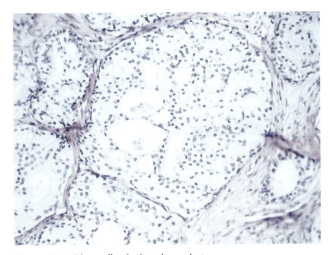

Figure 7.9. *Clear cell cribriform hyperplasia.*

Atypical adenomatous hyperplasia (atypical hyperplasia; small acinar atypical hyperplasia; adenosis; atypical adenosis)

Atypical adenomatous hyperplasia (AAH) is a localized proliferation of small acini within the prostate that may be mistaken for carcinoma (Fig. 7.10).[46–48] Small acinar proliferations in the prostate form a morphological continuum, ranging from benign proliferations with minimal architectural and cytological atypia to those in which the degree of atypia is such that they are easily recognized as well-differentiated adenocarcinoma. The proliferations are distinguished easily at widely spaced points of the spectrum; however, no abrupt changes are apparent along the continuum. The greatest difficulty in distinguishing AAH from carcinoma is with lesions containing nucleoli intermediate in size between benign and malignant. To accommodate this borderline group, the author recommends separating small acinar proliferations into AAH (probably benign) and atypical small acinar proliferation of uncertain significance (possibly benign, but having some features of carcinoma). Importantly, lesions in the category of 'atypical small acinar proliferation of uncertain significance' may have enlarged nucleoli, but they maintain a fragmented basal cell layer, similar to that with AAH. Furthermore, these lesions generate considerable discordance among observers. In view of the uncertainty of the nature of these lesions, some pathologists may prefer a more noncommittal term such as 'atypical small acinar proliferation, not further classified'.

AAH varies in incidence from 19.6% (TURP specimens) to 24% (autopsy series in 20–40-year-old men).[48,49] It can be found throughout the prostate, but is usually present near the apex and in the transition zone and periurethral area.[48]

Separation of AAH and cancer

AAH is distinguished from well-differentiated carcinoma by the following: (1) inconspicuous nucleoli; (2) infrequent crystalloids; (3) fragmented basal cell layer, as seen with basal-cell-specific antikeratin antibodies. All measures of nucleolar size allow separation of AAH from adenocarcinoma, including mean nucleolar diameter, largest nucleolar diameter and percentage of nucleoli greater than 1 μm in diameter. There is apparently widespread acceptance of Gleason's criterion of nucleolar diameter greater than 1 μm for separating well-differentiated cancer (Gleason primary grades 1 and 2) from other proliferative lesions.[50]

Despite the utility of these features, the absolute distinction between AAH and carcinoma is still problematic in some cases, particularly in those cases that are classified as atypical small acinar proliferation of uncertain significance. Other morphological features are not useful in distinguishing AAH from adenocarcinoma, including lesion shape, circumscription, multifocality, average acinar size, variation in acinar size and shape, chromatin pattern and the amount and tinctorial quality of the cytoplasm. Both lesions contain acidic mucin in the majority of cases.[51,52]

Immunohistochemistry of AAH

Immunohistochemistry is often useful in the diagnosis of AAH. The basal cell layer is characteristically discontinuous and fragmented in AAH, but absent in cancer, a feature that can be demonstrated in routine formalin-fixed sections with basal cell-specific antikeratin (high-molecular-weight keratin antibodies 34βE12).

Clinical significance of AAH

Three significant unanswered questions remain regarding AAH. First, does 'atypical small acinar proliferation of uncertain significance' represent

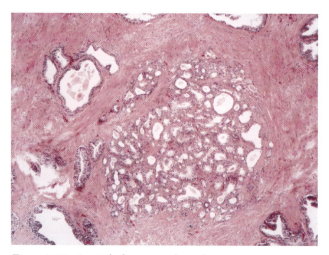

Figure 7.10. *Atypical adenomatous hyperplasia.*

underdiagnosed adenocarcinoma? Six of eight cases in one study created considerable diagnostic discord among the participants.[46] Critics could reasonably argue that the lack of concordance for this lesion indicates that it is not a distinct entity but merely a reflection of our uncertainty; in addition, the criteria for distinguishing this lesion from AAH and cancer may be difficult to apply in practice.

Second, does Gleason primary grade 1 adenocarcinoma represent overdiagnosed adenocarcinoma? These lesions are uncommon; most would agree that Gleason primary grade 2 adenocarcinoma (infiltrating acini) is malignant, but what is the true biological potential of the uniform circumscribed proliferation of Gleason primary grade 1 adenocarcinoma? At present, the author considers this to be malignant, following the suggestion of Gleason and others.

Third, is AAH a precursor of adenocarcinoma? AAH has been proposed as a premalignant lesion of the prostate because of the following: increased incidence in association with carcinoma (15% in 100 prostates without carcinoma at autopsy, and 31% in 100 prostates with cancer at autopsy); topographic relationship with small-acinar carcinoma; age peak incidence that precedes that of carcinoma; increasing AgNOR count; increased nuclear area and diameter; and a proliferative cell index that is similar to that of small-acinar carcinoma but significantly higher than that of normal and hyperplastic prostatic epithelium. Some authors claim that the link between cancer and AAH is an epiphenomenon and that the data are insufficient to conclude that AAH is a premalignant lesion.[53,54] It has also been suggested that AAH may be related to the subset of cancers that arise in the transition zone in association with BPH.[4,55] Although the biological significance of AAH is uncertain, its light-microscopic appearance and immunophenotype allow it to be separated from carcinoma.

In the author's opinion, when AAH is encountered in prostatic specimens, all tissue should be embedded and made available for examination; serial sections of suspicious foci may be useful. Unfortunately, needle biopsy specimens and cytological specimens frequently fail to show the suspicious focus on deeper levels, confounding the diagnostic dilemma. The identification of AAH should not influence or dictate therapeutic

decisions; however, the clinical importance of these lesions is not understood, and close surveillance and follow-up appear to be indicated, particularly for cases considered as atypical small acinar proliferation of uncertain significance.

Sclerosing adenosis

Sclerosing adenosis of the prostate, originally described as adenomatoid or pseudoadenomatoid tumour, consists of a benign circumscribed proliferation of small acini set in a dense spindle cell stroma (Fig. 7.11).[56–62] It is an incidental finding in TURP specimens for BPH, present in about 2% of specimens; rare cases are associated with elevated serum PSA levels. Sclerosing adenosis is usually solitary and microscopic, but may be multifocal and extensive.

The acini are predominantly well formed and of small to medium size, but may form minute cellular nests or clusters with abortive lumens. The cells lining the acini display a moderate amount of clear to eosinophilic cytoplasm, often with distinct cell margins. The basal cell layer may be focally prominent and hyperplastic, particularly in acini thickly rimmed by paucicellular hyalinized stroma. In some areas, the acini merge with the exuberant stroma composed of fibroblasts and loose ground substance. There is usually no significant cytological atypia of the epithelial cells or stromal cells, but some cases may show moderate atypia.

Sclerosing adenosis can be distinguished from adenocarcinoma by the following: its distinctive

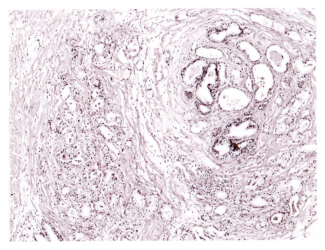

Figure 7.11. *Sclerosing adenosis.*

fibroblastic stroma, which is rarely seen in carcinoma; benign cytology, with epithelial cells and stromal cells that lack the prominent nucleomegaly and nucleolomegaly usually seen in prostatic carcinoma; hyalinized periacinar stroma, occasionally seen in sclerosing adenosis; intact basal cell layer; frequent association with BPH; and immunophenotype of S-100 protein and actin immunoreactivity.

The unique immunophenotype of sclerosing adenosis is a valuable diagnostic clue in distinguishing it from adenocarcinoma. The basal cells show positivity for S-100 protein and muscle-specific actin, unlike normal prostatic epithelium or carcinoma; consequently, sclerosing adenosis is considered a form of metaplasia. The basal cell layer is intact or fragmented and discontinuous in sclerosing adenosis, as demonstrated with immunohistochemical stains for high-molecular-weight keratin 34βE12, compared with absence of staining in carcinoma. PSA and PAP are present with secretory luminal cells. Acid mucin stain may also be of value in separating sclerosing adenosis from carcinoma; however, acid mucin is not specific for malignancy.

Ultrastructural studies confirm the presence of myoepithelial differentiation in sclerosing adenosis, with collections of thin filaments and dense bodies.[58]

Verumontanum mucosal gland hyperplasia

This is an uncommon form of small acinar hyperplasia which mimics well-differentiated adenocarcinoma.[63] It is invariably small (less than 1 mm in diameter), often multicentric and limited anatomically to the verumontanum, utricle, ejaculatory ducts, and adjacent prostatic urethra and ducts. The acini are small and closely packed, with an intact basal cell layer and small uniform nuclei and inconspicuous nucleoli. The basal cells display immunoreactivity for high-molecular-weight keratin, and are S-100 protein negative. This lesion is rare in needle biopsies, and is almost never sampled in TURP because of the sparing of the verumontanum by this procedure.

Hyperplasia of mesonephric remnants

Hyperplasia of mesonephric remnants in the prostate and periprostatic tissues is a rare and benign mimic of adenocarcinoma which is usually identified in TURP specimens. According to Gikas et al.,[64] it shares many features with mesonephric hyperplasia of the female genital tract, including apparent infiltration of the stroma and neural spaces, a lobular arrangement of small acini or solid nests lined by a single cell layer, prominent nucleoli and eosinophilic intratubular material.

Two histopathological patterns have been described, both with a lobular pattern and cuboidal cell lining. One pattern consists of small acini that contain colloid-like material, reminiscent of thyroid follicles. The lining consists a single layer of cuboidal cells without significant cytological atypia. The second pattern consists of small acini or solid nests of cells with empty lumens, reminiscent of nephrogenic metaplasia. Unlike prostate cancer, the acini of prostatic mesonephric remnants contain a small amount of cytoplasm, and this may be the most useful diagnostic finding. In addition, the acini may be atrophic or exhibit micropapillary projections lined by cuboidal cells. Prominent nucleoli are occasionally observed, compounding the diagnostic confusion.

The acini display immunoreactivity for keratin 34βE12, but not for PSA and PAP. One of the original cases was misdiagnosed as adenocarcinoma, resulting in unnecessary prostatectomy.

Summary

BPH is one of the most common diseases in elderly men, but its aetiology and pathogenesis remain uncertain. The pathological features of BPH are well defined and heterogeneous, and include varying amounts of epithelium, smooth muscle and fibrous stroma. The correlation of pathological findings and clinical symptoms is weak, although recent evidence suggests that men with symptomatic BPH have a significantly higher proportion of stroma than men with asymptomatic BPH. The tissue elements in BPH may respond differently to various forms of therapy. Numerous interesting and unusual pathological variants of BPH have been described that mimic adenocarcinoma clinically and pathologically.

References

1.   Isaacs J T, Brendler C B, Walsh P C. Changes in the metabolism of dihydrotestosterone in the hyperplastic human prostate. J Clin Endocrinol Metab 1983; 56: 139–145

2. Berry S J, Coffey D S, Walsh P C, Ewing L L. The development of human benign prostatic hyperplasia with age. J Urol 1984; 132: 474–479

3. Claus S, Wrenger M, Senge T, Schulze H. Immunohistochemical determination of age related proliferation rates in normal and hyperplastic human prostates. Urol Res 1993; 21: 305–308

4. Bostwick D G, Cooner W H, Denis L et al. The association of benign prostatic hyperplasia and cancer of the prostate. Cancer 1992; 70: 291–301

5. Sanda M G, Beatty T H, Stautzman R E et al. Genetic susceptibility of benign prostatic hyperplasia. J Urol 1994; 151: 115–119

6. Partin A W, Sanda M G, Page W F et al. Concordance rates for benign prostatic disease among twins suggest hereditary influence. Urology 1994; 44: 646–650

7. Franks L M. Benign nodular hyperplasia of the prostate: a review. Ann R Coll Surg Engl 1954; 14: 92–106

8. McNeal J E. Origin and evolution of benign prostatic enlargement. Invest Urol 1978; 15: 340–345

9. McNeal J E. The pathobiology of nodular hyperplasia. In: Bostwick D G (ed) Pathology of the prostate. New York: Churchill Livingstone, 1990: 31–36

10. Geller J. Benign prostatic hyperplasia: pathogenesis and medical therapy. J Am Geriatric Soc 1991; 39: 1208–1216

11. Peters C A, Walsh P C. The effect of nafarelin acetate, a luteinizing-hormone-releasing hormone agonist, on benign prostatic hyperplasia. N Engl J Med 1987; 17: 599–604

12. Partin A W, Oesterling J E, Epstein J I et al. Influence of age and endocrine factors on the volume of benign prostatic hyperplasia. J Urol 1991; 145: 405–409

13. Gleason P E, Jones J A, Regan J S et al. Platelet derived growth factor (PDGF), androgens and inflammation: possible etiologic factors in the development of prostatic hyperplasia.

14. Steiner G, Gessl A, Kramer G et al. Phenotype and function of peripheral and prostatic lymphocytes in patients with benign prostatic hyperplasia. J Urol 1994; 151: 480–484

15. Helpap B. Histological and immunohistochemical study of chronic prostatic inflammation with and without benign prostatic hyperplasia. J Urol Pathol 1994; 2: 49–59

16. Egawa S, Ohori M, Uchida T et al. Nodular hyperplasia in the peripheral zone of the prostate gland. Br J Urol 1994; 74: 520–521

17. Hamper U M, Sheth S, Walsh O C et al. Stage B adenocarcinoma of the prostate: transrectal US and pathologic correlation of nonmalignant hypoechoic peripheral zone lesion. Radiology 1991; 180: 101–104

18. Oyen R H, Van de Voorde W M, Van Poppel H P et al. Benign hyperplastic nodules that originate in the peripheral zone of the prostate. Radiology 1993; 189: 707–711

19. Ohori M, Egawa S, Wheeler T M. Nodules resembling nodular hyperplasia in the peripheral zone of the prostate gland. J Urol Pathol 1994; 2: 223–233

20. Kawamura S, Takata K, Yoshia I, Matsui S. A case of giant prostatic hypertrophy. Hinyokika Kiyo 1984; 30: 1861–1866

21. Fishman J R, Merrill D C. A case of giant prostatic hyperplasia. Urology 1993; 42: 336–337

22. Ockerblad N F. Giant prostate: the largest recorded. J Urol 1946; 56: 81–82

23. Seppelt U. Correlation among prostate stroma, plasma estrogen levels and urinary estrogen excretion in patients with benign prostatic hypertrophy. J Clin Endocrinol Metab 1978; 47: 1230–1234

24. Shapiro E, Becich M J, Hartanto V et al. The relative proportion of stromal and epithelial hyperplasia is related to the development of symptomatic benign prostatic hyperplasia. J Urol 1992; 147: 1293–1297

25. Costa P, Robert M, Sarrazin B et al. Quantitative topographic distribution of epithelial and mesenchymal components in benign prostatic hypertrophy. Eur Urol 1993; 24: 120–123

26. Bartsch G, Muller H R, Oberholzer M, Rohr H P. Light microscopic sterological analysis of the normal human prostate and of benign prostatic hyperplasia. J Urol 1979; 122: 487–491

27. Jardin A, Bensadoun A, Tranbaloc P. Constitution de l'adenome prostatique et profil hormonal. In: Legrain M, Chatelain C (eds) Seminaire d'urologie. Paris: Masson, 1985: 11

28. Eble J N, Tejada E. Cost implications of sampling strategies for prostatic transurethral resection specimens: analysis of 549 cases. Am J Clin Pathol 1986; 85: 382

29. Murphy W M, Dean P J, Brasfield J A et al. Incidental carcinoma of the prostate. How much sampling is adequate? Am J Surg Pathol 1986; 10: 170–176

30. Rohr L R. Incidental adenocarcinoma in transurethral resection of the prostate. Partial versus complete microscopic examination. Am J Surg Pathol 1987; 11: 53–58

31. Vollmer R T. Prostate cancer and chip specimens: complete versus partial sampling. Hum Pathol 1986; 17: 285–290

32. Henson D E, Hutter R V P, Farrow G M. Practice protocol for the examination of specimens removed from patients with carcinoma of the prostate gland. A publication of the Cancer Committee, College of American Pathologists. Arch Pathol Lab Med 1994; 118: 779–783

33. Franks L M. Atrophy and hyperplasia in prostate proper. J Pathol Bacteriol 1954; 68: 617–621

34. Cheville J C, Bostwick D G. Post-atrophic hyperplasia of the prostate. A histological mimick of prostatic adenocarcinoma. Am J Surg Pathol 1995; 19: 1068–1076

35. Eble J N, Tejada E. Prostatic stromal hyperplasia with bizarre nuclei. Arch Pathol Lab Med 1991; 115: 87–89

36. Leong S S, Vogt P F, Yu G M. Atypical stroma with muscle hyperplasia of prostate. Urol 1988; 31: 163–167

37. Devaraj L T, Bostwick D G. Atypical basal cell hyperplasia of the prostate: immunophenotypic profile and proposed classification of basal cell proliferations. Am J Surg Pathol 1993; 17: 645–659

38. Grignon D J, Ro J Y, Ordonez N G et al. Basal cell hyperplasia, adenoid basal cell tumor, and adenoid cystic carcinoma of the prostate gland: an immunohistochemical study. Hum Pathol 1988; 19: 1425–1433

39. Cleary K R, Choi H Y, Ayala A G. Basal cell hyperplasia of the prostate. Am J Clin Pathol 1983; 80: 850–854

40. Dermer G B. Basal cell proliferation in benign prostatic hyperplasia. Cancer 1978; 41: 1857–1862

41. Bonkhoff H, Stein V, Remberger K. Multidirectional differentiation in the normal, hyperplastic, and neoplastic human prostate: simultaneous demonstration of cell-specific epithelial markers. Hum Pathol 1994; 25: 42–46

42. Maygarden S, Strom S, Ware J L. Localization of epidermal growth factor receptor by immunohistochemical methods in human prostatic carcinoma, prostatic intraepithelial neoplasia, and benign hyperplasia. Arch Pathol Lab Med 1992; 116: 269–273

43. Mellon K, Thompson S, Charlton R G et al. p53, c-erbB-2 and the epidermal growth factor receptor in the benign and malignant and malignant prostate. J Urol 1992; 147: 496–499

44. Ayala A G, Srigley J R, Ro J Y et al. Clear cell cribriform hyperplasia of prostate. Am J Surg Pathol 1986; 10: 665–672

45. Frauenhoffer E E, Ro J Y, El-Naggar A K et al. Clear cell cribriform hyperplasia of the prostate: immunohistochemical and flow cytometric study. Am J Clin Pathol 1991; 95: 446–453

46. Bostwick D G, Srigley J, Grignon D et al. Atypical adenomatous hyperplasia of the prostate: morphologic criteria for its distinction from well-differentiated carcinoma. Hum Pathol 1993; 24: 819–832

47. Bostwick D G, Algaba F, Amin M B et al. Consensus statement on terminology: recommendation to use atypical adenomatous

hyperplasia in place of adenosis of the prostate. Am J Surg Pathol 1994; 18: 1069–1070

48. Bostwick D G, Qian J. Atypical adenomatous hyperplasia of the prostate. Relationship with carcinoma in 217 whole-mount radical prostatectomies. Am J Surg Pathol 1995; 19: 506–518

49. Brawn P N, Speights V O, Contin J U et al. Atypical hyperplasia in prostates of 20 to 40 year old men. J Clin Pathol 1989; 42: 383–386

50. Gleason D F. Atypical hyperplasia, benign hyperplasia, and well-differentiated adenocarcinoma of the prostate. Am J Surg Pathol 1985; 9: 53–67

51. Epstein J I, Fynheer J. Acidic mucin in the prostate: can it differentiate adenosis from adenocarcinoma? Hum Pathol 1992; 23: 1321–1325

52. Goldstein N S, Qian J, Bostwick D G. Mucin expression in atypical adenomatous hyperplasia of the prostate. Hum Pathol 1995; 26: 887–891

53. Epstein J I. Adenosis vs. atypical adenomatous hyperplasia of the prostate. Am J Surg Pathol 1994; 18: 1070–1071

54. Srigley J R. Small-acinar patterns in the prostate gland with emphasis on typical adenomatous hyperplasia and small-acinar carcinoma. Semin Diagn Pathol 1988; 5: 254–257

55. Helpap B. The biological significance of atypical hyperplasia of the prostate. Virchows Arch [A] 1980; 387: 307–317

56. Chen K T K, Schiff J J. Adenomatoid prostatic tumour. Urology 1983; 21: 88–89

57. Collina G, Botticelli A R, Martinelli A M et al. Sclerosing adenosis of the prostate. Report of three cases with electronmicroscopy and immunohistochemical study. Histopathology 1992; 20: 505–510

58. Grignon D J, Ro J Y, Srigley J R et al. Sclerosing adenosis of the prostate gland. A lesion showing myoepithelial differentiation. Am J Surg Pathol 1992; 16: 383–391

59. Hulman G. 'Pseudoadenomatoid' tumor of prostate. Histopathology 1989; 14: 317–323

60. Jones E C, Clement P B, Young R H. Sclerosing adenosis of the prostate gland. A clinicopathologic and immunohistochemical study of 11 cases. Am J Surg Pathol 1991; 15: 1171–1180

61. Sakamoto N, Tsuneyoshi M, Enjoji M. Sclerosing adenosis of the prostate. Histopathologic and immunohistochemical analysis. Am J Surg Pathol 1991; 15: 660–667

62. Young R H, Clement P B. Sclerosing adenosis of the prostate. Arch Pathol Lab Med 1987; 11: 363–366

63. Gagucas R J, Brown R W, Wheeler T M. Verumontanum mucosal gland hyperplasia. Am J Surg Pathol 1995; 19: 30–36

64. Gikas P, Del Buono E A, Epstein J I. Florid hyperplasia of mesonephric remnants involving prostate and periprostatic tissue: possible confusion with adenocarcinoma. Am J Surg Pathol 1992; 16: 454–459

65. Greene D R, Wheeler T M, Egawa S, Carter S, Weaver R P, Seardino P T. Relationship between clinical stage and histological zone of origin in early prostate cancer: morphometric analysis. Br J Urol 1991; 68: 499–509

8

Bladder responses to obstruction
J. D. McConnell

Bladder outlet obstruction

The partially obstructed urethra, detrusor muscle and central nervous system function interact to produce the group of symptoms known collectively as 'prostatism', which may significantly reduce the quality of life of ageing men. There are several mechanisms by which benign prostatic hyperplasia (BPH) may cause obstruction, such as a prominent median lobe of the prostate acting as a ball valve, a dynamic obstruction related to the contractile properties of prostate smooth muscle, a static obstruction resulting from the enlarged prostate enveloping the prostatic urethra, or a restricted surgical capsule. Each of these mechanisms is clinically feasible and components of each are likely to be present in most instances of lower urinary tract obstruction due to BPH. The result is a raised intravesical pressure and a reduction in flow, which lead to the gradual development of secondary changes in the muscle itself.

Effect of obstruction on the bladder

Gross anatomical, histological, cellular and molecular alterations in the bladder wall (Fig. 8.1), which result from obstruction of the urethra, impair its function and add to the symptomatology of BPH.[1–3] Hypertrophy of the detrusor muscle in the early phases of outflow obstruction allows a compensatory increase in detrusor pressure in order to maintain flow in the presence of increased outflow resistance. With persistent obstruction, however, decreased compliance in the bladder wall and impaired emptying occur, owing to the deposition of increasing amounts of extracellular matrix (ECM), e.g. collagen (Fig. 8.2).[4,5] Acute urinary retention may occur during this process and may be related to bladder failure, as well as to a sudden increase in uroflow obstruction. The alteration in ECM expression is probably the predominant pathophysiological feature in long-term obstruction. During the early phases of obstruction, however, alteration in smooth muscle contractile function is likely. In addition, the probable source of ECM production in both the normal and abnormal bladder is the smooth muscle cells of the detrusor itself.

It is hypothesized that obstruction induces a phenotypic modulation in the detrusor smooth muscle cell. This initially alters the contractile function of the cell and eventually affects the expression of ECM. The following discussion focuses on the alteration in smooth muscle contractile protein expression in the early phases of obstruction.

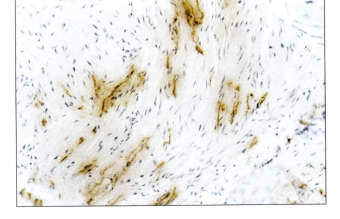

Figure 8.1. *Acetylcholinesterase-containing (presumptive parasympathetic) nerve fibres in the bladder.*

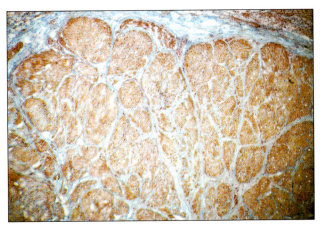

Figure 8.2. *Detrusor smooth muscle bundles infiltrated by collagen.*

Animal physiological studies

Animals were used to study the effects of early short-term obstruction on gene expression, as they provide a better illustration of events than human tissue.[3,6] A rabbit model of obstruction, which involved the partial ligation of the adult rabbit urethra, resulted in a significant increase (four to fivefold) in bladder mass, secondary to smooth muscle hypertrophy; bladder emptying and force production per cross-sectional area were decreased, however.[7] The increase in bladder mass was mainly due to cellular hypertrophy (increase in single cell size).[8] In theory, the increase could have been due to hyperplasia (an increase in cell number) or polyploidy (the formation of large cells with multiple nuclei). Polyploidy may occur in vascular smooth muscle in response to spontaneous hypertension;[9,10] true hyperplasia has been demonstrated in certain rat aorta hypertensive models.[11] In the present model, no evidence was found for an increase in cellular DNA content or an increase in number of proliferating cells, as based on single-cell DNA measurements and flow cytometry. Hyperplasia might yet be involved in the increased muscle mass seen in a younger animal with an obstructed urethra, as the above studies were conducted in adult rabbits.

Bladder emptying is impaired, despite the significant increase in muscle mass produced in animal models of short-term obstruction.[7] Furthermore, higher force is produced in whole-thickness strips of obstructed rabbit bladder than in control strips.[7] When force is adjusted for the increased muscle mass (force per cross-sectional area), however, a significant impairment in the stress-generating capabilities of muscle is evident.[12] In theory, this decrease could be due either to a decreased activation of force-generating units per cross-sectional area, or to a decrease in the number of such units. The final step in the activation of the contractile elements was studied in order to rule out the former possibility.

Myosin light-chain phosphorylation

An increase in the level of intracellular calcium and its subsequent binding to calmodulin precedes the contraction of smooth muscle.[13] The enzyme myosin light-chain kinase, on activation by the calcium–calmodulin complex, phosphorylates the myosin light chain (MLC), leading to the activation of myosin adenosine triphosphatase (ATPase) activity and crossbridge cycling. Cell shortening and force generation result.[14–16] The decrease in activation of the contractile elements within the cell could be due to alterations in signal transduction, downregulation of cholinergic receptors, or loss of cell–cell contact. The ultimate effect of each of these abnormalities is an impairment in MLC phosphorylation. This final step in smooth muscle cell activation was studied, therefore, to determine whether upstream regulatory elements are involved in obstruction-induced bladder hypertrophy.

The response of MLC phosphorylation to a variety of stimuli was found to be the same in smooth muscle isolated from obstructed and control rabbit bladders.[12] This suggests that altered contractility in this animal model was not due to upstream regulatory elements. It is thought likely that signal transduction abnormalities have a role in detrusor instability, the other common secondary feature of obstruction.

Myosin protein studies

The activation of myosin ATPase activity by the calcium–calmodulin complex leads to the contraction of smooth muscle. The ATP-dependent interactions between myosin and actin that follow produce a sliding motion along the thick and thin filaments present within the cell, resulting in shortening and force generation. Myosin, a hexameric molecule, is composed of two myosin heavy chains (MHCs) and two pairs of MLCs. Two isoforms (SM1 and SM2) are produced from a single smooth muscle MHC gene via alternative splicing mechanisms.[17–19] The two isoforms differ in molecular weight by approximately 4000 Da and their ratio is developmentally regulated.[18]

The total amount of MHC protein in obstructed rabbit bladders, as well as the ratio between the two isoforms, was studied using qualitative gel electrophoresis. A decrease in the total amount of MHC per cross-sectional area was recorded;[20] this effect has also been observed in the rat model of obstruction.[3] It is apparent that MHC expression does not increase in proportion to the hypertrophy of the smooth muscle cell resulting from increasing load (obstruction). The effect is a decrease in number of myosin thick filaments per cross-sectional area. The decrease in myosin content is in direct proportion to the decrease in force generation per cross-sectional area.

There is a slight predominance of the SM2 (lower molecular weight) isoform of MHC in the normal adult rabbit bladder. However, a significant shift towards SM1 predominance at the protein level takes place 2–3 weeks after the onset of obstruction.[20] This would suggest that obstruction-induced hypertrophy produces an alteration in alternate splicing of the MHC gene product, in addition to downregulation of MHC expression.

Expression of the myosin heavy chain

The transcription of total rabbit smooth muscle MHC and the individual isoforms was studied using Northern blot and S1 nuclease protection assays.[21] A high constitutive level of MHC expression exists in the normal rabbit bladder, which is significantly downregulated shortly after onset of obstruction and is barely detectable by the third week; a significant shift towards SM1 expression can also be demonstrated.[21] It is interesting to note that the predominant SM1 expression pattern is also seen in dedifferentiated smooth muscle cells in culture and during foetal development of the rabbit bladder. This would suggest that obstruction-induced hypertrophy in the rabbit model is linked to the dedifferentiation of the smooth muscle cell.

Caldesmon expression in the smooth muscle cell

Caldesmon is another important regulatory protein in the smooth muscle cell; it maintains the 'latch state' of the smooth muscle, as well as being involved in modulating contraction.[22,23] Two isoforms of caldesmon exist within smooth muscle: a high-molecular-weight form (h-caldesmon) is present in normal smooth muscle, and a low-molecular-weight form (l-caldesmon) is present in fibroblasts and smooth muscle cells in culture. Studies show that obstruction induces expression of l-caldesmon,[24] suggesting, yet again, that obstruction induces smooth muscle dedifferentiation.

Conclusions

Studies using a rabbit model of obstruction show that significant smooth muscle hypertrophy is induced when load is increased and that this is associated with a downregulation of MHC expression. This effect obviously contributes to the decreased smooth muscle contractility seen in this model. Moreover, obstruction-induced hypertrophy results in the development of a dedifferentiated smooth muscle phenotype. In other systems, for example atherosclerotic vessels, the dedifferentiation exhibited is also associated with significant alterations in ECM expression. It is quite possible that obstruction of the bladder induces dedifferentiation of the smooth muscle cell, resulting in alterations in ECM expression and contractility, and finally altered bladder performance and decreased compliance.

References

1. Susset J G. Effects of aging and prostatic obstruction on detrusor morphology and function. In: Hinman C (ed). Benign prostatic hypertrophy. New York: Springer-Verlag, 1985: 653–665
2. Luutzeyer W, Hannapel J, Schafer W. Sequential events in prostatic obstruction. In: Hinman C (ed) Benign prostatic hypertrophy. New York: Springer-Verlag, 1985: 693–700
3. Malmqvist U, Arner A, Uvelius B. Cytoskeletal and contractile proteins in detrusor smooth muscle form bladder outlet obstruction: a comparative study in rat and man. Scand J Urol Nephrol 1991; 25: 261–267
4. Susset J G, Servot-Viguir D, Lamy F et al. Collagen in 155 human bladders. Invest Urol 1978; 16: 204–215
5. Gosling J A, Dixon J S. Structure of trabeculated detrusor smooth muscle in cases of prostatic hypertrophy. Urol Int 1980; 35: 3351–3372
6. Malkowicz S B, Wein A J, Elbadawi A et al. Acute biochemical and functional alterations in the partially obstructed rabbit urinary bladder. J Urol 1986; 136: 1324–1329
7. Levin M R, Longhurst P A, Monson F C et al. Effect of bladder outlet obstruction on the morphology, physiology, and pharmacology of the bladder. Prostate 1990; 3(suppl): 9–26
8. Pettaway C A, Murphree S, McConnell J D. The response of detrusor smooth muscle nucleus to obstruction. J Urol 1990; 143: 367A
9. Owens G K, Schwartz S M. Alterations in vascular smooth muscle mass in the spontaneously hypertensive rat: role of cellular hypertrophy, hyperploidy and hyperplasia. Circ Res 1982; 51: 280–289
10. Owens G K, Rabinovitch, Schwartz S M. Smooth muscle cell hypertrophy versus hyperplasia in hypertension. Proc Natl Acad Sci USA 1981; 78: 7759–7763
11. Arner A, Uvelius B. Force–velocity characteristics and active tension in relation to content and orientation of smooth muscle cells in aortas from normotensive and spontaneously hypertensive rats. Circ Res 1982; 50: 812–821
12. Cher M L, Kamm K E, McConnell J D. Stress generation and myosin phosphorylation in the obstructed bladder. J Urol 1990; 143: 355A
13. Murphy R A, Aksoy M O, Dillon P F et al. The role of myosin light chain phosphorylation in regulation of the crossbridge cycle. Fed Proc 1983; 42: 51–56
14. Aksoy M O, Murphy R A, Kamm K E. Role of Ca^{2+} and myosin light chain phosphorylation in regulation of smooth muscle. Am J Physiol 1982; 242: C109–116
15. Dillon P F, Aksoy M O, Driska S P, Murphy R A. Myosin phosphorylation and crossbridge cycle in arterial smooth muscle. Science 1098; 211: 495–497

16. Kamm K E, Stull J T. Regulation of smooth muscle contractile elements by second messengers. Annu Rev Physiol 1989; 51: 299–313

17. Beckers-Bleukx G, Maréchal G. Detection and distribution of myosin isozymes in vertebrate smooth muscle. Eur J Biochem 1985; 152: 207–211

18. Rovner A S, Thompson M M, Murphy R A. Two different heavy chains are found in smooth muscle myosin. Am J Physiol 1986; 250: C861–870

19. Nagai R, Kuro-o M, Babij P, Periasamy M. Identification of two types of smooth muscle myosin heavy chain isoforms by cDNA cloning and immunoblot assay. J Biol Chem 1989; 264: 9734–9737

20. Abernathy B B, Kadesky K T, McConnell J D. Myofilament protein alterations in the obstructed rabbit bladder. J Urol 1988; 139: 195A

21. Cher M L, Lin V K, McConnell J D. Myosin gene expression in obstruction-induced bladder hypertrophy. J Urol 1991; 145: 310A

22. Sobue K, Kanda K, Tanaka T, Ueki N. Caldesmon: a common actin-linked regulatory protein in the smooth muscle and non-muscle contractile system. J Cell Biochem 1988; 337: 317–325

23. Lash J A, Sellers J R, Hathaway D R. The effects of caldesmon on smooth muscle heavy actomeromyosin ATPase activity and binding of heavy meromyosin to actin. J Biol Chem 1986; 262: 16155–16160

24. Lin V K, Lee I L, McConnell J D. Expression of l-caldesmon in obstruction-induced bladder hypertrophy. J Cell Biol 1991; 115: 1380a

9

Molecular genetics of benign prostatic hyperplasia
M. C. W. Völler J. A. Schalken

Introduction

Benign prostatic hyperplasia (BPH) occurs in the majority of ageing males: the incidence of BPH is low in the fourth decade of life and steadily increases to a prevalence of almost 100% in men aged 90 years.[1] Although almost all men develop BPH histologically, only half of them will develop a macroscopic enlargement of the prostate and ultimately 25% of these patients need surgery to alleviate urinary obstruction.[2]

BPH is the most common neoplastic disease in man, yet the exact aetiology of BPH is unknown. It has been well established that age and hormones are important factors in the development of BPH.[3] Ageing, and a functional testis, are the two prerequisites for the development of this disease. The molecular basis of BPH development is only poorly understood. Interest has been focused on the role of growth factors in the pathogenesis of BPH. In the prostate, many growth factors are involved in autocrine or paracrine interactions. Furthermore, they mediate the effect of androgens and they have a critical role in maintenance of the epithelial–stromal balance. Some of these molecular changes are similar to those seen in prostate cancer, which raises again the question of whether BPH can be a precursor lesion for prostate cancer. The hypothesis would imply that clonal genetic changes occur in BPH development; the role of genetic changes in the development of BPH has, therefore, recently gained more attention. Both molecular changes and genetic changes in BPH development are discussed in this chapter.

Molecular endocrinology and BPH development

Growth, development, maintenance and function of the prostate gland are androgen dependent.[4–7] Removal of testosterone by castration leads to prostatic involution and subsequent administration of exogenous androgens leads to regrowth of the prostate to its original size.[8,9] The fact that men who fail to produce androgens by genetic failure, or by castration before puberty, do not develop BPH, indicates that androgens play a crucial part in this disease.[2]

In the prostate, testosterone is converted to 5-alpha-dihydrotestosterone (DHT) by 5 alpha-reductase, which is located on the nuclear membrane. DHT is the active intracellular androgen and it elicits its biological activity by binding to the nuclear androgen receptor (AR) protein. This complex (DHT–AR) can bind to a specific DNA sequence, thereby initiating or inhibiting the expression of genes involved in growth-regulatory pathways or the production of secretory products such as prostatic specific antigen (PSA). However, in vitro tissue culture experiments have shown that androgens do not stimulate prostatic epithelial cell growth directly, whereas growth factors such as epidermal growth factor (EGF) and transforming growth factor-alpha (TGFα) stimulate prostatic epithelial cell proliferation directly.[7] Thus, it appears that DHT is not directly responsible for epithelial growth. Nevertheless, a role for androgens seems likely in the pathogenesis of BPH because DHT is essential for growth in vivo and because BPH and prostate cancer do not develop in men who are castrated before puberty.

It is hypothesized that androgens provide the 'switching on' of proliferative processes,[7] with a certain level of androgens needed to initiate proliferation. However, this effect is permissive rather than causal, and other intermediary growth regulators that act at cellular levels are necessary.

Oestrogens originate from testosterone and the adrenal androgen androstenedion, through conversion by the peripheral aromatase enzyme system. Evidence that oestrogens are involved in the pathogenesis of BPH has been obtained in experimental animal models. In young castrated dogs, administration of oestrogens combined with androgens induces BPH,[6] which is related to an oestrogen-mediated increase in oestrogen receptor (ER) and AR levels. Furthermore, administration of androstenedion induces stromal hyperplasia in the prostates of the dog and monkey.[10,11] This is in line with the reported localization of the ER in the stromal compartment of the prostate.[12]

In human males over 50 years of age there is a slight increase in oestrogen levels, leading to an increased free-oestradiol/free-testosterone ratio that may promote the development of prostatic adenoma and the clinical symptoms of bladder outflow obstruction.[7] In BPH patients, higher free testosterone and oestrogen levels have been detected.[13] Other possible effects of oestrogens are inhibition of the rate of programmed cell death, leading to prostate enlargement,[4] and contractile effects leading to urinary obstruction.[14]

Paracrine and autocrine interactions in BPH

It is now apparent that there is an important biological interaction between the prostatic stroma and the epithelium. Several studies have shown that, during embryonic development of the prostate, inductive signalling processes between the stoma and the epithelium occur.[15,16] Under the influence of androgens and — to some extent — oestrogens, stromal cells produce factors that regulate epithelial cell growth and differentiation. Several growth factors may be involved, among which the members of the epidermal growth factor family (EGF and TGFα), fibroblast-like growth factor family [basic FGF (bFGF) and kerakinocyte growth factor (kGF or FGF-7)], transforming growth factor-beta family (TGFβ) and insulin-like growth factor family (IGF-I and -II) are the most important.

The members of the EGF family appear to be universal stimuli for epithelial cell growth. A high concentration of EGF is detected in human prostatic fluid[17] and proliferation of prostatic epithelial cells (PECs) can be stimulated by EGF. The expression of the EGF-receptor (EGF-R) in the epithelial cells has been demonstrated by immunohistochemistry[18] and is confined predominantly to the basal cells. It is not yet clear whether EGF and EGF-R levels differ in normal, BPH and tumour tissue. Yan et al.[19] did not observe a difference between the level of EGF and TGFα in

prostatic tissue extracts obtained from patients with BPH or cancer.

The first evidence that FGFs are important in the regulation of prostatic growth came from studies that showed that conditioned medium, derived from prostatic fibroblasts, was mitogenic in PECs.[20,21] Furthermore, overexpression of the int-2 gene product, which is also a member of the FGF family, in transgenic mice leads to epithelial hyperplasia.[22] In addition, the level of bFGF has been reported to be elevated in BPH, compared with normal prostate.[23] However, in vitro no response is seen when normal PECs are stimulated with purified aFGF or bFGF.

Another member of the FGF family, kGF or FGF-7, is produced by prostatic fibroblasts in culture in an androgen-dependent manner and is mitogenic in cultures of normal PECs.[19] The growth-enhancing effects of kGF in epithelial cell cultures can be reversed by adding TGFβ, indicating that both growth factors probably are involved in regulating epithelial growth.[24]

In general, TGFβ is considered to be an inhibitor of epithelial cell growth. In the prostate, TGFβ also acts as an inhibitor of proliferative processes[25,26] and is involved in apoptosis. Thus, TGFβ can regulate prostatic epithelial cell growth by restraining the growth-stimulatory effects of EGF and FGF. A loss of sensitivity of epithelial cells for TGFβ or other properties of TGFβ as inducing stromal cell proliferation could contribute to the development of BPH.

Other growth factors that are probably important in the homoeostasis of the prostate are members of the IGF family. Cultured PECs express the IGF-I receptor[27] and they are stimulated by purified IGF-I or IGF-II. However, IGF-I and IGF-II have not been detected in conditioned medium of PECs, indicating that autocrine regulation is unlikely. Recent studies have shown that cultured prostatic fibroblasts produce IGF-II, which may imply the existence of a paracrine regulation of prostatic epithelial growth.[28] Other proteins that are involved in the mitogenic effects of the IGFs are the IGF-binding proteins (IGF-BPs). The precise mechanism of action is still unclear but they probably are involved in the control of the availability of IGFs for interaction with their receptors.[28,29]

Genetic basis of BPH

The possibility of predisposing a laboratory animal to prostate epithelial hyperplasia similar to BPH by transgenetics[22] has indicated that genetic changes can play a part in the development of this disease. The germ-line introduction of the *int*-1 oncogene, a member of the FGF family, under control of an MMTV promoter, resulted in benign epithelial proliferation in the mammary and prostate gland. It is noteworthy that this is, so far, the only available rodent model system for the study of BPH.[30] Recently, the first reports became available on the possible genetic susceptibility to BPH development in humans. Sanda and colleagues[31] performed a case–control study of men with early onset of BPH. A sixfold increased risk of undergoing prostatectomy for BPH was found for brothers of males who had undergone prostatectomy for BPH, when compared with controls. The concordance rate for BPH among twins also suggests a hereditary influence in the development of BPH.[32] The putative genes involved in the predisposition to BPH have not yet been characterized. It is not clear whether these genetic events are similar to or differ from those found in prostate cancer.

It has been well established that the development of prostate cancer is a multistep process.[33] However, the precise molecular events are largely unknown and it is not clear if there is a genetic relation between BPH and prostate cancer. Two different models have been postulated for the development of BPH in relation to prostate cancer (Fig. 9.1). The first model states that there are some similar events in the induction of BPH or cancer; the second model predicts that different events lead to either BPH or prostate cancer. The results of Partin et al.[34] who examined the nuclear matrix proteins in human normal prostate, BPH and prostate cancer, support model I. No proteins were found that were exclusively expressed in, or absent from, BPH tissue compared with normal prostate and prostate cancer. Only one protein was specific for prostate cancer. This would suggest that BPH and/or prostate cancer share the same early events and that, in the progression to cancer, additional events occur.

Allelic loss on chromosome 8p is a frequent event in human prostate cancer.[35] Loss of heterozygosity (LOH) analysis by microsatellite polymerase chain reaction on microdissected prostate tissue[36] revealed 8p loss in

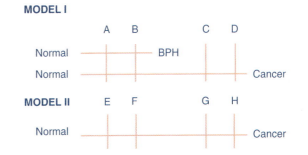

Figure 9.1. *Models of the development of BPH: relation to cancer development. (From ref. 32 with permission.)*

prostatic intraepithelial neoplasia and BPH lesions,[37] which corroborates a precursor function for these lesions. However, the frequency of 8p loss was very low, which might be explained by the fairly large amount of contaminating stromal cells, assuming that the genetic change occurs in the epithelial cells. Another genetic change that is often seen in prostate cancer is allelic loss of chromosome 13q, the region to which the retinoblastoma gene is mapped. Interestingly, in one of ten BPH samples studied by Phillips and colleagues,[38] the Rb1 gene was deleted. Again, there was a low frequency of LOH, but similar to that seen in prostate cancer.

Summary and conclusions

The molecular basis of BPH development is still poorly understood. The stromal–epithelial interactions seem to have a crucial role and more insight needs to be obtained on the complicated balance between growth-stimulatory and growth-inhibitory processes. These are androgen and oestrogen dependent, and together they regulate normal prostatic growth and maintenance of the prostate to a certain size (Fig. 9.2). In the development of BPH, one can hypothesize that there is either an overexpression of growth-stimulatory factors such as EGF and/or FGF, and/or a decreased expression of TGFβ resulting in an imbalance that brings about an enlargement of the prostate. Furthermore, the heterogeneity of the cells in the prostate, as well as the regional stromal–epithelial interactions, have to be considered in relation to the pathogenesis of BPH.

The more recent realization that there can be a genetic predisposition to BPH, and the anecdotal

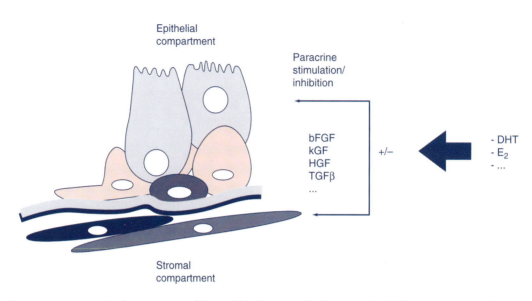

Figure 9.2. *Paracrine interactions in the prostate; candidate soluble factors involved in stromal epithelial interactions and relation to endocrine modulation.*

findings that allelic loss can be found in BPH processes, indicate a clonal origin of the disease. The most provocative hypothesis that now emerges is that BPH could, in fact, serve as a precursor lesion for prostate cancer. It should be noted that only in a small proportion of the lesions analysed has supportive evidence been obtained, in small-scale studies. Nevertheless, these recent findings indicate that the disease can have a very heterogeneous origin.

References

1. Bostwick D G, Cooner W H, Denis L et al. The association of benign prostatic hyperplasia and cancer in the prostate. Cancer 1992; (suppl 70): 291–301
2. Meares E M, Sant G R. Differentiele diagnose van prostaatziekten. London: Gower Medical Publishing, 1992
3. Isaacs J T, Coffey D S. Etiology and disease process of benign prostatic hyperplasia. Prostate 1989; (suppl 2): 33–50
4. Coffey D S, Berry S J, Ewing L L. An overview of current concepts in the study of benign prostatic hyperplasia. In: Rodgers C H, Coffey D S, Cunha G R et al. (eds) Benign prostatic hyperplasia II. NIH Publ. No 87-2881, US Dept Health, Human Serv. Bethesda: NIH, 1987: 1–13
5. Coffey D S. The structure and function of the prostate gland and the sex accessory tissues in prostate cancer. In: Khoury S, Chatelain C, Murphy G, Denis L (eds) Proc FIIS. Paris: FIIS, 1990: 70–103
6. Coffey D S, Walsh P C. Clinical and experimental studies of benign prostatic hyperplasia. Urol Clin North Am 1990; 17: 461–475
7. Griffiths K, Akaza H, Eaton C L et al. Regulation of prostatic growth. In: Cockett A T K, Khoury S, Aso Y et al. (eds) The 2nd International Consultation on Benign Prostatic Hyperplasia (BPH). Jersey, Channel Islands: SCI, 1993: 49–75
8. Bruchovsky N, Lesser B, Vandoorn E, Craven S. Hormonal effects on cell proliferation in rat prostate. Vitam Horm 1975; 33: 61–102
9. Isaacs J T. Antagonistic effect of androgen on prostatic cell death. Prostate 1984; 5: 545–557
10. El Etreby M F, Habenicht U-F. Experimental induction of stromal hyperplasia in prostate of castrated dogs treated with 4-androstene-3,17-dione. Effect of aromatase inhibitor 4-hydroxyandrostene-3,17-dione. In: Rodgers C H, Coffey D S, Cunha G R et al. (eds) Benign prostatic hyperplasia. NIH Publ. No 87-2881, US Dept Health, Human Serv. Bethesda: NIH, 1987: 303–310
11. Habenicht U-F, Schwartz K, Neumann F, El Etreby M F. Induction of oestrogen related hyperplastic changes in the prostate of the Cynomolgus monkey (Macaca fascicularis) by androstenedione and its antagonization by the aromatase inhibitor 1-methyl-androsta-1,4-diene-3,17-dione. Prostate 1987; 11: 313–326
12. Krieg M, Klotzl G, Kaufman J, Voigt K D. Stroma of human benign prostatic hyperplasia: preferential tissue for androgen metabolism and oestrogen binding. Acta Endocrinol (Copenh) 1981; 96: 422–432
13. Partin A W, Oesterling J E, Epstein J I et al. Influence of age and endocrine factors on the volume of benign prostatic hyperplasia. J Urol 1991; 145: 405–409
14. Khanna O M P. Effect of nonautonomic drugs on the vesical neck. In: Hinman F (ed) Benign prostatic hypertrophy. Berlin: Springer-Verlag, 1983: 384–404
15. Cunha G R, Chung L W K, Shannon J M et al. Hormone induced morphogenesis and growth: role of mesenchymal–epithelial interactions. Recent Prog Horm Res 1983; 39: 559–595
16. Cunha G R, Donjacour A A, Cooke P S et al. The endocrinology and developmental biology of the prostate. Endocr Rev 1987; 8: 338–362
17. Gregory H, Willshire I R, Kavanagh J P et al. Urogastrone-epidermal growth factor concentrations in prostatic fluid of normal individuals and patients with benign prostatic hypertrophy. Clin Sci 1986; 70: 359–363
18. Maddy S Q, Chisholm G D, Hawkins R A, Habib F K. Localization of epidermal growth factor receptors in the human prostate by biochemical and immunocytochemical methods. J Endocrinol 1987; 113: 147–153

19. Yan G, Fukabori Y, Nikolaropoulos S et al. Heparin-binding keratinocyte growth factor is a candidate stromal to epithelial cell andromedin. Mol Endocrinol 1992; 6: 2123–2128

20. Kabalin J N, Peehl D M, Stamey T A. Clonal growth of human prostatic epithelial cells is stimulated by fibroblasts. Prostate 1989; 14: 251–263

21. Eaton C L. Growth factors, oncogenes and prostate cancer. Rev Endocr Rel Cancer 1992; 40: 5–12

22. Muller W J, Lee F S, Dickson C et al. The int-2 gene product acts as an epidermal growth factor in transgenic mice. EMBO J 1990; 9: 907–913

23. Mori H, Maki M, Olshi K et al. Increased expression of genes for basic fibroblast growth factor type β-2 in human benign prostatic hyperplasia. Prostate 1990; 16: 71–80

24. Story M T, Hopp K A, Meier D A et al. Influence of transforming growth factor beta 1 and other growth factors on basic fibroblast growth factor level and proliferation of cultured human prostate-derived fibroblasts. Prostate 1993; 22: 183–197

25. Kyprianou N, Isaacs J T. Expression of transforming growth factors in the rat ventral prostate during castration induced programmed cell death. Mol Endocrinol 1989; 3: 1515–1522

26. Wilding G, Valverius E, Knabbe C, O'Elmann E P. Role of transforming growth factor β in human prostate cancer cell growth. Prostate 1989; 15: 1–12

27. Cohen P, Peehl D M, Lamson G, Rosenfield R G. Insulin-like growth factors (IGFs), IGF receptors, and IGF binding proteins in primary cultures of prostatic epithelial cells. J Clin Endocrinol Metab 1991; 73: 401–407

28. Cohen P, Peehl D M, Baker B et al. Insulin-like growth factor axis abnormalities in prostatic stromal cells from patients with benign prostatic hyperplasia. J Clin Endocrinol Metab 1994; 79: 1410–1415

29. Cohen P, Graves H C, Peehl D M et al. Prostate specific antigen (PSA) is an insulin-like growth factor binding protein 3-like protease found in seminal plasma. J Clin Endocrinol Metab 1992; 75: 1046–1053

30. Tutrone R F Jr, Ball R A, Ornitz D M et al. Benign prostatic hyperplasia in a transgenic mouse: a new hormonally sensitive investigatory model. J Urol 1993; 149: 633–639

31. Sanda M G, Beaty T H, Stutzman R E et al. Genetic susceptibility of benign prostatic hyperplasia. J Urol 1994; 152: 115–119

32. Partin A W, Page W F, Lee B R et al. Concordance rates for benign prostatic disease among twins suggest hereditary influence. Urology 1994; 44: 646–650

33. Carter H B, Piantadosi S, Isaacs J T. Clinical evidence for and implications of the multistep development of prostate cancer. J Urol 1990; 143: 742–746

34. Partin A W, Getzenberg R H, CarMichael M J et al. Nuclear matrix protein patterns in human benign prostatic hyperplasia and prostate cancer. Cancer Res 1993; 53: 744–746

35. Bergerheim U S R, Kunimi K, Collins V P, Ekman P. Deletion mapping of chromosomes 8, 10 and 16 in human prostatic carcinoma. Genes Chromosomes Cancer 1991; 3: 215–220

36. Wolman S R, Macoska J A, Micale M A, Sakr W A. An approach to definition of genetic alterations in prostate cancer. Diagn Mol Path 1992; 13: 192–199

37. Macoska J A, Trybus T M, Sakr W A et al. Fluorescence in situ hybridization analysis of 8p allelic loss and chromosome 8 instability in human prostate cancer. Cancer Res 1994; 54: 3824–3830

38. Phillips S M, Barton C M, Lee S J et al. Loss of the retinoblastoma susceptibility gene (RBI) is a frequent and early event in prostatic tumorigenesis. Br J Cancer 1994; 70: 1252–1257

Epidemiology

II

10

Population-based studies of benign prostatic hyperplasia*
H. A. Guess

Introduction

A thorough understanding of benign prostatic hyperplasia (BPH) requires a knowledge not only of its pathophysiology but also of its epidemiology. Until recently, most epidemiological information about BPH had come from studies involving only men who had sought treatment for BPH. Such studies make it difficult to separate factors related to seeking treatment from factors related to other measures of disease progression. In addition, they do not provide information on the full spectrum of disease or of early findings, since they are limited to men in whom the clinical manifestations have progressed far enough to lead them to seek medical attention. To provide more complete information requires *population-based* studies, which involve representative sampling from a geographically defined population.

Population-based studies of BPH can contribute to medical knowledge in at least three areas.[1] First, there is the need to establish community-based normal ranges of symptom scores and commonly used diagnostic tests. A proper evaluation of any test requires that the study population includes a sufficiently broad spectrum of diseased and non-diseased individuals.[2] Studying only men seen in urology clinics can lead to optimistic estimates of sensitivity and specificity that are later proved to be incorrect when the test is applied to men with milder disease in a general practice setting.[2,3] Studies to establish community-based normal ranges of tests also provide information on the community prevalence of symptoms and other measures of BPH. This information is useful in characterizing the amount of morbidity attributable to BPH.

Second, it is important to determine how symptoms and other factors influence both the decision to seek treatment and the choice of treatment. Barry has shown that differences in individual patient preferences are important in making rational choices of treatments.[4] Such information is also useful in estimating how practice guidelines may affect utilization of medical services.[5]

A third potential contribution of long-term community-based studies is to provide information on outcomes from a representative sample of a defined population rather than only from patients treated at particular health-care facilities. What may appear to be intervention-related or hospital-related variation in outcomes may be variation in the magnitude and form of patient selection bias. Selection bias in non-population-based studies is often impossible to control by co-morbidity adjustments, because factors that bring patients to a particular facility or that lead to the choice of one type of treatment over another are often not adequately reflected in medical records or in any other readily available data source.[6–9] It is the lower potential for selection bias that makes community-based studies of disease natural history preferable to natural history studies conducted in referral populations.[10] Studies of BPH natural history are discussed in Chapter 11.

In this chapter, several population-based studies of urinary symptoms and health status related to BPH that have been undertaken recently are reviewed. Many of these studies are still ongoing and further publication of results will be forthcoming in the next few years. This chapter can do no more than to acquaint readers with the study designs and some initial results. An overview of the sampling methods is given in the Appendix. One of these studies is a national survey of urinary symptoms and quality of life among French men; the others involve community-based studies in Denmark, Japan, Netherlands, Scotland and the United States. The emphasis here is on newer studies and recent results. For more comprehensive reviews of BPH epidemiology the reader is referred to several recent review articles.[11–14]

---

*Portions of this chapter were adapted from Guess,[14] with permission.

French national survey

To date, it appears that there has been only one nationwide urological symptom survey conducted in any country. Sagnier and colleagues conducted a survey of urinary symptoms and quality of life in a nationally representative probability sample of 2011 French men aged 50–80 years, using a French translation of the American Urological Association Symptom Index (AUASI).[15–19] This French symptom score has been accepted as the French language version of the International Prostate Symptom Score (I-PSS).[16]* In the survey, information was collected by household interview, in which 12 525 dwellings had to be contacted to obtain the above sample size. The authors noted that a calculation of the true response rate in this study is not possible, since the sampling unit (dwellings) and the reporting units (subjects) were different and the eligibility status of subjects who were not at home at the time of the initial contact is not known. However, one accepted definition of response rate is the ratio of the number of completed interviews divided by the number of known eligible units in the sample.[20] By that definition, the response rate was 53%.

After exclusion of patients with prostate cancer, 7% of the subjects reported having undergone prostate surgery and an additional 8% reported having received a diagnosis of BPH. Among those with no history of surgery or prostate cancer, 19% had no symptoms, 67% had mild symptoms (I-PSS range 1–7), 13% had moderate symptoms (I-PSS 8–19) and 1% had severe symptoms (I-PSS 20+). The proportion with moderate to severe symptoms approximately doubled with each decade of age. Nocturia and repeat voiding within 2 h were the most prevalent symptoms.

The index formed by the American Urological Association (AUA) questions on bother due to urinary symptoms (referred to here as the AUA Bothersomeness Index) was the best determinant of each subject's level of worry about urinary conditions and the degree to which urinary symptoms interfered with daily life. Urgency was by far the most bothersome symptom among men who reported one or more urinary symptoms, followed by wet underclothes, re-voiding within 10 min and nocturia. Intermittency and weak stream appeared to be less bothersome. The AUA Bothersomeness Index was highly correlated to the I-PSS ($r = 0.85$, $p<0.001$).

The authors estimated that, in 1992, approximately 1.14 million French men had moderate to severe urinary symptoms. They noted that previous studies in other populations had yielded higher percentage prevalence estimates, probably owing to differences in sampling design and diagnostic criteria. In particular, the prevalence of moderate to severe urinary symptoms (I-PSS of 8 or more) in France was somewhat similar to that in Scotland but was considerably lower than that in Olmsted county (Fig. 4 in ref. 21). This large difference in age-specific symptom prevalence is in contrast to findings in two population-based studies that the age-specific incidence of initial prostatectomy for BPH in Olmsted County, Minnesota[22] is nearly identical to that in Lyon, France across all age groups.[23]

Community-based studies

Copenhagen, Denmark survey

Jensen and colleagues conducted a survey of urological symptoms and urinary flow rates based on a randomly drawn sample of 200 men aged 50 years and older, with an age distribution representative of the metropolitan population of Copenhagen, Denmark.[24] The final sample consisted of 121 men, representing a 61% response rate. Of these men, 17% were considered to have prostatism, which was defined as the presence of self-reported voiding problems unrelated to dysuria or haematuria. Only limited relationships between symptom scores and urinary flow rate were found and there was considerable overlap in urinary flow rates between those who did and those who did not meet the above definition of prostatism. The authors concluded that, no matter what flow rates are chosen as the cutoff limits of normal, urinary flow-rate measurements are not an efficient means of confirming a clinical impression of prostatism. A similar conclusion as to the relative non-

---

*In the initial article describing prevalence of symptoms,[17] the authors referred to their symptom score as the AUASI. In a subsequent article describing the impact of symptoms on quality of life,[18] the same symptom score was referred to as the International Prostate Symptom Score. For the sake of consistency, their symptom score is henceforth referred to as the International Prostate Symptom Score.

specificity of urinary flow-rate measurements was found by Girman.[25]

Forth Valley, Scotland study

Garraway and colleagues conducted a study of urinary symptoms in four villages in the Forth Valley of Scotland.[26-30] As in the Olmsted County study discussed below, only men 40–79 years of age with no history at baseline of prostate cancer, prostate surgery or other specified conditions that could interfere with normal voiding function were eligible to participate. This study used a definition of BPH based on a prostate size of more than 20 g plus (1) a maximum urinary flow rate less than 15 ml/s and/or (2) lower urinary tract symptoms in excess of a specified level. This study provided data documenting that the prevalence of BPH among apparently healthy men in the community was higher than had previously been reported,[26] increasing from 14% of men in their forties to 43% of men in their sixties.

About one-half of men with BPH, compared with one-quarter of men without BPH, reported some interference with one or more of the seven living activities on a scale developed and validated by Epstein and discussed below.[31] Among men of working age (40–64 years), 17% of those with BPH, compared with 3% of those without BPH, reported interference most or all of the time.[29] Men with BPH had more anxiety and depression, less vitality and self-control, and more worry and embarrassment about urinary dysfunction than did men without BPH.[30] In a 1-year follow-up of this cohort, the authors noted that a longer period of observation was needed to determine the extent to which a consistent pattern of urinary symptomatology exists in untreated BPH and whether interference with living activities continues to progress over time.[28]

Olmsted County study

Study design

The Olmsted County study (OCS) of urinary symptoms and health status among men is a community-based study of 2115 randomly selected Caucasian male residents of Olmsted County, Minnesota, USA, between 40 and 79 years of age with no history of prostate surgery, prostate cancer or any of a specified list of conditions known to affect voiding function.[32] At the baseline evaluation, completed in 1991, all men had urinary flow-rate measurements and completed the symptom and quality of life questionnaire previously validated by Epstein and colleagues.[31]

This questionnaire covers frequency of urinary symptoms, bother due to urinary symptoms, worries and concerns about urinary problems and prostate cancer, interference in living activities due to urinary symptoms, sexual functioning and general psychological well-being. The questionnaire pre-dates the AUASI but includes questions on urinary symptoms that have nearly identical wording to the AUASI and permit computation of AUASI scores. The scale to measure BPH-specific interference with daily activities is based on seven questions regarding the extent to which urinary symptoms interfere with the following: (1) drinking fluids before travelling; (2) drinking fluids before going to bed; (3) driving for 2 h without stopping; (4) getting enough sleep at night; (5) going to places that have no toilet; (6) playing outdoor sports such as golf; and (7) going to the cinema, theatre or church. Each question is scored from 0 (none of the time) to 4 (all of the time). Thus, a composite score describing the extent of interference with living activities can be calculated by adding the responses, with possible scores ranging from 0 to 28. This questionnaire has been used not only in the OCS but also in the Forth Valley, Scotland study[26-30] and the Shimamaki-mura, Japan study.[33,34]

Additional information obtained on all men in the OCS includes access to and use of health care, physician consultation during the past year for urinary problems, insurance status, family income, current medications, alcoholic and non-alcoholic beverage intake, smoking history, marital status, personal medical history, family medical history and other demographic information.

The OCS includes biennial post-based follow-up questionnaires on the full cohort through 1996, with planned longer-term follow-up studies of medical care utilization and outcomes using the medical records database of the Rochester Epidemiology Project. A randomly chosen subset of approximately one-quarter of the OCS cohort (about 475 men) also had a baseline urological evaluation that included the following: digital rectal examination, prostate size determined by transrectal ultrasound, residual urine measurements by abdominal ultrasound, urinalysis, serum creatinine, prostate-specific antigen (PSA) determination and serum storage. The 3-year follow-up clinical evaluation has recently been completed and a 5-year follow-up is planned.

Initial results

Publications to date from the baseline phase of the study have included reports on the following: BPH symptom prevalence;[32] impact of urinary symptoms on quality of life;[35] comparison of symptoms and their impact on living activities in Scottish and American men;[36] relationships among symptoms, prostate volume and peak urinary flow rate;[37] community-based age-specific reference ranges for urinary flow rates;[25] community-based age-specific reference ranges for PSA;[38] health-care-seeking behaviour for urinary symptoms;[39] the relationship between health-care-seeking behaviour and worry and embarrassment from urinary symptoms;[40] cigarette smoking and prostatism;[41] family history in association with prostatism;[42] factors associated with discordance between the frequency and the extent of bother in urinary symptoms;[43] the potential impact of BPH practice guidelines on health-care utilization;[5] comparison of prevalence rates and health-care-seeking behaviour of survey responders and non-responders;[44] effect of several different recruitment strategies on survey response rates;[45] and the role of community-based studies in evaluating treatment effects in BPH.[1] Although some of these findings have been discussed previously, it is worth summarizing some of the published findings here.

Health-related quality of life and symptoms of BPH.
Girman and colleagues[35] found that men with moderate to severe voiding symptoms had about four to six times more bother and interference with daily activities and twice the level of worry experienced by men with mild symptoms. This study also confirmed original clinic-based studies,[19] in which an AUASI of 8 or more was found to differentiate men with and without some degree of bother due to urinary symptoms. These results show that moderate to severe urinary symptoms have a significant impact on patients' lives in terms of the degree of bother, worry, interference with living activities and psychological well-being. The results also provide further support for the validity of an AUASI (or I-PSS) score of 8 as defining the lower limit of moderate symptoms.

Health-care-seeking behaviour and urinary symptoms.
Even though symptom severity is an important determinant of health-care-seeking behaviour for treatment of urinary symptoms, it is neither sensitive nor specific as a predictor of health-care-seeking behaviour.[39] Worsening of symptoms over the past year was found to be a statistically significant independent predictor of health-care-seeking behaviour, even after controlling for symptom severity. This suggests that perception of change for the worse is an additional determinant of health-care-seeking behaviour. Age was found to be the most highly predictive determinant of health-care-seeking behaviour. This implies that there are unidentified age-related factors, other than symptoms or patient demographics, which influence health-care-seeking for urinary symptoms. Identification of such factors may help account for at least some of the large amount of variation that has been found in BPH treatment patterns, both within the United States and between European countries.[39]

Relationship among symptoms, prostate volume and peak urinary flow rate.
Most previous studies of the relationships among symptoms, prostate volume and peak flow rates have been conducted as clinic-based studies. To determine how these relationships would apply in a community-based study, an analysis of baseline data from the OCS was conducted based on data from 466 men.[37] Age was found to explain only about 3% of the variability in symptom scores, while prostate volume and peak flow rate explained only an additional 10%. However, the odds of moderate to severe symptoms, adjusting for age, were 3.5 times higher for men who had prostate volumes above 50 ml than for those who did not. The correlation between prostate volume and AUASI was 0.185, which was similar in magnitude to the correlation of prostate volume and urinary flow rate of -0.214, but lower in magnitude than the correlation between symptoms and peak flow rate of -0.35. Because of the large number of patients involved, all of these correlations were statistically significant ($p < 0.001$). The correlations between physiological measurements and symptoms, though relatively weak, are stronger than the correlations of 0.09–0.14 found in clinic-based studies and are roughly compatible with correlations between physiological measures and symptoms in other chronic diseases.[46]

Urinary flow-rate norms. An example of the value of obtaining population-based age-specific normal ranges of parameters commonly used to evaluate treatment effects is given by studies of urinary flow rates. Normal ranges for urinary flow rates have often been based on selected groups of patients from clinics or referral practices. On the basis of such information, urinary flow rates of less than 12 ml/s have been identified as indicative of obstruction.[47] However, the *median* value of the maximum urinary flow rate among the 268 randomly selected history-negative men aged 70–79 years in the OCS was found to be 12 ml/s.[1,25] Clinical evaluation of the randomly chosen one-quarter sample of the OCS found no man who was judged to require treatment. These results suggest that flow rates in the range of 12 ml/s may have poor specificity as indicators of obstruction, especially in older men. This result is consistent with earlier findings of Jensen and colleagues in a Danish population-based study, discussed above.[24]

Shimamaki-mura, Japan study

A community-based cohort study of urological symptoms and health status is being conducted in Shimamaki-mura, a small fishing village on the west coast of the island of Hokkaido in northern Japan, using a study design very close to that used in the OCS. Symptoms, urinary flow rates, prostate size measurements, hormonal measurements and serum PSA measurements have been obtained on 274 men between 40 and 79 years of age, as part of the baseline phase of this study.[33] In this study the age-specific prevalence of moderate to severe symptoms was somewhat higher than that in Olmsted County.[33] Peak urinary flow rates were somewhat higher in Japanese men than in American men (21.3 ± 0.6 ml/s vs 17.2 ± 0.4 ml/s, $p<0.0001$), although the estimated rate of decline with increasing age was greater for Japanese men than for American men (3 ml/s per decade of age for Japanese men compared with 1 ml/s for American men). The American men had larger prostates than the Japanese men, even after adjusting for weight, height and age. The increase in prostate size with increasing age was about 6 cm^3 per decade of age in the American population compared with about 3 cm^3 per decade of age in the Japanese population.[34]

Maastricht study

A survey of urinary symptoms and physician visits was conducted in all 2734 male patients aged 55 years and older, registered in ten general practices in Maastricht, Netherlands.[48] Responses were obtained from 1692 subjects, yielding a response rate of 64%. The authors noted that all Dutch inhabitants are registered with local general practices, so this survey was considered to represent a sample of the general male population of Maastricht. The symptom questionnaire used in this study was based on that of Boyarsky but differed from that used in the OCS and the Forth Valley, Scotland study. Hence direct comparisons are problematic, although the authors noted symptom prevalences within the same general range as in Scotland and lower than in Olmsted County. The percentage of men with physician visits for urinary conditions within the past 5 years (25%) appears to be considerably higher than the percentage of men in Olmsted County or Scotland consulting a physician for urinary conditions within the past 1 year (approximately 6%). The authors concluded that more information is needed to identify determinants of health-care-seeking behaviour for urinary symptoms.

Washtenaw County study

This study involved a probability sample of 802 community-dwelling men aged 60 years and older in Washtenaw County, Michigan (65% response rate). Approximately 20% of the men reported having had prior prostate surgery at baseline. Among those with no history of surgery at baseline, 35% reported at least one of six symptoms of voiding difficulty, while 15% reported two or more symptoms.[49] The six symptoms were hesitancy, straining, weak stream, interrupted stream, need to void twice to empty the bladder completely, or use of a catheter in the past 6 months. Non-urological conditions related to the presence of moderate to severe symptoms of prostatism included the use of sedatives or tranquillizers, arthritis, poor health status and transient ischaemic attacks. In follow-up surveys taken 1 year and 2 years later, substantial remissions and exacerbations were noted in the absence of any treatment. In each of the two follow-up years approximately 3% of men with no history of prostate surgery underwent prostatectomy.

Summary

Recent population-based studies in several different countries have confirmed that mild urinary symptoms are very common among men aged 50 years and older. While moderate to severe urinary symptoms are clearly less common than mild symptoms, their prevalence shows considerable variability among surveys. One consistent finding among studies in Olmsted County, in Scotland and in France is that symptoms classified as mild (I-PSS≤7) are associated with little bother, whereas those classified as moderate (I-PSS 8–19) and severe (I-PSS 20–35) are associated with increasingly higher levels of bother.[18,25,36] Increasing symptoms are clearly associated with greater interference with living activities and with poorer scores on many indices of health-related quality of life. The relative non-specificity of urinary flow-rate measurements has been confirmed in several population-based studies.[24,25] While correlations among symptoms, prostate size and urinary flow rates are relatively low, they are in the same general range as correlations between measures of other chronic diseases.[37] Symptom frequency and symptom bother together explain only a small proportion of the variation in health-care-seeking behaviour for treatment of urinary symptoms.[39] Ongoing population-based studies of urinary symptoms have made substantial contributions to epidemiological knowledge of BPH. However, it is evident that the results obtained to date have mainly served to identify areas in which knowledge is especially lacking. Further research is needed to understand factors related to patient decision-making and health perceptions in this disease.

Appendix: sampling methods used in BPH population studies

One method of obtaining a representative sample from a geographically defined population is to attempt to enrol all eligible members of the population. This approach is useful only when the geographically defined population is a small community. One example where this technique was used was in the small fishing village, Shimamaki-mura, on the island of Hokkaido, Japan. A closely related approach, which also works only for small communities, is to attempt to enrol all eligible patients in all primary care practices serving a community. For this approach to yield a truly population-based study, it is necessary that essentially all eligible residents of the community be registered with these practices and that all urological care be referred through the primary care practices. This approach was used in studies in the Forth Valley, Scotland and in a part of Maastricht, Netherlands.

When the population is too large to make it feasible to enrol all eligible residents, it is necessary to base the study on a sample from the defined population. A truly population-based study should be based on a *probability sample*, which is one in which every eligible resident of the population has a known, non-zero probability of being included in the sample.[50] Statistics based on such samples can be extrapolated to provide unbiased estimates, of known precision, of quantities in the geographically defined population from which they were drawn. One example of such a study is the OCS. In this study the sample was an age-stratified random sample, so that within each 5-year age stratum (e.g. 40–44, 45–49, and so on) every single eligible resident had an equal probability of being sampled. The sampling was conducted from a list that included over 90% of all residents of the county in the age range of interest.

When there is no complete listing of all residents of the defined population, the techniques for drawing a probability sample approach the problem in a series of stages. For national surveys the sampling first samples geographic regions, then localities within the regions, then blocks or land tracts within the localities, and then households within each block or tract. At each stage the sampling probability is known and so the results can be extrapolated back to produce national estimates of known precision. The response rate can also be calculated, according to accepted rules.[20,50] This is the method of probability sampling used in the French national survey of urinary symptoms and quality of life.[17]

References

1. Guess H A, Jacobsen S J, Girman C J et al. The role of community-based longitudinal studies in evaluating treatment effect — example: benign prostatic hyperplasia. Med Care 1995; 33: AS26–35

2. Ransohoff D F, Feinstein A R. Problems of spectrum and bias in evaluating the efficacy of diagnostic tests. N Engl J Med 1978; 299: 926–930

3. Kulka R A, Schlenger W E, Fairbank J A et al. Validating questions against clinical evaluations: a recent example using diagnostic

interview schedule-based and other measures of post-traumatic stress disorder. In: Fowler F J Jr (ed) Health survey research methods — conference proceedings. DHHS Publication No. (PHS) 89-3447. Hyattsville: National Center for Health Services Research and Health Care Technology Assessment, US Department of Health and Human Services, 1989: 29–34

4. Barry M J, Mulley A G Jr, Fowler F J, Wennberg J W. Watchful waiting vs immediate transurethral resection for symptomatic prostatism. The importance of patients' preferences. JAMA 1988; 259: 3010–3017

5. Jacobsen S J, Guess H A, Girman C J et al. Diagnosis and treatment guidelines for benign prostatic hyperplasia: potential impact in the community. Arch Intern Med 1995; 155: 477–481

6. Melton L J III. Selection bias in the referral of patients and the natural history of surgical conditions. Mayo Clin Proc 1985; 60: 880–889

7. Ballard D J, Duncan P W. Role of population-based epidemiologic surveillance in clinical practice guideline development. Forum methodology manual for guideline development. Hyattsville: Agency for Health Care Policy and Research, 1995

8. Ballard D J, Bryant S C, O'Brien P C et al. Referral selection bias in the Medicare hospital mortality prediction model: are centers of referral for Medicare beneficiaries necessarily centers of excellence? Health Serv Res 1994; 28: 771–784

9. Anderson C. Measuring what works in health care [News and Comment]. Science 1994; 263: 1080–1082

10. Ellenberg J H, Nelson K B. Sample selection and the natural history of disease — studies of febrile seizures. JAMA 1980; 243: 1337–1340

11. Barry M J. Epidemiology and natural history of benign prostatic hyperplasia. Urol Clin North Am 1990; 17: 495–507

12. Boyle P, McGinn R, Maisonneuve P et al. Epidemiology of benign prostatic hyperplasia: present knowledge and studies needed. Eur Urol 1991; 20(suppl 2): 3–10

13. Guess H A. Benign prostatic hyperplasia: antecedents and natural history. Epidemiol Rev 1993; 14: 131–153

14. Guess H A. Epidemiology and natural history of benign prostatic hyperplasia. Urol Clin North Am 1995; 22: 247–261

15. Sagnier P P, Macfarlane G, Richard F et al. Adaptation et validation en langue française du score international des symptômes de l'hypertrophie bénigne de la prostate. Prog Urol 1994; 4: 532–540

16. Sagnier P P, Macfarlane G, Richard F et al. Adaptation and cultural validation in French language of the International Prostate Symptom Score and Quality of Life Assessment. In: Cockett A T K, Khoury S, Aso Y et al. (eds) Proc 2nd International Consultation on Benign Prostatic Hyperplasia. Paris 27–30 June 1993. Paris: SCI, 1993: 144–147

17. Sagnier P P, Macfarlane G, Richard F et al. Results of an epidemiological survey employing a modified American Urological Association Index for benign prostatic hyperplasia in France. J Urol 1994; 151: 1266–1270

18. Sagnier P P, Macfarlane G, Teillac P et al. Impact of symptoms of prostatism on bothersomeness and quality of life of men in the French community. J Urol 1995; 153: 669–673

19. Barry M J, Fowler F J, O'Leary M P et al. The American Urological Association symptom index for benign prostatic hyperplasia. J Urol 1993; 148: 1549–1557

20. Frankel L R. On the definition of response rates. A special report of the CASRO task force on completion rates. Port Jefferson, New York: Council of American Survey Research Organizations, 1982

21. Guess H A. Prevalence of benign prostatic hyperplasia in community surveys. In: Garraway W M (ed) The epidemiology of prostate disease. Heidelberg: Springer-Verlag, 1995: 121–131

22. Stephenson W P, Chute C G, Guess H A et al. Incidence and outcome of surgery for benign prostatic hyperplasia among residents of Rochester, Minnesota: 1980–87: a population-based study. Urology 1991; 38(suppl 1): 32–42

23. Teboul F, Ecochard R, Colin C et al. Descriptive analysis of a series of operations for prostatic adenomas in inhabitants of Lyon, France, in 1988. Eur Urol 1991; 20(suppl 2): 18–21

24. Jensen K M, Jorgensen J B, Mogensen P et al. Some clinical aspects of uroflowmetry in elderly males. A population survey. Scand J Urol Nephrol 1986; 20: 93–99

25. Girman C J, Panser L A, Chute C G et al. Natural history of prostatism: urinary flow rates in a population-based study. J Urol 1993; 150: 887–892

26. Garraway W M, Collins G N, Lee R J. High prevalence of benign prostatic hypertrophy in the community. Lancet 1991; 338: 469–471

27. Garraway W, McKelvie G, Rogers A, Hehir M. Benign prostatic hypertrophy influences on daily living in middle-aged and elderly men. In: Guiliani L, Puppo P (eds) Urology. Bologna: Monduzzi Editore, 1992: 161–164

28. Garraway W M, Armstrong C, Auld S et al. Follow-up of a cohort of men with untreated benign prostatic hyperplasia. Eur Urol 1993; 24: 313–318

29. Garraway W M, Russell E B, Lee R J et al. Impact of previously unrecognized benign prostatic hyperplasia on the daily activities of middle-aged and elderly men. Br J Gen Pract 1993; 43: 318–321

30. Tsang K K, Garraway W M. Impact of benign prostatic hyperplasia on general well-being of men. Prostate 1993; 23: 1–7

31. Epstein R S, Deverka P A, Chute C G et al. Validation of a new quality of life questionnaire for benign prostatic hyperplasia. J Clin Epidemiol 1992; 45: 1431–1445

32. Chute C G, Panser L A, Girman C J et al. The prevalence of prostatism: a population-based survey of urinary symptoms. J Urol 1993; 150: 85–89

33. Tsukamoto T, Kumamoto Y, Masumori N et al. Prevalence of prostatism in Japanese men in a population-based study with comparison to a similar American study. J Urol 1995; 154: 391–395

34. Tsukamoto T, Kumamoto Y, Masumori N et al. Japanese men have lower increase in prostate growth and greater decrease in peak urinary flow rate with age than American men. J Urol, in press

35. Girman C J, Epstein R S, Jacobsen S J et al. Natural history of prostatism: impact of urinary symptoms on quality of life in 2115 randomly selected community men. Urology 1994; 44: 825–831

36. Guess H A, Chute C G, Garraway W M et al. Similar level of urologic symptoms have similar impact in Scottish and American men — though Scots report less symptoms. J Urol 1993; 150: 1701–1705

37. Girman C J, Jacobsen S J, Guess H A et al. Natural history of prostatism: relationship among symptoms, prostate volume, and peak urinary flow. J Urol 1995; 153: 1510–1515

38. Oesterling J E, Jacobsen S J, Chute C G et al. Serum prostate-specific antigen in a community-based population of healthy men. Establishment of age-specific reference ranges. JAMA 1993; 270: 860–864

39. Jacobsen S J, Guess H A, Panser L A et al. A population-based study of health-care-seeking behaviour for treatment of urinary symptoms — the Olmsted County Study of urinary symptoms and health status among men. Arch Fam Med 1993; 2: 729–735

40. Roberts R O, Rhodes T, Panser L A et al. Natural history of prostatism: worry and embarrassment from urinary symptoms and health-care-seeking behaviour. Urology 1994; 43: 621–628

41. Roberts R O, Jacobsen S J, Rhodes T et al. Cigarette smoking and prostatism: a biphasic association? Urology 1994; 43: 797–801

42. Roberts R O, Rhodes T, Girman C J et al. Family history of prostatism. Am J Epidemiol 1995, in press

43. Jacobsen S J, Girman C J, Guess H A et al. Natural history of prostatism: factors associated with discordance between frequency and bother of urinary symptoms. Urology 1993; 42: 663–671

44. Panser L A, Chute C G, Larson-Keller J J et al. Comparison of prevalence rates and health-care-seeking behaviour among survey responders and non-responders: the Olmsted County study of urinary symptoms and health status among men. Am J Epidemiol 1993; 138: 642

45. Panser L A, Chute C G, Girman C J et al. Response rates in a prospective cohort study: effect of several recruitment strategies. Ann Epidemiol 1994; 4: 321-326

46. Wilson I B, Cleary P D. Linking clinical variables with health-related quality of life — a conceptual model of patient outcomes. JAMA 1995; 273: 59–65

47. Cockett A T, Barry M J, Holtgrewe H L et al. Indications for treatment of benign prostatic hyperplasia. The American Urological Association Study. Cancer 1992; 70(suppl 1): 280–283

48. Wolfs G G M C, Knottnerus J A, Janknegt R A. Prevalence and detection of micturition problems among 2,734 elderly men. J Urol 1994; 152: 1467–1470

49. Diokno A C, Brown M B, Goldstein N, Herzog A R. Epidemiology of bladder emptying symptoms in elderly men. J Urol 1992; 148: 1817–1821

50. Levy P S, Lemeshow S. Sampling of populations: methods and applications. New York: Wiley, 1991: 17–18

Overview and definition of BPH

Benign prostatic hyperplasia (BPH) is an extraordinarily common disease of older men. In the United States alone, 329 000 transurethral prostatectomies were performed in 1990.[1] Despite a modest decline in the number of operations since 1987, prostatectomy is still the second most common major operation, after cataract surgery, performed on Medicare-aged men. About 1.2 million office visits, primarily for BPH, were made to urologists in 1990,[2] and literally millions of older men experience symptoms attributable to BPH. Most men manage these symptoms for years, using simple lifestyle modifications, which when supervised by a physician, are part of a strategy termed 'watchful waiting'.[3]

Despite the high prevalence of BPH, the natural history of this condition has been described in the medical literature for only a small fraction of these men. Epidemiological study of BPH has been difficult, in part, because there are no widely accepted standardized diagnostic criteria.[4,5] BPH, at the histological level, refers to prostatic cellular proliferation which may be detected, at clinical level, as prostatic enlargement on digital rectal examination (DRE) or imaging studies. Prostatic enlargement, in turn, may produce characteristic lower urinary tract symptoms or evidence of physiological obstruction on urodynamic measurement. The prevalence of BPH, or how many men in the population at a given time have the condition, varies widely, depending upon which of these features are incorporated into the case definition. Guess[6] has summarized this point in Figure 11.1, which reveals that, although the prevalence of BPH increases with age, regardless of which of several case definitions are used, within each age group there is dramatic

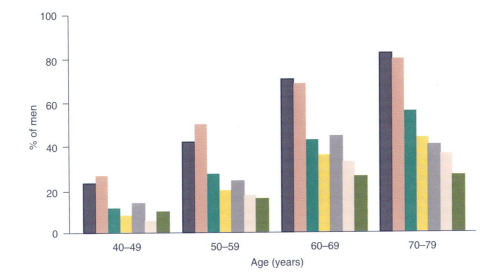

Figure 11.1. *Age-specific prevalence of BPH according to clinical features incorporated into the case definition. Bar 1 (■): pathologically defined BPH from a compilation of five autopsy studies. Bar 2 (■): Clinically defined BPH based on both history and DRE in the Baltimore Longitudinal Study of Aging (BLSA). Bar 3 (■): BPH defined by DRE alone in the BLSA. Bar 4 (■): BPH defined by DRE in a compilation of life insurance examinations. Bar 5 (■): BPH defined by symptoms, DRE and urinary flow rates in a Scottish community. Bar 6 (■): BPH defined by symptoms, DRE and urinary flow rates in Rochester, Minnesota. Bar 7 (■): BPH defined by transrectal ultrasonography in a mass screening study in Japan. (Adapted from ref. 6, with permission.)*

variation in the prevalence of BPH, depending upon how it is defined. Even in the same population[7,8] (bars 2 and 3), simply changing the case definition produces as much as a twofold variation in the age-specific prevalence of BPH. Interpretation of natural history studies, therefore, will depend on which features are used to define cases of BPH.

Natural history studies

Natural history refers to the progression of a disease over time without treatment. Studies of the natural history of BPH can help clinicians inform their patients about the possible outcomes of BPH and the frequencies with which these outcomes might occur. In addition, the effectiveness of different treatments for BPH can be judged only with respect to their contribution to a difference in outcomes beyond what can be expected with time alone. Prospective cohort studies best describe the natural history of BPH. Ideally, individuals representative of the population of interest are identified at a well-defined inception point in their illness and followed for outcomes defined by objective criteria.[9] Placebo arms of clinical trials can also provide information on the course of an untreated disease. However, subjects in these trials tend to be less representative of the general population, and placebo treatment may well have some measurable clinical effect.[10] Most of the relatively sparse evidence on the natural history of BPH comes from cohort studies of men presenting to urologists or primary care physicians. Studies of BPH defined at presentation to a physician probably miss a considerable period in the natural history of the condition but can provide valuable information. However, such data need to be interpreted with caution. Studies of disease natural history based on patients presenting for medical care are likely to be subject to selection bias, which can vary in complex ways because patients differ in their threshold for bringing symptoms to the attention of physicians, primary care physicians differ in their testing and referral thresholds, and urologists differ in their thresholds to perform surgery.[11–13] Observed variations in outcomes in non-population-based studies may be at least partly due to variation in patient selection.[14] Guess[14] has shown that the distribution of 'normal'

values for urinary flow rates or prostate-specific antigen (PSA), for example, obtained in a community-based study is very different from that of values obtained in clinic-based studies or from placebo arms of randomized trials. Our understanding of the natural history of BPH will be influenced not only by the way in which the condition is defined but by how patients are found for inclusion in studies.

For men with BPH, urinary symptoms primarily produce the morbidity of the condition. Urologists report that about 30% of prostatectomies are performed solely for the relief of symptoms, and symptom relief is at least one of the indications for surgery in over 90% of operations.[15] Patients considering treatment may want to know whether their symptoms will become worse, stay the same or improve over time. Patients and their doctors may also be concerned about the possibility of acute urinary retention, renal failure, serious urinary tract infection, bladder decompensation or urinary tract calculi. Clinicians may also want to know whether symptoms, urodynamic findings or other clinical features can predict the need for prostatectomy.

Natural history of urinary symptoms in men with BPH

Several cohort studies have followed men after presentation to a physician with apparent BPH. In the first such study, Clarke[16] retrospectively examined the outcomes of 36 men who were felt to have definite BPH but did not have absolute indications for surgery at baseline. The diagnosis was based on symptoms, rectal examination and cystoscopic findings. These men had a mean age of 64 years, had symptoms for an average of 3 years before presentation, and had records describing about 3.5 years of follow-up. Over this period, 25 of the men had symptomatic improvement lasting about 2 years, and 31 men had either symptomatic improvement or stable symptoms over almost 3 years. At the end of the follow-up period, 12 men had undergone prostatectomy. The indications for prostatectomy were not clearly defined.

Craigen and colleagues[17] described 212 men with a mean age of 70 years who presented to 59 general practitioners in the United Kingdom with 'any symptoms related to their bladder function', presumably suggesting BPH. The case definition was not further specified. Men with evidence of prostate cancer were excluded. Of the 212 men, 89 presented with acute urinary retention and 123 presented with 'prostatic symptoms' but without retention. The patients were followed by their general practitioners on a sporadic basis for more than 6 years, although fewer than 100 men were followed beyond the first year. After 4–7 years of follow-up, 29 of 60 men who had not undergone prostatectomy in the interim had no urinary symptoms. This proportion was similar for men with and without acute retention when first seen. The specific nature of the urinary symptoms and how they changed over time was not specified.

Birkoff and colleagues[18] reported outcomes for a small cohort of 26 men with prostatism but without absolute indications for surgery. These highly selected men had declined treatment with experimental drugs for BPH but were followed up none the less at 3- to 6-month intervals for 3 years. Clearly defined criteria were used to describe the degree of symptoms at baseline and in follow-up. At the end of 3 years, seven men (27%) had improvement in symptoms, four (15%) were unchanged and 15 (58%) were worse.

Ball and colleagues[19] reported outcomes for a group of British men less highly selected than the men in the Birkoff series. They studied 107 men seen at a urology practice for symptoms suggesting BPH and who, for unspecified reasons, did not initially undergo prostatectomy. The men were contacted 5 years after their initial presentation to determine outcomes in the interim. These men had a mean age of 62 years at baseline; 53 had evidence of bladder outflow obstruction by simultaneous pressure–flow studies. Ten men had subsequently undergone prostatectomy. Of the 97 men who did not have surgery, 16 (17%) felt that their overall symptoms had worsened, 50 (52%) felt that they were about the same and 31 (32%) thought that their symptoms had improved over 5 years. Whereas about half the men in this series who had symptoms suggestive of BPH were not found to have urodynamic parameters consistent with physiological obstruction, all ten men who had surgery in the interim (two for acute retention and eight for worsened symptoms) were in fact urodynamically obstructed as judged by their baseline pressure–flow studies. Although the case definition of

BPH in this study included men without objective physiological evidence of bladder outflow obstruction, this series is closer to an inception cohort than Birkoff's series and suggests a slower progression of symptoms over time, with more than two-thirds of men having stable or improved symptoms over 5 years.

Diokno and colleagues[20] studied the prevalence and progression of bladder-emptying symptoms by interviewing a random sample of 802 men aged 60 years and older living in Washtenaw County, Michigan. Men who had used a urinary catheter or who had three or more lower urinary tract symptoms (including a weak stream, hesitancy, pushing or straining, or an interrupted stream) were defined as having severe symptoms, men with two symptoms were defined as having moderate symptoms and men with only one symptom were defined as having mild symptoms. After 1 year, 68% of the men were re-interviewed. Again, most men's symptoms had waxed and waned. Of men with no bladder-emptying symptoms at baseline, 12% had developed mild symptoms, 3% moderate symptoms and 1% severe symptoms 1 year later. Of men with severe symptoms at baseline, 23% had no symptoms, 17% had mild symptoms and 11% had moderate symptoms 1 year later.

Placebo arms of randomized trials of pharmacological agents for the treatment of BPH have also provided information on the natural history of symptoms.[4,10] Table 11.1 displays symptom data from selected clinical trials that include patients treated with placebo. In these trials, 10–70% of men had symptomatic improvement over 1 month to 1 year of follow-up. Symptom improvement may have been due to a tendency for BPH symptoms to improve spontaneously over the short term, as well as to the effect of placebo treatment itself. Although these trials were all a year, or considerably less, in duration, the natural history of symptoms in placebo-treated patients is consistent with the evidence from observational studies that there is considerable variability in the progression of symptoms in men with BPH. The results also underscore the importance of including placebo control-treatment arms in any evaluation of new treatment modalities for BPH.

Table 11.1. *Results of placebo arms in selected randomized clinical trials of pharmacological interventions for symptomatic BPH*

Reference	Duration (weeks)	Number (placebo)	Response (%)*		
			Worse	Same	Better
Abrams (1977)	26	29	14	52	34
Geller (1979)	20	33	0	42	58
Hedlund (1983)	4	20	20	10	70
Resnick (1983)	52	22	5	59	36
Carbin (1990)	12	27	19	70	11
Kawabe (1990)	4	54	2	42	56
Jardin (1991)	26	132	0	27	73

*Responses are patients' global assessments of symptom change. The listed references can be found in ref. 57. (Adapted from ref. 57 with permission.)

Risk for prostatectomy in men with BPH

The Craigen series[17] provides some information on the rate of prostatectomy in men presenting with probable BPH. The cumulative incidence of prostatectomy over time was calculated using a life-table analysis to account for different durations of observation due to death or loss to follow-up. Cumulative incidence refers to the proportion of new prostatectomy cases occurring in a population over a specified period. For men presenting with acute retention, the cumulative incidence of prostatectomy was projected to be 60% at 1 year and 80% at 7 years; for men presenting without retention, the cumulative incidence of prostatectomy was projected to be 35% at 1 year and 45% at 7 years. The indications for prostatectomy in these men were not specified, and no combinations of symptoms or rectal examination findings at baseline were significantly associated with prostatectomy.

In the Diokno series,[20] the risk of prostatectomy for all men in the cohort was about 3% per year. About two-thirds of men who underwent prostatectomy over 2 years of follow-up had BPH symptoms at baseline. The symptoms of urinating more than once, interrupted stream, hesitancy and straining were all associated with subsequent prostatectomy during 2 years of follow-up. Although these associations were adjusted for age and overall health status, it is not clear to what extent individual symptoms are independent predictors of incident prostatectomy.

The Baltimore Longitudinal Study on Aging (BLSA) has also provided information on risk factors for

undergoing prostatectomy.[7,8] Symptom questionnaires and physical examinations have been administered to 1057 men in the BLSA cohort without a baseline history of prostatectomy or prostate cancer over up to 30 years of follow-up. Multivariate proportional hazards regression analysis was used to predict prostatectomy, controlling for both variable length of follow-up and all factors that may be associated with prostatectomy. In this study, increasing age was the predominant risk factor for undergoing prostatectomy. Of specific symptoms sought by the BLSA questionnaire, change in the size and force of the urinary stream and a sensation of incomplete emptying were both, independently, positively associated with prostatectomy. Prostatic enlargement on rectal examination was also independently associated with prostatectomy. Of 464 men with none of these risk factors, only 3% eventually required surgery. For 303 men with one risk factor, the cumulative incidence of surgery was 9%; for 178 men with two risk factors it was about 16%; and for 112 men with all three, about 37%. Table 11.2 demonstrates that the risk for prostatectomy is a function both of age and the presence of risk factors. Men over the age of 70 without risk factors have more than six times the risk of prostatectomy after 10 years as do men in their 40s; the risk increases to 11-fold in the presence of risk factors. The BLSA findings can be compared with a similar analysis in the Veteran Affairs Normative Aging Study (VANAS).[21] In the VANAS, the experiences of 1868 men aged 49–68 years without prostate cancer were analysed after 20–25 years of follow-up. Only the symptoms of nocturia and hesitancy emerged as independent predictors of prostatectomy; prostatic

Table 11.2. *Age-specific predicted cumulative incidence of prostatectomy over 10 and 20 years for men in the Baltimore Longitudinal Study of Aging with or without risk factors**

| | Cumulative incidence of prostatectomy (%) | | | |
| | No risk factors | | Risk factors | |
Patient age (years)	10 years	20 years	10 years	20 years
40–49	2	4	3	13
50–59	2	9	7	24
60–69	9	22	16	39
70+	13	–	34	41

*Any obstructive symptoms and prostatic enlargement on DRE. (Adapted from ref. 8 with permission.)

enlargement on physical examination was not associated with having undergone surgery. Risk factors for surgery for BPH were also sought in a study of 16 219 men at least 40 years old who were members of Kaiser Permanente of Northern California (a major prepaid health plan).[22] Subjects were given a multiphasic health check-up that included questions about urological symptoms. After a mean of 12 years of follow-up, 1027 men had undergone surgery for BPH. Using multivariate proportional hazards regression analysis, a variety of factors including age and five urological symptoms (dysuria, loss of bladder control, trouble starting urination, nocturia and slow urine stream) were associated with risk of surgery for BPH.

These studies all used different case definitions for BPH, methods for selection of patients and ascertainment of risk factors and indications for prostatectomy. Despite these cautions, these studies reinforce the impression that an increasing burden of urinary symptoms as men age is an important source of morbidity in BPH as well as an important determinant of incident prostatectomy.

Complications of BPH

Progression of urodynamic parameters

There is very little information on the natural history of basic urodynamic parameters in men with BPH. In the Ball series,[19] 64 of the original 107 men had urinary flow rates measured after 5 years of follow-up. The mean peak flow rate fell from 13.1 to 11.9 ml/s, and only six men had a decrease greater than 1.2 standard deviations on the Siroky[23] nomogram (felt to represent evidence of a significant within-patient increase in urethral

resistance). Only three of these patients actually perceived a diminution in urine flow.

Drach and colleagues[24] calculated a decrease in flow rate due to normal ageing of about 2.1 ml/s per decade. This decrement seemed to be blunted in patients with bladder outlet obstruction and low baseline flow rates. The distribution of flow rates as a function of age and voided volume in a community-based population has recently been described by Girman and colleagues.[25] Longitudinal follow-up of these men should considerably enhance our understanding of changes in uroflow over time.

Acute urinary retention

Acute urinary retention is a relatively common complication of BPH and in the United States is the indication for surgery in 25–30% of patients.[15,26] As with progression of urinary symptoms, the rate of acute retention varies dramatically among studies. In the Craigen series,[17] the cumulative incidence of acute retention using life-table analysis was projected to be 10% at 7 years, or 0.015 episodes of retention per person-year. In the Birkoff series,[18] nine of 26 patients developed ten episodes of acute retention over an unspecified length of follow-up. The acute retention rate, assuming each patient had 3 years of follow-up (the minimum period), may have been as high as 0.13 per person-year. The acute retention rate was much lower in the Ball series,[19] where only two of 107 patients had acute retention over 5 years. If the ten patients who had a prostatectomy did so halfway through the follow-up period, on average, then the incidence of acute retention was about 0.004 episodes per person-year.

Even among the 53 patients who were classified as urodynamically obstructed at baseline, the acute retention rate was still only 0.008 episodes per person-year. Among men in the placebo arm of the phase III clinical trials of finasteride (Proscar), the incidence of acute urinary retention was about 0.02 per person-year (H. Guess, personal communication). These incidence rates translate into 10-year risks of acute retention that vary widely, from as low as 4% (using data from all patients in the Ball series) to as high as 73% (using data from the Birkoff series).

Patients and clinicians may want to know what to expect after a first episode of acute retention. Although most patients undergo immediate prostatectomy, a few series have reported on the untreated course in these men. In the Craigen series,[17] 55% of patients had a prostatectomy within 3 months of their episode of acute retention, but 20% had not, even 7 years after presentation. In another series, 73% of 59 Danish men who presented to an emergency department with acute urinary retention due to BPH had recurrent retention within a week.[27] In a more recent series, 72% of 60 men with acute urinary retention due to BPH had an unsuccessful voiding trial.[28] The probability of a successful trial did not depend on whether the catheter was removed immediately or after 24 or 48 h. Bladder volume at the time of initial catheter insertion was the strongest predictor of a successful voiding trial: 15 of 34 men with a volume of less than 900 ml had a successful trial, as opposed to two of 26 men with a volume of more than 900 ml. Of 17 men with a successful voiding trial, none had recurrent acute retention over the next 6 months; six of these underwent prostatectomy for severe symptoms, six had minor symptoms and five were asymptomatic. None of these series indicate whether a longer period of catheter drainage and bladder decompression would result in a higher proportion of successful voiding trials. Longer drainage might be helpful, both to allow resolution of oedema if there is prostatic infarction,[29] and to allow recovery of bladder contractility.

Chronic renal failure due to obstructive uropathy

Although chronic renal failure is a feared complication of urinary obstruction in BPH,[30,31] its true frequency is not well defined. None of the patients in the natural history series reviewed in this chapter developed obstructive uropathy, but the small numbers of patients in these studies would not allow a low but clinically important rate of chronic renal failure to be measured. Case reports document that this complication can occur with minimal BPH symptoms.[32] In series of patients coming to prostatectomy, six of 345 men in Israel had evidence of 'occult progressive renal damage',[33] and 27 of 379 men in Britain had plasma creatinine values above 2.26 mg/dl.[30] In a New Zealand survey of patients admitted to a urology service with the clinical diagnosis of BPH, 35 of 2171 men had a blood urea nitrogen level above 60 mg/dl.[34] At the Boston VA Medical Center, 17 of 100 cases of community-acquired acute renal failure identified over a 17-month period were due to urinary obstruction; 11 of these were attributed to BPH.[35] A survey of admissions to a urological unit in Britain over an 11-year period found that 25% of admissions for acute renal failure were due to obstruction; 14% of these were due to BPH.[36] None of these studies allows estimation of the incidence of renal insufficiency in men with BPH, but they imply that BPH is associated with a small but important fraction of this complication. Research is needed to define better the risk of renal failure due to urinary obstruction. Optimal monitoring strategies for detection of renal insufficiency at a reversible stage in men being managed with watchful waiting remain to be determined.

Serious urinary tract infection

As with chronic renal failure due to obstructive uropathy, the risk of urinary tract infection, especially serious upper tract infection with urosepsis, is not well defined among men with BPH. Recurrent urinary tract infection is the indication for prostatectomy in about 12% of cases in the United States.[15] Although many elderly men with a serious urinary tract infection have bladder outlet obstruction, most men with bladder outlet obstruction do not have serious urinary tract infections; the probability of this complication among men with BPH is probably relatively low. Serious urinary tract infections were not reported in any of the patients in the natural history series reviewed in this chapter.

Bladder decompensation

There is concern that delayed surgical intervention in men with symptomatic BPH may lead to irreversible bladder decompensation. Biopsy samples from trabeculated, chronically obstructed bladders show dense connective tissue deposition.[37,38] Experimental bladder outlet obstruction in animal models also leads to bladder hypertrophy and connective tissue deposition.[39,40] However, there is evidence that the bladder fibrosis seen in older men is a normal consequence of ageing and may not be a consequence of bladder outlet obstruction, as similar changes are seen in older women.[41] In addition, about half of men with bladder outlet obstruction show uninhibited bladder contractions on filling cystometry,[42,43] presumably secondary to obstruction. These findings may sometimes disappear after prostatectomy.

Clinical research studies have not provided supporting evidence that delayed intervention for bladder outlet obstruction leads to irreversible bladder damage and a 'loss to cure'. Even men with evidence of severe bladder decompensation appear to improve after prostatectomy.[32] For example, Jones and colleagues[44] followed 32 men with high-pressure chronic retention of urine for a mean of 43 months after prostatectomy. These men had residual volumes of 320–2690 ml and a mean creatinine clearance of 53 ml/min. Bladder biopsy samples from 23 patients revealed muscular hypertrophy, bladder fibrosis and a reduced density of acetyl cholinesterase-containing nerve fibres. At follow-up, 25 of 32 men had residual volumes less than 200 ml, and the mean creatinine clearance had risen to 83 ml/min. All but one of the men had at least an initial improvement in renal function, although three eventually deteriorated from recurrent obstruction (two due to prostate cancer). Undoubtedly, it is preferable to intervene with prostatectomy before patients get to this late point in the natural history of BPH. Again, however, the appropriate strategy of periodic monitoring to prevent poor outcomes among men with symptomatic BPH has not been defined.

Urinary tract calculi

The prevalence of urinary tract calculi in men with BPH has been best defined by Grosse[45] in a large autopsy series of German men and women. Bladder stones were about eight times more frequent in the men with histological evidence of BPH at autopsy (3.4 vs 0.4%); kidney and ureter stones occurred with nearly equal frequency in men with or without evidence of BPH (6.0 and 5.7%, respectively). BPH appears to predispose to bladder, but not kidney, stones.

Recent data on the natural history of BPH

Review of the few available studies of the natural history of BPH suggests that, in most men, symptoms of bladder outlet obstruction wax and wane considerably over time, but probably progress slowly over years. The risks of symptom progression or complications of BPH, and the risk factors for prostatectomy, remain incompletely defined. There is insufficient information available to recommend an evidence-based clinical protocol for watchful waiting for men with symptomatic BPH. No true inception cohorts of men identified at an early, uniform point in the disease have been identified and followed for sufficient periods. Studies have not used clearly specified case definitions, and methods for measuring symptomatic outcomes have not been clearly specified or validated. The fact that the projected 10-year risk of acute retention varies between 4 and 73% among studies highlights the marked uncertainty about the course of untreated BPH.

Veterans Administration Cooperative Study of transurethral resection of the prostate

Two studies currently under way or recently completed have addressed some of these concerns and are beginning to provide data that will refine our understanding of the natural history of BPH. The first is a Veterans Administration Cooperative Studies Program clinical trial[46] comparing immediate transurethral prostatectomy with a strategy of watchful waiting among male veterans with BPH of sufficient severity to come to the attention of a urologist. The case definition of BPH in this study included men with moderate symptoms of BPH and in whom their urologist would consider performing prostatectomy. Patients were excluded from the study at baseline if they were less than 55 years old; had previous prostate surgery or irradiation; were non-ambulatory; or if they had primary or obstructive azotaemia, refractory urinary tract infection, prostate or bladder cancer, a post-void residual of more than 350 ml, a low total score on a BPH rating algorithm (incorporating findings from cystoscopy, the symptom interview and bladder ultrasonography)[47] or a serious medical co-morbidity. After randomization, about half of the men were followed carefully for 3 years without initial surgery. Both symptoms and urodynamic parameters were measured. Patients were followed for specific 'treatment failures' or for crossover to prostatectomy. Treatment failures included death, repeated or intractable urinary tract infection, residual urine of more than 350 ml as assessed by bladder ultrasound, progression to azotaemia (defined as a doubling of the baseline serum creatinine concentration or a concentration higher than 3.0 mg/dl), the development of bladder stones secondary to infection, new persistent incontinence requiring the use of a pad or device, or a symptom score of 24 points or more at one follow-up visit or of 21 points or more at two consecutive visits.

Watchful waiting was assigned to 276 men. Their mean age was 66 years, mean residual urine volume 113 ml, mean peak urine flow rate 12.5 ml/s, mean symptom score 14.6 points (scale range: 0 = none, 27 = severe), and mean bother from urinary difficulties 46.3 (scale range 0–100, with higher scores corresponding to less bother[48]). Follow-up was 94% complete in men assigned to watchful waiting. Over 3 years of follow-up, 65 men (24%) assigned to watchful waiting crossed over to prostatectomy after randomization at a steady rate of about eight per 100 person-years. Of men assigned to watchful waiting, 47 (17%) suffered a treatment failure, causing 20 of these men to go on to prostatectomy. The most common reason for treatment failure resulting in prostatectomy was high residual urinary volume (11 men). Acute retention resulting in prostatectomy occurred in five cases; overall, eight men assigned to watchful waiting had acute retention, giving an incidence rate of 0.01 per person-year. Only one patient on watchful waiting developed azotaemia. Treatment failure resulting in prostatectomy occurred in eight men due to a high symptom score. Over 40% of men assigned to watchful waiting who were most bothered by urinary difficulties at baseline (score of 55 or less) had improved bother scores after 3 years of follow-up, while about 30%

of men who were least bothered by urinary difficulties at baseline also had improved bother scores. However, among men assigned to watchful waiting, the rate of crossover to surgery over 3 years of follow-up was twice as high in men with high baseline scores for bother from urinary symptoms as for those with low baseline scores (31 vs 16%). In men assigned to watchful waiting who did not crossover to surgery, bother from urinary difficulties improved by 14% in men who were most bothered by urinary symptoms at baseline but worsened by 6% in men who were least bothered at baseline. Peak urinary flow rate remained essentially unchanged over 3 years in men assigned to watchful waiting. For men who were bothered by symptoms of BPH, prostatectomy resulted in a much greater improvement than watchful waiting. Nevertheless, few men assigned to watchful waiting suffered adverse events and many had some improvement over 3 years without surgery.

Shared Decision-Making Program cohort

The second ongoing study providing data on the natural history of BPH recruited subjects to view an interactive computer and video disk-based educational program for men who are facing a treatment decision for BPH.[49] This Shared Decision-Making Program (SDP) was developed by the Patient Outcome Research Team (PORT) for prostatic diseases[50] and has been incorporated into five urological practices in North America. From 1990 to 1993, the first version of the SDP presented the choice between prostatectomy and watchful waiting. Beginning in 1993, a second version of the program also included the options of drug treatment with alpha-blockers or finasteride and balloon dilatation of the prostate.

Starting in 1990, urologists at these sites were encouraged to refer patients in whom they had made a diagnosis of BPH, and whom they considered to be candidates for elective prostatectomy, to view the program before a definite treatment decision was made. The case definition of BPH was thus a clinical diagnosis by a urologist in a man affected enough by his symptoms to be considered for surgical intervention. Men referred by their urologists to view the SDP completed a baseline questionnaire regarding symptom status and quality of life; in addition, their medical records were abstracted to obtain any basic medical and urological data that might have been collected in the course of their 'usual care'. After the baseline evaluation and program viewing, patients collaborated with their urologists to make a decision about treatment. Patients have been followed annually by a mailed questionnaire to reassess symptom status and to enquire if additional treatments for BPH had been given or if complications of BPH, such as acute retention, had developed.

In the early years of the study, symptom severity was measured with a self-administered five-question index developed and validated by the Maine Medical Assessment Program (MMAP) for an outcome study of prostatectomy.[26] The MMAP index has questions covering frequency and intermittency of urination, straining, post-void dribbling and dysuria; responses on a five-point frequency scale are summed to yield a total score with a range from 5 to 25 points. This scale can be divided into mild (5–8 points), moderate (9–12 points) or severe (13–25 points) ranges. When the American Urological Association (AUA) Symptom Index became available,[51] this instrument was added to the baseline and follow-up questionnaires. AUA Symptom Index scores have been shown to correlate closely with MMAP scores ($r = 0.88$) in the same patients.[52]

As of November 1993, 810 men had completed the baseline evaluation. Of these, 43% were less than 65 years old and 28% were more than 70 years old. The MMAP score was in the mild range in 28% of the men, moderate in 49% and severe in 23%. One-year outcome data for 612 men are displayed in Table 11.3. Of men with MMAP scores in the mild range, 6% eventually had surgery; 18% of men with symptoms in the moderate range had surgery; and 34% of men with severe symptoms at baseline ultimately had surgery during the first year of follow-up. As has been seen in previous studies, the change in symptom status over time varied considerably. For example, among men who chose watchful waiting, 11% with symptoms in the mild range at baseline had severe symptoms at follow-up, whereas 4% of men with severe symptoms at baseline had only mild symptoms 1 year later. In addition, of men who chose watchful waiting, only 1% reported an episode of acute urinary retention during the follow-up year.

Summary

BPH is an extraordinarily common medical problem among older men. Despite the high prevalence of BPH, the natural history of only a small fraction of these men has been described in the medical literature. Understanding of the natural history of BPH has been impeded by the lack of a standardized epidemiological definition of BPH, and of its symptoms and complications, and by the lack of true inception cohorts of men followed from an early point in their disease process. Many men with symptoms of BPH do not seek medical attention and clearly must be following a self-imposed regimen of watchful waiting. Symptoms of BPH

Table 11.3. *Twelve-month outcomes after viewing the program for 612 men enrolled in the SDP cohort*

| Outcome | Initial symptom index | | |
	Mild (n=166)	Moderate (n=310)	Severe (n=136)
Surgery within 3 months	6 (4)*	33 (11)	34 (25)
Surgery between 3 and 12 months	3 (2)	21 (7)	12 (9)
Symptom status at 12 months for non-surgical patients:			
Mild	95 (57)	69 (22)	15 (11)
Moderate	55 (33)	136 (44)	35 (26)
Severe	7 (4)	51 (16)	46 (29)
	(100)	(100)	(100)

*Percentages in parentheses. (Adapted from ref. 57 with permission.)

wax and wane, but appear to progress over time, with an apparently small risk of serious complications. However, the safety and effectiveness of watchful waiting, as well as the appropriate strategy of follow-up visits and testing for men in a watchful waiting programme, have not been fully resolved.

Incomplete knowledge of the natural history of BPH has contributed, to some degree, to the controversies that surround the indications for interventions in this condition. This controversy, in turn, has contributed to three- to fourfold variations in the rate of prostatectomy among small, sometimes adjoining, geographical areas both in the United States[53,54] and among countries.[55] This variation phenomenon has engendered opportunities in outcomes research;[56] these and other studies of BPH currently under way will help to clarify our understanding of the epidemiology and natural history of this condition.

Acknowledgements

The assessments of BPH natural history included in this chapter were funded by AHCPR grant number HS 08397. We are indebted to Harry A. Guess MD PhD for helpful comments on an earlier version of this chapter.

References

1. Graves E. Detailed diagnoses and procedures, National Hospital Discharge Survey 1990. In: Vital and health statistics, Vol 13. Hyattsville: National Center for Health Statistics, 1992: 117

2. Woodwell D. Office visits to urologists: United States, 1989–90, National Ambulatory Medical Care Survey. In: Advance data from vital and health statistics, No 234. Hyattsville: National Center for Health Statistics, 1992: 1–12

3. Barry M, Mulley A, Fowler F, Wennberg J. Watchful waiting vs. immediate transurethral resection for symptomatic prostatism: the importance of patients' preferences. JAMA 1988; 259: 3010–3017

4. Barry M. Epidemiology and natural history of benign prostatic hyperplasia. Urol Clin North Am 1990; 17: 495–507

5. Guess H. Epidemiology and natural history of benign prostatic hyperplasia. In: Chisholm G (ed) Handbook of benign prostatic hyperplasia. New York: Raven Press, 1994: 1–18

6. Guess H. Benign prostatic hyperplasia: antecedents and natural history. Epidemiol Rev 1992; 14: 131–153

7. Arrighi H, Guess H, Metter E, Fozard J. Symptoms and signs of prostatism as risk factors for prostatectomy. Prostate 1990; 16: 253–261

8. Arrighi H, Metter E, Guess H, Fozard J. Natural history of benign prostatic hyperplasia and risk of prostatectomy: the Baltimore Longitudinal Study of Ageing. Urology 1991; 38: s4–s8

9. Laupacis S, Wells G, Richardson W, Tugwell P. User's guide to the medical literature V. How to use an article about prognosis. JAMA 1994; 272: 234–237

10. Isaacs J. Importance of the natural history of benign prostatic hyperplasia in the evaluation of pharmacologic intervention. Prostate 1990; 3: 1s–7s

11. Ellenberg J, Nelson K. Sample selection and the natural history of disease — studies of febrile seizures. JAMA 1980; 243: 1337–1340

12. Melton I L. Selection bias in the referral of patients and the natural history of surgical conditions. Mayo Clin Proc 1985; 60: 880–889

13. Ballard D, Bryant S, O'Brien P et al. Referral selection bias in the Medicare hospital mortality prediction model: are centers of referral for Medicare beneficiaries necessarily centers of excellence? Health Serv Res 1994; 28: 771–784

14. Guess H, Jacobsen S, Girman C et al. The role of community-based longitudinal studies in evaluating treatment effects — example: benign prostatic hyperplasia. Med Care 1994; 50: 1–2

15. Mebust W, Holtgrewe H, Cockett A et al. Transurethral prostatectomy: immediate and postoperative complications: a comparative study of 13 participating institutions evaluating 3,885 patients. J Urol 1989; 141: 243–247

16. Clarke R. The prostate and the endocrines: a control series. Br J Urol 1937; 9: 254–271

17. Craigen A, Hickling J, Saunders C, Carpenter R. The natural history of prostatic obstruction: a prospective survey. J R Coll Gen Pract 1969; 18: 226–232

18. Birkoff J, Wiederhorn A, Hamilton M, Zinsser H. Natural history of benign prostatic hypertrohy and acute urinary retention. Urology 1976; 7: 48–52

19. Ball A, Feneley R, Abrams P. The natural history of untreated 'prostatism'. Br J Urol 1981; 53: 613–616

20. Diokno A, Brown M, Goldstein N, Herzog A. Epidemiology of bladder emptying symptoms in elderly men. J Urol 1992; 148: 1817–1821

21. Epstein R, Lydick E, DeLabry L, Vokonas P. Age-related differences in risk factors for prostatectomy for benign prostatic hyperplasia: the VA Normative Ageing Study. Urology 1991; 38: 59–62

22. Sidney S, Quesenberry J C, Sadler M et al. Risk factors for surgically treated benign prostatic hyperplasia in a prepaid health care plan. Urology 1991; 38(suppl 1): 13–19

23. Siroky M, Olsson C, Krane R. The flow-rate nomogram: II. Clinical correlation. J Urol 1980; 123: 208–210

24. Drach G, Layton T, Binard W. Male peak urinary flow rate: relationship to voided volume and age. J Urol 1979; 122: 210–214

25. Girman C, Panser L, Chute C et al. National history of prostatism: urinary flow rates in a community-based study. J Urol 1993; 150: 887–892

26. Fowler F, Wennberg J, Timothy R et al. Symptom status and quality of life following prostatectomy. JAMA 1988; 259: 3018–3022

27. Breum L, Klarskov P, Munck L et al. Significance of acute urinary retention due to infravesical obstruction. Scand J Urol Nephrol 1982; 16: 21–24

28. Taube M, Gajraj H. Trial without catheter following acute retention of urine. Br J Urol 1989; 63: 180–182

29. Spiro L, Labay G, Orkin L. Prostatic infarction: role in acute urinary retention. Urology 1974; 3: 345–347

30. Sacks S, Aparicio S, Began A et al. Late renal failure due to prostatic outflow obstruction: a preventable disease. Br Med J 1989; 298: 156–159

31. Bishop M. The dangers of a long urological waiting list. Br J Urol 1990; 65: 433–440

32. Ghose R, Harinda V. Unrecognized high pressure chronic retention of urine presenting with systemic arterial hypertension. Br Med J 1989; 298: 1626–1628

33. Mukamel E, Nissenkorn I, Boner G, Servadio C. Occult progressive renal damage in the elderly male due to benign prostatic hypertrophy. J Am Geriatr Soc 1979; 27: 403–406

34. Beck A. Benign prostatic hypertrophy and uraemia. A review of 315 cases. Br J Surg 1989; 298: 156–159

35. Kaufman J, Dhakal M, Patel B, Hamburger R. Community-acquired acute renal failure. Am J Kidney Dis 1991; 17: 191–198

36. Chisholm G. Obstructive nephropathy. Functional abnormalities and clinical presentation. Proc R Soc Med 1970; 63: 1242–1245

37. Gosling J, Dixon J. The structure of the trabeculated detrusor smooth muscle in cases of prostatic hypertrophy. Urol Int 1980; 35: 351–355

38. Gilpin S, Gosling J, Barnard J. Morphological and morphometric studies of the human obstructed, trabeculated urinary bladder. Br J Urol 1985; 57: 525–529

39. Dixon J, Gilpin C, Gilpin S et al. Sequential morphologic changes in the pig detrusor in response to chronic partial urethral obstruction. Br J Urol 1989; 64: 385–390

40. Levin R, Longhurst P, Monson F et al. Effect of bladder outlet obstruction on the morphology, physiology, and pharmacology of the bladder. Prostate 1990; 3: 9s–26s

41. Lepor H, Sunaryadi I, Hartano V, Shapiro E. Quantitative morphometry of the adult human bladder. J Urol 1992; 148: 414–417

42. Dorflinger T, Frimodt-Moller P, Bruskewitz R et al. The significance of uninhibited detrusor contractions in prostatism. J Urol 1985; 133: 819–821

43. Christensen M, Bruskewitz R. Clinical manifestations of benign prostatic hyperplasia and indications for therapeutic intervention. Urol Clin North Am 1990; 17: 509–516

44. Jones D, Gilpin S, Holden D et al. Relationship between bladder morphology and long-term outcome of treatment in patients with high pressure chronic retention of urine. Br J Urol 1991; 67: 280–285

45. Grosse H. Frequency, localization, and associated disorders in urinary calculi. Analysis of 1671 autopsies in urolithiasis. Z Urol Nephrol 1990; 83: 469–474

46. Wasson J, Reda D, Bruskewitz R et al. A comparison of transurethral surgery with watchful waiting for moderate symptoms of benign prostatic hyperplasia. N Engl J Med 1994; 332: 75–79

47. Madsen P, Iverson P. A point system for selecting operative candidates. In: Hinman F (ed) Benign prostatic hypertrophy. New York: Springer-Verlag, 1983: 763

48. The Department of Veterans Affairs Cooperative Study of Transurethral Resection for Benign Prostatic Hyperplasia. A comparison of quality of life with patient reported symptoms and objective findings in men with benign prostatic hyperplasia. J Urol 1993; 150: 1696–1700

49. Kasper J, Mulley A, Wennberg J. Developing shared decision-making programs to improve the quality of health care. Qual Rev Bull 1992; 18: 183–190

50. Wennberg J. On the status of the Prostate Disease Assessment Team. Health Serv Res 1990; 25: 709–716

51. Barry M, Fowler F, O'Leary M et al. The American Urological Association Symptom Index for benign prostatic hyperplasia. J Urol 1992; 148: 1549–1557

52. Barry M, Fowler F, O'Leary M et al. Correlation of the American Urological Association Symptom Index with self-administered versions of the Madsen–Iverson, Boyarsky, and Maine Medical Assessment Program Symptom Indexes. J Urol 1992; 148: 1558–1563

53. Chassin M, Brook R, Park R. Variations in the use of medical and surgical services by the Medicare population. N Engl J Med 1986; 314: 285–290

54. Wennberg J. Dealing with medical practice variations: a proposal for action. Health Affairs 1984; 3: 6–32

55. McPherson K, Wennberg J, Hovind O, Clifford P. Small area variations in the use of common surgical procedures: an international comparison of New England, England and Norway. N Engl J Med 1982; 307: 1310–1314

56. Blumenthal D. The variation phenomenon in 1994. N Engl J Med 1994; 331: 1017–1018

57. Barry M. Natural history of untreated benign prostatic hyperplasia. In: Garraway M (ed) The epidemiology of prostate disease. Heidelberg: Springer-Verlag, 1994

Evaluation

III

12

Evaluating symptoms and functional status
M. P. O'Leary M. J. Barry

Measuring symptoms in BPH

Benign prostatic hyperplasia (BPH) is one of the most common conditions affecting the ageing male. The effects of BPH on voiding function, however, vary greatly from patient to patient and thus make measuring its impact a challenging task. Ideally, any kind of measurement should be both precise (reliable) and accurate (valid). Precise measurements are reproducible when the underlying phenomenon being measured does not change; accurate measurements measure what they are supposed to measure correctly. Clinicians are familiar with measurements of anatomical or physiological phenomena using devices that may be as simple as a ruler or as complicated as a multichannel urodynamic monitor. These sorts of measurements give clinicians a sense of objectivity and 'hardness'. However, in many cases the experience of illness from a patient's perspective — which tends to be dominated by symptoms, worry and functional limitation — is not so easily measured. To some clinicians, measurements of these phenomena with questionnaires are inherently subjective and 'soft'. However, methods are available to develop more precise and accurate measures of general feelings of well-being, symptoms of illness and adequacy of functioning, and the resultant measurements are being used more frequently in both practice and research.[1]

Measurement in urological practice

In urology, measurements of prostate size, uroflow, residual volume, serum creatinine and prostate-specific antigen levels, all are part of day-to-day care. Nevertheless, it is largely symptoms that bring patients to a urologist, and that lead the urologist to decide what therapy, if any, is appropriate. There has, therefore, been increasing interest in improving the measurement of symptoms in urology.[2,3] Uniform and consistent measures among patients allow clinicians to compare patients, to monitor the progression of disease, and may enhance the efficiency of communication between physician and patient.

Potential uses of symptom measurements

The methods used for developing a symptom (or any health status) measure, and for assessing the reliability and validity of that measure, may differ depending on the planned use of the measurement. Kirshner and Guyatt have distinguished among discriminative, predictive and evaluative measurement instruments.[4] Discriminative measurements are designed to distinguish between individuals or groups on some characteristic in the absence of a gold standard. Predictive measurements are used to classify individuals into groups when some gold standard is available to confirm the classification but may be too risky or expensive to use routinely. Discriminative and predictive measurements relate to the tasks of diagnosis or screening in clinical practice. Finally, evaluative measurements are used to measure longitudinal change in a patient characteristic over time, as in the tasks of assessing prognosis or the response to treatment.

An instrument may be developed for many purposes, but clarity about the intended purposes is important in discussing its utility. For example, responsiveness to important changes in patient condition is critical for an evaluative measurement, but irrelevant for discriminative or predictive purposes.

When questionnaires are used to measure a patient characteristic such as health status, multiple questions are often used to get a more detailed picture of the patient's situation. When multiple questions address the same patient characteristic, as documented by intercorrelation among the items, patient responses will often be combined into an index. A multi-item index can generate a score that is both more reproducible when patients are stable and more responsive to change with treatment. One would not want to combine unrelated items (such as questions about sexual and urinary function); at the same time, too close a relationship among items in an index suggests redundancy. Shorter (parsimonious) question sets are advantageous in terms of respondent burden, but may be less reliable and risk ignoring important facets of the characteristic of interest.

A broad set of response categories for individual questions may help to discriminate among subjects and improve sensitivity to change, but too many categories can confuse subjects and result in a deterioration in reliability. Ideal questions should have a response appropriate for every subject (*collectively exhaustive*), but only one category appropriate for each subject (*mutually exclusive*).

Instruments for measuring urinary symptom severity

A number of instruments have been developed and used to measure urinary symptom severity among men with BPH. The two used most extensively in the past have been the Boyarsky and Madsen–Iversen indices.[5,6] From a psychometric perspective, the best-validated instrument used in the past may have been the Maine Medical Assessment Program (MMAP) Symptom Index, which was used in an outcomes study of prostatectomy conducted by community urologists in Maine.[7] Other, less well known instruments have been described by Bardsley and colleagues, and Hald and colleagues.[8,9] More recently, the Measurement Committee of the American Urological Association (AUA) developed and validated an AUA Symptom Index, which has enjoyed increasing use in both clinical practice and research.[10] Concurrently, investigators at Merck Research Laboratories developed and validated a symptom questionnaire for use in their phase III trial of finasteride.[11] The starting point for instruments developed to measure symptoms in men with BPH has been a list of questions that clinicians have long felt reflect important manifestations of this condition. These lower urinary tracts symptoms (a term many prefer to 'prostatism')[12] are daytime frequency, nocturia, hesitancy, intermittency, terminal dribbling, urgency, a weak stream, dysuria and a sense of incomplete emptying. However, there is considerable debate about the fine points of this symptom roster. For example, does dysuria imply 'pain', 'burning' or simply 'discomfort'? Is urge incontinence a separate symptom, or simply endstage urgency? Questions may ask how often a symptom happens (its frequency), or how bad it is when it happens (its severity); these two dimensions of symptoms are intercorrelated.

Some urinary symptom questionnaires have been divided into 'obstructive' and 'irritative' subsets, based on the perception of underlying pathophysiology. Obstructive symptoms (most commonly hesitancy, intermittency, terminal dribbling, a weak stream and a sense of incomplete emptying) have been felt to be due to the direct effect of bladder outlet obstruction, whereas irritative symptoms (most commonly frequency, nocturia, urgency and dysuria) have been felt to be attributable to secondary uninhibited detrusor contractions. In truth, neither physiological nor psychometric data provide much support for this well-entrenched dichotomy.[10,12]

What follows is a description of the three most widely used indices — the Boyarsky, the Madsen–Iversen and the AUA [or International Prostate Symptom Score (I-PSS)].

In 1977, Boyarsky and colleagues published the results of a consultation by an ad hoc group of urologists with United States Food and Drug Administration officials regarding guidelines for protocols for the evaluation of the efficacy of pharmacological treatments for BPH.[5] This landmark paper presented a list of important symptoms to be assessed in study protocols, along with a set of recommended response categories (Table 12.1). Although subsequently developed symptom indices have resulted in important improvements and have been better validated from a psychometric perspective, the Boyarsky Index is the conceptual parent of all subsequent questionnaires. Clearly, given the auspices under which it was developed, the Boyarsky Index was intended for evaluative, rather than discriminant or predictive, purposes. No distinction between irritative and obstructive subscores was recommended.

A number of concerns can be raised about the Boyarsky Index. First, the authors did not recommend a mode of administration of the questions (self versus interviewer), and the symptoms were simply listed, without a text specifying how the questions were to be phrased. As a result, different investigators have certainly asked these questions in different ways, reducing the potential for valid comparisons among

Table 12.1. *The Boyarsky Symptom Index (total score range 0–27 points)*

Symptom	Score	Intensity of symptom
Nocturia	0	Absence of symptom
	1	Subject awakened 1 time each night because of need to urinate
	2	Subject awakened 2–3 times each night because of need to urinate
	3	Subject awakened 4 or more times each night because of need to urinate
Frequency	0	Subject urinates 1–4 times daily
	1	Subject urinates 5–7 times daily
	2	Subject urinates 8–12 times daily
	3	Subject urinates 13 or more times daily
Hesitancy	0	Occasional hesitancy (occurs in 20% or fewer of subject's attempts to void)
	1	Moderate hesitancy (occurs during 20–50% of subject's attempts to void)
	2	Frequent hesitancy (occurs more than 50% of the time, but not always, and may last up to 1 min)
	3	Symptom always present, lasts for 1 min or longer
Intermittency	0	Occasional intermittency (occurs in 20% or fewer of subject's attempts to void)
	1	Moderate intermittency (occurs during 20–50% of subject's attempts to void)
	2	Frequent intermittency (occurs more than 50% of the time, but not always, and may last up to 1 min)
	3	Symptom always present, lasts for 1 min or longer
Terminal dribbling	0	Occasional terminal dribbling (occurs in 20% or fewer of the subject's voiding)
	1	Moderate terminal dribbling (occurs during 20–50% of the subject's voiding)
	2	Frequent terminal dribbling (occurs more than 50% of the time but not always)
	3	Symptom always present, dribbling lasts for 1 min or more, wets clothing
Urgency	0	Absence of symptom
	1	Occasionally difficult for subject to postpone urination
	2	Frequently difficult (more than 50% of the time) to postpone urination and may rarely lose urine
	3	Always difficult to postpone urination and subject sometimes loses urine
Impairment of size and force of stream	0	Absence of symptoms
	1	Impaired trajectory
	2	Most of the time size and force are restricted
	3	Subject urinates with great effort and stream is interrupted
Dysuria	0	Absence of symptoms
	1	Occasional burning sensation during urination
	2	Frequent (more than 50% of the time) burning sensation during urination
	3	Frequent and painful burning sensation during urination
Sensation of incomplete voiding	0	Absence of symptom
	1	Occasional sensation of incomplete emptying of bladder after voiding
	2	Frequent (more than 50% of the time) sensation of incomplete voiding
	3	Constant and urgent sensation and no relief upon voiding

(From ref. 5 with permission.)

studies. Furthermore, the response frames tend to mix frequency and severity, so that categories do not always appear to be mutually exclusive and collectively exhaustive. For example, a subject who always has terminal dribbling but never for more than 1 min would have difficulty in selecting the appropriate response from the available choices. In addition, response frames are constructed asymmetrically, so that some questions (on nocturia, urgency, weak stream, dysuria and incomplete emptying) require an absence of symptoms to achieve the lowest score, while others (on hesitancy, intermittency and terminal dribbling) permit a low level of symptoms to achieve the lowest score. As a result, investigators need to be cautious in making conclusions about the relative impact of treatments on individual symptoms measured with this instrument. Finally, no data were provided on its reliability, validity and responsiveness.

The Madsen–Iversen Index (Table 12.2) was published in 1983 as part of a point system for selecting candidates for prostatectomy.[6] Although the publication was terse, the instrument was apparently intended for use both to select men for surgery (discriminative/predictive) and to assess their response to prostatectomy (evaluative). The point values assigned to responses were arbitrary. The authors did not recommend calculation of irritative and obstructive subscores, but did suggest that total scores could be divided again arbitrarily into mild (< 10 points), moderate (10–20 points) and severe (> 20 points) ranges, with moderate and particularly severe symptoms providing a stronger rationale for surgical intervention.

Like the Boyarsky paper, this publication provides no guidance about how the questions should be worded, or how the questionnaire should be administered. The differential weighing of questions does not have an empirical basis, nor does the different number of response categories among questions. The inclusion of terminal dribbling as part of the spectrum of incontinence is also curious. Finally, although data from a small study correlating symptom score with the presence or absence of physiological obstruction and response to surgery were provided, no data on reliability or other aspects of validity or responsiveness were presented.

Recognizing the limitations of previously published indices, a measurement committee appointed by the AUA developed and validated the AUA Symptom Index.[10,13] The primary purpose of the AUA Index was evaluative; the index was to be used as an outcome measurement in a study of different treatment strategies for BPH.[14,15] However, implicit in the development and validation of the AUA Index was a discriminative purpose — to distinguish between men more or less

Table 12.2. *The Madsen–Iversen Symptom Index (score range 0–27 points)*

Symptom	Score	Symptom intensity
Stream	0	Normal
	1	Variable
	3	Weak
	4	Dribbling
Voiding	0	No strain
	2	Abdominal strain or Crede
Hesitancy	0	None
	3	Yes
Intermittency	0	None
	3	Yes
Bladder emptying	0	Don't know or complete
	1	Variable
	2	Incomplete
	3	Single retention
	4	Repeated retention
Incontinence	0	None
	3	Yes (including terminal dribbling)
Urge	0	None
	1	Mild
	2	Moderate
	3	Severe (incontinence)
Nocturia	0	0–1 time
	1	2 times
	2	3–4 times
	3	> 4 times
Diuria	0	q > 3 h
	1	q 2–3 h
	2	q 1–2 h
	3	q < 1 h

(From ref. 6 with permission.)

bothered by their urinary condition. This discriminative ability resulted in the later incorporation of the index into BPH practice guidelines in the United States. However, it must be emphasized that the AUA Index was not developed to distinguish among men with urinary symptoms due to different pathophysiological processes, to discriminate among men with or without physiological evidence of bladder outlet obstruction, or to serve as a general measure of urinary symptom severity among patients (including women) with various causes of lower urinary dysfunction.

The methods used for developing and validating the AUA Symptom Index have been described in detail.[10] A self-administered questionnaire was desired to avoid potential problems of interviewer bias. Briefly, previous instruments were examined and questions were selected with rewording as necessary; Merck Research Laboratories also kindly provided copies of their BPH questionnaire for this phase of the study. Candidate questions were reviewed by both urologists and patients for clarity and completeness. A preliminary questionnaire had 15 items covering nine symptoms; subjects were asked to consider symptom level over the last month in answering the questions (as symptoms can wax and wane from day to day).

In a first validation study, men with a clinical diagnosis of BPH (without prior surgery) from three

Table 12.3. *The AUA Symptom Index (score range 0–35 points)*

	Response (score)					
Question	Not at all	Less than 1 time in 5	Less than half the time	About half the time	More than half the time	Almost always
1. Over the past month or so, how often have you had a sensation of not emptying your bladder completely after you finished urinating?	0	1	2	3	4	5
2. Over the past month or so how often have you had to urinate again less than 2 h after you finished urinating?	0	1	2	3	4	5
3. Over the past month or so, how often have you found you stopped and started again several times when you urinated?	0	1	2	3	4	5
4. Over the past month or so, how often have you found it difficult to postpone urination?	0	1	2	3	4	5
5. Over the past month or so, how often have you had a weak urinary stream?	0	1	2	3	4	5
6. Over the past month or so, how often have you had to push or strain to begin urination?	0	1	2	3	4	5
	None	1 time	2 times	3 times	4 times	5 times
7. Over the past month, how many times did you most typically get up to urinate from the time you went to bed at night until the time you got up in the morning?	0	1	2	3	4	5

(From ref. 10 with permission.)

urological practices and men without urinary problems in a general medical practice self-administered the questionnaire on two separate occasions a week apart, and were debriefed about the items by a research assistant or nurse. On the basis of these data, a modified, shortened questionnaire was re-evaluated in the same settings, and subjected to a test of responsiveness by administration to BPH patients before and 1 month after prostatectomy. The final seven-item questionnaire, the AUA Symptom Index, is presented in Table 12.3.

The items in the index are highly intercorrelated, with a Cronbach's alpha statistic of 0.86, which provides a strong rationale for summing the answers on individual items into a total score. One-week test–retest reliability of overall scores was excellent with a correlation coefficient of 0.92. AUA scores correlated well with subjects' global ratings of the magnitude of their urinary problem, as well as with scores on the Boyarsky and Madsen–Iversen indices, providing evidence of the 'construct validity' of the index. Although AUA scores discriminated well between BPH and control subjects in the validation studies, this task was not challenging, as the latter group was younger and did not include men with other urological problems that can be confused with BPH. Finally, the AUA score was responsive when a group of men underwent prostatectomy: the mean score dropped from 17.6 points preoperatively to 7.1 points 4 weeks postoperatively. The two symptoms not included in the AUA Index were terminal dribbling and dysuria. Data from the validation study indicated that responses to questions about these symptoms were less strongly related to patients' global ratings of their degree of urinary difficulty, less strongly correlated with the seven items that were included in the index, and had the same distributions in BPH and control subjects. No psychometric basis could be found for differential weighting of the seven questions, or for calculating obstructive and irritative subscores.

Recently, Sagnier and colleagues have described a process of linguistic validation that they followed to obtain a translation of the AUA Index for use in France.[16] This methodology is an appropriate model for translation of the AUA Index into other languages; either the original English or French language version of the index may serve as a template for such efforts.

The AUA Symptom Index is enjoying wider use in clinical research and practice. The International Consultation on BPH, held under the auspices of the World Health Organization, has recommended the use of the seven items in the AUA Index, along with one of the BPH-specific quality of life questions used in the original validation study, as the I-PSS.[17] Recently, practice guidelines were released by a multidisciplinary panel supported by the US Agency for Health Care Policy and Research, focusing on the management of men with BPH;[18] again, use of the AUA Symptom Index was recommended. In a recent survey of a sample of 500 American urologists conducted in 1993 (less than 1 year after publication of the AUA Index), 95% of respondents reported that they were familiar with the index, and 60% of those familiar with it reported using it to evaluate and follow patients with BPH.[19]

A number of appropriate concerns have been raised about the AUA Index, particularly regarding its use outside the areas for which it was intended. A primary concern has been the role of the AUA Index in the diagnosis of BPH — in particular, whether the index can discriminate men with urinary symptoms due to other pathophysiological conditions from men with BPH, or men with greater from lesser degrees of physiological obstruction. A number of papers describing similar AUA scores among groups of men and women highlight the potential non-specificity of the AUA Index,[20–22] a point that was made in the paper describing the original validation. It is important to stress that this observation is not relevant to the purposes for which the index was designed; scores on the index clearly *can* separate men with BPH before and after treatment, or with differing degrees of bother from their urinary condition.

Correlation of symptoms with anatomical and physiological variables

An interesting issue in the debate about the utility of symptom measurements among men with BPH is the relationship of symptom severity to anatomical and physiological variables that might also reflect BPH severity. The weak relationships of symptoms with prostate size, uroflow and data from simultaneous pressure–flow studies have long been recognized.[23–26]

However, to study the true relationships among variables, precise measurements are necessary; measurement error attenuates and can obscure clinically important relationships.

Given the documentation precision of the AUA Index for measuring symptoms, this issue was readdressed among about 200 men enrolled in the AUA's BPH Treatment Outcomes Pilot Study, the study for which the index was developed.[27] Although there were weak but statistically significant relationships between post-void residual volume and answers to the question about incomplete emptying, and between peak and average uroflow and answers to the question about a weak stream, there was no relationship between overall symptom severity and any of the anatomical or physiological variables measured (Table 12.4). This study also documented a highly significant relationship between symptom severity and measurements of overall quality of life, while anatomical and physiological variables, as one would expect, had no relationship to the quality-of-life measurements.

This study could not determine whether the lack of correlation between symptoms and the anatomical and physiological variables was due to the fact that these measurements simply address unrelated phenomena, or whether there was a problem with the precision of the

Table 12.4. *Relationship of AUA symptom scores to other measures of BPH severity and overall quality of life in the BPH Treatment Outcomes Pilot Study*

Variable	Pearson correlation coefficient with AUA symptom score	p value
Peak flow rate	−0.07	0.27
Average flow rate	−0.13	0.08
Post-void residual[†]	0.01	0.84
Prostate size[†]	−0.09	0.22
Prostate-specific antigen	−0.06	0.43
General health[‡]	−0.37	0.0001
Activity[‡]	−0.29	0.0001
Mental health[‡]	−0.29	0.0001

*n varies from 181 to 196 for individual comparisons owing to occasional missing data on individual items. [†]As measured by transabdominal ultrasonography. [‡]Based on general health, activity and mental health indices where higher scores indicate better overall health. (Adapted from ref. 27 with permission.)

latter measurements.[28–31] Some data exist that do raise questions about the precision of such anatomical and physiological measurements. Pending additional study, it is clear that measures of symptom severity cannot serve as proxies for anatomical and physiological measurements, or vice versa.

Utility of symptom measurements in clinical practice and research

In the office setting, the AUA Index can, and should, be administered as part of the initial patient evaluation. There is considerable controversy about which additional tests should be used to confirm a diagnosis of BPH, and in what settings they should be used.[32,33] Nevertheless, once a diagnosis of BPH is made, patients with symptom scores in the mild range (seven points or fewer) are rarely bothered by their condition and seldom need active treatment. On the other hand, many men with higher symptom scores will not be sufficiently bothered to merit treatment, either. In the process of therapeutic decision-making, the AUA Index merely serves to help initiate a discussion about how intrusive the patient finds his symptoms. The urologist can work with the patient to determine what risks, if any, he would accept to try to reduce them.

A major rationale for the inclusion of the AUA Index in research protocols is to permit comparisons among studies. The recently published report from the BPH Guideline Panel noted that heterogeneity in methods of symptom measurement among studies in the literature posed real problems in evaluating the comparative effectiveness of different BPH therapies.[18] The established reliability of the AUA Index, combined with its responsiveness, should facilitate detection of clinically important differences in symptom severity attributable to either time or treatment.

Once a treatment strategy is selected, whether 'watchful waiting' or an active treatment modality, the AUA Index can be periodically readministered to assess patient response more objectively. However, in individual patients, some variability in score can be expected based on chance variation alone. In fact, despite excellent test–retest reliability, when only two measurements are available for a patient, increases or decreases in AUA scores of up to five points could easily be due to chance.[34] Clinicians using AUA scores to monitor patients serially might well be advised to base decisions on the average of two baseline scores, and the average of two scores at follow-up, to reduce the effect of chance variation. The same point applies to other serial measurements in individual patients, such as measurements of peak uroflow or prostate-specific antigen.

Need for further research on symptom measurement

Further research is needed to clarify the utility of symptom measurement in general, and the AUA Index in particular, in clinical practice and research. Currently, the authors are conducting a randomized trial of interviewer-administration versus self-administration of the index. If the results are equivalent, the index could be administered by an interviewer to visually impaired or illiterate men. A Spanish language version of the AUA Index for use in the United States is undergoing validation.

Another important area for further research is the development of disease-specific health status measures for men with BPH. Such measures focus on how urinary symptoms affect the activities, mental health and general health perceptions of BPH patients and are being designed as a bridge between symptoms and overall health. The authors have recently developed and validated two companions to the AUA Index that should allow a more complete assessment of the significance of symptoms to individual patients, as well as providing a more global attempt to quantify how symptoms affect patients' daily lives.[35] Other groups have also developed instruments that can be integrated with measurement of symptom severity to provide a more detailed evaluation of the true impact of BPH.[36,39]

Finally, groups are working on the question of the relationship between urinary symptoms and physiological measurements of BPH severity, particularly variables that can be extracted from simultaneous pressure–flow studies.[38] The International Continence Society is currently conducting a major study to relate symptoms and urodynamic findings,[23] although preliminary data suggest that the urodynamic data collected on these study patients correlated poorly with symptom scores.[39]

Conclusions

Clinicians have tried, and will continue to try, to measure symptom severity in men with BPH as objectively as possible, as the report of symptoms and the degree of discomfort vary greatly from patient to patient. To date, the AUA Index is the most useful measurement tool in this endeavour. Additional research will further clarify its role and help us to understand better the utility of symptom measurement in men with this common condition.

Acknowledgements

This work was supported in part by Grant No. HS 08397 from the Agency for Health Care Policy and Research.

References

1. Fowler F J, Barry M J. Quality of life assessment for evaluating benign prostatic hyperplasia treatments. Eur Urol 1993; 24: 24–27
2. Barry M J, Fowler F J. The methodology for evaluating the subjective outcomes of treatment for benign prostatic hyperplasia. Adv Urol 1993; 6: 83–99
3. O'Leary M P, Barry M J, Fowler F J. Hard measures of subjective outcomes: validating symptom indexes in urology. J Urol 1992; 148: 1545–1548
4. Kirshner B, Guyatt G. A methodological framework for assessing health indices. J Chron Dis 1985; 38: 27–36
5. Boyarsky S, Jones G, Paulson D F et al. A new look at bladder neck obstruction by the Food and Drug Administration regulators: guidelines for investigation of benign prostatic hypertrophy. Trans Am Assoc Genitourin Surg 1977; 68: 29–32
6. Madsen P O, Iversen P. A point system for selecting operative candidates. In: Hinman F Jr (ed) Benign prostatic hypertrophy. New York: Springer-Verlag, 1983: 763–765
7. Fowler F J, Wennberg J E, Timothy R P et al. Symptom status and quality of life following prostatectomy. JAMA 1988; 259: 3018–3022
8. Bardsley M J, Venning P M, Cham C W et al. A self-administered patient questionnaire in the assessment of symptoms before and after prostatectomy. Br J Urol 1992; 69: 375–380
9. Hald T, Nordling J, Andersen J T et al. A patient weighted symptom score system in the evaluation of uncomplicated benign prostatic hyperplasia. Scand J Urol Nephrol 199; 138 (suppl): 59
10. Barry M J, Fowler F J, O'Leary M P et al. The American Urological Association symptom index for benign prostatic hyperplasia. J Urol 1992; 148: 1549–1557
11. Bolognese J A, Kozloff R C, Kunitz S C et al. Validation of a symptoms questionnaire for benign prostatic hyperplasia. Prostate 1992; 21: 247–254
12. Abrams P. New words for old: lower urinary tract symptoms for 'prostatism'. Br Med J 1994; 308: 929–930
13. Barry M J, Fowler F J, O'Leary M P et al. Correlation of the American Urological Association Symptom index with self-administered versions of the Madsen–Iversen, Boyarsky and Maine medical assessment program indexes. J Urol 1992; 148: 1558–1563

14. Cockett A T K, Barry M J, Holtgrewe H L et al. Indications for treatment of benign prostatic hyperplasia. Cancer 1992; 70: 280–283

15. Holtgrewe H L. An American Urological Association prospective, randomized clinical trial in the treatment of benign prostatic hyperplasia. Cancer 1992; 70: 351–354

16. Sagnier P P, McFarlane G, Richard F et al. Results of an epidemiological survey using a modified American Urological Association symptom index for benign prostatic hyperplasia in France. J Urol 1994; 151: 1266–1270

17. Cockett A T, Aso Y, Denis L et al. Recommendations of the International Consensus Committee concerning: 1. Prostate symptom score and quality of life assessment. In: Cockett A T K, Khoury S, Aso Y et al. (eds) Proceedings, The 2nd International Consultation on Benign Prostatic Hyperplasia (BPH), Paris, June 27–30, 1993. Jersey, Channel Islands: Scientific Communication International Ltd, 1994: 553–555

18. McConnell J D, Barry M J, Bruskewitz R C et al. Benign prostatic hyperplasia: diagnosis and treatment. In: Clinical Practice Guideline, No. 8. Rockville, Md: US Department of Health and Human Services, 1994: 99–103

19. Gallup Poll Organization Inc. Practicing urologists survey. Baltimore: American Urological Association, 1993

20. Chai T C, Belville W D, McGuire E J, Nyquist L. Specificity of the American Urological Association voiding symptom index comparison of unselected and selected samples of both sexes. J Urol 1993; 150: 1710–1713

21. Chancellor M B, Rivas D A. American Urological Association Symptom Index for women with voiding symptoms: lack of index specificity for benign prostatic hyperplasia. J Urol 1993; 150: 1706–1708

22. Lepor H, Machi G. Comparison of AUA symptom index in unselected males and females between fifty-five and seventy-nine years of age. Urology 1993; 42: 36–40

23. Abrams P. Urodynamics and the International Continence Society come of age. Br J Urol 1993; 72: 527–529

24. Andersen J T. Benign prostatic hyperplasia: symptoms and objective interpretation. Eur Urol 1991; 20: 36

25. Chapple C R. Correlation of symptomatology, urodynamics, morphology and size of the prostate in benign prostatic hyperplasia. Curr Opin Urol 1993; 3: 5

26. Frimodt-Moller P C, Jensen K M E, Iverson P et al. Analysis of presenting symptoms in prostatism. J Urol 1984; 132: 272–276

27. Barry M J, Cockett A T K, Holtgrewe H L et al. Relationship of symptoms of prostatism to commonly used physiological and anatomical measures of the severity of benign prostatic hyperplasia. J Urol 1993; 150: 351

28. Birch N C, Hurst G, Doyle P T. Serial residual volumes in men with prostatic hypertrophy. Br J Urol 1988; 62: 571–575

29. Bruskewitz R C, Iversen P, Madsen P O. Value of postvoid residual urine determination in evaluation of prostatism. Urology 1982; 20: 602–604

30. Golomb J, Lindner A, Siegel Y, Korczak D. Variability and circadian changes in home uroflowmetry in patients with benign prostatic hyperplasia compared to normal controls. J Urol 1992; 147: 1044–1047

31. Matzkin H, Van Der Zwaag R, Chen Y et al. How reliable is a single measurement of urinary flow in the diagnosis of obstruction in benign prostatic hyperplasia? Br J Urol 1993; 72: 181–186

32. Abrams P. Editorial: In support of pressure flow studies for evaluating men with lower urinary tract symptoms. Urology 1994; 44: 153

33. McConnell J D. Editorial. Why pressure–flow studies should be optional and not mandatory studies for evaluating men with benign prostatic hyperplasia. Urology 1994; 44: 156

34. Barry M J, Girman C J, O'Leary M P et al. Using repeated measures of symptom score, uroflow, and prostate specific antigen in the clinical management of prostate disease. J Urol 1995; 153: 99–103

35. Barry M J, Fowler F J, O'Leary M P et al. Measuring disease-specific health status in men with benign prostatic hyperplasia. Med Care 1995; 33: 145–155

36. Epstein R S, Deverka P A, Chute C G et al. Urinary symptoms and quality of life questions indicative of obstructive benign prostatic hyperplasia: results of a pilot study. Urology 1991; 38: 20–26

37. Epstein R S, Deverka P A, Chute C G et al. Validation of a new quality of life questionnaire for benign prostatic hyperplasia. J Clin Epidemiol 1992; 45: 1431–1445

38. Chancellor M B, Rivas D A, Keeley F X et al. Similarity of the American Urological Association symptom index among men with benign prostatic hyperplasia (BPH), urethral obstruction not due to BPH and detrusor hyper-reflexia without outlet obstruction. Br J Urol 1994; 74: 200–203

39. Hofner K, Tan H, Krah H et al. The correlation between mechanical outflow obstruction and ICS and Boyarsky symptom scores in BPH patients. Société Internationale D'Urologie, 1994: abstr 539

13

Clinical assessment: digital rectal examination
L. J. Denis

Introduction

The clinical assessment or diagnostic work-up of patients presenting with symptoms of prostatism concerns the evaluation of four interrelated concepts that comprise the symptom complex of prostatism. These four concepts include: voiding symptoms in any patient over the age of 50 (commonly referred to as prostatism), the presence of detectable benign prostatic hyperplasia (BPH), the presence of obstruction in the micturition process, and possibly the presence of a dysfunction or failure of the detrusor muscle, caused by the hyperplasia and/or resulting obstruction. Although the clinical assessment of prostatism is described in considerable detail in a standard work of Marion, published in 1921,[1] it is not even considered worthy of a chapter in another equally famous standard work, edited by Hinman.[2] The suspected reason for the latter omission is probably the fact that clinical assessment and digital rectal examination (DRE) had no direct relation to the diagnosis of BPH and the outcome of treatment. Fittingly, Brendler as editor of the section on the evolution of BPH and history of treatment, refers to the chapter's merit in illustrating past mistakes and keeping us humble.

The growing awareness of the problem of BPH reaching epidemic proportions due to ageing of the world's population has led to International Consultations on Benign Prostatic Hyperplasia, in which all aspects of the disease have been re-examined for the current priorities for optimal health care, based on available peer review data.[3]

Clinical assessment

Clinical history

The patient with infravesical obstruction, secondary to BPH, will present to his physician complaining of a number of irritative and/or obstructive symptoms in his urinary stream. The symptoms are extremely variable and do not always bother the patient, and the decrease in size and force of his urinary stream has to be queried specifically by the physician. One of the important achievements of the International Consultations has been the establishment of the International Prostate Symptom Score (I-PSS) and quality-of-life assessment, based on seven questions. This I-PSS, described in detail in Chapter 12, is strongly recommended not only for the initial interview of the patient but also during and after treatment in order to monitor treatment response. An additional, complete medical history is vital to the initial diagnosis and should focus on a number of items to narrow the diagnosis to BPH (Table 13.1). Particular attention should be paid to synchronous complaints of impotence, vague perineal and testicular pains (especially in younger patients), and the presence or absence of the patient's wife at the consultation and her specific contribution to the anamnesis. In the opinion of the author, the reason for the consultation is very important. The main reasons are either symptoms that are bothersome, or anxiety about symptoms that are not bothersome, or anxiety

Table 13.1. *Information required to narrow the clinical diagnosis of patients with voiding problems to BPH*

Age of the patient
Sexual problems
General health issues, especially diabetes
Previous surgical procedures, especially those involving the genitourinary tract
Previous urological treatment
Previous treatment of BPH or prostate cancer
History suggestive of a neurological disorder
Medications, currently taken by the patient, able to affect bladder function
Patient's mental and physical fitness
Careful description of the usual urinary stream of the patient

caused by media information. It is attempted to avoid the latter problem in the region of Flanders by including the subject of prostatism in the yearly preventive health check by the general practitioner. Last, but not least, the duration of the symptoms can point to fairly benign congestion of the prostate by lifestyle problems such as alcohol abuse, extreme fatigue, sexual aberrations, constipation or haemorrhoids. Appropriate measures for decongestion have been largely ignored in the medical literature; phytotherapy may have a role in this context.

Physical examination

The physical examination starts with the observation of how the patient walks into the consultation room, sits down and addresses the subject. The author notes the patient's speech and pattern of thought and his ability to answer questions on his symptoms for confirmation. For the physical examination itself, the focus is on inspection of the abdomen and palpation for superficial lymph node masses. Scars on the abdomen reveal previous surgery. An overdistended bladder should not be ignored as a midline suprapubic renitent mass in patients that dribble urine and have no specific complaints. Blood pressure is taken in both the recumbent and standing positions; once the patient is standing up, he is asked to drop his pants. This gives the clinician the chance to look at the underwear of the patient, confirming or negating post-micturition dribbling. The presence of inguinal hernia is checked and the genitals, including retraction of the foreskin, are examined. The patient is then asked to bend over with his elbows on the table in order that examination of the anus and a DRE can be performed. A number of positions have been proposed for a correct DRE examination, including standing, lying on one side, lying in the lithotomy position, or the elbow–knee position. The most important point is that the patient is relaxed to allow easy inspection and adequate penetration of the rectum. Whenever there is the slightest doubt about the palpation of possible indurations, the DRE is repeated as a bimanual examination, pushing the prostate with one hand towards the examining index finger. After the DRE, the physical examination is completed by a focused neurological examination, paying special attention to the tone of the anal sphincter; the bulbocavernosus

reflex is not elicited, as the DRE by itself is already a cause of embarrassment for a number of patients. A check of motor and sensory function of the lower extremities is useful to complete the examination, gives the patient a chance to discuss the findings of the DRE and enables the vascular status of the lower limbs to be evaluated in the context of subsequent surgery.

Digital rectal examination

The anatomical position of the prostate, between the bladder neck and the external sphincter, allows easy palpation of its posterior wall by the finger. DRE has been used to evaluate the prostate gland with regard to its approximate size, consistency, shape, symmetry and induration suggestive of prostate cancer. For all practical purposes, DRE is used to diagnose macroscopic BPH and to evaluate its extent, and to palpate for asymmetry and, especially, zones of induration that arouse the suspicion of prostate cancer. Unfortunately, DRE is only moderately effective in estimating the extent of BPH and diagnosing small cancers. Its value lies in its speed, low cost and the advantage that most cancers arise in the peripheral zone (posterior lobe) of the prostate; however, the small tumours that arise in the transition zone (inner prostate) will not be detected by palpation. Nevertheless, DRE is a most sensitive method for the diagnosis of palpable prostate abnormalities but lacks specificity for prostate cancer.[4]

With regard to the estimation of prostate size by DRE, it should be noted that the size of the prostate gland in itself does not correlate with the severity of the symptoms, judged by subjective or objective scoring methods.[5] This lack of relationship between the extent of the hyperplasia and obstructive pathology is a logical sequence of the surgical anatomy of the prostatic lobes in cases of BPH. BPH arises as spherical masses of adenomyofibromatous tissue from the glands lining the prostatic urethra. Its shape is that of lobes that vary according to their original location and the resistance of the true prostate and vesical neck. Randall[6] described five major types of lobar hyperplasia, presented in Table 13.2. It is clear that bilateral lobar hyperplasia is more easily detected than the early solitary posterior commissural hyperplasia and solitary subcervical hyperplasia. It is noteworthy that the latter forms result in the early peak before the age of 60, followed by a

Table 13.2. *Incidence of types of BPH according to surgical anatomy*

Type	Description	n
1	Simple bilateral lobar hyperplasia	32
2	Solitary posterior commissural hyperplasia	31
3	Bilateral and commissural hyperplasia	38
4	Solitary subcervical lobar hyperplasia	67
5	Bilateral and subcervical lobar hyperplasia	48

(From ref. 6 with permission.)

peak in the seventh decade for bilateral lobar hyperplasia. Bilateral lobar hyperplasia is easily felt by the index finger on DRE. Bilateral enlargement is generally the rule but asymmetry is not always an indication of prostate cancer. This growth continues but remains enclosed in its false and its true prostate capsule. Posteriorly, the lobes usually touch, protruding as a spherical mass with a loss of the median sulcus near the apex. The solitary posterior commissural hyperplasia may, in its early stage, be represented by the so-called median bar. It is mainly diagnosed in younger men, with 80% occurring before the age of 60 years. DRE is usually non-specific. This explains, of course, the controversy about the correlation between the age of the patient, maximum flow rate (Q_{max}) and the estimated prostate weight.[7] Simonson et al. evaluated prospectively 199 patients with BPH who underwent prostatectomy; as a general trend, the flow rate decreased with increasing age but there was no significant correlation between the weight of the prostate and the age of the patient.[7] In contrast, the author noted in 1800 patients in the Antwerp screening programme for prostate cancer that the weight of the prostate increased with every 5 years of life. These observations are supported by the establishment of age-specific reference ranges for serum prostate-specific antigen (PSA) in a community-based population of healthy men.[8] These observations are also in accord with the detailed observations of Franks on the autopsy incidence of BPH: at each decade the percentage of men without BPH decreased compared with the previous decade; by the age of 80, 53% of the patients had macroscopic BPH.[9] In addition, the probability of prostatic surgery for BPH in the subsequent decade increases by age, as demonstrated by Lytton et al.: the probability at age 50 was 1.4% and,

respectively at age 60 and 70, 4.7 and 6.8%.[10] Nevertheless, even if there is an overall relationship between size and symptoms, this certainly does not apply to the individual patient. Furthermore, the estimated size by rectal examination and the actual weight after surgery revealed a poor correlation, as demonstrated by Bissada et al.[11] By contrast, a much better correlation has been reported between prostate size determined at surgery, predicted by transrectal ultrasonography (TRUS).[12] In conclusion, DRE will provide only a rough estimate of prostate volume, which is sufficient to enable the appropriate therapeutic intervention to be selected but is inadequate for use in clinical studies involving prostate size.

The second reason for performing DRE on a patient with BPH is the ability of the index finger of the urologist to detect indurations or suspicious asymmetry of the gland. Termed in Latin 'palpatio per anum', this is still the cornerstone of any diagnostic work-up for prostate cancer. It is hard to imagine that we have improved very much on this examination in the last century. Any doubt is erased on reading the description by Marion in 1921 of the macroscopic pathology of the intracapsular disease or its extension including the invasion of the regional lymph nodes.[1] His description of DRE to make a differential diagnosis from BPH is still worth reading:

Prostate cancer is generally easy to differentiate from BPH. The consistency of the prostatic mass is distinctive and, rather than elastic, hard and almost always irregular. The form instead of being regular rounded is frequently uneven. Finally, instead of feeling a distinctive border, one feels a continuation with the surrounding tissues, many times on the superior and external borders. Sometimes the mass is regular and limited but hard as wood. This is cancer. Sometimes one feels no mass but a simple hard nodule without precise delineation in the tissue.

The diagnosis becomes delicate when one deals with an early cancer and is only characteristic by the feeling of a few hard nodules in a mass that has all the specifications of BPH. They may be BPH but are very suspicious, especially if they do not disappear by rectal massage. The diagnosis in the early stage of the disease is very delicate and even experienced urologists are sometimes obliged to reserve their diagnosis for a certain time.

The figures reported by Marion,[1] that 9% of his patients with voiding problems had prostate cancer, and confirmed by Albarran and Hallé,[13] who reported that 14% of their patients had cancer on histological examination, make a perfect link with the results published by Cooner in his landmark study, in which 16% of his patients with voiding problems had prostate cancer.[14] This result contrasts sharply with the report by Faul, in a screening study of German men over 45 years of age, in which the overall detection rate was 0.1%.[15] These contrasts merely testify to patient selection and possibly the expertise of the examiner in performing the DRE. Consider first the selection of patients: the significance of a localized nodularity during the DRE is well recognized but, in Jewett's classic example,[16] only 50% of the lesions palpated by the clinical expert and considered suggestive of carcinoma were actually cancer on biopsy. The degree of suspicion of the feeling of any induration during careful DRE plays some part, as shown in Table 13.3, which is adapted from results obtained by arbitrary, open perineal biopsy on 300 unselected patients,[17] and shows that the correlation between the degree of induration and age and extent of tumour leaves room for an arbitrary decision. The authors of this paper concluded that prostate cancer could be predicted by DRE in only 23% of patients, while a lesser degree of induration was present in 66% of prostate cancer cases diagnosed by biopsy. Thus, it is clear that the selection of patients based on symptoms and age, and the clinical impression of the examining physician, correlate with the positive predictive value (PPV) of DRE. Hence, it is no surprise that confirmation of prostate cancer by needle biopsy, initially based on abnormal DRE findings, ranges from 18 to 100%.[18] Recent confirmation of these figures was provided in a study by Cooner et al,[19] in which patients

presenting with symptoms to a urological practice had a DRE performed by two urologists who had to be in agreement for any patient to be assigned to the DRE-negative group. Of 2634 men aged 50–89 years, a suspicious DRE was noted in 32% and one-third had a positive biopsy irrespective of their level of PSA. This detection rate decreased considerably in a self-referred population of 2131 men, where only 1.45% had an initial abnormal DRE, resulting in a PPV of 25% and where 6.8% of the diagnosed cancers were clinically localized.[20] From a population of 6734 volunteers older than 50 years, responding to an open invitation, 15% had an abnormal DRE and one-fifth had cancer diagnosed in a routine sextant biopsy, resulting in a detection rate of 3.2% and a PPV of 21% for DRE.[21] Several studies, reviewed by Bentvelsen and Schröder,[22] confirmed a detection rate for prostate cancer in men over 50 years of age by DRE ranging from 0.13 to 3.2%, depending on the type of patient studied, with a PPV ranging from 22 to 39%. This is about the maximum that can be expected from a physical examination to detect induration as an expression of prostate cancer in the early stages of the disease. However, the 'bottom line' is that up to 25% of cancers are still detected by DRE in men with normal serum PSA levels, which is why most cancer research organizations, including the American Cancer Society and the Flemish Advisory Council for Cancer Prevention, recommend an annual DRE for all men over 50 years of age. A suspicious DRE should at least be followed by a serum PSA determination and, if available, TRUS both for diagnosis and to guide biopsies.

Table 13.3. *Correlation of induration* with age and extent of tumour in 39 patients*

No. of cases in groups	Degree of induration[†]		
	0	1–2	3
Group I (limited to the prostate)	4	18	4
Group II (extraprostatic)		7	4
Group III (other organs)		1	1
Average age (years)	51.5	58.1	67.2

*Rock-hard induration was present in 23% of cases confirmed by biopsy, but at least a slight induration was present in 66% of the confirmed cases of cancer. †Degree of induration: 0: no induration; 1–2: some induration, 3: rock-hard induration. (Adapted from ref. 17 with permission.)

These recommendations are followed by the majority of practising urologists in the USA. On being surveyed, 99.8% agreed that DRE should be incorporated in the routine physical examination of an asymptomatic 55-year-old man and, furthermore, 91.3% thought that DRE should be repeated each year.[23] In the USA, this practice was also found to be followed by 97% of family practitioners and interns engaged in detecting early cancers.[24] In the survey, a second question was posed about inter-observer and intra-observer variability in the description of DRE findings, and whether DRE performed by family practitioners was less able to discriminate prostate cancer than DRE performed by trained urologists. In a screening programme in Antwerp, the author observed a lack of expertise in the reporting and description of DRE performed by family practitioners. Closer scrutiny indicated that this was mainly due to a lack of experience and of proper training of medical students in carrying out routine DRE. The lack of expertise was apparent in studies evaluating the performance of properly trained general practitioners when compared with urologists.

The conclusion is that DRE is still a first, basic examination for patients and screening subjects alike, but is ineffective as a single screening test and is not sufficiently accurate for appropriate prostate cancer staging.

Other clinical assessments

To complete the clinical assessment, the urine should be analysed by examination of a spun sediment or by using a Dipstix test. The results, of course, have no bearing on the diagnosis of BPH but haematuria and/or leucocyturia will prompt more appropriate tests.

It is rare nowadays to see a patient in the industrialized nations with renal insufficiency due to BPH. However, a standard assessment is to measure serum creatinine in all patients. The purpose is to find the 10–15% of patients with decreased renal function. PSA estimation, of course, in conjunction with DRE, enhances prostate cancer detection. Prostate biopsies should be considered if either the PSA cutoff is greater than 4 ng/ml or the DRE gives rise to a suspicion of cancer.[21]

Conclusions

Clinical assessment in patients with prostatism is fairly straightforward, and symptoms, an appropriate medical history and DRE together provide the mandatory requirements to diagnose BPH. Recommended tests to assure the safety of the patient before invasive therapy are the measurement of residual urine and uroflow pressures. This simplistic approach follows, of course, the duck principle: if it flies, walks and talks like a duck, it must be a duck. Unfortunately, this dictum is not always true in real life, and special investigations are needed in cases of BPH where more aggressive therapy is contemplated.

References

1. Marion G (ed) Traité d'urologie II. Paris: Masson, 1921: 1050 pp
2. Hinman F Jr (ed) Benign prostatic hypertrophy. New York: Springer-Verlag, 1993: 1077 pp
3. Cockett A T K, Khoury S, Aso Y et al. (eds) Proceedings 2nd International Consultation on Benign Prostatic Hyperplasia (BPH). Jersey, Channel Islands: Scientific Communication International Ltd, 1993: 672 pp
4. Guinan P, Bush I, Ray V et al. The accuracy of the rectal examination in the diagnosis of prostate carcinoma. N Engl J Med 1980; 303: 499–503
5. Chute C G, Guess H A, Panser L A et al. The non-relationship of urinary symptoms, prostate volume and uroflow in a population based sample of men. J Urol 1993; 149: 356A
6. Randall A (ed) Surgical pathology of prostatic obstruction. Baltimore: Williams and Wilkins, 1931
7. Simonson O, Moller-Madsen B, Dorflinger T et al. The significance of age on symptoms and urodynamic and cystoscopic findings in benign prostatic hypertrophy. Urol Res 1987; 15: 355–358
8. Oesterling J, Jacobson S, Chute C et al. Serum prostate specific antigen in a community-based population of health men: establishment of age specific reference ranges. JAMA 1993; 270: 860–864
9. Franks L M. Benign nodular hyperplasia of prostate: review. Ann R Coll Surg Engl 1954; 14: 92–106
10. Lytton B, Emery J M, Harvard B M. The incidence of benign prostatic hypertrophy. J Urol 1968; 99: 639–645
11. Bissada N K, Finkbeiner A E, Redman J F. Accuracy of preoperative estimation of resection weight in transurethral prostatectomy. J Urol 1976; 116: 201–202
12. Watanabe H. Natural history of benign prostatic hypertrophy. Ultrasound Med Biol 1986; 12: 567–571
13. Albarran, Hallé (eds) Hypertrofie et néoplasies épithéliales de la prostate. Arm Mal Org Gen Urin 1900; Feb/March
14. Cooner W H, Mosley B R, Rutherford C L Jr et al. Prostate cancer detection in a clinical urological practice by ultrasonography, digital rectal examination and prostate specific antigen. J Urol 1990; 143: 1146–1152
15. Faul P. Experience with the German annual preventive check-up examination. In: Jacobi G H, Hohenfellner R (eds) Prostate cancer. Baltimore: Williams and Wilkins, 1982: 57–70
16. Jewett J J. Significance of the palpable prostatic nodule. JAMA 1956; 160: 838–839

17. Hudson P B, Finkle A L, Hopkins J A et al. Prostatic cancer IX. Early prostatic cancer diagnosed by arbitrary open perineal biopsy among 300 unselected patients. Cancer 1954; 7: 690–703

18. Brawer M K. The diagnosis of prostatic carcinoma. Cancer 1993; 71: 899–905

19. Cooner W H. Rectal examination and ultrasonography in the diagnosis of prostate cancer. Prostate 1992; 4(suppl): 3–10

20. Chodack C W, Keller P, Schoenberg H W. Assessment for screening for prostate cancer using the digital rectal examination. J Urol 1989; 141: 1136–1138

21. Catalona W J, Richie J P, Ahmann F R et al. Comparison of digital rectal examination and serum prostate specific antigen in the early detection of prostate cancer: results of a multicenter clinical trial of 6,630 men. J Urol 1994; 151: 1283–1290

22. Bentvelsen F M, Schröder F H. Modalities available for screening for prostate cancer. Eur J Cancer 1993; 29a: 804–811

23. Thompson I M, Zeidman E J. Current urological practice: routine urological examination and early detection of carcinoma of the prostate. J Urol 1992; 148: 326–330

24. American Cancer Society. 1989 Survey of physicians' attitudes and practices in early cancer detection. CA 1990; 40: 77–80

14

Prostate-specific antigen and cancer assessment
C. T. Lee J. E. Oesterling

Introduction

Prostate-specific antigen (PSA) is a single-chain glycoprotein of 237 amino acids and four carbohydrate side chains.[1] It has a molecular weight of approximately 34 kilodaltons (kDa).[2] The complete gene encoding the PSA molecule has been sequenced and localized to chromosome 19.[3] Functionally, PSA is an organ-specific, kallikrein-like, serine protease produced by prostatic epithelial cells lining the acini and ducts of the prostate gland.[4,5] It is expressed in both benign and malignant processes involving epithelial cells of the prostate. Under normal physiological conditions, it is secreted into the lumina of the prostatic ducts, is present in the seminal plasma in high concentration, and is known to cause liquefaction of the seminal coagulum.[6] Without question, this marker has revolutionized the diagnosis and staging of prostate cancer and may be the most useful tumour marker in oncology today.

Currently, it is the best biomarker for prostate cancer that clinicians have available. Nevertheless, it is not perfect, in that it is organ specific but not disease specific; it can not, therefore, always reliably differentiate benign from malignant prostate disease. Furthermore, it can not differentiate clinically significant from clinically insignificant prostate cancers on an individual basis. For these reasons, investigators continue their study of proteins such as TURP-27 (ref. 7) or PD41 (ref. 8) that may have future utility in differentiating benign prostatic hyperplasia (BPH) from prostate cancer, 7E11-C5 (ref. 9), which may have utility in immunolocalization of soft tissue and bony metastatic disease, and PR92 (ref. 10), which may have utility in the prediction of prostate cancer prognosis.

Issues concerning early detection of prostate cancer

Screening

Screening refers to the application of a test to the general population. Early detection refers to the application of a test to a select population seeking medical attention wish to be evaluated after being informed of the issues. There are several criteria for disease screening: (1) the disease must be an important health problem; (2) there must be a recognizable early stage; (3) treatment at an early stage should be more beneficial than treatment at a later stage; (4) the screening test should be convenient and generally tolerable to patients; (5) adequate facilities should exist for diagnosis and treatment; and (6) the screening cost must be acceptable to society.

Much controversy has arisen regarding the early detection of prostate cancer. The current recommendation by the American Cancer Society, the American Urological Association and the American College of Radiology is that men over 50 years of age should undergo an annual digital rectal examination (DRE) and serum PSA determination for the purpose of detecting early prostate cancer.[11,12] Annual screening should begin at the age of 40 years in African-American men or in patients with a known family history of prostate cancer.

Most would agree that prostate cancer represents an important and common disease with a great burden of morbidity and mortality, particularly as the second leading cause of cancer death in men.[13] Enthusiasm for early detection of this disease has arisen from a well-known fact regarding prostate cancer — that all prostate cancer begins as a tumour confined to the prostate. If men with organ-confined prostate cancer undergo radical prostatectomy, they can essentially be cured of their disease and have a survival rate equivalent to that of age-matched men without prostate cancer.[14] In contrast, prostate cancer that is no longer organ confined is incurable. With this in mind, many currently feel that the only means of prevention of prostate cancer-related mortality is to detect the cancer at an early, organ-confined stage and initiate definitive therapy.

Sceptics regarding early detection of prostate cancer often fear that early detection will be cost-inefficient and will lead to an increase in the number of clinically insignificant tumours identified (as autopsy studies have shown that 11% or more of American men older than 50 years have histological evidence of prostate cancer).[15] In addition, many are concerned about the suboptimal sensitivity, specificity and predictive value of DRE, PSA and transrectal ultrasound (TRUS), and the impact of lead- and length-time bias. There is also a potential for increased prostatic biopsies with increased false positives causing economic and emotional burden.

Although many of these concerns are well founded, Smith and Catalona[16] have presented evidence to suggest that PSA-based screening produces a dramatic shift towards earlier-stage prostatic cancer in which 96–99% of the tumours are clinically localized, 40% are not palpable, and 70% are pathologically organ confined. Furthermore, 97% of these detected cancers have histological features associated with aggressive cancer, affirming that PSA screening detects clinically important and potentially life-threatening prostate cancer.[16] In addition, Benoit and Naslund[17] make an interesting comparison between the overall screening cost per prostate cancer detected in men aged 50–69 years (US$2372) and the overall screening cost per breast cancer detected in women aged 50–69 years (US$10 975).

Currently, it is not clear whether screening or early detection of prostate cancer will significantly affect patient survival. The prostate, lung, colorectal and ovarian (PLCO) cancer screening trial of the National Cancer Institute[18] will include 74 000 men and 74 000 women aged 60–74 years. This study is designed to determine whether screening for prostate cancer followed by appropriate treatment will save lives. It has a design power of 90% to determine a 20% reduction of prostate cancer mortality with screening efforts.

The T1c stage of prostate cancer

PSA has been in widespread clinical use since 1987. Since that time, PSA has been used as a marker to measure tumour recurrence after therapy, and more recently as a marker for early detection of prostate cancer. As a result there has been an increasing number of patients with prostate cancer who have an elevated serum PSA level and an unremarkable DRE. These PSA-detected cancers are classified at T1c in the TNM staging system[19] and B0 in the revised Whitmore–Jewett staging system.[20] Table 14.1 shows a comparison between the TNM and the revised Whitmore–Jewett staging systems.

In an effort to define better the characteristics of T1c tumours, Oesterling and colleagues[21] conducted a review of 208 patients with T1c prostate cancer that was detected on prostate biopsy because of an elevated serum PSA value (Hybritech, Tandem-R PSA assay). The preoperative and pathological characteristics of these patients were compared with those of an equal number of randomly selected stage T2a or T2b prostate cancer patients. All subjects were treated with radical prostatectomy. In comparing the preoperative characteristics of the two groups, the median age and the distribution of preoperative tumour grade showed no difference. There was, however, a significantly higher median serum PSA level (10 ng/ml) in the T1c group than in the T2a,2b group (6.7 ng/ml; $p<0.001$). In comparing the pathological characteristics of the two groups, multiple factors were analysed, including mean cancer volume, tumour focality, Gleason score, DNA ploidy, pathological stage, surgical margins and predominant tumour location, none of which were significantly different. Mean gland size, however, was 57 g in the T1c group and 47 g in the T2a,2b group; this difference was statistically significant ($p<0.001$). From these results the authors concluded that the pathological characteristics of the cancers were very similar in both patient groups. Thus, T1c cancers should not be regarded as insignificant. Those patients with a clinical stage T1c prostate cancer warrant therapeutic consideration and should be managed similarly to those with clinical stage T2a and T2b prostate cancers.

Epstein and associates[22] examined the preoperative and pathological parameters in 157 men with clinical stage T1c disease who underwent radical prostatectomy. These results were compared with those in 64 men with clinical stage T1a disease and 439 men with clinical stage T2 cancers (both groups also were treated with

Table 14.1. *Comparison of TNM and Whitmore–Jewett staging systems for clinically localized prostate cancer*

Stage		
TNM	Whitmore–Jewett	Description
TX	*	Tumour cannot be assessed
T0	*	No evidence of tumour
T1a	A1	Tumour found incidentally at TURP (<5% of resected tissue)
T1b	A2	Tumour found incidentally at TURP (>5% of resected tissue)
T1c	B0	Non-palpable tumour identified because of an elevated serum PSA value †
T2a	B1	Tumour involvement is less than or equal to one-half of a lobe
T2b	B1	Tumour involvement is more than one half of a lobe, but not both lobes
T2c	B2	Tumour involves both lobes
T3a	C1	Unilateral extracapsular extension
T3b	C1	Bilateral extracapsular extension
T3c	C2	Tumour invades one or both seminal vesicles
T4a	*	Tumour invades the bladder neck, external sphincter or rectum
T4b	*	Tumour invades the levator muscles or is fixed to the pelvic side wall

*No corresponding stage. †In the TNM staging system, the tumour should not be visible on transrectal ultrasonography. (From ref. 21 with permission.)

radical prostatectomy). Tumour burden was classified as insignificant if the volume was less than 0.2 cm³ and confined to the prostate, with a Gleason score of less than 7. All other tumour burden was felt to be significant, and was classified as minimal if 0.2–0.5 cm³ in volume, confined to the prostate, with a Gleason score less than 7; moderate if over 0.5 cm³, with capsular penetration and a Gleason score less than 7; or advanced if there was capsular penetration, a Gleason score of 7 or more, or positive margins, seminal vesicle invasion or lymph node involvement. Using these criteria, 16% of the subjects had insignificant disease and 84% had significant disease (10% minimal, 37% moderate and 37% advanced). These findings were intermediate between those found in clinical stages T1a and T2. The authors, like Oesterling and colleagues, concluded that non-palpable tumours detected by elevated serum PSA values are significant and deserve definitive treatment.

Similarly, Scaletscky et al.[23] examined 142 men who underwent radical prostatectomy for clinical stage T1c disease; they considered a tumour burden of 1 cm³ or above to be significant. Using this criterion they determined that 93 of 142 men (65%) displayed a significant disease state. The authors advocated treatment of stage T1c tumours in view of these data.

PSA and diagnosis

The glycoprotein

PSA was originally identified in seminal plasma in 1971 by Hara and associates,[24] and was later isolated and purified by Li and Beling.[3] In 1979, Wang and co-workers[2] isolated the same glycoprotein from human prostate tissue and were the first to refer to it as 'prostate-specific antigen'. In 1980, Papsidero et al.[25] developed a serological test to measure human serum levels of PSA.

The quantity of PSA in the serum is determined by commercial immunoassays that use monoclonal antibodies (MAbs) to identify epitopes on the PSA molecule. The most frequently used assays in the United States are the Tandem-R PSA and Tandem-E PSA assays (Hybritech, Inc., San Diego, CA) and the IMx PSA assay (Abbott Laboratories, Abbott Park, IL). The Tandem-R PSA and Tandem-E PSA assays both use two murine MAbs directed at separate epitopes on the PSA molecule. The IMx PSA assay is a monoclonal–polyclonal assay. For all three assays, the age-specific reference ranges (see Table 14.2) are applicable.[26] Most recently, an enhanced reverse transcriptase–polymerase chain reaction (PCR) assay[27] has also been described as a more sensitive and specific means of serum PSA

Table 14.2. *Age-specific reference ranges for serum prostate-specific antigen (PSA)*

Age (years)	Serum PSA* (ng/ml)	PSA density* (ng/ml/ml)
40–49	0.0–2.5	0.0–0.08
50–59	0.0–3.5	0.0–0.10
60–69	0.0–4.5	0.0–0.11
70–79	0.0–6.5	0.0–0.13

*Upper limits are defined as the 95th percentile. (Modified from ref. 26 with permission.)

detection. This type of assay may prove to be an effective modality for detecting micrometastases that are not identifiable by standard methods.

The half-life of PSA was determined by Stamey et al.[28] to be 2.2 ± 0.8 days, and later by Oesterling et al.[29] to be 3.2 ± 0.1 days. Because of the long half-life of this glycoprotein, it may take several weeks for serum levels to return to baseline levels after prostatic manipulation or to an undetectable value after retropubic radical prostatectomy. Oesterling et al.[30] showed that neither flexible nor rigid cystoscopy significantly changes serum PSA. In the same study, they showed that prostate biopsy causes an immediate median elevation in serum PSA of 7.9 ng/ml and requires a median of 15 days to return to baseline levels. In addition, transurethral resection of the prostate (TURP) causes a median elevation in PSA of 5.9 ng/ml and a median of 17 days is required for the PSA value to return to baseline following this procedure. Neal et al.[31] have shown that prostatitis causes elevations in serum PSA, possibly as a result of cell death and inflammatory disruption of epithelial cells and the normal physiological barriers that routinely keep PSA within the prostatic ductal system.

Effect of DRE on serum PSA

In a prospective, randomized controlled trial, Chybowski et al.[32] showed that the median serum PSA (Hybritech assay) elevation caused by DRE was 0.4 ng/ml. This represented a statistically but not clinically significant increase in the serum PSA level. The authors concluded that the serum PSA concentration in the immediate post-DRE period is accurate and would not compromise clinical use of the marker. Yuan et al.[33] similarly found that DRE had no significant effect on PSA. Prostatic massage produced serum PSA elevations in three of 20 (15%) patients and TRUS produced elevations above pre-TRUS serum PSA in four of 36 (11%) patients; the elevations, however, were not statistically significant. The authors concluded that DRE, prostatic massage and TRUS all have minimal effects on serum PSA levels in most patients.

These studies show that the serum PSA value is accurate and reliable after DRE, TRUS, prostatic massage or cystoscopic examination. However, PSA is significantly elevated after prostatic needle biopsy, TURP or episodes of prostatitis. Clinicians should therefore delay obtaining serum PSA levels for at least 4–6 weeks after such procedures/events to avoid spurious results. There appears to be no diurnal variation of PSA or significant PSA changes after ejaculation,[34] although the latter is the subject of ongoing studies by several investigators.

Prostate-specific antigen density

Because PSA is not specific to prostate cancer, there can be considerable overlap in the serum PSA concentrations between patients with early prostate cancer and BPH. The sensitivity of serum PSA ranges from 57 to 79%, and the specificity ranges from 59 to 68%;[35] thus, it can be difficult to distinguish patients with BPH from those with prostate cancer. Benson and co-workers[36,37] have described the concept of PSA density (PSAD), which represents the serum PSA concentration divided by the volume of the prostate gland as determined by TRUS. They have presented evidence to support a role for PSAD in the differentiation of BPH from prostate cancer.[36] Furthermore, they have shown that PSAD can be used to stratify the risk of cancer in patients with mild elevations of serum PSA (4.1–10.0 ng/ml, Hybritech assay).[37]

In another review,[38] 3140 men between the ages of 50 and 89 underwent prostatic evaluation with DRE, TRUS of the prostate and serum PSA. The authors concluded that PSAD or routine prostatic biopsy is not warranted in patients with a PSA of less than 4.0 ng/ml and a normal DRE. In addition, if the PSA is more than 20.0 ng/ml, the patient should undergo prostatic biopsy regardless of the DRE, given a 65% cancer detection rate. (PSAD does not contribute significantly to the detection rate in men with these higher PSA values and is therefore not recommended.) They do advocate the use of PSAD in patients with a PSA value between 4.1 and 20. The prostate volume determination is felt to be important in this group, since statistically significant differences were noted in PSAD values, but not PSA values, between cancer and BPH groups. Seemingly, the PSAD would allow the clinician to make an informed decision as to whether a biopsy is warranted.

Figure 14.1 is a probability plot that uses PSAD to predict the likelihood of a positive biopsy. The authors recommend clinical observation, DRE and serial serum PSA for a patient with a PSAD of 0.15 or less and a normal DRE. For patients with a normal DRE and a PSA greater than 0.15, the authors advocate proceeding with a prostate biopsy.

In contrast to this report, Brawer and colleagues[39] reviewed 218 men (median age 67 years) undergoing systematic random prostatic needle biopsy. They examined the ability of PSA and PSAD to distinguish benign and malignant disease; in addition, they studied the ability of the two to predict biopsy results. They were unable to show any advantage of PSAD over PSA alone in predicting the presence of prostate cancer. In fact, PSA was superior to PSAD in predicting biopsy results in patients with a normal DRE. Neither test was able reliably to distinguish benign disease from malignant disease in patients with serum PSA values between 4.1 and 10.0 ng/ml.

Catalona and associates[40] have questioned the suggested PSAD upper limit of normal (0.15). They prospectively studied 4962 men, average age 63 years. Subjects were evaluated by DRE and PSA. If the serum PSA was greater than 4 ng/ml and/or DRE was suspicious, the patient underwent four (quadrant) TRUS-guided prostatic biopsies in addition to biopsies of suspicious areas on DRE and/or TRUS. In evaluating the PSAD for patients with intermediate PSA levels (4.1–9.9), a PSAD cutoff of 0.15 had a specificity of 81% and an unacceptably low sensitivity of 52%. The majority (93%) of the tumours missed with this PSAD cutoff were clinically significant. If a PSAD cutoff of

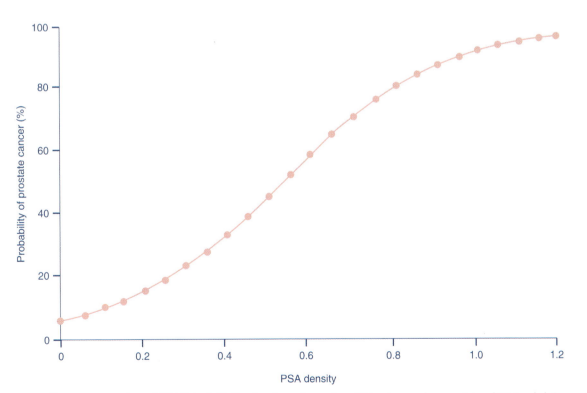

Figure 14.1. *Discriminant analysis of PSAD (ng/ml/ml) values for patients whose PSA values are between 4.1 and 10.0 ng/ml. It examines only those patients who underwent prostate biopsy (either abnormal transrectal ultrasound or abnormal digital rectal examination). (From ref. 38 with permission.)*

0.15 had been used as an indication for prostatic biopsy, nearly half of the tumours would have been missed. The authors recommended that men in this group should undergo biopsy based upon PSA concentration rather than on the PSAD determination.

PSAD appears to have some utility in distinguishing BPH from prostate cancer, and in identifying those patients with prostate cancer who have mildly elevated or intermediate PSA levels and normal DRE. However, Oesterling et al. have shown that PSAD does not provide additional clinical information over PSA, when age-specific reference ranges are used.[41] Despite the ability of PSAD to identify unapparent but clinically significant cancers in some patients, concerns still remain regarding reproducibility of density determinations in relation to volume measurements with TRUS and variations in normal prostate sizes, as well as the significant differences in stromal-to-epithelial ratios between prostates.

Currently, the authors conclude that there is no significant role for PSAD in the early detection of prostate cancer, especially when age-specific reference ranges are used.

Prostate-specific antigen velocity

PSA velocity (PSAV) is defined as the change in serum PSA over time. This concept was developed in an effort to improve the ability of the clinician to distinguish BPH from malignant prostatic disease, in addition to improving the identification of men with prostate cancer destined to progress. The rationale for developing such a concept would be to use serial PSA concentrations in a meaningful way to evaluate a patient, thus avoiding the interrelated variables of PSA concentration, BPH volume, cancer volume and cancer differentiation.[42] As the amount of benign epithelium increases or the cancer volume increases, the PSA concentration increases. However, poorly differentiated cancers produce less PSA than well-differentiated cancers when equal volumes of each are compared.[42] Thus, these variables may make the interpretation of a single PSA somewhat difficult.

In a retrospective study, Carter and associates[43,44] reviewed prostatic evaluation and treatment in 54 men who were part of the Baltimore Longitudinal Study of Aging. A group of 20 men with a histological diagnosis of BPH and a group of 20 men with a histological diagnosis of prostate cancer were compared with a control group of 16 men without prostatic disease. When the PSAV was calculated, the investigators found a significant difference in the age-adjusted rate of change in PSA between the groups, with that for cancer being greater than that for BPH, which, again, was greater than that for controls ($p<0.01$). (Figure 14.2 shows the exponential changes in the cancer group, and the non-linear changes in the BPH group. The mean change in PSA for the control group did not differ significantly from zero.)

A PSAV of at least 0.75 ng/ml per year resulted in correct identification of 72% of the cancer subjects (sensitivity 72%) and correct identification of 92% of the BPH subjects (specificity 90%). The authors concluded that PSAV was a potentially useful tool in distinguishing benign and malignant prostate disease. In addition, PSAV might be helpful in much earlier detection of prostate cancer in men with a normal DRE and a normal PSA.

In a prospective study of 376 cancer-free men, Oesterling and associates[45] examined the rate of change

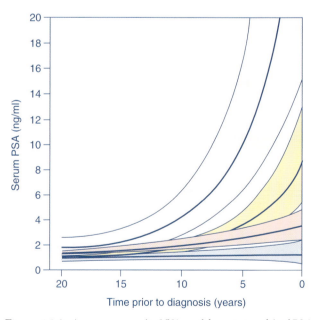

Figure 14.2. *Average curves (± 95% confidence intervals) of PSA levels (ng/ml) as a function of years before diagnosis for three diagnostic groups (■, BPH; ■, local/regional cancer; , metastatic cancer) and a control group ( ); based on observed data (n = 54). (From ref. 43 with permission.)*

in serum PSA over a period of at least 12 months. They found a very wide variation in both the serum PSA concentration and PSAV across all age ranges; in addition, approximately 25–33% of patients without clinical evidence of cancer had more than a 20% increase in the serum PSA concentration during 1 year. Similarly, Carter and associates[46] suggested that there is great variability in PSA measurements made a few months apart. If PSAV is to have clinical value, therefore, the present authors advocate obtaining PSA determinations at least 1 year apart, and using at least three determinations to calculate the velocity value.

Free versus complexed PSA

Discrepancies in serum PSA levels between different immunoassays can quickly make the evaluation process quite confusing. Discrepancies may be due to different forms of PSA in circulation or the ability of assays to detect these different forms. Whether an assay utilizes monoclonal or polyclonal antibody conjugates may also affect the selection of varying forms.[47] In addition, protein binding kinetics may favour smaller molecules and, therefore, rapid assay may tend to detect these molecules preferentially.

PSA exists in serum predominantly in a complexed form, bound to either alpha-1-antichymotrypsin (ACT, MW 58 kDa), or to alpha-2-macroglobulin (AMG, MW 725 kDa).[48,49] Figure 14.3 shows the free and complexed

forms of PSA. ACT and AMG are two major extracellular protease inhibitors, referred to as serpins. Purified PSA is known to form stable complexes with ACT and AMG in vitro.[48] The complexed form of PSA and ACT (PSA–ACT) inactivates the protease effects of PSA. This complex does not prevent immunoassays from detecting PSA, because the ACT molecule does not cover important PSA epitopes. In contrast, when PSA forms a complex with AMG, its epitopes become covered by the enclosing action of the AMG. This enclosure of PSA prevents exposure of its epitopes and therefore inactivates its protease function as well as preventing its detection by immunoassays. Therefore, free PSA and PSA–ACT are able to be detected by assays.

Antibodies are used in commercial assays to identify epitopes of PSA. Monoclonal antibodies recognize a specific epitope that is present on free and complexed PSA. Polyclonal antibody conjugates, however, may include a subpopulation that binds to the same region of PSA to which ACT binds. Thus, free PSA would only be bound by the subpopulation, as ACT would block the epitope, resulting in preferential binding of free PSA and a skewed response.[50] Differences in kinetics between commercial assays can also lead to discrepancy in detection. Because of its small size (approximately 30 kDa), PSA may have the potential to react faster than PSA–ACT (approximately 100 kDa). Thus, in rapid non-equilibrium assays there might be a higher response to free PSA.[50]

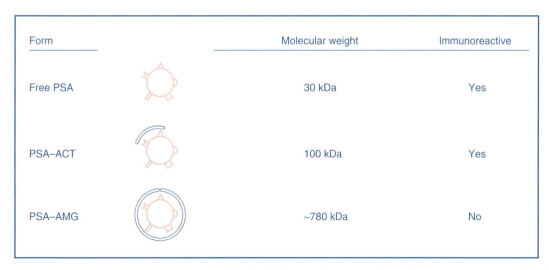

Form		Molecular weight	Immunoreactive
Free PSA		30 kDa	Yes
PSA–ACT		100 kDa	Yes
PSA–AMG		~780 kDa	No

Figure 14.3. *Forms of PSA in serum: PSA–ACT, PSA complexed to alpha-1-antichymotrypsin (ACT); PSA–AMG, PSA complexed to alpha-2-macroglobulin (AMG). (From ref. 50 with permission.)*

Graves[51,52] has described PSA assays that have equimolar response and skewed response. The equimolar assay is dependent on the concentration of PSA present. A skewed-response assay is dependent upon PSA concentration and the ratio of free PSA to PSA–ACT in the sample; the skewed response may therefore measure PSA forms disproportionately. The clinical significance of these differences has yet to be determined but, because of assay discrepancies, many currently advocate the standardization of PSA detection.[53]

There has been speculation concerning heterogeneity of PSA among pathological conditions, which might be manifest as differing patterns of serum binding of PSA forms. Christensson et al.[54] examined serum samples from 265 consecutive patients with prostatic disease; 121 had prostate cancer (mean age of 74 years) and 144 had BPH (mean age 72 years). They used three different assays to study free and complexed levels of PSA in the serum of both categories of patients: one assay measured free PSA, a second measured complexed PSA (PSA–ACT), and a third measured total PSA (free plus complexed). The found that complexed PSA was the predominant form in all sera. In addition, the complexed-to-total ratio was significantly ($p<0.0001$) higher in patients with prostate cancer than in patients with BPH. Free PSA constituted a significantly smaller fraction in cancer patients than in patients with BPH ($p<0.0001$). They were unable to find a direct correlation between serum PSA and serum ACT.

Similarly, Lilja and co-workers[55] found a median of 18% free PSA in carcinoma and 28% free PSA in BPH. Stenman and co-workers[56] reported 40% free PSA in prostate cancer in comparison to 60% in BPH, as well as a significantly higher proportion of serum PSA complexed to ACT in patients with prostate cancer as opposed to those with BPH. These corroborating observations support the concept that there is a lower free-to-total PSA ratio or a higher complex-to-total PSA ratio in the serum of prostate cancer patients. This concept may create a mechanism to improve the diagnostic specificity of PSA further by examining its various forms.

Oesterling et al.[57] have established age-specific reference ranges for free (F), complexed (C) and total (T) PSA, seen in Table 14.3. These investigators are prospectively studying a cancer-free cohort of 426 men in order to determine the clinical utility of free and complexed PSA forms in the detection of early prostate cancer. Currently, the clinical utility remains to be defined. It may also be that the ratio of the molecular forms, F/T, C/T and F/C, will have clinical importance. The free-to-total PSA ratio may particularly increase the ability of PSA to distinguish early prostate cancer accurately from BPH.[54] This issue will probably be clarified with the development of a recently designed dual-label, monoclonal–monoclonal, immunofluorometric assay for the simultaneous measurement of both free and total PSA serum levels as well as of the value of the free-to-total PSA ratio.[58,59]

Age-specific reference ranges of PSA

Clinicians have used a general PSA reference range of 0.0–0.4 ng/ml as a normal result. If an elevated level has returned, further evaluation by TRUS and/or prostate biopsy has been carried out. This may not be the appropriate range for all men, as this single range does not account for age difference or normal variations in prostatic volume.

The normal ageing prostate undergoes histological hyperplastic changes of the epithelial cells. These changes result in increased prostate size and increased levels of PSA production, as 1 g BPH gives rise to 0.2 ng/ml PSA in the serum.[28] Increased PSA levels in ageing prostates may also be influenced by prostatic ischaemia or infarction, chronic subclinical prostatitis, prostatic intraepithelial neoplasia, and loss of normal physiological barrier integrity and a leakage of PSA into capillaries and lymphatics.

Table 14.3. *Age-specific reference ranges for free (F), complexed (C) and total (T) PSA*

Molecular form of PSA	Age-specific reference range (ng/ml)			
	40–49 years	50–59 years	60–69 years	70–79 years
F	0.5	0.75	1.0	1.5
C	1.5	2.0	2.5	3.5
T	2.5	3.5	4.5	6.5

(From ref. 57 with permission.)

Oesterling and co-workers[26] critically reviewed this issue in a prospective study of 471 White men aged 40–79 years who had no evidence of prostatic cancer by DRE, PSA determination (Tandem-R PSA) or TRUS. These investigators attempted to define a relationship between serum PSA concentration, prostatic volume (as determined by TRUS), PSAD and patient age. Pearson product–moment correlation coefficients were used to measure associations between serum PSA concentration and age, prostate volume and age, PSA and prostate volume, and PSAD and age. The Pearson product–moment correlation (r) is a parametric statistical method designed to measure the extent to which pairs of measurements are associated. Table 14.4 shows a breakdown of the patient population and median data for these parameters by age group. There were direct correlations between PSA and age ($r=0.43$; $p<0.0001$) (Fig. 14.4), prostatic volume and age ($r=0.43$; $p<0.0001$), PSA and prostatic volume ($r=0.55$; $p<0.0001$), and PSAD and age ($r=0.25$; $p<0.0001$). Age ranges were grouped by 10-year intervals from 40 to 79 years of age. The 95th percentile was used as the upper limit of normal for PSA concentration and PSAD, and the 2.5–97.5th percentile range was considered normal for prostate volume, within each 10-year range. Table 14.4 reflects the age-specific median values and ranges for serum PSA, prostate volume and PSAD.

Table 14.4. *Median values of serum PSA concentration, prostate volume and PSA density, by age*

Parameter	Age group (years)			
	40–49	50–59	60–69	70–79
No. of patients	165	144	94	68
Serum PSA (ng/ml)	0.7 (0.5, 1.1)*	1.0 (0.6, 1.4)	1.4 (0.9, 3.0)	2.0 (0.9, 3.2)
Prostate vol. (ml)	23.5 (20.4, 29.0)	30.7 (23.0, 37.1)	34.6 (28.0, 43.7)	35.4 (29.6, 51.4)
PSA density (ng/ml)	0.03 (0.02, 0.04)	0.03 (0.02, 0.05)	0.05 (0.03, 0.07)	0.05 (0.03, 0.08)

*Numbers in parentheses indicate the 25th and 75th percentiles.
(From ref. 26 with permission.)

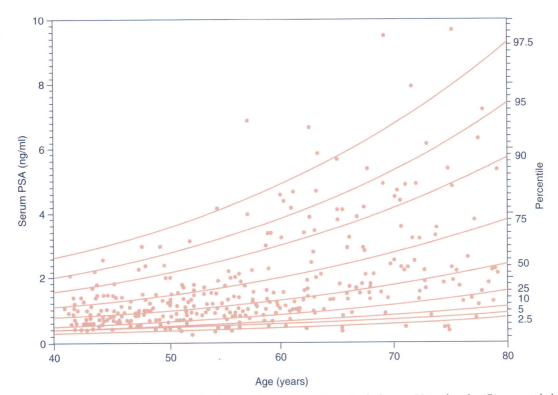

Figure 14.4. *Serum PSA concentration as a function of patient age. Scattergram of the individual serum PSA values for 471 men, with the curves for the 2.5th, 5th, 10th, 25th, 50th, 75th, 90th, 95th and 97.5th percentiles. (From ref. 26 with permission.)*

Dalkin and associates[60] have defined upper limits of normal PSA levels after examining 5220 men without evidence of prostate cancer. They determined normal serum PSA levels to be 3.7 ng/ml for men aged 50–54 years, 4.0 ng/ml for those of 55–59 years, 5.4 ng/ml for 60–64 years, 6.2 ng/ml for 65–69 years, and 6.6 ng/ml for 70–74 years. Feneley and colleagues[61] studied 200 men with symptoms of bladder outlet obstruction using DRE, serum PSA determination and TRUS. Patients without evidence of prostate cancer demonstrated a statistically significant correlation between prostate volume and age, and PSA and age. These authors favoured the use of an age-adjusted PSA reference range applied to the investigation of symptomatic prostatic disease.

Collins et al.[62] examined the relationship between PSA levels, prostate volume and age in 472 men (40–79 years, mean age 60 years) who underwent PSA determination, DRE and TRUS as part of a survey of BPH. None of these subjects had prostate cancer. The authors noted that age and prostate volume influenced PSA levels independently. They concluded that further study was needed to determine the sensitivity and specificity of age-adjusted PSA levels in association with DRE and TRUS in the detection of prostate cancer. Additional evidence in support of age-adjusted reference ranges has been put forward by Crawford and colleagues[63] upon examination of data obtained during Prostate Cancer Awareness Week, 1993. Similarly, Dalkin and associates[64] have provided additional evidence to support this concept.

Recently, the selection of optimal PSA cutoffs for early detection of prostate cancer was reviewed. Catalona and associates[65] conducted a multicentre prospective clinical trial involving 6630 men aged 50 years or more. These men underwent serum PSA determination and DRE. Biopsies were performed if the PSA level was greater than 4.0 ng/ml or if the DRE was suspicious for cancer. Sensitivity, specificity, and positive and negative predictive values were compared in varying age groups and varying PSA ranges. They did not find a significant difference in total cancers detected and total biopsies avoided. Although there were differences in the number of cancers detected in varying age populations, the authors concluded that there is no need for age-adjusted PSA reference ranges.

The current authors advocate the use of age-specific reference ranges for PSA determinations. Prostate cancer does not have the same clinical significance for men of all ages. In view of this, a constant predictive value for PSA across all ages need not be maintained and should not be an objective. With advancing age, the prevalence of prostate cancer increases, but the biological threat to life diminishes. As a result, the true goal is to increase the sensitivity of PSA in younger men with an extended life expectancy (men who can truly benefit from definitive treatment) and to increase the specificity of PSA in older men with a limited life expectancy (men who are less likely to benefit from aggressive medical intervention). The age-specific reference ranges for serum PSA do exactly this, making PSA a more clinically useful tumour marking for the detection of early prostate cancer.

Effect of finasteride on serum PSA

In the quest to find medical treatment for BPH, finasteride was developed. Finasteride is a synthetic 4-azasteroid compound that competitively inhibits 5-alpha-reductase, an enzyme that converts testosterone to dihydrotestosterone (DHT).[66] The indications and effects of finasteride are discussed in depth in Chapter 22.

In general, the effect of finasteride is a median decrease of 20% in the size of the prostate gland after 6 months' treatment.[67] Gormley and co-workers[68] also analysed the effect of finasteride on BPH and serum PSA level in 895 men from 40 to 83 years of age in a multicentre, double-blind study: they noted a 50% decrease in PSA levels in patients receiving 5 mg/day by 3 months, and a 48% decrease in those receiving 1 mg/day, also by 3 months; the PSA levels of the placebo group did not change significantly.

Guess and co-workers[69] undertook further review of the North America phase III multicentre clinical trial of finasteride in the treatment of men with symptomatic BPH. The authors determined that percentage reduction in PSA induced by finasteride did not appear to be influenced by the age of the patient. They reviewed the men found to have prostate cancer while receiving a 5 mg daily dose of finasteride, either during the initial 12 months (n=1) or during the subsequent 12 months, when all patients were administered 5 mg finasteride daily (n=14). The median percentage decrease in PSA concentration, from before therapy to the time of cancer diagnosis, was 36%. Finasteride did not appear to have a greater effect on PSA of malignant origin than PSA of benign origin.

Clinicians should have an increased suspicion for prostate cancer when a patient on finasteride therapy has not had the expected 50% decline from the baseline serum PSA level. There are, however, patients whose PSA levels may not be appropriately decreased, secondary to non-compliance. A serum DHT level can provide objective evidence of compliance and should reflect a 60% decrease after 6 months of finasteride therapy.[67] It is important to have a baseline level before initiation of finasteride therapy.

Diagnostic algorithm for the detection of prostate cancer

In view of the recent developments in PSA and its use as a diagnostic marker, Oesterling and colleagues[41] have proposed a diagnostic algorithm to aid clinicians in providing the most thorough, yet cost-effective, evaluation of the prostate gland. They recommend restricting evaluation of the prostate to men aged 50 years or older, with a life expectancy of 10 years or more, in view of the slow-growing nature of prostate cancer. That recommendation implies that elderly or debilitated patients with a less than 10-year life expectancy should not be subjected to either a serum PSA determination or a DRE for the purpose of detecting early prostate cancer. In contrast, they advocate aggressive and early evaluation, beginning at age 40, for individuals at high risk for the development of prostate cancer, including African-American men and those with a family history of prostate cancer.

Table 14.5 demonstrates this algorithm. If the serum PSA is less than or equal to the age-specific range (see Table 14.2) and the patient has an unremarkable DRE, the patient should be followed with yearly PSA levels and DRE. If the PSA level is greater than the age-specific range and the DRE is unremarkable, TRUS should be performed, together with an accompanying biopsy of visible lesions; in addition, a systematic sextant biopsy of remaining prostatic tissue should be performed, taking care to gain tissue from the transition zone. If the DRE is remarkable, the patient should

Table 14.5. *Algorithm for the use of age-specific PSA reference ranges and DRE to detect clinically significant prostate cancers at an early, curable stage*

PSA*	DRE	Diagnostic action
≤ Age-specific range	Negative	Annual PSA and DRE
> Age-specific range	Negative	TRUS: biopsy visible lesions; sextant biopsy of remaining prostate, with two cores containing transition zone tissue
Any value	Positive	TRUS: biopsy palpable and visible lesions; sextant biopsy of remaining prostate

*Tandem-R or IMx PSA assay. (From ref. 41 with permission.)

undergo TRUS, regardless of the PSA level; at the time of TRUS, a biopsy of the palpable nodules and hypoechoic lesions should be performed; in addition, a systematic sextant biopsy of the remaining prostate gland should be carried out.

PSA and staging

Kleer and Oesterling[70] have demonstrated a direct relationship between serum PSA and tumour volume. However, overlap in serum PSA levels between stages has resulted in the inability of PSA to predict pathological stage reliably on an individual basis. The predictive power of PSA, however, can be enhanced with the combination of other factors such as clinical stage (assessed by DRE) and tumour grade (via prostatic biopsy).

Most recently, in a retrospective study of 945 untreated prostate cancer patients with a mean age of 66 years, Kleer and colleagues[71] used multivariate regression analysis to show that local clinical stage and tumour grade significantly enhance the predictive power of PSA to determine pathological stage. They used these preoperative parameters to construct probability plots that would estimate the likelihood of an individual having histological disease that displayed organ confinement, capsular penetration, seminal vesicle invasion, positive surgical margins or lymph node involvement. They concluded that these estimates would assist clinicians in recommending the most appropriate therapy and also in planning surgical approaches to ensure complete tumour resection with reduced compromise to normal function. Similarly, Partin and co-workers[72] also used logistic regression analysis to show that serum PSA (Hybritech assay), preoperative Gleason score and clinical stage, in combination, were able to predict final pathological stage.

Blackwell and colleagues[73] undertook a prospective analysis of 311 previously untreated men with prostate cancer with clinical stages T1cN0 (n=19), T2aN0 (n=271) and T3N0 (n=21) (see Table 14.1 for the TNM classification system for prostate cancer). They assessed the PSA cancer density (PSACD; serum PSA times cancer volume divided by prostate volume) and demonstrated a significantly stronger correlation of PSACD with pathological stage than PSA level alone or PSAD with stage. However, in this study the cancer and prostatic volumes were obtained from the surgical specimen after radical retropubic prostatectomy, making the results rather difficult to apply to preoperative situations. Nevertheless, these data do suggest that preoperative quantification of cancer volume (currently imprecise using standard imaging methods) and prostate volume (probably by TRUS) may provide a promising combination of variables that will be highly predictive of pathological stage. The authors do suggest the use of endorectal coil magnetic resonance imaging as a future means of assessing prostatic cancer volume more precisely.

Eliminating the staging bilateral pelvic lymphadenectomy using PSA

Many urologists will perform open or laparoscopic pelvic lymphadenopathy for patients with clinically localized prostate cancer in order to stage the patient accurately and therefore advise on the most definitive and effective therapy.

Danella and co-workers[74] have found that the incidence of lymphatic metastases in patients with clinically localized prostate cancer is 5.7%. Bluestein and colleagues[75] have attempted to demonstrate a reasonable means of predicting which patients are most likely to have positive pelvic nodes. In a retrospective study, they looked at 1632 patients, ranging in age from 38 to 83 years with a mean of 66 years, who had localized prostate cancer and underwent bilateral pelvic

lymphadenopathy. None of these men had received preoperative therapy. Univariate and multivariate logistic regression models were used to predict the probability of positive pelvic lymph nodes as a function of patient age, prior TURP, PSA (Hybritech Tandem-R assay), primary Gleason grade and local clinical stage. Neither patient age nor TURP was significant in predicting positive pelvic lymph nodes. Gleason grade, PSA and clinical stage all had a positive correlation with the presence of pelvic lymph node metastases ($p<0.001$ for each).

Using the logistic regression model to analyse all three variables, they were able to predict the probability of a patient having positive lymph nodes, as seen in Table 14.6. They further proposed that a conservative false-negative rate of 3% would be acceptable. Table 14.6 shows the combined clinical stage, tumour grade and PSA level that would yield a 3% false-negative rate. The authors recommend eliminating pelvic lymphadenectomy in patients with equal or lower serum PSA levels, and the appropriate corresponding stages/grades as seen in Table 14.6. If this recommendation had been applied to their patient population, 406 patients would not have undergone bilateral pelvic lymphadenectomy. Among these 406 patients, three actually had microscopic positive lymph nodes, representing a false-negative rate of less than 1%. These results suggest that 25–30% of patients with

Table 14.6. *Combinations of local clinical stage, primary Gleason grade and serum PSA to yield a false-negative rate of 3% for positive lymph nodes*

Local clinical stage	Primary Gleason grade	Serum PSA* (ng/ml)
T1a–T2b (A1–B1)	1 and 2	17.1
	3	8.0
	4 and 5	4.2
T2c (B2)	1 and 2	4.1
	3	2.0
	4 and 5	1.0
T3a (C1)	1 and 2	1.4
	3	0.7
	4 and 5	0.3

*Patients with lower serum PSA values have a false-negative rate of less than 3%. (From ref. 75 with permission.)

clinically localized disease may be spared pelvic lymph node dissection when PSA is used in combination with tumour grade. In support of these results, in a retrospective study of 945 men, Kleer and colleagues[71] found PSA to be the best single predictor of positive lymph node status. By including local clinical stage, as determined by DRE, and tumour grade, as determined by biopsy specimen, there was a significant enhancement of the predictive power of PSA.

This type of predictability could have important implications in prevention of patient morbidity from lymphadenectomy and in health care dollar expenditure, as the mean total cost of open pelvic lymphadenectomy is US$8185 and that of laparoscopic dissection is US$9449.[76]

Eliminating the staging radionuclide bone scan using PSA

Standard staging evaluation for prostate cancer has included DRE, serum PSA, serum prostatic acid phosphatase (PAP) and a radionuclide bone scan. For many patients a staging radionuclide bone scan may no longer be necessary. Investigators have recently assessed the ability of PSA to be a positive predictor of bone-scan findings.

Chybowski and co-workers[77] looked at 521 randomly selected patients in a retrospective study. These patients, ranging from 44 to 92 years of age with a mean age of 70 years, all had untreated prostate cancer. All patients were assessed with DRE (establishing clinical stage), prostate biopsy or TURP (establishing tumour grade), serum acid phosphatase, PAP, PSA and radionuclide bone scan. The investigators attempted to correlate these factors with bone-scan findings. Local clinical stage, tumour grade, acid phosphatase, PAP and PSA all correlated positively with the incidence of a positive bone scan, each with $p<0.0001$. However, using receiver operating characteristic (ROC) curves, PSA was found to be the best in predicting the results of a radionuclide bone scan. Figure 14.5 is a probability plot, based on ROC curve data, that demonstrates the relationship between serum PSA and the likelihood of positive bone-scan findings. No patient with a serum PSA concentration less than or equal to 15 ng/ml had a positive bone scan. Only one man had a PSA of less than 20 ng/ml (18.2 ng/ml) and a positive scan. The

false-negative rate for a serum PSA of 20 ng/ml or less was calculated as 0.3%, with the lower and upper 95% confidence limits being 0.1 and 1.8 ng/ml, respectively. The observed false-negative rate for a PSA of 10 ng/ml or less was 0.0, with confidence limits of 0.0–1.2 ng/ml.

Multivariate logistic regression anaysis was used to predict whether these variables in combination would improve the power of PSA to predict bone-scan findings. Only clinical stage and acid phosphatase contributed slightly (but not significantly) to the overall predictive power of PSA. The authors concluded that radionuclide bone scans are unnecessary in the staging evaluation of previously untreated prostate cancer patients who have no skeletal symptoms and a serum PSA value of 10 ng/ml or less.

In confirmation of these findings, Oesterling et al.[78] retrospectively reviewed 852 patients with newly diagnosed untreated prostate cancer and a serum PSA concentration of less than 20 ng/ml. A correlation of multiple factors with bone-scan findings, again revealed serum PSA — irrespective of tumour grade and local clinical stage — to be the best predictor of bone-scan results. Of the 852 patients, 66% had PSA concentrations of 10 ng/ml or less, 20% had PSA concentrations from 10.1 to 15.0 ng/ml, and 14% had values of from 15.1 to 20 ng/ml. Only seven (0.8%) patients had a positive bone scan; five of these patients (71%) had appreciable skeletal symptoms relating to the location of positive findings on the bone scan. There was, however, one patient who had no skeletal symptoms, a PSA concentration of less than 10.0 ng/ml and a positive bone scan. The observed false-negative rate for a PSA of 10.0 ng/ml or less was 0.5, with 95% lower and upper confidence limits of 0.1 and 1.6 ng/ml.

These studies show that very few patients with serum PSA concentrations of less than 20 ng/ml, and only rarely those with PSA concentrations of 10 ng/ml or less, have skeletal metastases. It is, therefore, unnecessary to use a radionuclide bone scan in staging the asymptomatic, newly diagnosed, previously untreated prostate cancer patient with a PSA concentration of 10 ng/ml or less. This group represents a substantial number of patients, since 39% of men presenting with newly diagnosed prostate cancer have a PSA of 10 ng/ml or less.[79] Oesterling and co-workers[78] examined the economic implications of eliminating the

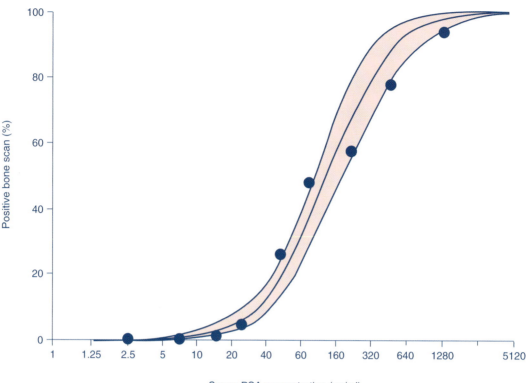

Figure 14.5. *Probability plot. Predicted percentage of newly diagnosed, untreated prostate cancer patients with positive bone scans (solid line) based on a logistic regression model using a natural logarithm of serum PSA concentration. Confidence limits (95%) for predicted percentages also are shown (shaded area). Solid circles denote observed percentages based on PSA groupings determined by cutoff points of 5, 10, 20, 40, 80, 160, 320 and 640 in 521 patients. (From ref. 77 with permission.)*

radionuclide bone scan in this group of patients and calculated a potential saving of 38 million US health care dollars annually.[79]

Summary

PSA is currently the most important, accurate and clinically useful tumour marker for prostate cancer. PSA can be effectively used to diagnose, stage and monitor the prostate cancer patient. To improve the sensitivity and specificity of PSA, factors such as rate of change, prostate volume and age have been considered in combination with PSA, thereby creating PSAV, PSAD and age-specific PSA reference ranges, respectively. These factors have assisted in distinguishing benign from malignant prostatic disease. Finasteride will decrease PSA levels by 50% within 6 months, and therefore the clinician must consider this reduction when interpreting PSA-related variables. The previously mentioned diagnostic algorithm (Table 14.5) is a useful and efficient guide for clinicians to utilize for the detection of cancer.

Staging based on PSA level alone is inexact. However, the combination of tumour grade (by prostatic biopsy), clinical stage (by DRE) and, potentially, cancer and prostatic volumes, all enhance the power of PSA to predict final pathological stage. PSA is a very good predictor of positive lymph node status, enhanced by clinical stage and tumour grade, and can thus be used to eliminate pelvic lymphadenectomy according to the guidelines in Table 14.6. In addition, staging radionuclide bone scans can be eliminated in asymptomatic, previously untreated prostate cancer patients with serum PSA levels of 10 ng/ml or less.

Additional understanding of the biomolecular and physiological properties of PSA will probably improve the ability to detect clinically significant tumours using this parameter. The issue of increased levels of complexed PSA being associated with malignant disease as opposed to BPH may offer insight into improved detection. Further development of immunoassay techniques may prove to be clinically significant.

In view of the usefulness of PSA, the present authors advocate obtaining a serum level as part of the standard evaluation for men with the diagnosis of BPH. Symptoms of prostatism and prostate cancer often overlap, and therefore the clinician must be active in discerning the two processes. In men aged 50 years or more with a 10-year life expectancy, and in those aged 40 years or more with an increased risk for prostate cancer, minimum assessment must include a history, DRE and a serum PSA level. PSA is clearly important in prostate cancer assessment and additionally may be used in the early detection of prostate cancer.

References

1. Lundwall A, Lilja H. Molecular cloning of human prostate specific antigen cDNA. FEBS Lett 1987; 214: 317–322
2. Wang M, Valenzuela L, Murphy G et al. Purification of a human prostate specific antigen. Invest Urol 1979; 17: 159–163
3. Li T, Beling C. Isolation and characterization of two specific antigens of human seminal plasma. Fertil Steril 1973; 24: 134–144
4. Lilja H. A kallikrein-like serine protease in prostatic fluid cleaves the predominant seminal vesicle protein. J Clin Invest 1985; 76: 1899–1903
5. Oesterling J. Prostate specific antigen: a critical assessment of the most useful tumor marker for adenocarcinoma of the prostate. J Urol 1991; 145: 907–923
6. Schellhammer P, Wright G Jr. Biomolecular and clinical characteristics of PSA and other candidate prostate tumor markers. Urol Clin North Am 1993; 20: 597–606
7. Wright G Jr, Beckett M, Lipford G et al. A novel prostate carcinoma-associated glycoprotein complex (PAC) recognized by monoclonal antibody TURP-27. Int J Cancer 1991; 47: 717–725
8. Beckett M, Lipford G, Haley C et al. Monoclonal antibody PD41 recognizes an antigen restricted to prostate adenocarcinomas. Cancer Res 1991; 51: 1326–1333
9. Horoszewicz J, Kawinski E, Murphy G. Monoclonal antibodies to a new antigenic marker in epithelial prostatic cells and serum of prostatic cancer patients. Anticancer Res 1987; 7: 927–936
10. Kim Y, Robinson D, Manderino G et al. Molecular characterization of the epitope in prostate and breast tumor-associated PR92 antigen. Cancer Res 1989; 49: 2379–2382
11. Mettlin C, Jones G, Averette H et al. Defining and updating the American Cancer Society guidelines for the cancer-related checkup: prostate and endometrial cancers. CA 1993; 43: 42–46
12. American Urological Association. Early detection of prostate cancer and use of transrectal ultrasound. In: American Urological Association 1992 Policy Statement Book, Vol. 4. Baltimore: American Urological Association, 1992: 20
13. Boring C, Squires T, Tong T, Montgomery S. Cancer statistics, 1994. CA 1994; 44: 7–26
14. Jewett H. Radical perineal prostatectomy for palpable, clinically localized, non-obstructive cancer: experience at the Johns Hopkins Hospital 1909–1963. J Urol 1980; 124: 492–494
15. Halpert B, Sheehan E, Schmalhorst W, Scott R. Carcinoma of the prostate. A survey of 5,000 autopsies. Cancer 1963; 16: 737–742
16. Smith D, Catalona W. The nature of prostate cancer detected through prostate specific antigen based screening. J Urol 1994; 152: 1732–1736
17. Benoit N, Naslund M J. An economic rationale for prostate cancer screening. Urology 1994; 44: 795–803
18. Gohagan J, Prorok P, Kramer B, Cornett J. Prostate cancer screening in the prostate, lung, colorectal and ovarian cancer screening trial of the National Cancer Institute. J Urol 1994; 152: 1905–1909
19. Schroder F, Hermanek P, Denis L et al. The TNM classification of prostate cancer. Prostate 1992; 4S: 129–138
20. Stormont T, Farrow G, Myers R et al. Clinical stage B_0 or $T1_C$ prostate cancer: nonpalpable disease identified by elevated serum prostate-specific antigen concentration. Urology 1993; 41: 3–8
21. Oesterling J, Suman V, Zincke H, Bostwick D. PSA-detected (clinical stage T1c or B_0) prostate cancer: pathologically significant tumors. Urol Clin North Am 1993; 20: 687–693
22. Epstein J, Walsh P, Carmichael M, Brendler C. Pathologic and clinical findings to predict tumor extent of nonpalpable (stage T1c) prostate cancer. JAMA 1994; 271: 368–374
23. Scaletscky A, Koch M, Eckstein C et al. Tumor volume and stage in carcinoma of the prostate detected by elevations in prostate specific antigen. J Urol 1994; 152: 129–131
24. Hara M, Koyanagi Y, Inoue T, Fukuyama T. Some physico-chemical characteristics of gamma-seminoprotein, an antigenic component specific for human seminal plasma. Nippon Hoigaku Zasshi 1971; 25: 322–324
25. Papsidero L, Wang M, Valenzuela L et al. A prostate antigen in sera of prostatic cancer patients. Cancer 1980; 40: 2428–2432
26. Oesterling J, Jacobsen S, Chute C et al. Serum prostate-specific antigen in a community-based population of healthy men: establishment of age-specific reference ranges. JAMA 1993; 270: 860–864
27. Katz A, Olsson C, Raffo A et al. Molecular staging of prostate cancer with the use of an enhanced reverse transcriptase–PCR assay. Urology 1994; 43: 765–775
28. Stamey T, Yang N, Hay A et al. Prostate-specific antigen as a serum marker for adenocarcinoma of the prostate. N Engl J Med 1987; 317: 909–916
29. Oesterling J, Chan D, Epstein J et al. Prostate specific antigen in the preoperative and postoperative evaluation of localized prostatic cancer treated with radical prostatectomy. J Urol 1988; 139: 766–772
30. Oesterling J, Rice D, Glenski W, Bergstralh E. Effect of cystoscopy, prostate biopsy, and transurethral resection of prostate on serum prostate-specific antigen concentration. Urology 1993; 42: 276–282
31. Neal D Jr, Clejan S, Sarma D et al. Prostate specific antigen and prostatitis: effect of prostatitis on serum PSA in the human and nonhuman primate. Prostate 1992; 20: 105–111
32. Chybowski F, Bergstralh E, Oesterling J. The effect of digital rectal examination on the serum prostate specific antigen concentration: results of a randomized study. J Urol 1992; 148: 83–86
33. Yuan J, Coplen D, Petros J et al. Effects of rectal examination, prostatic massage, ultrasonography and needle biopsy on serum prostate specific antigen levels. J Urol 1992; 147: 810–814
34. Glenski W, Klee G, Bergstralh E, Oesterling J. Prostate-specific antigen: establishment of the reference range for the clinically normal prostate gland and the effect of digital rectal examination, ejaculation, and time on serum concentrations. Prostate 1992; 21: 99–110
35. Cupp M, Oesterling J. Prostate-specific antigen, digital rectal examination, and transrectal ultrasonography: their roles

in diagnosing early prostate cancer. Mayo Clin Proc 1993; 68: 297–306

36. Benson M, Whang I, Pantuck A et al. Prostate specific antigen density: a means of distinguishing benign prostatic hypertrophy and prostate cancer. J Urol 1992; 147: 815–816

37. Benson M, Whang I, Olsson C et al. The use of prostate specific antigen density to enhance the predictive value of intermediate levels of serum prostate specific antigen. J Urol 1992; 147: 817–821

38. Seaman E, Whang M, Olsson C et al. PSA density (PSAD): role in patient evaluation and management. Urol Clin North Am 1993; 20: 653–663

39. Brawer M, Aramburu E, Chen G et al. The inability of prostate specific antigen index to enhance the predictive value of prostate specific antigen in the diagnosis of prostatic carcinoma. J Urol 1993; 150: 369–373

40. Catalona W, Richie J, DeKernion J et al. Comparison of prostate specific antigen concentration versus prostate specific antigen density in the early detection of prostate cancer: receiver operating characteristic curves. J Urol 1994; 152: 2031–2036

41. Oesterling J, Cooner W, Jacobsen S et al. Influence of patient age on the serum PSA concentration: an important clinical observation. Urol Clin North Am 1993; 20: 671–680

42. Partin A, Carter H, Chan D et al. Prostate specific antigen in the staging of localized prostate cancer: influence of tumor differentiation, tumor volume and benign hyperplasia. J Urol 1990; 143: 747–752

43. Carter H B, Pearson J, Metter J et al. Longitudinal evaluation of prostate specific antigen levels in men with and without prostate disease. JAMA 1992; 267: 2215–2220

44. Carter H, Pearson J. PSA velocity for the diagnosis of early prostate cancer: a new concept. Urol Clin North Am 1993; 20: 665–670

45. Oesterling J, Chute C, Jacobsen S et al. Longitudinal changes in serum PSA (PSA velocity) in a community-based cohort of men. J Urol 1993; 149: 412A (abstr)

46. Carter H B, Pearson J, Wacliwew X et al. PSA variability in men with BPH. J Urol 1994; 151: 312A

47. Vessella R, Lange P. Issues in the assessment of PSA immunoassays. Urol Clin North Am 1993; 20: 607–619

48. Christensson A, Laurell C B, Lilja H. Enzymatic activity of prostate-specific antigen and its reactions with extracellular serine proteinase inhibitors. Eur J Biochem 1990; 194: 755–763

49. Lilja H. Significance of different molecular forms of serum PSA: the free, noncomplexed form of PSA versus that complexed to α1-antichymotrypsin. Urol Clin North Am 1993; 20: 681–686

50. Hybritech, Inc. Why might different PSA assays yield discrepant results on the same patient? Prostate-Specific Antigen Clinical Brief 1994; 3(1)

51. Graves H. Standardization of immunoassays for prostate-specific antigen: a problem of prostate-specific antigen complexation or a problem of assay design? Cancer 1993; 72: 3141–3144

52. Graves H. Issues on standardization of immunoassays for prostate-specific antigen: a review. Clin Invest Med 1993; 16: 416–425

53. Stamey T. Second conference on international standardization of prostate specific antigen immunoassays: September 1 and 2. Urology 1995; 45: 173–184

54. Christensson A, Bjork T, Nilsson O et al. Serum prostate specific antigen complexed to α1-antichymotrypsin as an indicator of prostate cancer. J Urol 1993; 150: 100–105

55. Lilja H, Christensson A, Dahlen U et al. Prostate-specific antigen in serum occurs predominantly in complex with alpha₁-antichymotrypsin. Clin Chem 1991; 37: 1618–1625

56. Stenman U-H, Leinonen J, Alfthan H et al. A complex between prostate-specific antigen and alpha-1-antichymotrypsin is the major form of prostate-specific antigen in serum of patients with prostatic cancer: assay of the complex improves clinical sensitivity for cancer. Cancer Res 1991; 51: 222–226

57. Oesterling J, Jacobsen S, Klee G et al. Free, complexed, and total serum PSA: establishment of age-specific reference ranges using newly developed immunofluorometric assays (IFMA). J Urol 1994; 151: 311A

58. Lilja H, Bjork T, Abrahamsson P et al. Improved separation between normals, benign prostatic hyperplasia (BPH) and carcinoma of the prostate (CAP) by measuring free (F), complexed (C) and total concentrations (T) of prostate specific antigen (PSA). J Urol 1994; 151(S): 400A

59. Mitrunen K, Pettersson K, Piironen T et al. Dual-label one-step immunoassay for simultaneous measurement of free and total prostate-specific antigen concentrations and ratios in serum. Clin Chem 1995; 41: 1115–1120

60. Dalkin B, Ahmann F, Southwick P, Bottaccini M. Derivation of normal prostate specific antigen (PSA) level by age. J Urol 1993; 149: 413A

61. Feneley M, McLean A, Webb J, Kirby R. Age-corrected prostate-specific antigen in symptomatic benign prostatic hyperplasia. J Urol 1994; 151: 312A

62. Collins G, Lee R, McKelvie G et al. Relationship between prostate specific antigen, prostate volume and age in the benign prostate. Br J Urol 1993; 71: 445–450

63. Crawford E. Report on the 1993 Prostate Cancer Awareness Week. J Urol 1994; 151: 71A

64. Dalkin B, Ahmann F, Kopp J. Prostate specific antigen levels in men older than 50 years without clinical evidence of prostatic carcinoma. J Urol 1993; 150: 1837–1839

65. Catalona W, Hudson M, Scardino P et al. Selection of optimal prostate specific antigen cutoffs for early detection of prostate cancer: receiver operating characteristic curves. J Urol 1994; 152: 2037–2042

66. Rasmusson G. Biochemistry and pharmacology of 5α-reductase inhibitors. In: Furr B, Wakeling A (eds) Pharmacology and clinical uses of inhibitors of hormone secretion and action. London: Baillière Tindall, 1987: 308–325

67. McConnell J. Current medical therapy for benign prostatic hyperplasia: the scientific basis and clinical efficacy of finasteride and alpha-blockers. In: Walsh P, Retik A, Stamey T, Vaughn E Jr (eds) Campbell's Urology, 6th ed. Update no. 3. Philadelphia: Saunders, 1992: 1–12

68. Gormley G, Stoner E, Bruskewitz R et al. The effect of finasteride in men with benign prostatic hyperplasia. N Engl J Med 1992; 327: 1185–1191

69. Guess H, Heyse J, Gormley G et al. Effect of finasteride on serum PSA concentration in men with benign prostatic hyperplasia: results from the North American phase III clinical trial. Urol Clin North Am 1993; 20: 627–636

70. Kleer E, Oesterling J. PSA and staging of localized prostate cancer. Urol Clin North Am 1993; 20: 695–704

71. Kleer E, Larson-Keller J, Zincke H, Oesterling J. Ability of preoperative serum prostate-specific antigen value to predict pathologic stage and DNA ploidy: influence of clinical stage and tumor grade. Urology 1993; 41: 207–216

72. Partin A, Yoo J, Carter H B et al. The use of prostate specific antigen, clinical stage and Gleason score to predict pathological stage in men with localized prostate cancer. J Urol 1993; 150: 110–114

73. Blackwell K, Bostwick D, Myers R et al. Combining prostate specific antigen with cancer and gland volume to predict more reliably pathological stage: the influence of prostate specific antigen cancer density. J Urol 1994; 151: 1565–1570

74. Danella J, DeKernion J, Smith R, Steckel J. The contemporary incidence of lymph node metastases in prostate cancer: implications for laparoscopic lymph node dissection. J Urol 1993; 149: 1488–1491

75. Bluestein D, Bostwick D, Bergstralh E, Oesterling J. Eliminating the need for bilateral pelvic lymphadenectomy in select patients with prostate cancer. J Urol 1994; 151: 1315–1320
76. Winfield H. Laparoscopy in urology. Urol Times 1993; 21: 6
77. Chybowski F, Larson-Keller J, Bergstralh E, Oesterling J. Predicting radionuclide bone scan findings in patients with newly diagnosed, untreated prostate cancer: prostate-specific antigen is superior to all other clinical parameters. J Urol 1991; 145: 313–318
78. Oesterling J, Martin S, Bergstralh E, Lowe F. The use of prostate-specific antigen in staging patients with newly diagnosed prostate cancer. JAMA 1993; 269: 57–60
79. Oesterling J. Using PSA to eliminate the staging radionuclide bone scan. Significant economic implications. Urol Clin North Am 1993; 20: 705–711

15

Flow rate and post-void residual issues
E. P. Arnold

Introduction

There are an increasing number of men in the over 60 years age group, and they are becoming ever more aware of men's health issues, in particular of lower urinary tract symptoms and of prostate cancer. The symptoms do not always give an accurate idea of the cause. Further investigations are indicated in order to be able to give proper and informed advice to the patient.

Symptoms can arise owing to mechanical obstruction by the size of the gland, or to functional obstruction arising from changes produced by contraction of the abundant smooth muscle at the bladder neck and within the prostate. The bulk of the prostate may produce sensory changes at the bladder base and contribute to sensory urgency or to a feeling of incomplete evacuation. In certain cases there may be no close correlation between the symptoms produced by the enlarging prostate and the degree of obstruction.[1,2]

Symptoms are heterogeneous and, although often grouped as 'obstructive' or 'irritative', they overlap and do not always correlate with obstruction as measured objectively. The terms 'obstructive' and 'irritative' would be best abandoned in favour of 'impaired voiding' or 'impaired storage', without assuming that the cause is understood.

Detrusor instability is common in patients with bladder outlet obstruction; its incidence rises with age even in the absence of obstruction and, indeed, rises also in women as age increases. It is often associated with symptoms of frequency, nocturia, urgency and urge incontinence. Relief of outlet obstruction does reduce the incidence of detrusor instability by about 30%,[3] but it persists in the remainder. Detrusor instability represents an increased excitability of the micturition reflex and its rising incidence in age might indicate an occult, or overt, neuropathy. In patients with known neurological disorders, such as multiple sclerosis or Parkinson's disease, detrusor overactivity is common and can give rise to symptoms difficult to distinguish from bladder outlet obstruction. Of course, it is the same age group in which prostatic enlargement is so common, and both problems can occur together. In this group of elderly men with neurological disorders it is essential to document obstruction before contemplating treatment.

Symptoms and symptom scores have been developed to grade and quantify the severity of symptoms. Their impact on the quality of life, and the degree of bother caused, are perhaps the most important questions in planning management strategies.

Good management demands accurate diagnosis for the following reasons:

1. To identify obstruction and to determine the site.
2. To assess the efficacy of any particular treatment strategy by tests done before and after the treatment.
3. To exclude prostate cancer; this has been addressed in Chapter 14.

The most widely accepted objective definition of obstruction is the demonstration of a low flow rate and a high pressure. Post-void residual (PVR) urine is considered to be the result of poor detrusor activity and its significance is addressed in the latter part of this chapter. To undertake pressure–flow studies in all those with urinary symptoms before offering treatment would be too time-consuming and costly for the resources available. However, the costs of the studies can be more than offset against savings made by avoiding surgery for the 30% of men who are not obstructed, despite having the same symptoms and flow rate records as those who are. This chapter attempts to assess the value of flow rate and PVR measurements in making the diagnosis of obstruction.

Flow rate

Self-assessment

The 'cast distance', popularized by schoolboys, is grossly inaccurate because it depends on the exit velocity at the external urethral meatus. A urethral stricture can cause a fine jet and a long cast distance without the flow rate changing, until the stricture has progressed to become almost completely occlusive. However, if a man has noticed that his stream is less forceful, he is usually right when this is measured. More commonly, the man might not have noticed any change in the stream because the slowing of the flow has come on so gradually. In any case, the symptom scores do not correlate with the flow rate measurements.[2]

Technical aspects

It has often been said that to evaluate voiding disorders, any self-respecting urology unit should have a flow meter, many different types of which are available. The majority are load cells or weight transducers that weigh the urine and then differentiate the rate of change of volume against time. Another popular type of flow meter directs the voiding urine on to a rotating disc with a ribbed edge that tends to slow the rate of spin and this is detected and electronically calibrated to a flow rate. The voided volume is subsequently calculated by integration of the flow curve. Electronic dipstick methods measure capacitance changes in a bimetallic strip as the volume of electrolyte-containing urine rises in a cylindrical container.

Most machines provide a printout and also some software to calculate and print such parameters as the maximum flow rate, average flow rate, voided volume and time. They are accurate within 1–5%, but artefacts occur due to 'splashing' and it is always necessary to correct these spikes and artefacts visually before accepting the machine's read out.[4] The machines should be calibrated regularly.[5]

Variability of flow rate

Learning effect

Anxiety can be aroused by the fear of not being able to hold on until the flow is done, from voiding in an unusual environment and from being anxious to do one's best. Such anxiety can cause a slower flow, presumably due to overactivity of the urethral striated muscle and its failure to relax, and perhaps to the adrenergic effects of increasing smooth muscle tone in the bladder neck and prostatic urethra. A learning effect

through repeated studies was noted by George and Slade.[6] This effect was not seen by Haylen et al.,[7] who showed no difference for maximum or average flow rates between first and second voids undertaken in a large number of men and women. Nor was it seen in a small group of 11 elderly men studied by Jensen et al.[8]

Individual variation

The patient should always be asked if he considers that his flow rate test was representative of his usual voiding. If there is any doubt, the test should be discarded and another arranged.

Siroky et al.[9] found that the variation in flow in a single asymptomatic individual voiding on multiple occasions was minimal and the probability that a flow rate will occur below −1 standard deviation (SD) is 0.159. They calculated that a change of 1.2 SD has a probability of only 2.5%. In the normal individual the flow rate varied by more than 1.2 SD in only three of 32 voids (9%).

However, variation of flow in patients with bladder outlet symptoms is often a feature of their history. Home uroflowmetry with multiple voids in more normal surroundings may give a better indication.[10] Golomb et al.[11] studied flow-rate variations by home uroflowmetry in 32 men with symptoms of obstruction, who did a mean of 14.9 tests, and 16 controls without symptoms, with a mean of 6.25 tests. They found that the men with obstruction varied their flow rates by more than 1 SD in 87.5%, and by more than 2 SD in 47%. The normal men had flows showing less variation but that still varied by more than 1 SD in 50%, and by more than 2 SD in 12.5%.

In an elderly population of incontinent men and women who underwent two urodynamic studies 2–4 weeks apart, the between-session variability of the flow rate was ± 4.7 ml/s, and the correlation coefficient was 0.44.[12] Similarly, the URA (which is a measure of obstruction; see Chapter 16) varied by ± 11.7 with a correlation coefficient of 0.61.[13] The results suggest that there is substantial long-term variability in voiding function, including urethral resistance.

Diurnal variation

Many patients say that their flow is worse at night, and this was borne out in the study done by Golomb et al.[11]

In their study the adjusted flow rate was lower in the home flowmetry studies done between midnight and noon than in the subsequent half-day. This variation was not seen in younger men.[14]

Bladder volume

The flow rate depends on volume voided and is slower than representative with volumes less than 150–200 ml.[15] Older men often have greater difficulty holding on to void this volume and hence volumes of 100 ml are not uncommon. When they do hold on deliberately, it does not always result in a representative voiding rate, and after going home they often have marked frequency. Because of this, some centres have developed 'Flow Clinics', at which patients are asked to drink plenty and to do three or four tests. In this way the proportion of men voiding less than 150 ml fell from 59 to 21%.[16]

Several workers studying flow patterns have developed nomograms and volume-independent variables. First, Drake[17] developed the idea of a 'corrected' peak flow rate derived by dividing maximum flow rate by the square root of bladder volume, itself measured as a sum of the volume voided and the residual urine volume. Second, the importance of using the initial bladder volume, rather than the voided volume alone (which would disregard the PVR), was emphasized by Siroky et al.[9] Using voided volume would result in an overestimate of voiding ability. Despite this, the measurement of PVR is considered unnecessary in the majority of cases unless the flow rate is normal or borderline. Siroky et al.[9] constructed a nomogram of flow rate against volume in a small group of young men, and expressed the variances in terms of a mean and standard deviations that paralleled the mean. None of the normals had values below –2 SD whereas, in a group of 53 men considered obstructed on clinical grounds, 52 had values below –2 SD.[18] The clinical diagnosis of obstruction was not validated by urodynamic studies, however.

Lim et al.[19] compared the reliability of the Bristol and Siroky nomograms against the objective criteria of obstruction using a URA of more than 29. They showed that the Siroky nomogram had poor specificity (30%) but good sensitivity (91%) in diagnosing obstruction. The Bristol nomogram had a specificity of 70% and a sensitivity of 53%. They concluded that if a precise diagnosis of obstruction is required, then pressure–flow studies must be performed. Schafer et al.[20] reported that only 75% of men considered to be obstructed in the Siroky nomogram were proven to be obstructed on pressure–flow studies.

Flow rates were slower with higher volumes in several studies.[5,15] Haylen et al.[7] constructed a Liverpool nomogram based on a large number of men and women. They found a strong correlation to voided volume of both maximum and average flow rate, but did not see any deterioration of flow rate in either sex with higher voided volumes. Pooling the results from 12 studies in 817 men from the age of 25 to 60 years showed the relation between flow rate and voided volume shown in Figure 15.1.[21] For voided volumes of more than 150 ml, Marshall et al.[22] used the slope of the curve of the flow rate versus volume voided, always including the point (0,0) (Fig. 15.2). They found that measuring this slope was useful in determining normal and impaired voiding, irrespective of the volume voided.

Age

Several studies have indicated that flow rate deteriorates with age.[7,15,22–25] The slower flows might well indicate increased incidence of obstruction in older men, but also could reflect lower voided volumes, probably due to

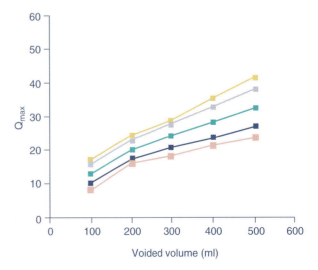

Figure 15.1. *Collected studies of relation between maximum flow rate (Q_{max}) and voided volume:* ■, *mean value;* ■, *+1 SD;* ■, *–1 SD;* ■, *minimum value;* ■, *maximum value. (Reproduced from ref. 20 with permission.)*

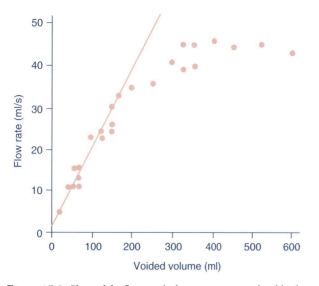

Figure 15.2. *Slope of the flow rate/volume curve extrapolated back to the origin; r = 0.963. (Reproduced from ref. 22 with permission.)*

detrusor instability, when flow rates have been shown to be slower. Impaired detrusor contractility due to ageing is another possible cause.

Jorgensen et al.[26] followed 61 men and repeated their studies 5 years later. They showed a significant fall in maximum flow rate and a drop in voided volume from 280 to 100 ml.

It is of interest that few men with obstruction, when observed longitudinally on a long surgical waiting list, actually go into acute retention. Ball et al.[23] showed that, of the 107 patients seen initially and reviewed again 5 years later, only two had gone into acute retention, and in the majority the symptoms had not worsened significantly with age.

Does the flow rate pattern help in the diagnosis of obstruction?

A reduced flow rate can be due to obstruction or to reduced bladder contractility. There is no way to distinguish these, apart from a pressure–flow study. Several variables have been developed from the flow rate curve and pattern in an attempt to discriminate.

Because the elderly with bladder outflow symptoms only rarely void volumes of more than 100–150 ml each time, this poses a difficulty in interpreting flow rates. To overcome this, various manipulations of the flow parameters have been used. Apart from the corrected flow rate, MUDI (male uroflow diagnostic interpretation)

variables developed by the Dantec Elektronik Company include: Q_{max} (the maximum flow rate), $Q_m 90$ (the mean flow rate for the middle 90% of the voided volume, but this does not account for residual urine), dl/dt40 (the velocity of detrusor contraction at 40 ml volume, calculated from flow rates at that point) and T_{desc} (the time from Q_{max} until 95% of the volume has been voided). Rollema et al.[27] performed these measurements on men considered to be obstructed on the basis of the Abrams–Griffiths nomogram[28] and the CLIM program, and applied it to small volumes of less than 100 ml with the results shown in Table 15.1. Even with this method, 22% were considered obstructed with maximum flow rate figures who were in fact, obstructed, and 18–30% were considered obstructed, using the three derived factors.

Patients with a flow rate of more than 15 ml, are less likely to have an obstruction confirmed by urodynamic studies than those with a flow of less than 5 ml/s. This does not exclude the small group of patients with symptoms who have normal flow rates at high pressure and who are obstructed.[29]

Is it then really necessary to do a pressure–flow study in each patient?

Neither the maximum flow rate nor any of the derivatives of the flow curve could predict the low pressure/low-flow syndrome.[30,31]

Andersen et al.[32] and Simonsen et al.[33] showed no relation between severity of symptoms of obstruction and maximum flow rate. A high flow rate of more than 15 ml/s does not preclude obstruction, and the patient with bothersome symptoms should be further investigated with pressure–flow studies.[34]

Jorgensen et al.[35] found that 17 of 134 men with lower urinary tract symptoms had a flow rate greater

Table 15.1. *MUDI variables measured on men considered to be obstructed on the basis of the Abrams–Griffiths nomogram and the CLIM program (volumes < 100 ml)*

	Q_{max}	$Q_m 90$	dl/dt40	T_{desc}
Sensitivity (%)	78	82	85	70
Specificity (%)	88	88	88	96

(From ref. 26 with permission.)

than 15 ml/s. There was a higher incidence of detrusor instability, a lower incidence of obstruction and a lower postoperative success rate in this group. Van Mastrigt[36] performed 109 pressure–flow studies and defined a group of 70 obstructed and 39 non-obstructed men on the basis of the URA being less than 29.[13,37] In relating this to the preoperative flow rates, it was found that 91% of those patients in whom the flow was less than 4.8 ml/s were obstructed. Conversely, those with a flow rate over 12 ml/s were usually not obstructed. The group between were impossible to discriminate and van Mastrigt recommended that they would need pressure–flow studies; however, this would mean that the numbers needing such studies could be rationalized to 53% of those with symptoms.

Can the flow rate predict the outcome of subsequent prostatectomy?

Abrams[38] indicated that patients having a prostatectomy had an overall success rate of 72%, the indications for prostatectomy having been based on symptoms and flow rates. He reported a less satisfactory outcome in those with normal preoperative flow rates than in those with low flow rates. Neal et al.[39] achieved a success rate of 75%. A proportion of those having an unsatisfactory result are not obstructed but have similar symptoms of frequency, nocturia, poor stream, urgency and the occasional urge incontinence. These symptoms could relate to detrusor instability;[40,41] another cause is the low-pressure/low-flow syndrome.

Where the preoperative flow rate was more than 15 ml/s, Jorgensen et al.[35] found a higher incidence of detrusor instability, a lower incidence of obstruction and a lower success rate from surgery. Jensen and colleagues[42,43] looked at the results of prostatectomy and

the preoperative flow rate. If the flow rate exceeded 15 ml/s, success was achieved in 70%, whereas the success rate was about 91% for those with flow rates less than 15 ml/s. The opposite conclusion was reached by Neal et al.,[41] who found that preoperative flow rates were not associated with the outcome of the operation; those with the higher flow rates did as well as those with lower flow rates.

Some patients with the low-flow/low-pressure syndrome considered to be due to an underactive detrusor, do get symptom relief after prostatectomy. Neal et al.[41] found 38/43 (88%) subjective success postoperatively in the high pressure group, compared with 13/34 (38%) in the low pressure group. In a group of 253 men undergoing urodynamic studies before prostatectomy, they found no clinical parameters that could identify men with voiding pressures at the high or low end of the range. However, several studies showed a reasonable outcome in patients with flow rates above 15 ml/s and high voiding pressures.[1,29]

In an analysis of the results of transurethral resection (TUR), Nordling[44] summarized three series, as shown in Table 15.2. Although there is a wide variation between these three studies, within each one the results of prostatectomy are worse in the unobstructed than in the obstructed group, but it was not possible to distinguish these groups by a preoperative flow rate.

Summary

Variations in individual flow rate support the suggestion that more than one flow rate test should be done and then corrected for bladder volume, either by various formulae of by use of nomograms.

From the flow rate it appears to be possible to separate those with impaired voiding from those who

Table 15.2. *Results of TUR in three series of men with or without preoperative obstruction*

Reference	No. of patients	No. unobstructed preoperatively	Percentage with symptomatic failure postoperatively	
			Obstructed	Not obstructed
Jensen et al.[42]	123	29	7	21
Neal et al.[41]	217	14	24	43
Rollema and van Mastrigt[37]	29	34	10	70

(From ref. 44 with permission.)

are normal. However, the flow rate does not discriminate those whose impaired voiding is due to obstruction from those in whom the cause is impaired detrusor contractility; neither does it distinguish those with symptoms and a high flow who also have high voiding pressures and are obstructed.

Post-void residual urine

Normal bladder emptying

The normal bladder is able to empty itself completely or to a negligible residual few millilitres, through a normal urethra. This is achieved by a bladder that continues to contract and a urethra that remains relaxed, until emptying is completed (Fig. 15.3). Di Mare et al.[45] noted that 78% of 46 normal males had residual urine of less than 5 ml and all had residual urine of less than 12 ml.

Techniques of measurement

Subjectively, the symptom of a feeling of incomplete emptying did correlate with the presence of PVR in one study.[32] However, in another study of 49 patients undergoing TUR, there was no relation between incomplete emptying and PVR.[46] Many men with chronic retention are quite unaware that they do not empty their bladders completely.

Abdominal examination can reveal a large non-painful bladder in chronic retention, but the PVR needs to be quite large before this can be palpated or percussed, depending on bodily habitus. Lesser volumes cannot be felt.

Catheterization might be considered the gold standard for measuring PVR. However, Stoller and Millard[47] demonstrated its inaccuracies, although these can be largely reduced by attention to detail in the technique of catheterization.

Indirect assessment of PVR can be performed by measurements taken from the post-void film of the intravenous urogram (IVU) or from abdominal ultrasound using a variety of formulae based on assumptions of a symmetrical shape of the bladder — rectangular or box shaped, or a pyramid. These methods have inherent inaccuracies but, because the clinical significance of small changes in bladder residual volume is unimportant, it seems that most of the methods for measuring ultrasound volumes are satisfactory.

Variability of PVR

Intra-individual variation

Anxiety affects the emptying ability, which is a well-known phenomenon in studies done in radiography departments using after-micturition film of the IVU. Similarly, patients in hospital, particularly women, but also men, have difficulty voiding when bedridden, and a residual is left that seems to predispose to infection in some of these patients. In a study by Birch et al.,[48] 30 men due for a TUR had three ultrasound examinations of PVR the day before surgery. Five different formulae were used. Wide variations from one void to the next were noted and two-thirds of the patients had significant variations in residual urine volume as measured by the different methods.[48] Bruskewitz et al.[46] also showed wide variations in 49 individual men and a lack of correlation with urodynamic parameters or symptoms. This wide intra-individual variation in PVR prior to TUR must make doubtful its value as a means of diagnosing obstruction.

Age

PVR appears to be a function of age in both sexes. Abrams and Griffiths[28] reported that 50% of men with lower urinary tract symptoms and in whom obstruction had been excluded by urodynamic testing had a PVR of more than 50 ml.

Pathogenesis of PVR

'Compensation' and 'decompensation'

The response of the bladder to obstruction of its outlet is to raise its pressure. This has been called 'compensation', implying increased strength of the detrusor to overcome the obstruction. This is now understood to be a misinterpretation. The detrusor pressure rises in obstruction because of the slower flow rate and the movement along the hyperbolic pressure–flow plot in accordance with the Hill equation. The bladder may continue to contract until it is empty (Fig. 15.4).

There is no evidence that the obstructed bladder compensates by contracting with greater force. Although the voiding pressure is high in obstruction, the bladder contracts at a slower contraction speed (Fig. 15.5) and the force is often unchanged or even slightly reduced.[49,50] Detrusor muscle strips from obstructed

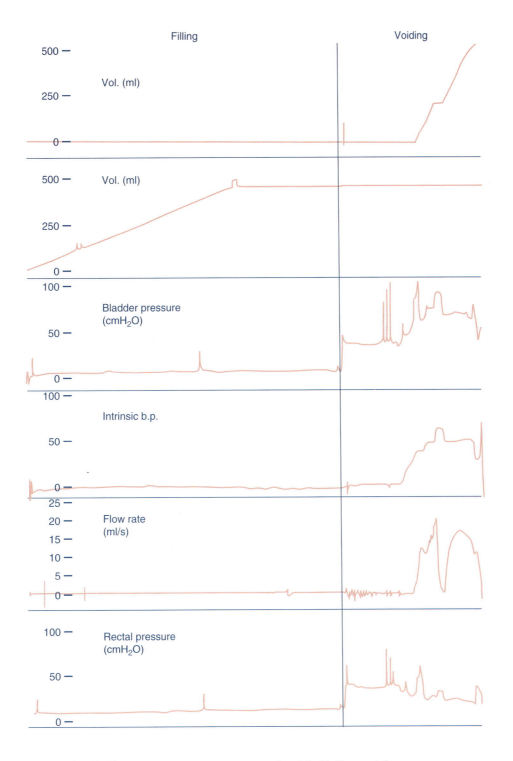

Figure 15.3. *Normal voiding and stable filling. Detrusor contraction is sustained until the bladder emptied.*

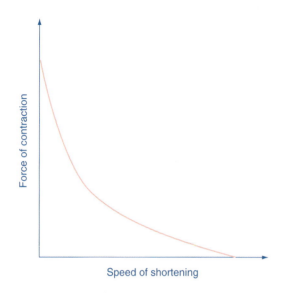

Figure 15.4. *Pressure–flow relation resembles force–velocity relation described by the Hill equation.*

patients showed a normal or near-normal force but a reduced velocity in the obstructed patients compared with the controls.[51] The slower velocity is possibly caused by structural and ultrastructural changes, with increase in non-contractile elements, smooth muscle atrophy and axonal degeneration as discussed by Elbadawi.[52]

Decompensation after a period of 'compensation' has been invoked to explain PVR and correlate it with left ventricular heart failure where the post-ejection volume fraction is a marker of the severity of heart failure.

Schafer[53,54] has suggested that PVR is caused by the limited amount of work the bladder is able to perform during any one voiding cycle.

Even those with high-pressure chronic retention are capable of strong detrusor contractions during voiding, even though the bladder volume may be distended to 1000 ml or more. After an initial strong burst of high pressure, the detrusor fades away before the bladder empties (Fig. 15.5).

Progress of obstruction leading to increasingly large residual urines, or to acute retention, happens relatively infrequently. Ball et al.[23] followed 107 patients with symptoms of obstruction, untreated for 5 years, and found no increase in residual urine in that time; only two patients went into acute retention.

Detrusor smooth muscle fatigue

Pressure–flow studies indicate that the bladder pressure initially is high and then falls away before the bladder is empty, and may leave residual urine. From this some have argued that the bladder muscle has 'fatigued'. While smooth muscle can maintain tension for longer than striated muscle, when continuously stimulated electrically in an organ bath, smooth muscle force falls away to around 20–30% of maximum.

Inactivation of micturition reflex

Another concept of why residual urine accumulates is that the micturition reflex may be switched off by afferents within the urethra, perhaps owing to the high pressure within it.[55] Sphincter-active voiding could also have this effect. However, Griffiths examined P/Q plots in patients with PVR and found that, almost invariably, the urethral opening pressure was lower towards the end of voiding than at the beginning, indicating relaxation of the urethra.[56]

PVR and neuropathy

Patients with spinal cord injuries and lesions above the spinal micturition reflex centre have a varying degree of detrusor–sphincter dyssynergia which will result in PVR, partly because of sphincter activity and partly because such sphincter activity can switch off the detrusor contraction reflex. Those with cauda equina or sacral root damage have a flaccid bladder and inability to excite a contraction voluntarily or reflexly. This will result in some voiding by straining, but rarely does this empty the bladder completely. Some patients with diabetes and autonomic neuropathy have large-capacity bladders that also empty incompletely.

Impaired detrusor contractility

This can coexist with an initially high voiding pressure and an overactive detrusor in the elderly.[57,58] Elbadawi[52] has documented the ultrastructural basis for this altered function to occur. He showed evidence of smooth muscle hyperplasia and some areas of muscle atrophy, neural disintegration and increased deposition of collagen and elastin in the bladder wall, all of which could contribute to reduced contractility and detrusor instability. Some of these changes have been seen in the ageing process. Because of these structural changes, the

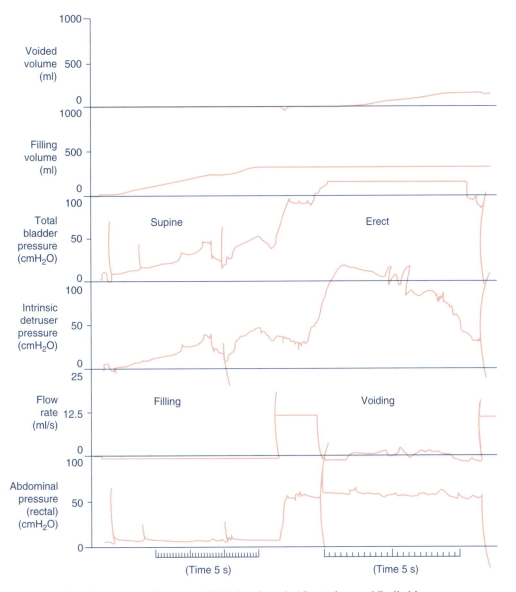

Figure 15.5. *High-pressure/low-flow prostatic obstruction. PVR left at the end of flow is due to a fall-off of detrusor pressure.*

muscle may not be able to shorten to the extent that it could formerly, with resulting inability to empty completely.

In summary, residual urine appears to be an abnormality of bladder function rather than a direct result of mechanical obstruction.

Chronic retention

This has been arbitrarily defined as a PVR of more than 300 ml.

Bladder compliance. The normal end filling pressure is equal to or less than 15 cmH$_2$O. In low-pressure chronic retention (LPCR) the end filling pressure is less than 25 cmH$_2$O. Such patients often have minimal 'obstructive' symptoms; they have a large floppy bladder and do less well after prostatectomy. The high-pressure chronic retention (HPCR) group, in whom the end filling pressure is more than 25 cmH$_2$O, are at risk of dilatation of the upper tracts and postobstructive renal failure. They do have a better success postoperatively and the upper tract dilatation often resolves after prostatectomy, unless permanent damage has ensued.[59]

Is LPCR due to detrusor contractility that has been impaired for many years, and is it the end result of the low-pressure/low-flow syndrome? Long-term studies have not yet been done to address this question but Neal's group has provided little support for the concept.[39]

A sensory problem? Diabetic patients often have large bladders and significant PVR and this has been ascribed to autonomic neuropathy.[60]

Parys et al.[61] found an increased sensory threshold in those with chronic retention when using electrical stimulation via the dorsal nerve of the penis, and at the bladder neck using a catheter-mounted electrode. They found normal somatic reflex latencies, however.

Clinical significance of PVR

PVR and outlet obstruction

PVR does not indicate obstruction, nor does its absence rule it out. No correlation has been demonstrated between flow rate and PVR.[1,62,63] Although some urologists still rely on PVR as an indication of obstruction and hence an indication for TUR, the PVR does not correlate with symptoms, prostatic size or urethral resistance.[64] This has been demonstrated also by Cetinel et al.,[65] who showed that 70% of those with urodynamically confirmed bladder outlet obstruction had a PVR of less than 50 ml. In another study, PVR did not correlate with the symptom of incomplete emptying, or with the peak flow rate, with the presence or absence of detrusor instability, or with the size of the gland.[46] Shoukry et al.[62] also showed that there was no correlation between PVR and urodynamic criteria of obstruction.

The absence of residual urine does not rule out obstruction, as was demonstrated by Turner-Warwick et al.[40] As shown in Figure 15.6, a large number of patients have no residual urine (or insignificant volumes) and yet have high pressure and the lowest of flows. Neal et al.[39] showed that weak pressures were uncommon (9.1%) and were not associated with a large PVR. Their data provide no support for the concept of PVR being a consequence of a weak detrusor.

Bruskewitz et al.[46] showed no correlation of PVR with uninhibited bladder contractions, although others have shown that there is a possible combination of detrusor overactivity of this type and poor detrusor contractility.

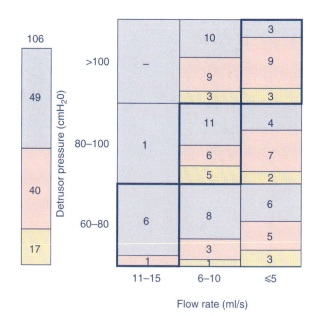

Figure 15.6. *Residual urine (▪, 0–30 ml; ▪, 30–200 ml; ▪, > 200 ml) related to severity of obstruction as judged by flow rate and detrusor pressures. (Adapted from ref. 40 with permission.)*

PVR and urinary tract infection

It has been a precept of urological thought that residual urine predisposes to urinary tract infection (UTI). In patients who have bladder outlet obstruction, infection is relatively uncommon. Hasner[66] showed no correlation between PVR and the incidence of UTI, nor did Bruskewitz et al.[46] or Hampson et al.[67] The incidence appears to be about 5–10%; however, no studies have compared the risk of UTI in those with and without residual urine.

PVR and results of surgery

The presence or absence of residual urine per se should not bear directly on the indications for prostatectomy.[40]

Although the association of residual urine with high voiding pressures is weak,[40] there is evidence that the residual urine does fall significantly by about 70% following successful prostatectomy — from a mean of about 100 ml to 30 ml.[41]

In looking at the success rate of surgery, Abrams et al.[68] showed an unsatisfactory outcome in low-pressure chronic retention in eight of 12 cases, whereas in those with high pressures an unsatisfactory result was found in one in nine. Neal et al.[41] reported an unsatisfactory outcome in approximately 29% of cases; this was associated with preoperative urge incontinence, a small prostatic size and a low voiding pressure. There was, however, no correlation of an unsatisfactory outcome with either maximum preoperative flow rate or PVR.

George et al.[59] examined 25 men with prostatism and a residual urine of more than 100 ml; in 21, normal upper tracts were preserved. High voiding pressures predicted a good result following TUR but, where the pressures were less than 70 cmH$_2$O during voiding, this produced a poor symptomatic response and also poor postoperative urodynamic findings.

After surgery for chronic retention, PVR decreased from a mean of 1141 ml (± 789) to a mean of 206 ml (± 268) postoperatively ($p<0.00006$).[69]

Acute retention

There is no single theory of the cause of acute retention. Overdistension due to increased diuretics or alcohol is a precipitating event in a patient developing acute retention on top of obstructive symptoms. Other factors include cold, pain, stress of many types and surgery. Alpha-adrenergic receptors in the urethra may be responsible in part. Caine and Perlberg[70] used alpha-adrenergic blockers with some success, presumably by reducing urethral and prostatic smooth muscle contractility. Detrusor instability, by causing urgency and frequency, may protect against acute retention by avoiding overdistension.

Where there are pre-existing symptoms of impaired voiding, the development of acute retention of urine is an indication for prostatectomy. If a catheter is passed to evacuate the bladder and is then removed, there is a high risk of the patient returning in retention. This is most likely within the first week, when 50% will again develop acute retention; this incidence arises to around 60% at the end of 4 weeks, and 68% by the end of 12 months. For patients able to void after an in–out catheter, if the flow rate is less than 5 ml/s, there is a 90% risk of repeat retention.[71]

Histological examination shows an increased incidence of infarction in the prostate removed subsequent to retention, compared with elective prostatectomy specimens; it may be that the oedema associated with the infarction suddenly increases the urethral resistance.

Practical issues

The justification for doing any test should depend on its ability to identify obstruction and to determine its site. This will then allow informed choice of any treatment strategy which can be retested after treatment.

There are two aspects to a successful outcome of any procedure: one is the symptomatic improvement, and the other is an objective improvement in parameters of obstruction for which the surgeon has done the procedure. Subjective success can occur within any measurable improvement in flow rate or pressure; the reverse is also true.

Definition of obstruction and use of flow rate

The only objective way of making a diagnosis of obstruction is to demonstrate the following (with apologies to Koch's postulates):

1. Slow flow rate.
2. Elevated detrusor pressure during voiding.
3. Narrow area on videocystourethrography.
4. Ablation of the narrow area that reverses the first three.

To undertake urodynamic studies in all those with symptoms of impaired storage/voiding would be time-consuming and costly, well beyond the resources of most urology departments worldwide. Cost–benefit analysis does indicate that, if resources of time, equipment and staff are available, savings can be made by operating on only those 70% of men with symptoms who have demonstrable obstruction.[72] However, for most units these resources are not available and it would, therefore, appear reasonable to adopt the following practical guidelines for patients with moderate to severe symptoms:

1. It is reasonable to measure the flow rate in all men before considering treatment options. Because of variation in flow rates, some have argued that two or three tests should be done.
2. If the flow rate is more than 15 ml/s, obstruction is unlikely. Symptoms may be due to detrusor instability. Urodynamic studies should be performed if the patient is bothered by the symptoms.

3. If the flow rate is less than 5 ml/s, the likelihood of obstruction is high and pressure–flow studies are probably not necessary.

4. Where the flow rate lies between 5 and 15 ml/s, pressure–flow studies are advisable in order to identify which patients are obstructed and which have the low-flow/low-pressure syndrome.

Guidelines for evaluation

Because flow rate measurements are readily available and have some predictive value in the diagnosis, the flow rate is *recommended* by the World Health Organization sponsored International Consultation on Benign Prostatic Hyperplasia (BPH), for the evaluation of patients with impaired voiding or storage functions of the bladder; however, it is considered only as an *optional* test in the *Clinical Practice Guidelines* for the diagnosis and treatment of BPH developed for the US Agency for Health Care Policy and Research.[21]

Guidelines, as such, while aiming to improve the overall standard of care, are the lowest common denominator of acceptable care and not of ideal care. Thoughts about optimum pathways for diagnosis and treatment do change — indeed, quite rapidly — so guidelines need frequent revision. Another concern about guidelines is the possible risk that those funding health care might restrict their funding to users of their accepted guidelines, and might refuse to fund or support any additional tests or any tests considered 'optional' or for clinical research purposes.

Measurement of the PVR is *recommended* by the International Consultation on BPH, although it would appear to be less easily justified, for the reasons discussed above. More information is needed on the risk of upper tract dilatation in those who have small or insignificant residual urine volumes.

If delays in treatment are a fact of life because of long waiting lists, it would seem prudent to assess upper urinary tracts by ultrasound, which is more sensitive in detecting upper tract dilatation than is measuring serum creatinine, a test recommended by both groups. For those with chronic retention and a palpably enlarged bladder that remains after voiding, the upper tracts should be checked by ultrasound before discussing treatment options aimed at improving bladder emptying. If other treatment options are considered in managing the outlet obstruction, measurement of the PVR should be included in the protocols. It is not enough to rely on symptoms alone: flow rates and urodynamic studies should be included to measure what has been achieved.

Who then should be treated?

Most urologists would agree that those patients who develop the complications of obstruction, such as acute or chronic retention, and postobstructive renal failure, bladder stones and recurrent urinary infections, should be treated. However, the majority present with symptoms. Priorities for selecting for treatment patients with bladder outlet obstruction could be developed if the risk factors for developing these complications were known, which, currently they are not. In particular, no information can apparently be gleaned from the symptoms, from the flow rate and its pattern, or from the PVR.

If obstruction remains untreated, is there any evidence of progressive detrusor failure or progressive detrusor instability? Detrusor instability does become more frequent with ageing, irrespective of obstruction, and may become more bothersome in producing urgency and urge incontinence. The observation that after prostatectomy detrusor instability improves in 30% of cases, indicates that the micturition reflex is less excitable after obstruction is treated, but obstruction is only one factor predisposing to reflex excitability.

Detrusor failure might develop or become progressive. Elbadawi[52] suggests that this is so, and that chronic fibrosis and elastosis causes separation of smooth muscle cells, which develop increased sarcolemmal dense bodies; there is also degeneration of intrinsic nerves. All these factors could cause reduced contractility due to obstruction. However, similar changes have been seen as a result of ageing.

Untreated, very few patients go into acute retention.[23] It is likely that the pathophysiology differs in acute and chronic retention, rather than that chronic retention is the end stage of decompensation. The concern remains as to which patients with high-pressure obstruction will develop poorly compliant bladders and high end filling pressures, and hence be at risk of upper tract dilatation and obstructive renal failure. Because the PVR varies within the same individual as well as according to the technique of assessing it, it remains impossible to predict who will go into chronic retention. There is no 'grand unifying theory', as Ball[73] points out, that would indicate progression from symptoms that are so variable on to acute or chronic retention. If the PVR is large and there is upper tract dilatation, then this should lead to prompt treatment; however, on the basis of symptoms and flow rate, it remains impossible to prioritize treatment.

References

1. Dorflinger T, Bruskewitz R C, Jensen K M E et al. Predictive value of low maximum flow rate in benign prostatic hyperplasia. Urology 1986; 27: 569–573

2. Rosier P F W M, Rollema H J, van der Beek C, Janknegt R A. Diagnosis of 'prostatism' relation between symptoms and urodynamic evaluation of obstruction and bladder function. Neurourol Urodyn 1992; 11: 399–400

3. Arnold E P. Bladder outlet obstruction in the male: a urodynamic analysis of the detrusor responses. University of London Ph.D. Thesis, 1980

4. Grino P B, Bruskewitz R, Blaivas J G et al. Maximum urinary flow rate by uroflowmetry: automatic or visual interpretation. J Urol 1993; 149: 339–341

5. Ryall R L, Marshall V R. Normal peak urinary flow rates obtained from small voided volumes can provide a reliable assessment of bladder function. J Urol 1982; 127: 484–488

6. George N J R, Slade N. Hesitancy and poor stream in younger men without outflow tract obstruction — the anxious bladder. Br J Urol 1979; 51: 506–510

7. Haylen B T, Ashby D, Sutherst J R et al. Maximum and average urine flow rates in normal male and female populations — the Liverpool nomograms. Br J Urol 1989; 64: 30–38

8. Jensen K M E, Jorgensen J B, Mogensen P. Reproducibility of uroflowmetry variables in elderly males. Urol Res 1985; 13: 237–239

9. Siroky M B, Olsson C A, Krane R J. The flow rate nomogram: I: Development. J Urol 1979; 122: 665–668

10. Hansen M V, Zdamowski A. The value of a patient-administered home flow test compared to office uroflowmetry in the evaluation of prostatism patients. Neurourol Urodyn 1994; 13: 452–453

11. Golomb J, Lindner A, Siegel Y, Koczak D. Variability and circadian changes in home uroflowmetry in patients with BPH compared to normal controls. J Urol 1992; 147: 1044–1047

12. Griffiths D J. Effects of bladder outlet obstruction. Prospectives 1992; 2: 1–8

13. Griffiths D J, von Mastrigt R, Bosch R. Quantification of method resistance during voiding, with special reference to the effects of prostatic size reduction on urethral obstruction due to BPH. Neurourol Urodyn 1989; 8: 17–27

14. Underberg Poulsen E, Kirkeby H J. Home monitoring of uroflow in normal male adolescents: relation between flow curve, voided volume and time of day. Scand J Urol Nephrol 1988; 114(suppl): 58–61

15. von Garrelts B. Micturition in the normal male. Acta Chir Scand 1957; 114: 197

16. Abrams P H. The urine flow clinics. In: Fitzpatrick J N (ed) Conservative treatment of BPH. Edinburgh: Churchill Livingstone, 1991: 33–43

17. Drake W M. The uroflowmeter: an aid to the study of the lower urinary tract. J Urol 1948; 59: 650–658

18. Siroky M B, Olsson C A, Krane R J. The flow rate nomogram: II. Clinical correlation. J Urol 1980; 123: 208–210

19. Lim C S, Reynard J, Abrams P. Flow rate nomograms. Their reliability in diagnosing bladder outflow obstruction. Proc ICS 1994; 74–75

20. Schafer W, Noppency R, Rubben H, Lutzeyer W. The value of free flow rate and pressure/flow studies in the routine investigation of BPH patients. Neurourol Urodyn 1988; 7: 219–221

21. McConnell J D, Barry M J, Bruskewitz R C et al. (eds) Benign prostatic hyperplasia: diagnosis and treatment. Clinical practice guidelines. AHCPR Publication No. 94-0582. Agency for Health Care Policy and Research, Public Health Service. Rockville, Md: US Department of Human Services, 1994

22. Marshall V R, Ryall R L, Austin M L, Sinclair G R. The use of urinary flow rates obtained from voiding volumes less than 150 mls in the assessment of voiding ability. Br J Urol 1983; 55: 28–33

23. Ball A J, Feneley R C L, Abrams P H. The natural history of untreated prostatism. Br J Urol 1981; 53: 613–616

24. Drach G W, Layton T, Bottaccini M R. A method of adjustment of male peak urinary flow rate for varying age and volume voided. J Urol 1982; 128: 960–962

25. Jorgensen J B, Jensen K M E, Bille-Brake N E, Mogensen P. Uroflowmetry in asymptomatic elderly males. Br J Urol 1986; 58: 390–395

26. Jorgensen J B, Jensen K M E, Mogensen P. Age-related variation in urinary flow variables and flow curve patterns in elderly males. Br J Urol 1992; 69: 265–271

27. Rollema H J, Ambergen A W, van den Ouden D. On-line uroflowmetry in males: clinical application to small (< 100 mls) voided volumes. Neurourol Urodyn 1989; 8: 407–408

28. Abrams P H, Griffiths D J. The assessment of prostatic obstruction from urodynamic measurements and from residual urine. Br J Urol 1979; 51: 129–134

29. Gerstenberg T C, Andersen J T, Klarskov P et al. High flow infravesical obstruction in men: symptomatology, urodynamics and the results of surgery. J Urol 1982; 127: 943–945

30. Gleason D M, Bottaccini M R, Drach G W, Layton T N. Urinary velocity as an index of male voiding function. J Urol 1982; 128: 1363–1367

31. Chancellor M B, Blaivas J G, Kaplan S A, Axelrod S. Bladder outlet obstruction versus impaired detrusor contractility: the role of uroflow. J Urol 1991; 145: 810–812

32. Andersen J T, Nordling J, Walter S. Prostatism. I. The correlation between symptoms, cystometric and urodynamic findings. Scand J Urol Nephrol 1979; 13: 229–236

33. Simonsen O, Moller-Madsen B, Dorflinger T et al. The significance of age on symptoms — urodynamic and cystoscopic findings in BPH. Urol Res 1987; 15: 355–358

34. Iversen P, Bruskewitz R C, Jensen K M E, Madsen P O. Transurethral prostatic resection in the treatment of prostatism with high urinary flow. J Urol 1983; 129: 995–997

35. Jorgensen J B, Jensen K M E, Mogensen P. Predictive value of uroflowmetry in prostatism. Neurourol Urodyn 1987; 6: 221–223

36. van Mastrigt R. Is it really necessary to do a pressure–flow study in each patient? Neurourol Urodyn 1993; 12: 419–420

37. Rollema H J, van Mastrigt R. Improved indication and follow-up in transurethral resection of the prostate using the computer program CLIM: a prospective study. J Urol 1992; 148: 111–116

38. Abrams P. Prostatism and prostatectomy: the value of urine flow rate measurement in the pre-operation assessment for operation. J Urol 1977; 117: 71–74

39. Neal D E, Styles R A, Powell P H, Ramsden P D. Relationship between detrusor function and residual urine, in men undergoing prostatectomy. Br J Urol 1987; 60: 560–566

40. Turner-Warwick R T, Whiteside C G, Arnold E P et al. A urodynamic view of prostatic obstruction and the results of prostatectomy. Br J Urol 1973; 45: 631–645

41. Neal D E, Ramsden P D, Sharples L et al. Outcome of elective prostatectomy. Br Med J 1989; 299: 762–767

42. Jensen K M E, Jorgensen J B, Mogensen P. Urodynamics in prostatism: I. Prognostic value of uroflowmetry. Scand J Urol Nephrol 1988; 22: 109–117

43. Jensen K M E. Clinical evaluation of routine urodynamic investigations in prostatism. Neurourol Urodyn 1989; 8: 545–578

44. Nordling J. Definition of prostatic urethral obstruction. Urol Res 1994; 22: 267–271

45. Di Mare, Fish S R, Harper J M, Politano V A. Residual urine in normal male subjects. J Urol 1966; 96: 180–181

46. Bruskewitz R C, Iversen P, Madsen P O. Value of post void residual urine determinations in evaluation of prostatism. Urology 1982; 20: 602–604

47. Stoller M, Millard R J M. The accuracy of a catheterised residual urine. J Urol 1989; 141: 15–16

48. Birch N C, Hirst G, Doyle P T. Serial residual urine volumes in men with prostatic hypertrophy. Br J Urol 1988; 62: 571–575

49. Griffiths D J. The mechanics of the urethra and of micturition. Br J Urol 1973; 45: 497–507

50. Williams J H, Turner W H, Sainsbury G M, Brading A F. Experimental model of bladder outflow tract obstruction in the guinea pig. Br J Urol 1993; 71: 543–554

51. Gilling P J, Arnold E P. Contractility of detrusor muscle from patients undergoing elective transurethral resection of the prostate. Proceedings of the Urological Society of Australasia AGM 1990. Br J Urol 1991; 400

52. Elbadawi A. BPH-associated voiding dysfunction: detrusor is pivotal. Contemp Urol 1994; 6: 21–38

53. Schafer W. Urethral resistance? Urodynamic concepts of physiological and pathological bladder outlet function during voiding. Neurourol Urodyn 1985; 4: 161–201

54. Schafer W. Analysis of active detrusor function during voiding with the bladder working function. Neurourol Urodyn 1991; 10: 19–35

55. Griffiths D J, Constantinou C, von Mastrigt R. Urinary bladder function and its control in healthy females. Am J Physiol 1986; 251: R225–R230

56. Griffiths D J. Residual urine, underactive detrusor function, and the nature of detrusor/sphincter dyssynergia. Neurourol Urodyn 1983; 2: 289–294

57. Resnick N M, Yalla S V. Detrusor hyperactivity with impaired contractile function. An unrecognised but common cause of incontinence in elderly patients. JAMA 1987; 257: 3076–3081

58. Ghoneim G M, Susset J G. Impaired bladder contractility in association with detrusor instability: underestimated occurrence in benign prostatic hyperplasia. Neurourol Urodyn 1988; 7: 230–231

59. George N J R, Feneley R C L, Roberts J B M. Identification of the poor risk patient with 'prostatism' and detrusor failure. Br J Urol 1986; 58: 290–295

60. Frimodt-Moller C. Diabetic cystopathy: epidemiology and related disorders. Ann Intern Med 1980; 92: 318–321

61. Parys B T, Machen D G, Woolfenden K A, Parsons K F. Chronic urinary retention — a sensory problem? Br J Urol 1988; 62: 546–549

62. Shoukry I, Susset J G, Elhillali M M, Dutartre D. Role of uroflowmetry in the assessment of lower urinary tract obstruction in adult males. Br J Urol 1975; 47: 559–566

63. Andersen J T. Prostatism III. Detrusor hyperreflexia and residual urine. Clinical and urodynamic aspects, and the influence of surgery on the prostate. Scand J Urol Nephrol 1982; 16: 25–30

64. Griffiths H J. An evaluation of the importance of residual urine. Br J Radiol 1970; 43: 409–413

65. Cetinel B, Turan T, Talat Z et al. Update evaluation of benign prostatic hyperplasia: when should we offer prostatectomy? Br J Urol 1994; 74: 566–571

66. Hasner E. Prostatic urinary infection. Acta Chir Scand 1962; 285 (suppl): 1

67. Hampson S J, Noble J G, Richards D, Milroy E J G. Does residual urine predispose to urinary tract infection? Br J Urol 1992; 70: 506–508

68. Abrams P H, Dunn M, George N. Urodynamic findings in chronic retention of urine and their relevance to the results of surgery. Br Med J. 1978; 2: 1258–1260

69. Styles R A, Ramsden P D, Neal D E. The outcome of prostatectomy on chronic retention of urine. J Urol 1991; 146: 1029–1033

70. Caine M, Perlberg S. Dynamics of acute retention in prostatic patients and role of adrenergic receptors. Urology 1977; 9: 399–403

71. Klarskov P, Andersen J T, Asmussen C F et al. Symptoms and signs predictive of the voiding patterns after acute urinary retention in men. Scand J Urol Nephrol. 1987; 21: 23–28

72. Nordling J. Views from international experts. Prospectives 1994; 7

73. Ball A J. Natural history of benign prostatic hyperplasia. Prospectives 1992; 3(2): 1–5

Urodynamics and benign prostatic hyperplasia

A. E. Te S. A. Kaplan

16

Introduction

The application of urodynamics in the evaluation of men with symptoms of prostatism remains controversial. In part, this is due to clinical differences between the symptoms that we commonly attribute to BPH and the presence or absence of mechanical bladder outflow obstruction as defined by urodynamics.[1-3] Because pressure–flow urodynamic studies remain as the most definitive method of documenting outflow obstruction, they serve as the best instruments to differentiate men whose symptoms are due to prostatic obstruction versus inherent bladder dysfunction.[1] However, within the realm of obtaining a diagnosis of BPH, do we need to diagnose obstruction? Is management of patients with symptoms of prostatism significantly altered by the knowledge that the patient has urodynamic evidence of outflow obstruction? Consequently, do patients with documented urodynamic outflow obstruction fare better after procedures designed to alleviate obstruction, i.e. prostatectomy, than those who do not?

Unfortunately there are few objective data of the natural history of untreated prostatism.[3,4] This is particularly true with regard to untreated 'urodynamic obstruction.' In addition, studies of the natural progression of BPH are hard to evaluate because of the poor correlation of symptoms with age of the patient, size of the prostate gland and urodynamic parameters such as uroflow, post-void residual and detrusor pressure.[3,5-12] Furthermore, progression of BPH in untreated patients with varying degrees of clinical manifestations has never been characterized in a large group of patients followed over long periods.

All these issues are reflective of the controversy involved in applying urodynamics to the diagnosis of BPH. However, it is valid to conclude that urodynamic studies continue to be a valuable tool in elucidating pathophysiological and therapeutic aspects of BPH. This chapter reviews various technical and clinical urodynamic issues, including their clinical diagnostic impact, indications for usage and clinical utility in the management of men with 'prostatism'.

Background

The relationship of voiding symptoms to bladder function and outlet obstruction is not simple. Although voiding symptoms often represent the clinical manifestations of inherent detrusor dysfunction and/or outlet obstruction, this relationship is not universal. 'Silent' obstructive uropathy secondary to BPH, for example, may occur without the patient experiencing significant voiding symptoms. Clinically, these symptoms are not 'prostate specific' and can often represent other 'non-prostatic' aetiologies such as impaired bladder contractility, detrusor instability, sensory urgency and vesical neck obstruction.[13-17] In fact, about 25–50% of men undergoing urodynamic investigation for prostatism symptoms do not have urodynamic evidence of obstruction.[16,18,19]

The authors recently completed a retrospective review of the records of over 2500 consecutive men with symptoms of prostatism who underwent synchronous video pressure–flow urodynamic studies between February 1982 and July 1994. For the 787 evaluable patients, the most common diagnosis was prostatic obstruction and detrusor instability (39%), followed by isolated prostatic obstruction (23%). Only 504 patients (64%) had demonstrable urodynamic evidence of prostatic urethral obstruction of which 318 (63%) had concomitant detrusor instability. For the group, 425 (54%) had detrusor instability; 181 (23%) had it as their sole diagnosis. Impaired detrusor contractility was noted in 134 patients (17%) patients; 49 (6%) of these had it as their only diagnosis. Finally, three (0.4%) patients had sensory urgency as the urodynamic aetiology of their symptoms.

To clarify the poor correlation between what a patient feels and what is occurring physiologically, uroflowmetry and multichannel urodynamics have been applied to provide a rational diagnostic approach to BPH. However, the suitability of urodynamics in assessing BPH has been confounded by controversies of both reproducibility and variability of results.[1–3] Furthermore, there is debate among leading urodynamic experts about which parameters to assess. In part, some of these differences are due to variability in technique, equipment, operator interpretation and philosophy, patient population and even quality of cooperation of the patient.[20,21] Therefore, issues of clinical validity and diagnostic utility have been subjects of controversies in the urological literature primarily because of a lack of true consistency between institutions, between operators and even between individual studies themselves.

Within the modern realm of urodynamics, there are few, if any, true controls or normal standards. Currently, urodynamic studies provide a meaningful understanding of bladder function and its potential relationship to outlet obstruction. More importantly, they are clinically useful in diagnosing subtle differential aetiologies of irritative and obstructive voiding symptoms, incontinence, urinary retention and the development of bladder outlet obstruction.[1–3,15] Their greatest clinical impact has been in elucidating voiding dysfunctional processes in patients with an underlying associated neurological process such as spina bifida, multiple sclerosis, diabetes and others in the face of BPH.[3,15,22–26] In addition, they have provided a more objective measurement of success in outcomes of BPH treatments whose previous yardsticks of success were based on subjective criteria.[26–30]

Cystometry

A simple but invasive urodynamic study is the cystometrogram (CMG). Technically, there are two types, the filling CMG and the voiding CMG. The term CMG generally refers to a filling CMG and can be performed with either a gas or liquid medium. The study is generally performed with a two-lumen catheter, one lumen to fill the bladder and the other to measure intravesical pressure. The filling CMG provides information regarding bladder capacity, presence of involuntary detrusor contractions (IDC), bladder

compliance and contraction pressures. However, the major limitation of simple cystometry is that the urodynamic diagnosis of bladder outlet obstruction can not be made.[15,31]

Data provided by several studies, including the authors' own, indicate that approximately 60% of men with symptoms of prostatism have IDC; postoperatively the incidence is 25–30%.[13,15,16,18,31–33] Although the presence of IDC may be associated with higher treatment failures after prostatectomy, there is currently no a priori method to predict which patients will have persistent IDC after therapy.[34,35] In addition, although a CMG may provide valuable information in patients with concomitant neurological conditions such as Parkinson's disease or diabetes, it is not as valuable as multichannel pressure–flow studies.[2,25] Currently, simple cystometry is not recommended by the American Urological Association BPH guidelines.[26]

Multichannel urodynamics and video multichannel urodynamics

Multichannel urodynamics are synchronous pressure–flow studies and are best suited to define bladder outlet obstruction. Simultaneous fluoroscopic video allows for visualization of the precise anatomical location of obstruction (prostatic obstruction vs vesical neck obstruction) in men with symptomatic prostatism (Fig. 16.1).[36] In addition, it can better define issues of impaired contractility, detrusor instability and sensory urgency.[15,23,37–39] It is particularly valuable in assisting in the differential diagnosis of patients with an associated underlying neurological or postoperative surgical condition. Essentially, it fills the diagnostic void left by simple uroflowmetry and cystometry. However, one caveat of pressure–flow studies is that there are significant combinations of detrusor pressures and flows that are diagnostically equivocal.

The principal role of multichannel urodynamics is to analyse the act of micturition. In other words, what is the detrusor function as measured by its generation of pressure in relation to its outlet resistance as defined by its flow? The association of an elevated voiding pressure with low peak urinary flow is the sine qua non of bladder outlet obstruction.[15,22] Reduced bladder pressure function or contractility is defined as low voiding

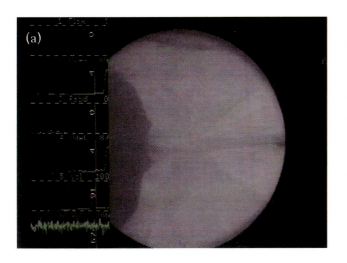

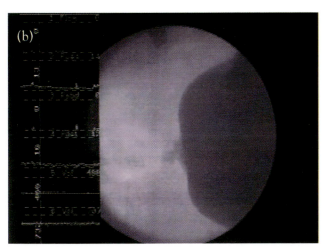

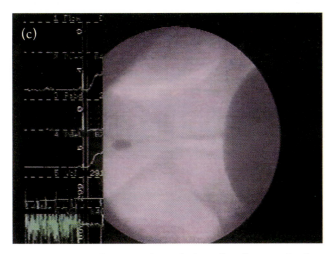

Figure 16.1. *Simultaneous video multichannel urodynamics (voiding cystourethrogram views): (a) patient with prostatic obstruction; (b) patient with impaired contractility; (c) patient with classic vesical neck obstruction. Note that (a) and (b) are indistinguishable radiographically but that (a) demonstrates a detrusor contraction (high detrusor pressure) whereas (b) does not.*

pressure in the presence of diminished flow ('low pressure, low flow').

One main advantage of the multichannel urodynamic study is its ability as a pressure–flow study to distinguish whether low urinary flow is secondary to obstruction and to impaired contractility. It also enables one to identify normal urinary flow and high detrusor contraction pressure due to obstruction. It also allows measurement of capacity, filling pressure, various parameters of a contraction and the presence of uninhibited contractions; observation of detrusor sphincter synergy and anatomical function; clarification of bladder function in the neurological patient; and a pretherapeutic assessment of bladder function that enables one to infer outcome prediction better. Thus, it has become an objective physiological tool with which to study patients with BPH.[6,15,19,40–44]

Methods and techniques

The standard multichannel urodynamic study consists of simultaneous synchronous real-time measurements of abdominal pressure, total intravesical pressure, a calculated detrusor pressure (total intravesical pressure minus abdominal pressure) and a urinary flow rate. In addition, other simultaneous measurements can be performed to provide additional information — electromyography (EMG) of the striated sphincter, video cystourethroradiographic imaging with voiding and urethral pressure profilometry.[15,45–48] A standard multichannel urodynamic flow recording is demonstrated in Figure 16.2. EMG, in the authors' practice, has little role as a diagnostic modality in patients with lower urinary tract symptoms; it has been reserved for those patients suspected of having external urethral contractions ('pseudodyssynergia') during voiding.[23] Urethral pressure profilometry (UPP) involves synchronous measurement of urethral and bladder pressure. Normally, the bladder and prostatic urethra are isobaric during voiding. The occurrence of a 'pressure drop' in the urethra suggests obstruction. Teleologically, UPP should be the optimal method of assessing outlet obstruction. However, because of difficulty in standardizing significant 'pressure drops', UPP has not been used routinely in men with BPH.[15]

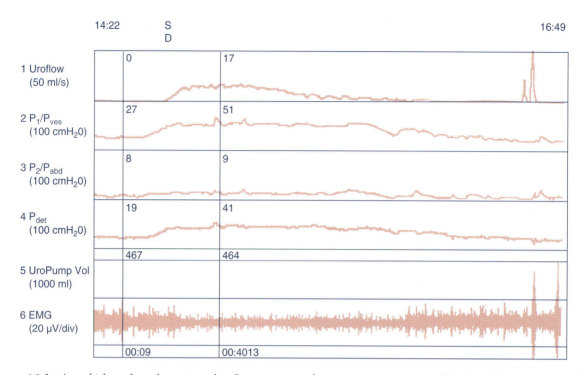

Figure 16.2. *A multichannel urodynamic study. Component simultaneous measurements include the following: (1) uroflowmetry; (2) P_1/P_{ves}=total intravesical pressure; (3) P_2/P_{abd}=abdominal pressure; (4) P_1–P_2/P_{det}=detrusor pressure; (5) volume infused; (6) electromyelography.*

Urodynamic quantitative analytical investigation of prostatic obstruction

As with all objective scientific instruments of measurement, standards of reference are important.[22] In considering the various techniques proposed to analyse prostatism, one must take into account the variability of urodynamic philosophies and operator preference utilized in each set of analytical studies. Specifically, issues as simple as catheter size (8–14 F), employment of suprapubic access, techniques of zeroing and type of EMG probe may cause differences in standards of reference of various individual laboratories and thus in interpretation of data. However, the basic concepts of diagnosis are the same.

In urodynamics, much attention has been given to both biomechanical engineering and mathematical modelling using theoretical dynamic states of voiding. Early efforts emphasized theories based on rigid tube physics.[48,49] These efforts evolved into complex equations analysing resistance coefficients/factors. These factors were then developed into elegant models to describe the complex relationships between detrusor pressure and flow, utilizing sophisticated computer analysis to simplify the process. Given the lack of fixed parameters to compare, a series of correlated parameters have been developed and studied.[48,50–54] Whereas the subjective definition of obstruction is easy to understand and identify, quantifiable standards for comparison have been difficult.

Detrusor pressure has been the subject of various cutoff criteria for obstruction in the low-flow state. This value has varied from 45 to 100 cmH$_2$O at the peak of urinary flow.[15,22,55] Because pressure is flow (force) against a resistance produced by an obstruction, one can theoretically calculate a resistance factor to define the cutoff for significant obstruction. Early endeavours tried to derive and describe this outlet or urethral resistance factor based on the rigid tube hydrodynamic theory described by Griffiths in 1975.[49] If the calculated factor exceeded a certain value, obstruction would be diagnosed. Applying a predefined resistance factor of 0.6, Bruskewitz et al. examined 46 patients treated for prostatism and found no significant changes in subjective or objective criteria in patients above or below the defined cutoff criteria.[56] This is not surprising, as the urethra is not a rigid tube.

Because the concept of simplifying urethral function to its cross-sectional area was attractive, it was the subject of many attempts to characterize outlet obstruction. However, as stated previously these attempts were based on a hydrodynamic basis of voiding; that is, the bladder outlet is similar to a rigid pipe with the urinary stream compared to laminar or turbulent flow. However, these models are limited by the following: (1) in a strict physical and mathematical sense, flow is neither turbulent nor laminar; (2) all resistance factors are calculated for a single point in the voiding cycle and thus do not reflect time-dependent flow changes. In addition, the urethra is elastic and distensible, and the flow-controlling zone is situated in the membranous urethra, as described by this rigid tube hydrodynamic theory.[50,57,58]

Although many have reported application of these resistance factors, some of which are still in use, it should be emphasized that the pathophysiological meanings of calculated values remain vague and hard to compare.[50,52,58] In obvious cases of high-pressure/low-flow states or low-pressure/high-flow states, the equation works well. However, in borderline cases, especially in preoperative evaluations, it has proved inadequate. Thus, the concept of these resistance factors based on rigid tube hydrodynamic theories was abandoned by the International Continent Society Standardization Committee in 1979.[58,59]

Additional attempts have been made to describe and interpret the voiding phase of the bladder through the characterization of the outlet alone and are achieved by quantifying 'resistance' or energy loss in the bladder outlet by factors based on advanced theoretical hydrodynamic understanding of micturition.[50] These efforts have involved developing conclusive biophysical models and have thereby derived advanced analytical procedures to assess characteristic features of voiding dynamics from pressure–flow recordings.[38,54,58,60]

These natural analytical extrapolations of the hydrodynamic concepts have encouraged many investigators to apply elegant mathematical models to characterize the complex interrelationship between detrusor pressure and uroflow.[54,57,58] To determine the adequacy of the detrusor contraction with respect to flow rate, several investigators have devised mathematical definitions of bladder outlet obstruction by calculating 'resistance coefficients'.[49–52,57,58] Because flow is dependent not only on outlet resistance but also on the power or pressure behind the resistance, this required investigators first to focus on techniques to assess the power of the bladder muscle or detrusor contractility.

The work of Griffiths describes a method to assess quantitatively the strength of detrusor contractions during any voiding where flow rate, detrusor pressure and residual urine are measured.[23,49,57,60] This is done by mathematically extrapolating a single point from the Hill curves, i.e. force versus contraction velocity. The parameters assessed include power [the product of detrusor pressure (P_{det}) and flow rate] and work (power integrated over time). Within a physiological range, maximum power increases with initial volume in the bladder as a function of the stretch created. This leads to an increase in peak flow with large volumes voided. However, when comparing power developed by the detrusor in bladders before and after prostatectomy, Schafer reported no differences.[50] He suggested that the overall contractile capability of the bladder is limited and well determined before surgery. However, Gleason looked at power at one point in time, either at maximal flow or maximal detrusor pressure, and reported a 20% increase after prostatectomy.[46] This suggests that, rather than a series of points, 'maximal' power may be a more important parameter. This is particularly true because power is volume dependent and is not constant for a constant contraction strength, falling to zero if the contraction is isovolumetric.

Detrusor contractility has also been defined by measurement of the 'bladder output relation', which is a mathematical relationship between pressure and flow based on the Hill model (an equation describing the relation between force and contraction velocity of a muscle). More recently, Griffiths has used the term WF, a factor dependent on detrusor pressure, uroflow, speed of detrusor contraction and bladder volume.[60–62] The advantage of such a model is that its two adjustable parameters — isovolumetric pressure and detrusor shortening velocity — are volume independent.

In the authors' laboratory, using a rabbit whole bladder in vitro model, changes in urethral resistance resulted in significant changes in both maximal power and WF.[63,64] It is noteworthy that detrusor pressure did not show variation with alteration of outlet resistance. Of interest, in a review of the urodynamic literature, Nielsen et al. reported considerable overlap in maximal intravesical detrusor pressure and intravesical detrusor opening pressure in men with and without obstruction.[58] It may be possible, therefore, to extrapolate that therapies that alter and reduce outlet resistance may result in changes in contractility parameters.

By utilizing the complex relationship between pressure, flow and outlet resistance during the dynamic function of voiding, biophysical models and advanced quantitative analytical techniques have been developed to study this complex relationship. These elegant models have sought to characterize and simplify this complex relationship to a quantitative value of comparison.

In the 1970s, Griffiths and colleagues introduced their urethral resistance relation, a graphical concept that analysed the relationship between detrusor pressure and flow during voiding to define the lowest resistance when the bladder outlet was passive or relaxed.[65–67] This

graphical relationship later evolved to a pressure–flow nomogram in 1979 by Abrams and Griffiths.[14] With this nomogram (Fig. 16.3), patients could be classified as obstructed, equivocal or unobstructed. In 1988, Jensen et al. classified a group of patients undergoing prostatectomy for 'prostatism' according to the nomogram.[17] Those classified as obstructed preoperatively became unobstructed postoperatively, on the basis of the nomogram and various other urodynamic parameters. Those unobstructed preoperatively remained unobstructed postoperatively without significant changes in other urodynamic parameters. These results validating the Abrams–Griffiths (AG) nomogram were similarly confirmed by Rollema and van Mastrigt in 1992.[68]

To advance further the concepts involved in the AG nomogram to a quantitative value of comparison, the analysis of the relationship between pressure, flow and outlet resistance evolved into a complex graphical quadratic equation that simplified this relationship into a variety of quantitative values for comparison. In some models, computer analysis was employed. The following is a brief description of various published models and quantitative parameters.

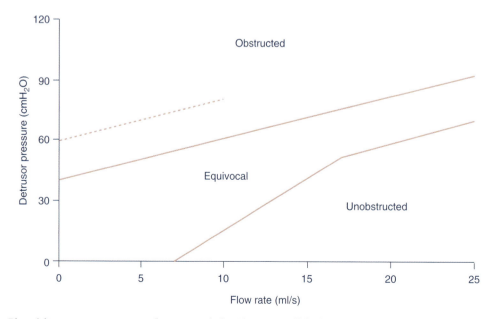

Figure 16.3. *Plot of detrusor pressure versus flow rate with the Abrams–Griffiths (AG) nomogram demonstrating pressure–flow regions of obstructed/equivocal/unobstructed relationships based on maximum pressure–flow recordings. Dotted line indicates extrapolation of an AG number: if P_{det} = 80 and Q_{max} = 10, AG no = 60.*

Schafer's model describes the urethra as a distensible tube with a flow-controlling zone in its proximal urethra.[11,48,50,62,69] A relationship between detrusor pressure and flow rate is described by the tube's distensibility and the size of the flow-controlling zone. It has been simplified to an estimated graphical relationship called PURR, the passive urethral resistance relationship. From this graphical description, an index quantifying obstruction is derived, termed the LPURR, the linear passive urethral resistance relation. LPURR is derived by looking up the position of a line segment that connects the point Q_{max},$p(Q_{max})$ with the point of lowest pressure during flow in a nomogram (Fig. 16.4).

As an extrapolation of this theory from the AG nomogram, Griffiths proposed the group-specific factor URA to characterize obstruction.[60] This parameter URA is estimated from the intersection of the quadratric urethral resistance relation with the pressure axis of the pressure–flow rate plot, basically connecting point Q_{max},$p(Q_{max})$ to the lowest pressure point during flow. A group-specific URA nomogram was then created (Fig. 16.4). From the nomogram, a simpler AG number can be extrapolated.[70] To obtain the AG number from the pressure–flow plot, a line is drawn through the $P_{det}Q_{max}/Q_{max}$ point, parallel to the upper line of the AG nomogram, to intersect with the pressure

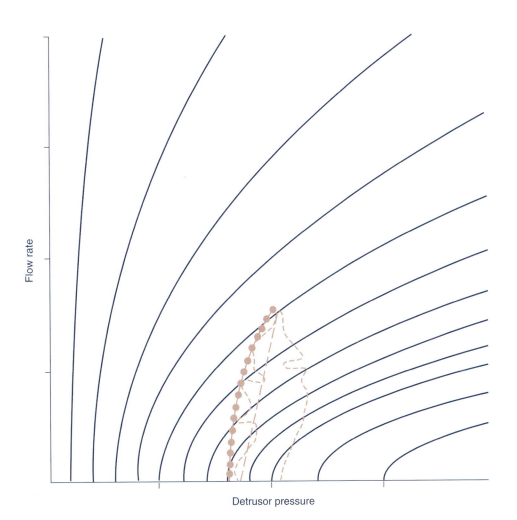

Figure 16.4. *Pressure–flow plot of a void and a demonstration of a graphical estimate of PURR (●—●—●), LPURR (— — — —) and URA of this void. The group-specific URA nomogram curves (———) are for values of 10 and are calculated on the basis of the formula: URA=p_{uo} (urethral opening pressure) = $[(1 + 4d\ Q_2 P_{det})\ 1/2{-}1]/(2d\ Q_2)$, where d= 0.00038. The pressure–flow void curve is shown as ------ .*

axis where an AG number is derived (Fig. 16.3). In 85 patients, Lim et al. compared AG number, URA and LPURR.[70] They found that agreement with AG number and URA is 94%, the agreement between AG number and LPURR is 98.2% and the agreement with URA and LPURR is 94.7%. Thus the three parameters appear to substantiate each other.

In an application utilizing computer analysis, van Mastrigt and Rollema developed a computer program, CLIM, to analyse detrusor pressure, flow rate signals during voiding and isometric detrusor pressure increase just before flow starts.[68,71,72] From this analysis, U/L, the maximum extrapolated rate of increase of isometric pressure, as well as URA, can be calculated. In addition, OBI, another quantification of urethral resistance can be calculated. Briefly, OBI is the parameter that fits the lowest part of a pressure–flow rate relation with a orthogonal polynomial.[73]

Recently, Kranse and van Mastrigt critically compared URA, LPURR, OBI, Q_{max} and pQ_{max} for quantification of bladder outlet obstruction.[74] Utilizing various alternative methods of comparing and classifying obstruction preoperatively and postoperatively, they critically analysed the sensitivity and specificity of each factor. They concluded that different classifications lead to different conclusions and that these parameters have a dependence on contractility that is not analysed and which affects their performance to measure obstruction.

In addition, Spangberg et al.[75,76] described a model based on computer analysis of pressure–flow data. Briefly, the model describes the flow-controlling zone in the urethra as it distends with increasing urethral pressure and calculates a urethral pressure/area relationship quantity. Its clinical usefulness still remains to be examined.

Finally, in 1988, Sarky and Blaivas[77,78] described a series of computer-generated parameters that added a time factor to the pressure–flow curve. This was translated into a bladder outlet conductance curve and a conductance factor was generated. Although this factor seems to be decreased in patients with outlet obstruction, its clinical validity remains to be determined.

As this brief description of these various models and parameters demonstrates, the state of quantitative urodynamic analysis and comparison of urodynamic data is still evolving and being assessed. Although the concepts are basic and useful in daily qualitative clinical application towards a urodynamic diagnosis, the quantitative techniques and parameters are at present all theoretical estimates of obstruction, as well as being too complicated and cumbersome for daily urodynamic patient examinations.

Despite these analytical limitations, the pressure–flow relationship may serve as the most widely clinically applicable measurable urodynamic parameter. In the study by Spangberg et al., 23 men were studied both pre- and postoperatively with sophisticated pressure–flow studies.[52] A host of 'contractility' and 'resistance' factors were measured, including the more standard detrusor pressure at maximum flow and maximal detrusor pressure. In this small population, conventional curve fitting of the pressure–flow plot allowed urodynamic estimation for quantifying obstruction, to determine whether detrusor pressure was adequate and to ascertain bladder function. Similarly, Jensen noted that utilization of obstructive parameters (catheterized flow of less than 12 ml/s and a peak detrusor pressure of more than 45 cmH$_2$0) lowered the failure rate after surgery from as high as 20% to 8% and increased the exclusion from surgery from 5% to 9%.[33] However, to date there have been no long-term follow-up pressure–flow analyses in symptomatic patients with prostatism who are left untreated, or those who are treated either surgically or pharmacologically.

Clinical application of urodynamic studies for BPH treatments

One important question that remains to be elucidated fully is the predictive value of urodynamic studies — specifically, their value in predicting which patient will benefit most from intervention and which will not improve after intervention. In particular, are urodynamic studies instrumental in providing information to obtain the best outcome, both symptomatically and objectively?

Studies utilizing urodynamics to predict outcome look at several urodynamic parameters and associated outcome success based on two general criteria — an objective measure such as flow rate and a subjective criterion such as patient satisfaction or improved symptomatology.

In 1979, Abrams et al. examined 152 men who underwent prostatectomy for BPH based on urodynamic testing.[13] Although the study did not specify the operative criteria or the process of operative decision-making, Abrams and colleagues reported 86% of patients improved, on the basis of Q_{max} and a decrease in voiding pressure. Subjectively, 88% of patients had improvement in their symptoms. In an earlier study, these authors reported that the inclusion of urodynamic testing in their operative criteria lowered their postoperative failure from 28% to 12%.[27] However, 28% is a higher surgical failure rate than that reported by others.[26]

The application of urodynamic pressure–flow studies to operative criteria is also advocated by Abrams and Griffiths,[14] who reported that 50% of patients could be correctly classified as obstructed and unobstructed, on the basis of Q_{max} alone. In addition, with detrusor pressure at Q_{max}, the diagnostic accuracy increased to 66%. The remaining one-third were assessed with pressure–flow plots and many of these demonstrated impaired contractility as a factor for their low-flow state.

If the addition of multichannel urodynamic testing appears to have improved diagnostic accuracy, is it possible to identify a population of patients who would most benefit from these studies without having to perform them on every patient to increase diagnostic accuracy? In 1988, Kuo and Tsai examined 50 patients urodynamically and by a general symptom analysis before and after prostatectomy.[79] Subjective outcome analysis was divided into good, fair and worse. They looked at the subjective outcome analysis of the prostatectomy based on selected preoperative urodynamic parameters such as different levels of Q_{max} and those with high-pressure obstruction, low-pressure obstruction and low-pressure/no obstruction (LPNOB). While they concluded that prostatectomy might be best for those with a Q_{max} less than 15 ml/s and those with high-pressure obstruction, the more interesting observation is the poor outcome in patients with a Q_{max} greater than 15 ml/s and those classified as LPNOB. Since failure rate in this group is high, does this identify a population with flows greater than 15 ml/s who would benefit from multichannel urodynamic testing to

identify them as LPNOB? Do these patients with poor subjective outcome fail after prostatectomy because their symptoms are due to involuntary contractions?

Recently, the application of sophisticated computer analysis of pressure–flow data has been used by many to analyse BPH and treatment efficacy.[80] Schafer et al. have applied these complex analyses better to define passive and dynamic urethral resistance measurement.[11,48,69] Using this model, they have identified patients with low Q_{max} who were not obstructed; objective improvement rates were 100% in the severely obstructed and less in the mildly obstructed. This model, as well as the CLIM model by Rollema and van Mastrigt, are also described and applied in order better to define obstruction and to improve the efficacy of BPH treatment through better urodynamic assessments.[71,72] However, in recent reports by Schafer et al.[20,21] in which manual urodynamic analysis was studied in order to examine issues of quality control and analysis as well as reproducibility, the application of automated computer analysis does not appear to be superior or acceptable because of lack of standards and issues of operator and patient variability.

Involuntary detrusor contraction (or detrusor instability) is a urodynamic entity that has become more important, especially with the recent trend to treat and monitor BPH with symptom scores. The prognostic significance of its presence preoperatively and its risk for persistence postoperatively has impact, especially if the goal of treatment is to improve symptom score. Currently, the presence of instability on a urodynamic assessment does not have good predictive value for its presence postoperatively. The authors recently reported their findings regarding 129 consecutive men, after prostatectomy (mean age 72 years) with voiding symptoms after transurethral resection of the prostate, whose urodynamic findings were retrospectively analysed with respect to symptoms, uroflow and synchronous video pressure–flow cystometry.[35] Obstruction was found in 38% of patients, impaired contractility in 25% and intrinsic sphincter deficiency in 8%. In 80 patients without neurological disorders, involuntary bladder contractions were detected in 50%; however, in 49 patients with neurological disorders, involuntary bladder contractions were detected in 76%. This difference was statistically significant. This study revealed the significance of involuntary contractions as a potential cause of treatment failure after prostatectomy.

Symptomatic, pathological, urodynamic and molecular expression of BPH

The ideal study of BPH would entail analysing the complex interrelationship of symptomatology, pathology, physiology and molecular biology of the progression of BPH and its response to therapy. Currently, it is a widely held belief that the development and persistence of symptoms in the untreated population is related to increasing severity of obstruction. It is believed that a proportion of symptoms, such as poor urinary stream and incomplete voiding, are directly related to an obstructive process itself; however, detrusor instability makes a significant contribution.

One current approach to examining the development instability focuses on the innervation of the bladder and prostate. One recent study suggests that the constant increased pressure produced by mild chronic obstruction causes an autonomic denervation injury that produces a state of supersensitivity in the target organ, resulting in new or persistent instability.[32] This concept of an autonomic denervation injury in the target organ is also consistent with the urodynamic finding of neuropathic changes in the diabetic bladder. Thus, numerous studies have combined analysis of the molecular expression of numerous biological factors with urodynamically documented findings in the animal model. These approaches have yielded a host of new questions to investigate. Does relief of obstruction allow for reinnervation to a normal state and thus for instability to resolve? Is there a point where reinnervation is not possible and instability remains persistent? These issues of urodynamics and molecular biology are speculative and warrant investigation. It is noteworthy that over 50% of those diabetic patients with voiding symptoms who undergo urodynamic testing have detrusor instability.[25] These patients are typical suspects for autonomic denervation injury in the bladder.

Conclusions

It is clear that, given our current understanding of BPH and its relationship to symptoms of prostatism and obstructive uropathy, the role of urodynamics as both a diagnostic tool and an instrument to assist in therapeutic management remains to be defined. Currently, urodynamic studies have provided an understanding of these three processes and their complex interaction. They are, at present, a tool best utilized in diagnosing obstruction. How prostatic obstruction interrelates to symptoms and progression toward obstructive uropathy and the concurrent development of BPH is still not well understood. It is through our increasing elucidation of molecular and neurological events occurring at the cellular level that we may understand further how prostatic growth leads to symptoms and bladder dysfunction. Prospective trials by both the International Continent Society and by the National Institutes of Health will help to define these relationships and determine the role and value of urodynamic studies in BPH. Finally, the integration of urodynamic physiology, clinical presentations and the molecular biological basis of BPH voiding dysfunctions will, it is hoped, elucidate and clarify a disease state that is currently elusive.

References

1. Abrams P. In support of pressure–flow studies for evaluating men with lower urinary tract symptoms. Urology 1994; 44: 153–155
2. McConnell J D. Why pressure–flow studies should be optional and not mandatory studies for evaluating men with benign prostatic hyperplasia. Urology 1994; 44: 156–158
3. McGuire E J. The role of urodynamic investigation in the assessment of benign prostatic hypertrophy. J Urol 1992; 148: 1133–1136
4. Ball A J, Feneley R C L, Abrams P H. The natural history of untreated prostatism. Br J Urol 1981; 53: 613–616
5. Andersen J T, Nordling J. Prostatism II. The correlation between cysto-urethroscopic, cystometric and urodynamic findings. Scand J Urol Nephrol 1980; 14: 23–27
6. Barry M J, Cockett A T, Holtgrewe H L et al. Relationship of symptoms of prostatism to commonly used physiological and anatomical measures of the severity of benign prostatic hyperplasia. J Urol 1993; 150: 351–358
7. Barry M J, Fowler F J Jr, O'Leary M P et al. The American Urological Association symptom index for benign prostatic hyperplasia. J Urol 1992; 148: 1549–1557
8. Barry M J, Fowler F J Jr, O'Leary M P et al. Correlation of the American Urological Association Symptom Index with self-administered versions of the Madsen–Iverson, Boyarsky and Maine Medical Assessment Program Symptom Indexes. J Urol 1992; 148: 1558–1563

9. Boyarsky S, Jones G, Paulson D F, Prout G R Jr. A new look at bladder neck obstruction by the Food and Drug Administration regulators; guide lines for the investigation of benign prostatic hypertrophy. Trans Am Assoc Genito-Urin Surg 1977; 68: 29.

10. Bruskewitz R C, Larsen E H, Madsen P O, Dorflinger T. 3-year followup of urinary symptoms after transurethral resection of the prostate. J Urol 1986; 136: 613–615

11. Schafer W, Rubben H, Noppeney R, Deutz F-J. Obstructed and unobstructed prostatic obstruction. A plea for urodynamic objectivation of bladder outflow obstruction in benign prostatic hyperplasia. World J Urol 1989; 6: 198–203.

12. Simonsen O, Moller-Madsen B, Dorflinger T et al. The significance of age on symptoms and urodynamic and cystoscopic findings in benign prostatic hypertrophy. Urol Res 1987; 15: 355–358

13. Abrams P H, Farrar D J, Turner-Warwick R T et al. The results of prostatectomy: a symptomatic and urodynamic analysis of 152 patients. J Urol 1979; 121: 640–642

14. Abrams P H, Griffiths D J. The assessment of prostatic obstruction from urodynamic measurements and from residual urine. Br J Urol 1979; 51: 129–134

15. Blaivas J G. Multichannel urodynamic studies in men with benign prostatic hyperplasia: indications and interpretation. Urol Clin North Am 1990; 17: 543–552

16. Coolsaet B R L A, Blok C. Detrusor properties related to prostatism. Neurourol Urodyn 1986; 5: 435

17. Jensen K M-E, Jørgensen J B, Mogensen P. Urodynamics in prostatism II. Prognostic value of pressure-flow study combined with stop-flow test. Scand J Urol Nephrol 1988; 114 (suppl): 72-77

18. Dean G E, Kaplan S A, Blaivas J G. The differential diagnosis of prostatism: a urodynamic survey. J Urol 1991; 145: 79A

19. Hellström P, Lukkarinen O, Kontturi M. Bladder neck incision or transurethral electroresection for the treatment of urinary obstruction caused by a small benign prostate? A randomized urodynamic study. Scand J Urol Nephrol 1986; 20: 187–192

20. Donovan J L, Abrams P, Schafer W. The International Continence Society study on BPH: urodynamic quality control and data analysis. J Urol 1994; 151: 294A

21. Kirchner-Hermanns R, Thorner M, Schafer W et al. Reproducibility of urodynamic data in BPH: influence of patient and investigator on data quality and analysis. J Urol 1994; 151: 295A

22. Abrams P, Blaivas J G, Stanton S L, Andersen J T. Standardization of terminology of lower urinary tract function. Neurourol Urodyn 1988; 7: 403–427

23. Griffiths D J, Scholtmeirer R J. Detrusor/sphincter dysynergia in neurologically normal children. Neurourol Urodyn 1983; 2: 27

24. Kaplan M H, Feinstein A R. The importance of classifying initial co-morbidity in evaluating the outcome of diabetes mellitus. J Chronic Dis 1974; 27: 387–404

25. Kaplan S A, Te A E. Bladder dysfunction in diabetes. Probl Urol 1992; 6: 659–668

26. McConnell J D, Barry M J, Bruskewitz R C et al. Benign prostatic hyperplasia: diagnosis and treatment. Clinical Practice Guideline No 8. AHCPR Publication 94-0582. Rockville: AHCPR, PHS, US Department of Health and Human Services, 1994

27. Abrams P H. Prostatism and prostatectomy: the value of urine flow rate measurement in the preoperative assessment for operation. J Urol 1977; 117: 70–71

28. Ball A J, Smith P J B. The long-term effects of prostatectomy: a uroflowmetric analysis. J Urol 1982; 128: 538–540

29. Kelly M J, Roskamp D, Leach G E. Transurethral incision of the prostate: a preoperative and postoperative analysis of symptoms and urodynamic findings. J Urol 1989; 142: 1507–1509

30. Scott F B, Cardus D, Quesada E M, Riles T. Uroflowmetry before and after prostatectomy. South Med J 1967; 60(2): 948–952

31. Jensen K M-E, Jørgensen J B, Mogensen P. Urodynamics in prostatism III. Prognostic value of medium-fill water cystometry. Scand J Urol Nephrol 1988; 114(suppl): 78–83

32. Cucchi A. The development of detrusor instability in prostatic obstruction in relation to sequential changes in voiding dynamics. J Urol 1994; 51: 1342–1344

33. Jensen K M-E, Andersen J T. Urodynamic implications of benign prostatic hyperplasia. Urologe [A] 1990; 29: 1–4

34. McLoughlin J, Gill K P, Abel P D, Williams G. Symptoms versus flow rates versus urodynamics in the selection of patients for prostatectomy. Br J Urol 1990; 66: 303–305

35. Olsson C A, Goluboff E T, Chang D T, Kaplan S A. Urodynamics and the etiology of post-prostatectomy urinary incontinence (PPI). J Urol 1994; 151: 326A

36. Kaplan S A, Te A E, Jacobs B Z. Urodynamic evidence of vesical neck obstruction in men with misdiagnosed chronic nonbacterial prostatitis and therapeutic role of endoscopic incision of bladder neck. J Urol 1994; 152: 2063–2065

37. George N J R, Feneley R C L, Roberts J B M. Identification of the poor risk patient with prostatism and detrusor failure. Br J Urol 1986; 58: 290–295

38. Glemain P, Buzelin J M, Cordonnier J P. New urodynamic model to explain micturition disorders in benign prostatic hyperplasia patients. Pressure–flow relationships in collapsable tubes, hydraulic analysis of the urethra and evaluation of urethral resistance. Eur Urol 1993; 24: 12–17

39. Neal D E, Styles R A, Powell P H, Ramsden P D. Relationships between detrusor function and residual urine in men undergoing prostatectomy. Br J Urol 1987; 60: 560–566

40. Andersen J T. Prostatism III. Detrusor hyperreflexia and residual urine. Clinical and urodynamic aspects and the influence of surgery on the prostate. Scand J Urol Nephrol 1982; 16: 25–30

41. Hald T. Urodynamics in benign prostatic hyperplasia: a survey. Prostate 1989; 2(suppl): 69–77

42. Haylen B T, Ashby D, Sutherst J R et al. Maximum and average urine flow rates in normal male and female populations: the Liverpool nomograms. Br J Urol 1989; 64: 30–38

43. Jensen K M-E. Clinical evaluation of routine urodynamic investigations in prostatism. Neurourol Urodyn 1989; 8: 545

44. Grino P B, Bruskewitz R, Blaivas J G et al. Maximum urinary flow rate by uroflowmetry: automatic or visual interpretation. J Urol 1993; 149: 339–341

45. Frimodt-Moller C, Hald T. Clinical urodynamics: methods and results. Scand J Urol Nephrol 1972; 6: 143

46. Gleason D M, Lattimer J K. The pressure flow study: a method for measuring bladder neck resistance. J Urol 1962; 87: 844

47. Jensen K M-E, Bruskewitz R C, Iversen P, Madsen P O. Predictive value of voiding pressures in benign prostatic hyperplasia. Neurourol Urodyn 1983; 2: 117

48. Schafer W. Principles and clinical application of advance urodynamic analysis of voiding function. Urol Clin North Am 1990; 17: 553–566

49. Griffiths D J. Urethral resistance to flow: the urethral resistance relation. Abbreviated report. Urol Int 1975; 30: 28

50. Schafer W. Urethral resistance? Urodynamic concepts of physiological and pathological bladder outlet function during voiding. Neurourol Urodyn 1985; 4: 161

51. Spangberg A, Terio H, Ask P, Engberg A. Quantification of urethral function based on Griffiths' model of flow though elastic tubes. Neurourol Urodyn 1989; 8: 29

52. Spangberg A, Terio H, Ask P, Engberg A. Pressure/flow studies preoperatively and postoperatively in patients with benign prostatic hypertrophy: estimation of the urethral pressure/flow relation and urethral elasticity. Neurourol Urodyn 1991; 10: 139–167

53. Susset J G. Resistance to flow in the lower urinary tract: clinical application. In: Hinman F Jr (ed) Hydrodynamics of micturition. Springfield: C. C. Thomas, 1981

54. Van Mastrigt R, Rollema H J. Urethral resistance and urinary bladder contractility before and after transurethral resection as determined by the computer program CLIM. Neurourol Urodyn 1988; 7: 226

55. Smith J C. Urethral resistance to micturition. Br J Urol 1968; 40: 125–156

56. Bruskewitz R C, Jensen K M-E, Iversen P, Madsen P O. The relevance of minimum urethral resistance in prostatism. J Urol 1983; 129: 769–771

57. Griffiths D J. Urodynamics: the mechanics and hydrodynamics of the lower urinary tract. Medical Physics Handbook 4. Bristol: Adam Hilger, 1980

58. Nielsen K K, Nordling J, Hald T. Critical review of the diagnosis of prostatic obstruction. Neurourol Urodyn 1994; 13: 201–217

59. Bates P, Bradley W E, Glen E et al. The standardization of terminology of lower urinary tract function. J Urol 1979; 121: 551–554

60. Griffiths D J, van Mastrigt R, Bosch R. Quantification of urethral resistance and bladder function during voiding, with special reference to effects of prostate size reduction on urethral obstruction due to benign prostatic hyperplasia. Neurourol Urodyn 1989; 8: 17

61. Griffiths D J, Constantinou C E, van Mastrigt R. Urinary bladder function and its control in healthy females. Am J Physiol 1986: 2: R251

62. Schafer W. Detrusor as the energy source of micturition. In: Hinman F Jr (ed) Benign prostatic hypertrophy. New York: Springer-Verlag, 1983; 450

63. Kaplan S A, Blaivas J G, Brown W C, Schuessler G. Parameters of detrusor contractility I: The effect of bladder volume and outlet resistance on Qmax, power and work in an in-vitro whole rabbit model. Neurourol Urodyn 1989; 8: 375–376

64. Kaplan S A, Brown W C, Chancellor M B et al. Parameters of detrusor contractility II. The effect of outlet resistance on the mechanical indices: power, work and WF. J Urol 1990; 143: 354

65. Griffiths D J. Hydrodynamics of male micturition. I. Therapy of steady state flow through elastic walled tubes. Med Biol Eng 1971; 7: 201–215

66. Griffiths D J. Hydrodynamics of male micturition. II. Measurement of stream parameters and urethral elasticity. Med Biol Eng 1971; 9: 589–596

67. Griffiths D J. The mechanics of the urethra and of micturition. Br J Urol 1973; 45: 497–507

68. Rollema H J, van Mastrigt R. Improved indication and followup in transurethral resection of the prostate using the computer program CLIM: a prospective study. J Urol 1992; 148: 111–116

69. Schafer W, Noppeney R, Rubben H, Lutzeyer W. The value of free flow rate and pressure/flow studies in the routine investigation of BPH patients. Neurourol Urodyn 1988; 7: 219–221

70. Lim C S, Reynard J, Cannon A, Abrams P. The Abrams–Griffith number: a simple way to quantify bladder outflow obstruction. Neurourol Urodyn 1994; 13: 475–476

71. Rollema H J, van Mastrigt R. Objective analysis of prostatism: a clinical application of the computer program CLIM. Neurourol Urodyn 1991; 10: 71–76

72. Rollema H J, van Mastrigt R, Janknegt R A. Urodynamic assessment and quantification of prostatic obstruction before and after transurethral resection of the prostate: standardization with the aid of the computer program CLIM. Urol Int 1991; 1(suppl): 52–54

73. Kranse M, van Mastrigt R. The derivation of an obstruction index from a three parameter model fitted to the lowest part of the pressure flow plot. J Urol 1991; 145: 261A

74. Kranse M, van Mastrigt R. A critical comparison of methods proposed for quantification of bladder outlet obstruction. Neurourol Urodyn 1993; 12: 267–272

75. Spangberg A, Terio H, Ask P. Pressure-flow studies in elderly without voiding problems: estimation of the urethral pressure/flow relation and urethral elasticity. Neurourol Urodyn 1990; 9: 123–138

76. Terio H, Spangberg A, Engberg A, Asp P. Estimation of elastic properties in the urethral flow controlling zone by signal analysis of urodynamic pressure–flow data. Med Biol Eng Comput 1989; 27: 314–321

77. Sarky M S, Blaivas J G. Functional types of prostatic obstruction. Neurourol Urodyn 1988; 7: 221–222

78. Sarky M S, Blaivas J G, Schussler G. Bladder outlet conductance: evolution, normal and obstructive patterns. Neurourol Urodyn 1988; 7: 223

79. Kuo H C, Tsai T C. The predictive value of urine flow rate and voiding pressure in the operative outcome of benign prostatic hypertrophy. Taiwan I Hsueh Hui Tsa Chih 1988; 87: 323–330

80. Van Mastrigt R, Kranse M. Automated evaluation of urethral obstruction. Urology 1993: 42: 216

17

Imaging and benign prostatic hyperplasia
D. Rickards

Introduction

All imaging modalities have a role in both imaging the prostate gland and the effect that prostate pathology has upon the rest of the urinary tract. Imaging is directed towards determining intraprostatic anatomy and measuring lower urinary tract function. Departments of radiology involved in such studies need the use of a flow-rate machine; to image post-micturition volumes without a flow rate is an almost meaningless exercise and a waste of resources.

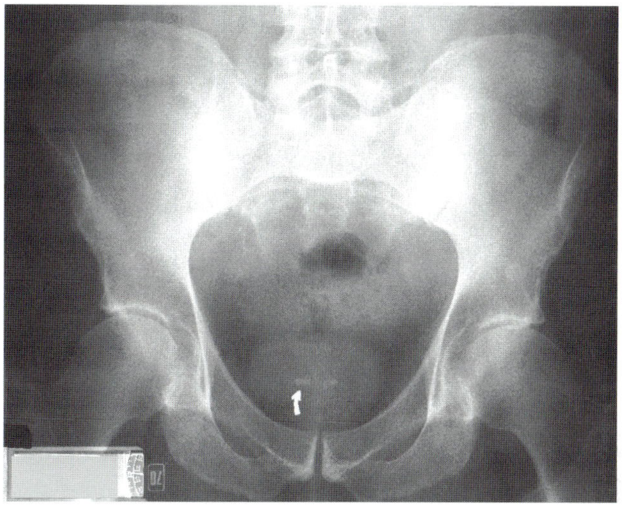

Excretory urography and BPH

Initial plain KUB (kidneys, ureters and bladder) films of the abdomen and pelvis may indicate the presence of prostatomegaly (Table 17.1).

A prostate soft tissue mass will be seen only with very large prostates. Corpora amylacea occur between the peripheral and central/transitional zones of the prostate, and appear as a curvilinear calcific line arching above the symphysis pubis or as a block-like calcification, and are usually bilateral (Fig. 17.1) but are occasionally unilateral. Such calcification is characteristic and, if seen above the symphysis, indicates that there is prostatomegaly. Sclerotic metastases due to prostate carcinoma may be seen in conjunction with benign prostatic hyperplasia (BPH). A large bladder shadow suggests chronic retention, possibly on the basis of BPH.

Following administration of contrast medium, the finding of upper tract dilatation down to the vesico-

Figure 17.1. *Plain film of the pelvis. There is calcification projected above the symphysis pubis (arrow) characteristic of corpora amylacea associated with BPH.*

ureteric junction is unusual except in high-pressure chronic retention of urine. Elevation of the bladder base by a soft tissue mass suggests prostatomegaly (Fig. 17.2), which is further evidenced by fish-hooking of the distal

Table 17.1. *Findings on KUB films in BPH*

1. Suprapubic soft tissue mass

2. Corpora amylacea extending above the symphysis pubis

3. Large bladder

4. Sclerotic bony metastases

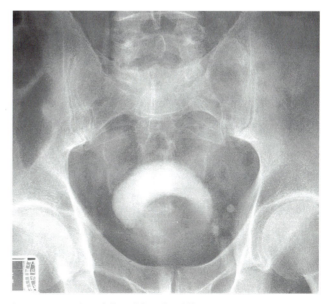

Figure 17.2. *Coned film of the pelvis following i.v. contrast. There is considerable elevation of the bladder base due to prostatomegaly.*

ureters, which can be slightly dilated (Fig. 17.3). The bladder outline may be crenated, suggesting hypertrophy and high-pressure voiding. The enlarged prostate can be seen as a vesical-filling defect, more commonly seen with so-called 'median lobes' which, in effect, are superior extensions of the central and transitional zones of the prostate. Small filling defects seen on the surface of the prostate represent prominent blood vessels, seen on cystoscopy to lie just beneath the bladder mucosa. Outflow obstruction due to BPH can be complicated by bladder stones which can be large, often laminated, usually single and radio-opaque (Fig. 17.4). Small and multiple acquired diverticula are further evidence of high-pressure voiding due to outflow obstruction and BPH. A large diverticulum that distends with

micturition and appears larger on the post-micturition film is another finding. The walls of such diverticula do not contain muscle and the bladder can decompress into these low-pressure sacs. Stones complicate diverticula because of stasis. Small stones are best seen on ultrasound.

Excretory urography for outflow obstruction should include a flow rate after the 20 min full-length film followed by an immediate post-micturition film. Assessment of the volume of post-micturition urine on such films is very inaccurate and is best described as large, moderate, minimal or none.

Urethrography and BPH

Ascending urethrography shows a normal anterior urethra. The posterior urethra in BPH will be attenuated and posteriorly displaced (Fig. 17.5), with elevation of the bladder base (Fig. 17.6). Clearly, the larger the BPH the more pronounced such findings. Splitting of contrast is a feature. Descending studies confirm these findings (Fig. 17.7), and provide additional information about the state of the bladder wall, bladder capacity, post-micturition residual and

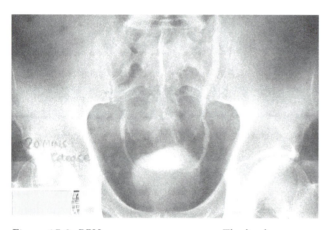

Figure 17.3. *BPH on an excretory urogram. The distal ureters are elevated and there is slight dilatation of the left distal ureter.*

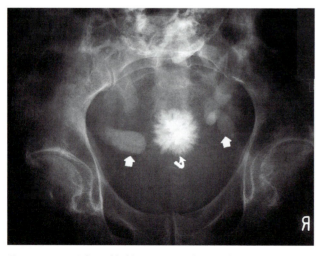

Figure 17.4. *A large bladder stone can be seen (curved arrow). In addition, there is gross dilatation of both distal ureters (arrows). This patient had high-pressure chronic retention due to BPH.*

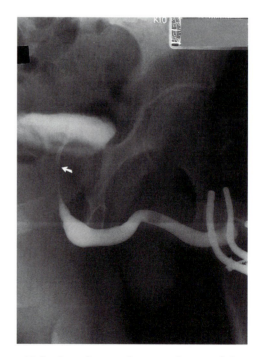

Figure 17.5. *Ascending urethrogram showing slight posterior displacement of the posterior urethra due to early BPH (arrow).*

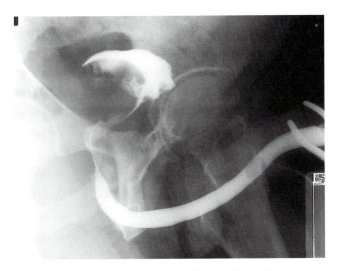

Figure 17.6. *Ascending urethrogram. There is a large soft tissue mass lesion invaginating the bladder base due to a large BPH.*

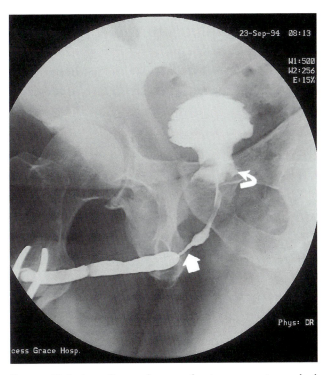

Figure 17.8. *Ascending urethrogram showing an anterior urethral stricture (arrow) following TURP for BPH (curved arrow).*

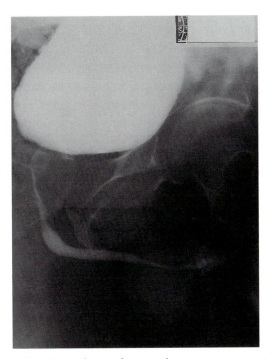

Figure 17.7. *Descending urethrogram showing gross attenuation of the posterior urethra and posterior displacement of the urethra due to BPH.*

vesicoureteric reflux. Surgery for BPH may be complicated by anterior urethral (Fig. 17.8) or sphincter stricture.

Computer tomography and BPH

Computed tomography (CT) is unable to differentiate the different zones of the prostate, which appears as a homogeneous structure, well defined and with an attenuation value of 25–30 Hounsfield units (HU). Glands involved in BPH appear larger, but still well defined and with a similar attenuation value (Fig. 17.9). Coexistent pathology in the bladder and distal ureters should be sought. There is no role for CT in the diagnosis of BPH.

Magnetic resonance and BPH

Magentic resonance (MR) imaging has been advocated as the imaging modality of choice for the prostate gland.[1] MR, unlike CT, can differentiate the zonal anatomy of the prostate using either surface or endorectal coils. Differing appearances in BPH have been reported and depend on the distribution and size of glandular tissue, as well as on the composition of the surrounding stroma.[2] Non-stromal hyperplasia is diagnosed when (a) the nodules in the central/transitional zone of the gland are characterized as having heterogeneous high signal intensity (Fig. 17.10) on T2-weighted images and peripheral enhancement on gadolinium-enhanced T1-weighted images, (b) a surgical capsule is present, or (c) the

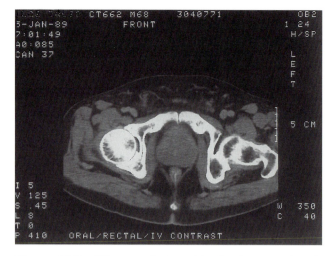

Figure 17.9. *CT scan of the pelvis showing an enlarged, homogeneous and well-defined prostate due to BPH. There is no differentiation of the zonal anatomy of the prostate.*

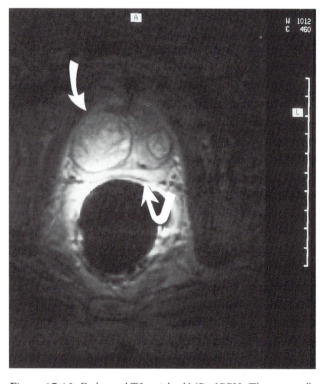

Figure 17.10. *Endorectal T2-weighted MR of BPH. There are well-defined nodules (arrow) in the central part of the gland suggesting non-stromal BPH. There is marked compression of the peripheral zone (curved arrow).*

central/transitional zone volume to total volume is greater than 0.75. When none of these findings are present, stromal BPH is diagnosed. The usefulness of this differentiation is relevant for predicting the reponse

of BPH to pharmacotherapy. Stromal hyperplasia has a large smooth muscle component and is more likely to respond to alpha-blockers.

Ultrasound and BPH

Transabdominal ultrasound and lower urinary tract dysfunction due to BPH

As an initial investigation in any patient with symptoms due to BPH, an ultrasound cystodynamogram (USCD) should be performed.[3] Bladder volumes are measured before and after micturition using the standard technique described by Poston,[4] in which the bladder volume in millilitres is 0.7HDW, where D is depth in the sagittal plane, H is maximum diameter in the sagittal plane and W is maximum transverse diameter in the transverse plane, all measurements being in centimetres. Voided volumes of less than 200 ml are of little clinical relevance. Over-full bladders are to be avoided, as such a state will inhibit micturition. Once the full bladder has been scanned and its volume measured, the patient voids into a standard flow rate machine, having been asked to void as normally as possible and not to try to impress with superimposed abdominal straining. Immediately after voiding, the bladder is rescanned and any residual measured . If there is a large residual (100 ml or more), the bladder should be rescanned after a second void and that residual assessed. The USCD provides both anatomical and physiological information (Tables 17.2 and 17.3). Prostate dimensions can be measured on suprapubic scanning, but are not accurate.

The following combinations can be identified:

Table 17.2. *Information gained from an USCD: anatomical*

Full bladder volume
Thickness of bladder wall
Distal ureteric anatomy
Intravesical filling defects, e.g. stone, ureterocoele, tumour
Bladder diverticula
Residual bladder volume
Relationship of the prostate to the base of the bladder
Perivesical anatomy

Table 17.3. *Information gained from an USCD: physiological*

Voided volume
Maximum flow rate
Average flow rate
Time to peak flow
Voiding time
Flow time

1. *Normal flow rate; complete bladder emptying; normal bladder wall.* A normal USCD does not exclude abnormalities of bladder function. Early prostate outflow obstruction is compensated for by the bladder generating higher voiding pressures to establish complete bladder emptying at normal flow rates. It will be in the later stages of bladder decompensation that flow rates will deteriorate and residual urine volumes will be seen. Instability (involuntary bladder contraction) will not be excluded.

2. *Low flow rate; complete bladder emptying.* This combination will be commonly seen in the following conditions:

   (a) *With hypertrophied bladder wall: outflow obstruction* (see above). The bladder wall may be thickened with elevation of the bladder base due to prostatomegaly (Fig. 17.11). Other causes of outflow obstruction, such as urethral stricture or bladder neck dyssynergia, cannot be excluded.

   (b) *With normal bladder wall: poor detrusor — partial detrusor failure.* A poorly functioning bladder without outflow obstruction is seen in women who are infrequent voiders (so-called cameloid bladders). It is also seen in males who have low-pressure chronic retention of urine and whose detrusor function has deteriorated. The bladder becomes chronically overdistended and the bladder muscle (detrusor) subsequently damaged. There will probably be elevation of the bladder base, but the bladder wall will be of normal thickness.

3. *High flow rate; complete bladder emptying; normal or hypertrophied bladder wall; no prostatomegaly.* This can be seen in normal subjects who augment micturition with abdominal straining. It is also seen in *detrusor*

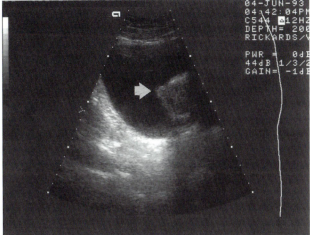

Figure 17.11. *Longitudinal scan of the bladder showing marked invagination of the bladder base (arrow) due to prostatomegaly.*

instability without obstruction. Such patients void with high pressures against a normal outflow tract that generates no increased resistance. Such bladders are referred to as 'super bladders'.

4. *Low flow rate; incomplete emptying; normal or hypertrophied bladder wall; prostatomegaly.* This is characteristic of *decompensated outflow obstruction*. The detrusor can generate sufficient pressure to overcome the outflow resistance for only so long; it decompensates and a residual is left. These patients characteristically feel the need to void a few minutes after the initial void as the detrusor recovers. The bladder wall is likely to be hypertrophied. This pattern is also seen in patients with *poor detrusors and no outflow obstruction*, who will have normal bladder walls.

5. *Intermittent flow rate; variable emptying; normal bladder wall.* Such flow patterns are characteristic of patients in whom voiding is predominately by abdominal pressure, the detrusor having all but failed. How much of a residual is left depends upon the effectiveness of the abdominal straining.

6. *No flow rate; no emptying; hypertrophied bladder wall.* This combination is seen in patients with neuropathic bladders and detrusor sphincter dyssynergia in whom voluntary voiding is usually not possible.

7. *Normal flow rate; large residual urines; hypertrophied bladder wall; dilated distal ureters.* This classic set of

findings occurs in high-pressure chronic retention of urine. This condition accounts for 10% of patients who present with chronic urinary retention and is important because renal function is likely to be impaired and chronic renal failure will ensue if treatment is not undertaken. The prostate in these patients is often not enlarged and the condition probably represents the end stages of bladder-neck obstruction.[5] The distal ureters will be seen to be symmetrically dilated.

The USCD is most useful in the follow-up of patients treated by transurethral resection of the prostate (TURP) for outflow obstruction due to BPH. As a diagnostic test, it is limited, being unable to differentiate between an overactive detrusor in the presence of obstruction and a normal patient. More invasive, but definitive, urodynamic studies will have to be performed. In the authors' unit, USCD is used as an initial test of lower tract function in all symptomatic patients. This gives some idea as to which patients need to proceed to formal urodynamic studies. It is extensively used to monitor the effect of treatment of any kind of lower tract obstruction, whether it be prostate mediated or due to urethral stricture. USCD also affords the advantage of defining other pelvic pathology that may be significant in determining the cause of lower tract function and pelvic pain.

Other pathology due to BPH that might be seen on USCD

Bladder diverticula are congenital or acquired.[6] Acquired diverticula are thin walled, contain very little muscle and are virtually always associated with outflow tract obstruction; 85% arise just lateral and superior to the ureteric orifice. They can achieve enormous sizes; calculi commonly form in them because of stasis and there is a 5% association between diverticula and transitional cell tumour.[7]

Ultrasonography (US) can rapidly confirm the presence of a diverticulum (Fig. 17.12) and can assess the extent to which it empties following micturition. In some, the diverticulum might transiently increase in size, as a functioning detrusor voids into it rather than through an obstructed lower tract. The position and size of the orifice can help preoperative planning. The most

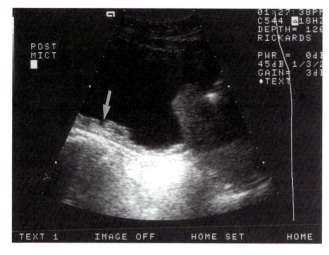

Figure 17.12. *Longitudinal scan of the bladder showing invagination of the bladder base and a thickened bladder wall with diverticula (arrow).*

important use of US is to detect complications, such as stone or tumour. It is not always possible to assess a diverticulum endoscopically.

Bladder stones appear as echogenic masses within the bladder that move with altered posture (Fig. 17.13). Bladder tumours can calcify, but do not move. Stones can be multiple and are always associated with outflow obstruction. If stones are seen, a USCD should be performed immediately, as well as assessment of the prostate. Stones complicating diverticula are common.

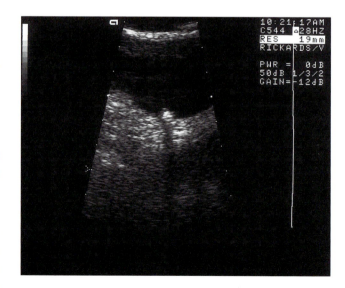

Figure 17.13. *Transverse scan of the bladder showing an echogenic focus (arrow) associated with acoustic shadowing due to a small bladder stone.*

Transrectal ultrasound and lower urinary tract dysfunction due to BPH

Technique

Accurate assessment of prostate volume requires scanning in two planes.[8] There is no linear correlation between prostate size and the degree of outflow obstruction. BPH can occur in the absence of any prostatomegaly with compression of the peripheral zones at the expense of the enlarging central part of the gland. Volume measurements are useful in deciding how patients might be treated, so are worth measuring. Huge prostates (in excess of 75 cm^3) might be considered for open prostatectomy and are unlikely to be considered for thermotherapy.

Posterior urethral imaging requires scanning of the prostate in the sagittal plane using a 7 MHz linear-array probe.[9,10] Such a configuration is available with biplane probes or dedicated linear-array probes. The present trend is for tight curved-array transducers that can be used for both transrectal and transvaginal work providing images of the prostate in an elongated forward-looking sagittal section — ideal for biopsy, but not for posterior urethral imaging. Prostate imaging is an integral part of assessing lower urinary tract function at rest before or during urodynamics.

Transrectal ultrasound (TRUS) can be performed as an investigative procedure of lower urinary tract abnormalities in the following ways:

1. *In combination with a renal US and a USCD.* These studies will provide all the functional information gained by the USCD plus:
   (a) prostate pathology;
   (b) prostate volume;
   (c) bladder neck configuration;
   (d) urethral position;
   (e) periurethral pathology.
2. *During micturition.* Patients find it difficult to micturate in either the left lateral decubitus position or when standing with a transrectal probe in their rectums. This is hardly surprising! The temptation is to overfill the patient's bladder by natural means by overhydrating the patient or through the administration of a diuretic; however, overfilling the bladder inhibits micturition and causes pain and bladder wall damage, and is to be avoided. It is not surprising that most papers on TRUS and urodynamics are on patients with neuropathic bladders who void spontaneously irrespective of what is within their rectums.[11,12] Additional information gained will be:
   (a) bladder neck function;
   (b) calibre of the posterior urethra;
   (c) posterior urethral pathology;
   (d) distal sphincter function;
   (e) posterior urethral emptying on interruption of micturition, the 'stop test'.[13]
   (f) course of the urethra.
3. *TRUS and bladder US prior to a full urodynamic study.* This has the potential of reducing the requirement for fluoroscopy to nothing, thus ridding the potential harm caused by radiation to the gonads, especially in young males. The only information that will not be seen is vesicoureteric reflux and anterior urethral pathology, although US is being promoted as the first line of investigation for that.

Normal TRUS appearances of the posterior urethra

At rest, the posterior urethra can usually be identified as two echogenic interfaces opposed to each other at the bladder neck with an echo-poor area anterior to it — the anterior fibromuscular stroma (Fig. 17.14). The urethra as it courses through the prostate assumes a very gentle curve until at the apex of the gland it is surrounded by the echo-poor distal sphincter mechanism where the subprostatic urethra takes a sharp turn anteriorly.

If the patient can initiate micturition while under continuous TRUS control, it is wise to record the event on video. As detrusor pressure increases, the prostate is displaced slightly inferiorly. Then the bladder neck starts to open, the posterior urethra fills with urine and the distal sphincter opens and micturition ensues. The posterior urethra is a thin-walled structure with a calibre of between 5 and 10 mm (depending on the rate at which the patient manages to micturate) and runs in almost a straight line through the prostate. The verumontanum can be identified towards the apex of the gland and marks the proximal aspect of the distal sphincter mechanism. When the patient is asked to stop micturition in mid-flow, the distal sphincter closes under voluntary control, the urine within the posterior urethra is milked back into the bladder through the

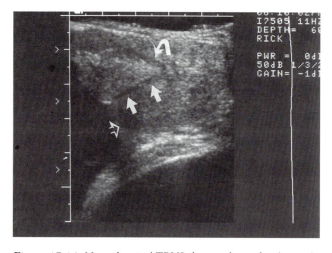

Figure 17.14. *Normal sagittal TRUS showing the urethra (arrows), ejaculatory duct (curved arrow) and anterior fibromuscular stroma (open arrow).*

and become more echogenic than normal (Fig. 17.16). The enlarged central part of the gland assumes varying echogenicities. Echogenic discrete adenomas can be mixed with predominately heterogeneous tissue and cystic degeneration is a feature (Fig. 17.17). Enlarged median lobes can be associated with apparently normal glands and are best seen on sagittal imaging. Colour Doppler scanning often reveals a marked increase in blood flow in the central and transitional zones of the gland (Fig. 17.18). Such a finding can alert the surgeon to a possible increase in haemorrhage and the possibility that thermotherapy will be less successful. The capsule of the gland should be intact.

In the early phases of BPH, the prostate may appear both clinically and on TRUS measurements to be of normal size because the enlarging adenoma compresses

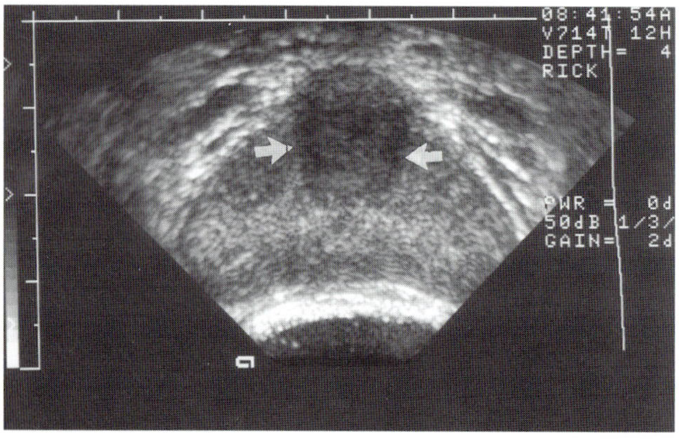

bladder neck and then the bladder neck closes, leaving the urethra totally empty.

TRUS and BPH

Early degrees of BPH produce an increase in the anteroposterior dimension of the prostate, normally less than 2.5 cm. This is due to enlargement of the transitional zones of the prostate (Fig. 17.15). The peripheral zones should be normal. As the prostate increases in size, the bladder base is elevated and, in very large glands, it may not be possible to insert the probe far enough into the rectum to image the base of the prostate. The peripheral zones become markedly compressed by the enlarging central part of the gland

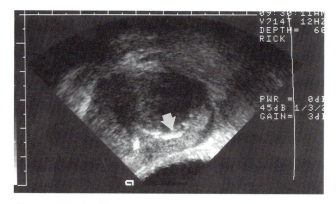

Figure 17.16. *Transverse axial TRUS of BPH. There is compression of the peripheral zones and corpora amylacea (arrow).*

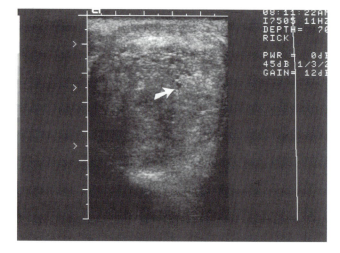

Figure 17.17. *Sagittal TRUS of a huge BPH. There is cystic degeneration (arrow).*

Figure 17.15. *Transverse axial TRUS of early BPH (between arrows). The peripheral zones are homogeneous.*

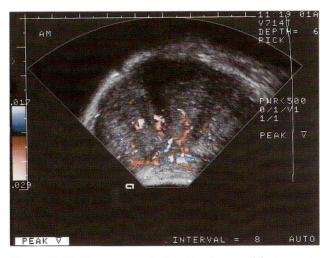

Figure 17.18. *Transverse axial colour Doppler scan of the prostate in BPH. There is considerable increased blood flow within the central part of the gland.*

the peripheral zones preferentially. This is more likely to happen when BPH occurs in the presence of bladder-neck obstruction where the prostate becomes trapped.

The following patterns will be seen:

1. *At rest:*
   (a) *Normal TRUS; normal USCD.* This combination excludes any significant degree of outflow obstruction due to BPH, but will not diagnose detrusor instability.
   (b) *Normal TRUS; low flow rate; variable bladder emptying.* This will be seen in those patients with poor detrusor function, detrusor failure where voiding is through abdominal straining, or where the obstruction is distal to the distal sphincter mechanism, e.g. urethral stricture.
   (c) *BPH on TRUS; normal USCD.* This is seen in the early stages of BPH where the increased resistance afforded by the outflow tract is overcome by increased voiding pressure maintaining normal flow rates.
   (d) *BPH on TRUS; low flow rates; complete emptying; hypertrophied bladder wall.* This combination is classic of outflow obstruction. The detrusor is able to generate sufficiently high pressures for long enough to ensure complete emptying.
   (e) *BPH on TRUS; low flow rates; incomplete emptying; hypertrophied bladder wall.* When seen, this combination is that of decompensated

outflow obstruction, where the bladder wall cannot generate sufficiently high pressures for long enough to ensure bladder emptying. The detrusor pressure falls and residual urine is left. As the detrusor recovers after a few minutes, the patient becomes aware of incomplete emptying and returns to empty his bladder. This is the classic symptom of 'pis-en-deux'.

   (f) *BPH on TRUS; low or intermittent flow rates; incomplete emptying; normal bladder wall.* This can occur in the late stages of outflow obstruction where larger and larger residuals are being formed, and the detrusor muscle decompensates and becomes thin walled. It will also be seen in those patients who in the presence of increasing obstruction do not compensate for it by generating higher bladder pressures and therefore bladder wall hypertrophy.

2. *During micturition.* The cardinal features seen on TRUS in patients with BPH during micturition are:
   (a) Attenuation of all or part of the posterior urethra.
   (b) Posterior displacement of the posterior urethra.
   (c) Lateral displacement of the posterior urethra.
   (d) Some trapping of contrast within the posterior urethra on interruption of micturition.

   All the above features depend upon the extent of BPH and bladder function. In practice, little is to be learned from these appearances except in early degrees of BPH where the prostate is near normal size and minor degrees of posterior displacement can be identified (Figs 17.19, 17.20). Trapping of urine is classically seen in bladder-neck disorders, but may be seen in BPH. It can be distinguished from bladder-neck pathology because there will be no distension of the posterior urethra. As the prostate increases in size, the urethra becomes more posteriorly displaced and more attenuated.

3. *Prior to urodynamics.* TRUS assessment before formal lower urinary tract urodynamics allows for interpretation of the urodynamics without the use of ionizing radiation to image the posterior urethra. In cases where cystometry suggests obstruction, TRUS will be able to determine whether the obstruction is at the level of the bladder neck, prostate or distal sphincter. Anterior urethral causes of obstruction

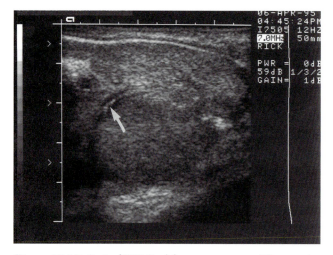

Figure 17.19. *Sagittal TRUS of the prostate at rest. The posterior urethra is posteriorly displaced due to BPH (arrow).*

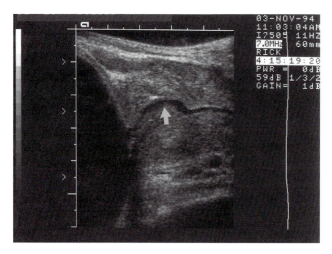

Figure 17.20. *Sagittal TRUS during micturition. There is posterior displacement and attenuation of the posterior urethra (arrow) due to BPH.*

will not be imaged, but significant strictures or other anterior urethral pathology will make catheterization prior to urodynamic studies difficult, if not impossible. Such pathology is best demonstrated by urethrography of prior urethral ultrasound.[14–17]

TRUS appearances of the prostate following treatment

The traditional surgical treatment by TURP for BPH is being challenged by less invasive treatments and ones that preserve the bladder neck and sexual function.

Surgery is the only effective method of treatment available for bladder-neck dyssynergia.

TRUS appearances following TURP

At TURP, the bladder neck and varying amounts of the central and transitional zones of the prostate are removed down towards the apex of the prostate gland, but not involving the distal sphincter mechanism (Fig. 17.21). TRUS following TURP will show the cavity produced by surgery, but failure to see a cavity does not necessarily imply that there is not one. For accurate assessment of the size of the cavity, the patient should have a full bladder and be asked to pass urine or strain in the attempt to do so, while the prostate is scanned continuously. Suprapubic compression of the full bladder will also extend what appear to be small or non-existent TURP cavities.

Postoperative stricture of the bladder neck will appear as a mid-prostatic cavity and a closed bladder neck (Fig. 17.22). Recurrent adenomas encroaching upon the operative cavity have appearances similar to those of preoperative benign tumours; for carcinoma to obstruct a cavity, it would have to be very extensive and would be obvious clinically.

Obstruction to the ejaculatory ducts is commonly seen following TURP and can cause perineal pain due to seminal vesiculitis. Dilatation of the ducts will be seen on TRUS. Postoperative haematuria is often caused by prominent vessels lining the TURP cavity;

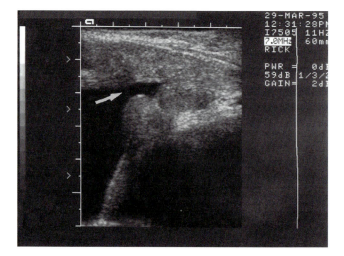

Figure 17.21. *Sagittal TRUS following TURP, showing a good cavity (arrow).*

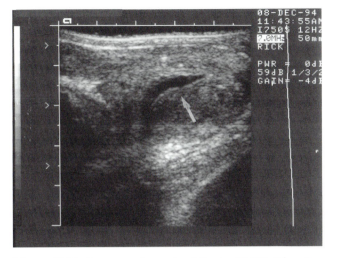

Figure 17.22. *Recurrent obstruction following TURP. There is a mid-prostatic cavity (arrow) and a bladder-neck stenosis.*

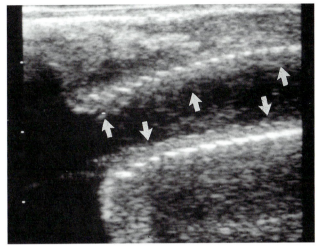

Figure 17.23. *Sagittal TRUS following insertion of a permanent metal stent in the treatment of BPH. The stent is placed exactly at the bladder neck and there is good urothelial coating of the stent (arrows).*

these will be identified on colour Doppler imaging. Incontinence following TURP is due either to distal sphincter damage or to underlying detrusor instability. Sphincter damage can be assessed with TRUS by compressing the full bladder and seeing the distal sphincter open up.

TRUS appearances following stent insertion for treatment of BPH

Temporary stents have a closely woven mesh that attenuates the ultrasound beam to such an extent that it is not possible to image the intrastent lumen or the relationship of the stent to the bladder neck — not that it is important to do so as the stents extend into the bladder by design. Assessment is best done by urethrography. The position of permanent stents is clearly defined by TRUS. For accurate scanning, the bladder needs to be partially full; this will allow for very accurate depiction of the relationship of the stent to the bladder neck. The position of the distal end of the stent and its relationship to the distal sphincter and apical prostatic tissue is then assessed. Postoperative incontinence may be due to pre-existing instability, instability as a result of instrumentation, or compromise of distal sphincter function because the stent is partly or wholly covering it. TRUS will help to differentiate between poor positioning and a functional abnormality.[18,19]

In the first few months following insertion, permanent stents invoke a hyperplastic reaction, but this settles within 6 months to leave a smooth urothelial covering of the stent (Fig. 17.23). The extent and uniformity of urothelium can be assessed by TRUS. Usually, the stent is covered by a uniform thickness (1–2 mm) of urothelium, leaving an adequate intrastent lumen. Occasionally, focal areas of overgrowth are seen. Colour Doppler imaging in the transverse axial or forward-looking sagittal planes allows for definition of the vascularity of the neourothelium.[20]

Misplacement of the stent at the bladder neck with free wires not in contact with urothelium is likely to lead to the wires becomimg encrusted. TRUS will demonstrate such free wires and show whether small stones are forming on them. Perineal pain following stent insertion may be due to the development of prostatic inflammatory disease, prostate abscess or blockage to the prostatic and ejaculatory ducts. TRUS will differentiate between these entities and point the clinician to the appropriate therapeutic course. Prolonged haematuria following stent insertion may be caused by prominent vessels supplying the urothelial covering; TRUS combined with colour Doppler imaging will demonstrate such vessels.

References

1. Lovett K J, Rifkin M D, McCue P A, Choi H. MR imaging characteristics of non-cancerous lesions of the prostate. JMRI 1992; 2: 35–39
2. Ishida J, Sugimura K, Okizuka H et al. Benign prostatic hyperplasia: value of MR imaging for detection of histological type. Radiology 1994; 190: 329–331

3. Boothroyd A E, Dixon P J, Christmas T J et al. The ultrasound cystodynamogram — a new technique. Br J Radiol 1989; 63: 331–332

4. Poston G L, Joseph A E A, Riddle P R. The accuracy of ultrasound in the measurement of changes in bladder volume. Br J Urol 1983; 55: 361–363

5. Holden D, George N, Rickards D et al. Renal pelvic pressures in human chronic obstructive uropathy. Br J Urol 1984; 56: 565–567

6. Millar A. The aetiology and treatment of diverticulum of the bladder. Br J Urol 1958; 85: 145–148

7. Fox M, Power R F, Bruce A W. Diverticulum of the bladder — presentation and evaluation in 115 cases. Br J Urol 1962; 34: 286–289

8. Jones D R, Roberts E E, Griffiths J G et al. Assessment of volume measurement of the prostate using per-rectal ultrasound. Br J Urol 1989; 64: 493–495

9. Brown M C, Sutherst J R, Murray A, Richmond D H. Potential use of ultrasound in place of X-ray fluoroscopy in urodynamics. Br J Urol 1985; 57: 88–90

10. Shabsigh R, Fishman I J, Krebs M. The use of transrectal longitudinal real-time ultrasonography in urodynamics. J Urol 1987; 138: 1416–1419

11. Shapeero L G, Friedland G W, Perkash I. Transrectal sonographic voiding cystourethrography: studies of neuromuscular bladder dysfunction. AJR 1983; 141: 83–90

12. Petritsch P, Colombo T H, Rauchenwald M et al. Ultrasonography of the urinary tract as an alternative to radiologic investigation in spinal cord injured patients. Eur Urol 1991; 20: 97–102

13. Abrams P H, Torrens M. Clinical urodynamics. Urol Clin North Am 1979; 6: 71–79

14. Perkash I, Friedland G W. Real time grey scale transrectal linear ultrasonography in urodynamic evaluation. Semin Urol 1985; 3: 49–59

15. Shabsigh R, Fishman I L, Krebs M. Combined transrectal ultrasonography and urodynamics in the evaluation of detrusor–sphincter dyssynergia. Br J Urol 1988; 62: 326–330

16. Bidair M, Tiechman J M H, Brodak P P, Juma S. Transrectal ultrasound urodynamics. Urology 1993; 42: 640–645

17. Heidenreich A, Derschum W, Bonfig R, Wilbert D M. Ultrasound in the evaluation of urethral stricture disease: a prospective study of 175 patients. Br J Urol 1994; 74: 93–98

18. Milroy E M, Chapple C R, Cooper J E. A new treatment for urethral stricture. Lancet 1988; 1: 1424–1427

19. Chapple C R, Milroy E M, Rickards D. Permanently implanted urethral stent for prostatic outflow obstruction in the unfit patient — preliminary report. Br J Urol 1990; 66: 58–65

20. Rickards D. Advances in ultrasound. In: Kirby R S, Hendry W F (eds) Recent advances in urology. London: Churchill Livingstone, 1993: 2–15

Role and interpretation of core biopsies in clinical benign prostatic hyperplasia

M. R. Feneley M. C. Parkinson

18

Introduction

Benign prostatic hyperplasia (BPH) is one of the most prevalent diseases in the ageing male population. It comprises nodular hyperplasia of epithelium, smooth muscle and fibroblasts in various proportions, with hypertrophy of these cells, especially those of the epithelium. These changes give rise to five growth patterns — fibromyoadenomatous, fibroadenomatous, muscular, fibromuscular and fibrous[1] (Fig. 18.1). Fibromyoadenomatous nodules are the most common but more than one pattern may be present within any single gland. Hyperplastic nodules are located in the transition zone that encircles the proximal segment of the prostatic urethra between the bladder neck and the verumontanum.[2–4] Only rarely are hyperplastic nodules identified in the gland periphery.[5] The development and progression of nodular hyperplasia is androgen dependent and its incidence increases with age. In a review of six post-mortem studies of the prostate, hyperplasia in the 31–40-year age group was found in only three series but was identified in 14–55% and 34–95% of the male post-mortem population in the 51–60 and 71–80 age groups, respectively.[6] As the prostate enlarges owing to progressive hypertrophy and hyperplasia, the peripheral zone is gradually compressed posteriorly into a rim with a somewhat variable anterior extent. However, a large gland is not necessarily the cause of 'prostatism'[7] and, despite the above figures based on tissue diagnosis, only one-quarter of middle-aged to elderly men (40–79 years) were found to be in need of assessment and treatment for BPH in a community study.[8]

Indications for biopsy

In a research context, prostatic biopsies have been taken from benign glands in order to correlate the content of the different tissue components with the presence of symptoms and response to various therapies. The background to these investigations includes the following. Symptoms of BPH are not directly and consistently associated with the volume of hyperplastic tissue.[9,10] Patients in whom BPH in transurethral resection (TUR) specimens is predominantly stromal (fibrous tissue and muscle) respond less well to surgery when evaluated urodynamically than do those patients in whom the major component is glandular.[11] Applying quantitative image analysis to prostatectomy and TUR specimens, a significantly higher stromal/epithelial ratio may be found in symptomatic hyperplasia than in asymptomatic hyperplastic glands.[12]

Biopsy assessment of tissue components within hyperplasia would be justified if treatment could be tailored to particular morphological patterns. For this to be achieved, the information derived from biopsy material must be representative of the whole process. This will depend on the extent of sampling, the degree of morphological heterogeneity and the size of the gland. Some studies have suggested that needle biopsies may be representative of the stromal content of BPH when compared with large tissue samples (as from open prostatectomy).[13] It has also been stated that one biopsy may reflect 'the nature of an adenoma'.[14] However, within that study (which compared the morphometric findings on a single biopsy, six biopsies and larger sections from retropubic prostatectomy), although the percentage of fibrous tissue and glandular epithelium was similar in these three groups, the value for smooth muscle was significantly lower and that for glandular tissue (epithelium and glandular spaces) significantly higher in the larger sections. Following the correlation between the success of alpha-1-adrenergic blockers and the muscle density in BPH,[15] and the facility of finasteride — a 5 alpha-reductase inhibitor — to improve uroflow by preferentially reducing the transition zone volume in patients with BPH,[16] it is interesting to speculate that the analysis of tissue content of transition zone biopsies may become more frequent. If the above relationship can be established in

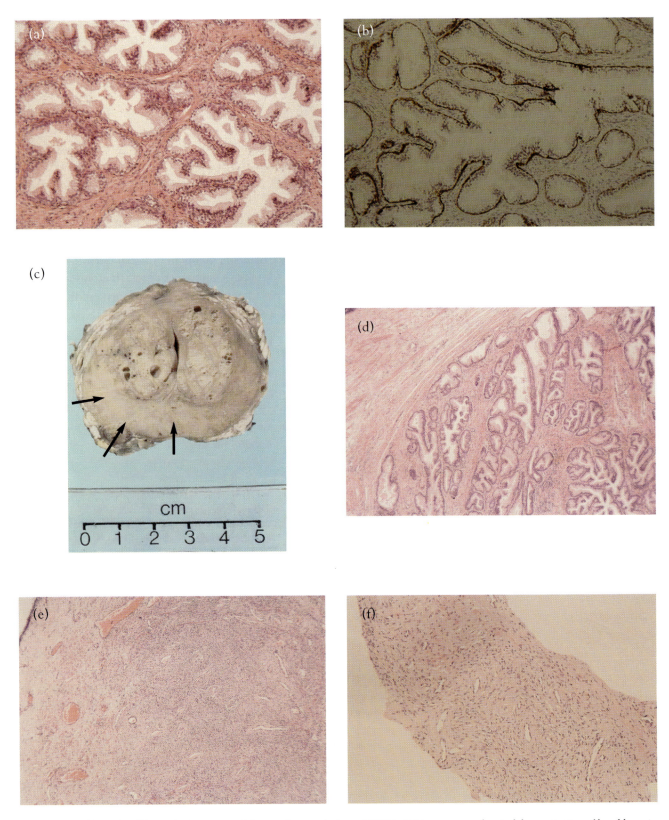

Figure 18.1. *Normal and hyperplastic prostate: (a) normal prostatic tissue (H&E); (b) immunocytochemical demonstration of basal layer in normal prostate (cytokeratin clone LP34); (c) transverse section of prostate showing hyperplastic nodules and coincidental peripheral cancer (arrowed); (d) edge of hyperplastic nodule — epithelium predominating (H&E); (e) hyperplastic stromal nodule in typical site adjacent to urethra (H&E); (f) hyperplastic stromal nodule in needle core (H&E).*

a larger series, transition zone biopsies may have a role in the management of BPH.

The commonest indication for biopsy assessment of a palpably benign prostate is the attempt to exclude adenocarcinoma. Prostate cancer is the second commonest cause of male cancer deaths in most industrialized nations, but is the leading cause of cancer mortality in American males, having exceeded lung cancer.[17] Like BPH, it is androgen dependent and incidence increases with age,[18] accordingly, both conditions commonly coexist (Fig. 18.1c). Digital rectal examination (DRE) undertaken in the evaluation of the lower urinary tract symptoms provides an opportunity to detect abnormalities associated with carcinoma[19] but, even within an apparently benign gland, malignancy may be extensive. Before the recent dramatic increase in the number of prostatic needle biopsies undertaken for early detection of malignancy, many patients presenting with clinical disease had locally advanced or metastatic disease at the time of its diagnosis.[20,21] Of patients with clinically localized palpable prostate cancer undergoing radical prostatectomy, around 50% have tumours that have extended beyond the prostate.[22] These facts provide the impetus to use prostatic biopsy as a method of case finding or early detection of cancer in patients presenting with clinical BPH.

Prostate-specific antigen (PSA) has become established as the most useful serum marker for prostatic malignancy and is increasingly used for screening or case finding among men over 50 years of age, as well as for detecting early-stage cancer in men with lower urinary tract symptoms.[23,24] It is a prostate-specific marker[25] expressed by normal and diseased tissue.[26] The currently recommended and widely accepted upper limit of normal for serum PSA is 4.0 ng/ml (Hybritech).[27] It is also elevated in various benign diseases including prostatitis (Fig. 18.2a,b), prostatic infarction (Fig. 18.2c) and approximately 25% of men with BPH,[28] and there is an increase with age that cannot be explained entirely by increasing prostatic volume.[29] In around 80% of men with a clinically benign gland and serum PSA between 4.0 and 10.0 ng/ml, cancer is not found on systematic needle biopsy.[30] Various refinements have been made to serum PSA measurements in an attempt to distinguish the elevation associated with benign disease from that caused by

carcinoma, including PSA density,[31] PSA velocity[32] and age-specific reference ranges,[29,33] but their reliability in clinical practice is yet to be established. More recently, it has been suggested that a low ratio of free to

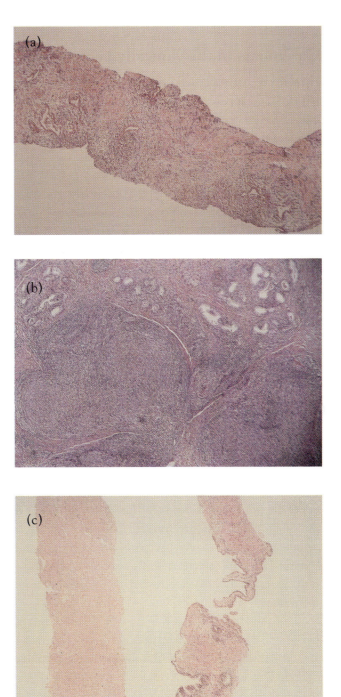

Figure 18.2. *Additional benign prostatic conditions possibly causing raised serum PSA: (a) acute and chronic prostatitis (H&E); (b) granulomatous prostatitis (H&E); (c) prostatic infarction (H&E).*

complexed PSA in serum may be a more accurate indicator of the presence of malignancy than total PSA in men with intermediate PSA levels, capable of reducing the number of negative biopsies in men with BPH by approximately one-third with minimal impact on the overall detection rate.[34]

Carcinoma in the clinically benign gland

Historically, the clinical importance of malignancy within an apparently benign gland has been a controversial subject for debate because of the notoriously unpredictable prognosis for the individual patient. The traditional presentation of these tumours at transurethral resection of the prostate (TURP) was particularly haphazard, dependent upon the need for surgery, the method of pathological examination[35] and, possibly, the extent of prostatic resection.[36] The prognosis associated with these cancers was highly variable and the need for subsequent treatment used to be largely based upon the morphological features of the tumour within the surgical specimen. In 1975, Jewett stated that patients with well-differentiated or focal tumours generally had a good prognosis, whereas those with less-differentiated or diffuse disease were at significant risk of progression.[37] Underlying the potential therapeutic importance of these so-called incidental carcinomas, tumours associated with good prognosis not requiring treatment were staged as A1 and those associated with significant risk of progression as A2. Although impalpable and diagnosed only after prostatectomy for benign disease, A2 tumours are generally considered to be clinically significant,[38] although older patients nevertheless may die from unrelated causes.[39] Compared with unilateral palpable tumours, they are more frequently of higher grade[40] and more commonly associated with pelvic lymph node metastases.[41]

The tendency for prostate cancer to arise in the peripheral zone and its multifocality may account for the difficulties associated with representative sampling at TURP, as well as discrepancies in prevalence. Focal malignant lesions may be multiple and their pattern of invasion may differ according to their site of origin within the prostate.[42] Greene and colleagues showed that nearly half of A1 (transition zone) tumours may be associated with additional peripheral zone cancers of greater volume.[43] In their study, some of these unsuspected peripheral cancers were associated with aggressive pathological features including extraprostatic or seminal vesicle invasion, in spite of their sometimes small volume.[44] Furthermore, peripheral zone cancers were usually of higher grade and more likely to have extended beyond the prostate than a transition zone malignancy of equivalent size. In the transition zone, correlation between volume and grade was weak and not statistically significant, whereas it was moderately strong in the peripheral zone. These findings suggest that, in patients with stage A cancer, either an additional unsuspected impalpable peripheral tumour or the originally detected transition zone tumour could be responsible for subsequent disease progression, underlining the importance of evaluating the peripheral zone even following the diagnosis of incidental carcinoma.

Prostatic needle biopsies are now commonly performed in patients with benign findings on DRE but a raised serum PSA in an attempt to exclude carcinoma, particularly when associated with lower urinary tract symptoms. A rarer indication for prostatic biopsy in patients with clinical evidence of BPH is included in the many protocols evaluating innovative treatments of BPH, especially when tissue for pathological examination is not obtained. Cancer detected in a palpably benign gland on needle biopsy commonly involves the peripheral zone,[45] and even when low grade may indicate the presence of biologically significant malignancy.[46]

Prevalence of carcinoma

Information regarding the prevalence of carcinoma among men in the community and in those presenting with symptomatic, clinically benign prostatic enlargement is available from a variety of sources. These include the results of necropsy studies in men dying from unrelated causes, the microscopic findings after TURP carried out for clinically benign disease and the findings from population screening for prostatic cancer.

The results of post-mortem surveys of prostatic carcinoma are shown according to age at death in Table 18.1. The incidence of prostatic carcinoma may be two

Table 18.1. *Incidence of prostatic carcinoma at post-mortem related to age*

Authors*	Year	Origin	No. of patients	Percentage of prostatic carcinoma by decade					Overall percentage CaP at > 40 years
				4th	5th	6th	7th	8th	
Moore[101]	1935	New York, USA	375	0	17	14	23	21	20
Andrews[102]	1949	Bristol, UK	142	0	4.9	5.3	18	32	12
Liavag[103]	1968	Ulleval, Sweden	340	0	8	20	24	30	26.5
Lundberg and Berge[†49]	1970	Malmo, Sweden	308	0	57	23.5	38.8	47.1	43

*In all the above series the prostates had been step sectioned at 4–5 mm intervals throughout the gland and whole mounts examined. Only one series (†) included 16 patients in whom carcinoma had been diagnosed during life.

to three times greater if systematic whole-mount sections rather than sections from random blocks are examined.[47–49] In the series included in the Table 18.1, therefore, the prostates have all been examined using whole-mount step sections at 4–5 mm intervals throughout the gland. The series did not include patients in whom carcinoma had been diagnosed during life, except that by Lundberg and Berge,[49] in which 16 patients were known to have prostatic carcinoma before autopsy. Metastases from the prostate carcinoma were not noted macroscopically in any of these studies.

When recording the incidence of adenocarcinoma at TURP carried out for apparently benign disease, the age range is set by the necessity for surgery. The relationship between sampling and the diagnosis of prostatic carcinoma is emphasized once again. In three series that included a minimum of 100 TURPs, on restricted sampling carcinoma was diagnosed in 7–8% but when all the tissue was processed a malignant diagnosis was made in 14–19%.[35,50,51] This latter figure was supported when carcinoma was found in 14.2% of 457 TURPs processed in their entirety.[52] Such cancers are, by definition, impalpable and — without the availability of serum PSA levels — clinically unsuspected. The majority are of transition zone origin, although some may represent extension of a peripheral tumour into the central gland resected at TURP.[53] The absence of malignancy at TURP does not exclude the presence of biologically significant peripheral zone malignancy, and this may account not only for the disparity between the prevalence of prostate cancer at post-mortem and the finding of malignancy at TURP but also for the unpredictable clinical significance of unsuspected tumours.

Cancer detection in urological practice was evaluated by Cooner and colleagues who undertook biopsies in men with abnormal transrectal ultrasound (TRUS).[23] Among 1807 men with symptoms or concern about prostate cancer, 15% were found to have cancer, 99% of these being of non-transition zone origin. This detection rate is consistent with the estimated prevalence of peripheral tumours. Of the men evaluated, 69% had a palpably benign prostate and, among these, only 5% were found to have cancer compared with 36% of those with an abnormal DRE. Of the impalpable tumours, 68% were associated with a PSA greater than 4.0 ng/ml. These findings are inevitably influenced by the limited accuracy of TRUS in cancer detection.[30]

In a recent study evaluating cancer detection in an invited screened population, Catalona and colleagues demonstrated cancer in 4.0% of 6630 men using DRE and PSA. In fact, biopsies were performed only in 68% of men advised to undergo this, which also indicates that patient compliance may be a problem.[30] Overall, 12% of the study population had a clinically benign gland associated with a raised PSA between 4.0 and 9.9 ng/ml and 15% had an abnormal DRE. Of organ-confined cancers, 44% were detected by PSA in a clinically benign gland. The positive predictive value of PSA between 4.1 and 9.9 ng/ml associated with a palpably benign gland was 21%, identical to that of a suspicious DRE.

TRUS is valuable in demonstrating the morphology and zonal anatomy of the prostate[54] and may also be used to estimate gland volume.[55] It is also used to examine ultrasonographic abnormalities that may be associated with malignancy[56] and permits calculation of PSA density, should this be employed as a criterion for biopsy. Under ultrasonographic guidance, prostatic tissue may be obtained from the peripheral or transition zone for microscopic assessment using a spring-loaded biopty gun.[57] Biopsies may also be taken from sites of palpable or ultrasonographic abnormalities and systematically from other regions of the prostate.[58]

Biopsy strategy

The selection of patients for prostatic biopsy as part of a cancer detection strategy depends upon the impact that a histologically proven malignancy will have upon the clinical management, and this will reflect the age and health of the individual patient. The number of prostatic biopsies taken from an individual with a clinically benign gland may depend upon the indication for biopsy and the opinions held within any particular centre. When DRE findings or TRUS scans are equivocal or suspicious, biopsies can be directed at the site of the abnormality, although additional systematic biopsies are commonly obtained and may demonstrate cancer in palpably benign isoechoic regions of the prostate. When elevated PSA is the indication for biopsy, multiple cores are usually taken from predetermined sites. Quadrant biopsies were performed in the multicentre study of early detection of prostate cancer.[30] In many centres, sextant biopsies are taken from the base, mid and apical areas of the gland bilaterally.[59–61] Certain centres advocate additional biopsies to a total of 10 or 12 per gland.[62,63]

For the purpose of cancer detection, biopsies are usually obtained from the peripheral zone at least initially, as this is not only the most common site of most palpable tumours[53] but also the most common site of malignancy within a palpably benign prostate in men with raised PSA.[45] Additional transition zone biopsies may be undertaken in an attempt to diagnose those carcinomas that would have been identified in the TUR specimen,[63] particularly when PSA levels are raised and previous peripheral zone biopsies have not demonstrated

malignancy; these tumours cannot be reliably detected by ultrasound owing to considerable inhomogeneity associated with the BPH itself.[64]

The site and number of biopsies necessary for the reliable diagnosis of early invasive malignancy is related to the importance of detecting small volume disease. McNeal et al[65] found that cancer volume was correlated with local invasion and metastatic potential, and that the capacity to metastasize was acquired by tumours greater than 1 cm^3. Epidemiological studies have also suggested that the capacity for malignant behaviour develops in tumours larger than 0.5 cm^3.[66] On this basis, tumours of this size are generally assumed to be clinically significant; furthermore, they can be detected by needle biopsy.[57] However, smaller tumours, particularly when less than well differentiated, may be capable of demonstrating malignant characteristics.[67,68] Studies have attempted to assess the possibility of predicting the volume, stage and grade of carcinoma from biopsy findings in order to avoid 'overtreating' patients with 'insignificant' disease. The detection of these insignificant tumours will also depend upon the proportion of such cancers in the biopsied population and this may vary between 2.3%[69] and 16%.[45] Although various models have been developed relating tumour volume to serum PSA,[70] ultrasound findings,[71] the extent of cancer in biopsy specimens,[72] and a combination of these,[73] their prospective accuracy and reproducibility between centres remains unproven.

Addressing the specific question of carcinoma detection in patients with elevated PSA levels but a benign gland on DRE, the following conclusions were made on the basis of 12 biopsies per gland:[63] in 37% of the patients the biopsies were invaded by adenocarcinoma; in one-third of the biopsies containing carcinoma, only the specimens from the transition zone (taken in addition to the usual sextant biopsies) were infiltrated by tumour. The importance of transition zone biopsies is further emphasized by the following facts: transition zone cancers are frequently impalpable as a result of their site and associated distortion caused by BPH; for similar reasons they are notoriously difficult to detect on TRUS — their incidence is variously reported as 4–16%,[74] 20–25%[75] and 30–40% in the 'central area' of the older post-mortem studies.[49]

Prostatic biopsy is not without morbidity, although major complications are rare.[76] Patients may experience a varying degree of haematuria, haemospermia or rectal bleeding. Urinary tract infection or bacteraemia may occur, particularly after transrectal procedures, even when prophylactic antibiotics are used.[77] Tumour seeding in the biopsy track is the subject of case reports[78,79] but is probably very uncommon.[80]

Histopathology

If DRE, imaging and microscopic findings are to be correlated, prostatic biopsies need to be labelled according to site of origin and processed separately. Several sections are cut from each biopsy, as examination of levels often clarifies the diagnosis. Sufficient tissue should remain in the block to allow special techniques to be performed.

The histopathological diagnoses fall into three major groups — benign, premalignant and malignant. Within the benign group a diagnosis of glandular hyperplasia is rarely made, as there is insufficient tissue to identify the nodular outline that distinguishes hyperplastic from normal glands (Fig. 18.1d). In contrast, the morphology of stromal hyperplasia is distinctive and may be diagnosed in the absence of a nodular margin (Fig. 18.1f). Stromal nodules are virtually restricted to the suburethral tissue (Fig. 18.1e). Included within the benign group are biopsies showing acute prostatitis, granulomatous prostatitis and occasionally an area of infarction (Fig. 18.2). The latter may be associated with squamous metaplasia of the epithelium at the edge of the necrotic tissue. These conditions are important as they may cause elevation of serum PSA.

As more prostatic biopsies are prompted by a raised serum PSA in the absence of localized pathology, the diagnosis of premalignant conditions, possibly adjacent to carcinoma, will increase in frequency. There are two putative premalignant prostatic acinar lesions — atypical adenomatous hyperplasia (AAH) (Fig. 18.3)[81,82] and prostatic intraepithelial neoplasia (PIN) (Fig. 18.4).[75,83–85] The former is an architectural abnormality composed of clusters of small acini, often within or related to a benign lobule. The relationship between AAH and adenocarcinoma is based on its similarity to the lower Gleason grades of carcinoma, its predominant occurrence in the transition zone and some evidence of its spatial association with invasive tumour. However, currently there is insufficient evidence for clinicians to treat such lesions as premalignant in terms of patient follow-up. The major importance of AAH lies in its potential morphological confusion on biopsy with adenocarcinoma Gleason grades 1 and 2 (see below).[86–89]

In contrast to AAH, PIN occurs within a normal, hyperplastic or atrophic architecture but has the cytological features of malignancy, which may be graded into three subgroups.[90,91] The relationship between PIN and adenocarcinoma is well established in terms of morphological identity, continuity, spatial distribution in the peripheral zone and peak age. With respect to a

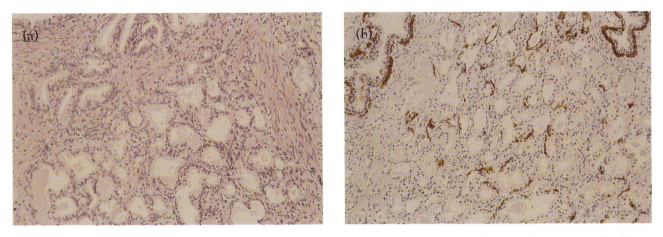

Figure 18.3. *Atypical adenomatous hyperplasia (AAH): (a) focus of closely packed small acini (H&E); (b) intermittent basal layer demonstrated immunocytochemically (adjacent level to (a), cytokeratin clone LP34).*

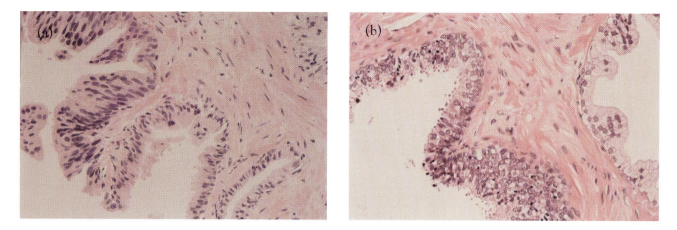

Figure 18.4. *Prostatic intraepithelial neoplasia (PIN): (a) low-grade PIN: stratification of luminal cells with large nuclei (upper left) and abrupt change to normal morphology (lower right) (H&E); (b) high-grade PIN: stratification of luminal cells, large nuclei showing loss of polarity and large nucleoli (left). Compare with normal acinus (right) (H&E).*

variety of biochemical markers PIN shows an intermediate position between benign prostatic epithelium and invasive adenocarcinoma.[92]

When high-grade PIN is found on biopsy in the absence of invasive carcinoma, concern relates to concomitant invasive carcinoma (sometimes adjacent to the biopsy site) as well as to the future development of malignancy. When patients with high-grade PIN (PIN grade 2 and 3) were re-biopsied, invasive carcinoma was diagnosed in 33–100%.[93–98] However, in those with low-grade PIN (PIN 1) the incidence of invasive carcinoma on re-biopsy was 13–19% — an incidence virtually identical to that found in patients whose initial biopsies did not show PIN.[93,99] These small series

indicate close follow-up with consideration of re-biopsy in patients with elevated PSA and high-grade PIN.

Diagnosis of adenocarcinoma on biopsy is made against the background of other abnormalities within the gland, which may resemble carcinoma either by forming small acini (Table 18.2) or showing cytological atypia (Table 18.3).

Distinction between well-differentiated adeno-carcinoma and the benign small acinar lesions (Table 18.2) is based on the presence of a double cell layer in the latter. If not apparent on haematoxylin and eosin (H & E) stain at high power, basal cells may be demonstrated by antibodies to high-molecular-weight cytokeratins.[81,89] Large nucleoli, intraluminal acid mucin and crystals are all more frequently seen in carcinoma but are also present in some cases of AAH.[81,88,89] Nephrogenic adenoma (Fig. 18.5e),

Table 18.2. *Small acinar lesions mimicking adenocarcinoma (Figs 18.3, 18.5)*

Lesion	Reference no.
Atypical adenomatous hyperplasia	86
Basal cell hyperplasia	104
Sclerosing adenosis	105
Atrophy	86,106
Urethral nephrogenic adenoma	107
Verumontanum glandular hyperplasia	108
Hyperplasia of mesonephric remnants	109
Seminal vesicle (normal structure)	86,106
Ejaculatory duct (normal structure)	86,106
Cowper's glands (normal structure)	86,106

Table 18.3. *Cytological abnormalities mimicking adenocarcinoma (Figs 18.4, 18.6)*

Abnormality	Reference no.
PIN	90,110
Clear cell cribriform hyperplasia	111
Atypical basal cell hyperplasia	112
Reactive duct/acinar epithelium adjacent to inflammation	113
Transitional cell carcinoma spreading within ducts and acini	114

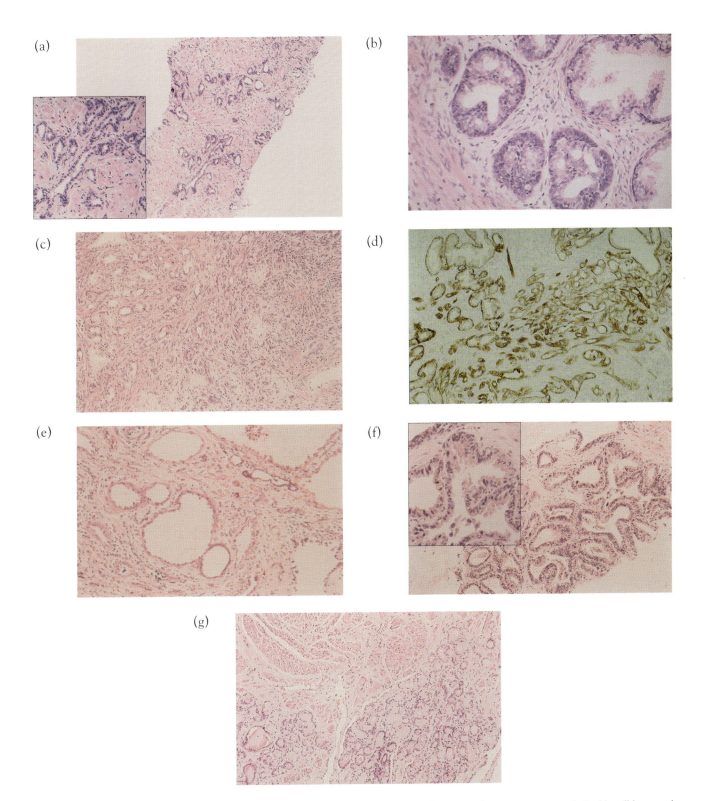

Figure 18.5. *Other small acinar lesions mimicking adenocarcinoma: (a) atrophy: duct/acinar configuration maintained, double cell layer and benign cytology (insert) (H&E); (b) basal cell hyperplasia: clusters of small acini in which darker staining basal cells predominate (H&E); (c) sclerosing adenosis: poorly circumscribed focus of small distorted acini, epithelial cell clusters and cords blending with the stroma (H&E); (d) sclerosing adenosis: basal layer demonstrated immunocytochemically (adjacent level to (c), cytokeratin clone LP34 — also positive with S100); (e) nephrogenic adenoma: a form of glandular metaplasia in transitional epithelium that may extend from urethra into prostate — acini lined by 'hobnailed' cells (H&E); (f) seminal vesicle: on biopsy, closely packed acini lined by pleomorphic cells. Insert demonstrates yellow/brown cytoplasmic pigment (H&E); (g) Cowper's glands (H&E from a radical cystectomy).*

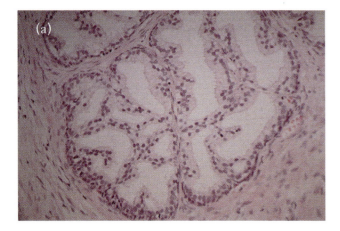

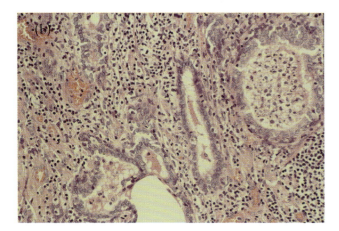

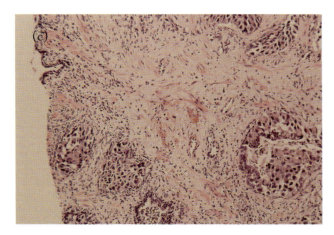

Figure 18.6. *Other cytological abnormalities mimicking adenocarcinoma: (a) cribriform hyperplasia: clear cell cytoplasm and architecture superficially resemble carcinoma, nuclei are benign and basal layer demonstrable (H&E); (b) reactive changes associated with inflammation: luminal cells are basophilic and include small nucleoli, basal layer is present (H&E); (c) transitional cell carcinoma arising in or extending into prostatic ducts/acini: large pleomorphic cells, lacking cohesion, PSA negative, between normal basal layer and inner residual PSA positive luminal cells (H&E).*

mesonephric remnants, seminal vesicle (Fig. 18.5f) and ejaculatory duct do not show positive staining with antibodies to PSA and prostatic acid phosphatase (PAP). In addition, the epithelium of ejaculatory duct, the verumontanum and seminal vesicle commonly include refractile brown/orange granules.

Differentiation between invasive carcinoma and other lesions showing a degree of cytological atypia (Table 18.3) is also dependent on the demonstration of an outer basal cell layer in the latter.[100] Transitional cell carcinomas spreading within ducts and acini do not contain PSA or PAP (Fig. 18.6c).

The prognosis for patients with malignancy within a palpably benign prostate is highly variable. For some, radical treatment may be curative but improved survival is yet to be demonstrated in any controlled trial. Following radical prostatectomy, the greater failure rate associated with seminal vesicle invasion, extraprostatic or specimen margin invasion and less-differentiated or larger-volume tumours indicates that some of these cancers do reduce host survival. The early natural history of prostate cancer and the importance of genetic and environmental factors on progression is poorly understood. At present, there are no morphological or biochemical criteria for reliably distinguishing tumours that will become the cause of clinical disease. Prospective, randomized controlled trials are required to determine a relationship between clinically diagnosed early prostate cancer and cancer-related death, and thereby provide a more secure basis upon which screening may be recommended.

References

1. Franks L M. Benign nodular hyperplasia of the prostate: a review. Ann R Coll Surg Engl 1954; 14: 92–106
2. McNeal J E. Normal histology of the prostate. Am J Surg Pathol 1988; 12: 619–633
3. McNeal J. Benign prostatic hyperplasia. Urol Clin North Am 1990; 17: 477–486
4. Price H, McNeal J E, Stamey T A. Evolving patterns of tissue composition in benign prostatic hyperplasia as a function of specimen size. Hum Pathol 1990; 21: 578–585
5. Ohori M, Egawa S, Wheeler T M. Nodules resembling nodular hyperplasia in the peripheral zone of the prostate gland. J Urol Pathol 1994; 2: 223–233
6. Petersen R O. Prostate and seminal vesicles. In: Petersen R O (ed) Urologic pathology. Philadelphia: Lippincott; 1992; 575–673
7. Abrams P. New words for old: lower urinary tract symptoms for 'prostatism'. Br Med J 1994; 308: 929

8. Garraway W M, Collins G N, Lee R J. High prevalence of benign prostatic hypertrophy in the community. Lancet 1991; 338: 469–471

9. Girman C J, Jacobsen S J, Guess H A et al. Natural history of prostatism: relationship among symptoms, prostatic volume and peak urinary flow rate. J Urol 1995; 153: 1510–1515

10. Rosier P F W M, de la Rosette J J M C H. Is there a correlation between prostatic size and bladder outlet obstruction? World J Urol 1995; 13: 9–13

11. Dorflinger T, England D M, Madsen P O, Bruskewitz RC. Urodynamic and histological correlates of benign prostatic hyperplasia. J Urol 1988; 140: 1487–1490

12. Shapiro E, Becich M J, Hartanto V, Lepor H. The relative proportion of stromal and epithelial hyperplasia is related to the development of symptomatic benign prostate hyperplasia. J Urol 1992; 147: 1293–1297

13. Deering R E, Bigler S A, King J et al. Morphometric quantitation of stroma in human benign prostatic hyperplasia. Urology 1994; 44: 64–70

14. Robert M, Coasta P, Bressolle R et al. Percentage area density of epithelial and mesenchymal components in benign prostatic hyperplasia: comparison of results between single biopsy, multiple biopsies and multiple tissue specimens. Br J Urol 1995; 75: 317–324

15. Shapiro E, Hatano V, Lepor H. The response to alpha blockade in benign prostatic hyperplasia is related to the per cent area density of prostate smooth muscle. Prostate 1992; 21: 297–307

16. Tewari A, Shinohara K, Narayan P. Transition zone volume and transition zone ratio: predictor of uroflow response to finasteride therapy in benign prostatic hyperplasia. Urology 1995; 45: 258–265

17. Coffey D S. Prostate cancer. An overview of an increasing dilemma. Cancer 1993; 71 (suppl): 880–886

18. Boyle P, Zaridze D G. Risk factors for prostate and testicular cancer. Eur J Cancer 1993; 29A: 1048–1055

19. Guinan P, Bush I, Ray V et al. The accuracy of the rectal examination in the diagnosis of prostate carcinoma. N Engl J Med 1980; 303: 499–503

20. Chisholm G D, Habib F K. Prostate cancer: experimental and clinical advances. In: Hendry WF (ed) Recent advances in urology and andrology, 3rd ed. Edinburgh: Churchill Livingstone, 1981: 212–232

21. Murphy G P, Natarajan N, Pontes J E et al. The national survey of prostate cancer in the United States by the American College of Surgeons. J Urol 1982; 127: 928–934

22. Chodak G W, Keller P, Schoenberg H W. Assessment of screening for prostate cancer using the digital rectal examination. J Urol 1989; 141: 1136–1138

23. Cooner W H, Mosley B R, Rutherford C L et al. Prostate cancer detection in a clinical urological practice by ultrasonography, digital rectal examination and prostate specific antigen. J Urol 1990; 143: 1146–1152

24. Catalona W J, Smith D S, Ratliff T L et al. Measurement of prostate–specific antigen in serum as a screening test for prostate cancer. N Engl J Med 1991; 324: 1156–1161

25. Wang M C, Valenzuela L A, Murphy G P, Chu T M. Purification of a human prostate specific antigen. Invest Urol 1979; 17: 159–163

26. Bostwick D G. Prostate-specific antigen: current role in diagnostic pathology of the prostate. Am J Clin Pathol 1994; 102: 531–537

27. Colberg J W, Smith D S, Catalona W J. Prevalence and pathological extent of prostate cancer in men with prostate specific antigen levels of 2.9 to 4.0 ng/ml. J Urol 1993; 149: 507–509

28. Lepor H, Owens R S, Rogenes V, Kuhn E. The detection of prostate cancer in males with prostatism. Prostate 1994; 25: 132–140

29. Oesterling J E, Jacobsen S J, Chute C G et al. Serum prostate-specific antigen in a community-based population of healthy men. Establishment of age-specific reference ranges. JAMA 1993; 270: 860–864

30. Catalona W J, Richie J P, Ahmann F et al. Comparison of digital rectal examination and serum prostate specific antigen in the early detection of prostate cancer: results of a multicenter clinical trial of 6,630 men. J Urol 1994; 151: 1283–1290

31. Benson M C, Whang I S, Pantuck A et al. Prostate specific antigen density: a means of distinguishing benign prostatic hypertrophy and prostate cancer. J Urol 1992; 147: 815–816

32. Carter H B, Pearson J D, Metter E J et al. Longitudinal evaluation of prostate-specific antigen levels in men with and without prostate disease. JAMA 1992; 267: 2215–2220

33. Dalkin B L, Ahmann F R, Kopp J B. Prostate specific antigen levels in men older than 50 years without clinical evidence of prostatic carcinoma. J Urol 1993; 150: 1837–1839

34. Catalona W J, Smith D S, Wolfert R L et al. Increased specificity of PSA screening through measurement of percent free PSA in serum. J Urol 1995; 153: 312 (abstr)

35. Murphy W M, Dean P J, Brasfield J A, Tatum L. Incidental carcinoma of the prostate. How much sampling is adequate? Am J Surg Pathol 1986; 10: 170–174

36. Sonda L P, Grossman H B, MacGregor R J, Gikas P W. Incidental adenocarcinoma of the prostate: the role of repeat transurethral resection in staging. Prostate 1984; 5: 141–146

37. Jewett H J. The present status of radical prostatectomy for stages A and B prostatic cancer. Urol Clin North Am 1975; 2: 105–124

38. Cantrell B B, Deklerk D P, Eggleston J C et al. Pathological factors that influence prognosis in stage A prostatic cancer: the influence of extent versus grade. J Urol 1981; 125: 516–520

39. Anderson G A, Lawson R K, Gottlieb M S. Quantitation of potentially undiagnosed incidental carcinoma of the prostate in patients treated non-surgically for benign prostatic hyperplasia. Br J Urol 1993; 72: 465–469

40. Golimbu M, Schinella R, Morales P, Kurusu S. Differences in pathological characteristics and prognosis of clinical A2 prostatic cancer from A1 and B disease. J Urol 1978; 119: 618–622

41. Donohue R E, Augspurger R R, Mani J H et al. Pelvic lymph node dissection: guide to patient management in clinically locally confined adenocarcinoma of prostate. Urology 1982; 20: 559–565

42. McNeal J E, Redwine E A, Freiha F S, Stamey T A. Zonal distribution of prostatic adenocarcinoma. Correlation with histologic pattern and direction of spread. Am J Surg Pathol 1988; 12: 897–906

43. Greene D R, Wheeler T M, Egawa S et al. Relationship between clinical stage and histological zone of origin in early prostate cancer: morphometric analysis. Br J Urol 1991; 68: 499–509

44. Greene D R, Wheeler T M, Egawa S et al. A comparison of the morphological features of cancer arising in the transition zone and in the peripheral zone of the prostate. J Urol 1991; 146: 1069–1076

45. Epstein J I, Walsh P C, Carmichael M, Brendler C B. Pathologic and clinical findings to predict tumor extent of nonpalpable (stage T1c) prostate cancer. JAMA 1994; 271: 368–374

46. Epstein J I, Steinberg G D. The significance of low-grade prostate cancer on needle biopsy. A radical prostatectomy study of tumor grade, volume, and stage of the biopsied and multifocal tumor. Cancer 1990; 66: 1927–1932

47. Kahler J E. Carcinoma of the prostate gland: a pathologic study. J Urol 1939; 41: 557–574

48. Baron E, Angrist A. Incidence of occult adenocarcinoma of prostate after 50 years of age. Arch Pathol 1941; 32: 787–793

49. Lundberg S, Berge T. Prostatic carcinoma. An autopsy study. Scand J Urol Nephrol 1970; 4: 93–97

50. Newman A J Jr, Graham M A, Carlton C E Jr, Lieman S. Incidental carcinoma of the prostate at the time of transurethral resection: importance of evaluating every chip. J Urol 1982; 128: 948–950

51. Vollmer R T. Prostate cancer and chip specimens: complete versus partial sampling. Hum Pathol 1986; 17: 285–290

52. Rohr L R. Incidental adenocarcinoma in transurethral resection of the prostate. Am J Surg Pathol 1987; 11: 53–58

53. McNeal J E, Price H M, Redwine E A et al. Stage A versus stage B adenocarcinoma of the prostate: morphological comparison and biological significance. J Urol 1988; 139: 61–65

54. Rifkin M D, Dahnert W, Kurtz A B. State of the art: endorectal sonography of the prostate gland. AJR 1990; 154: 691–700

55. Aarnink R G, Huynen A L, Giesen J B et al. Automated prostate volume determination with ultrasonographic imaging. J Urol 1995; 153: 1549–1554

56. Shinohara K, Wheeler T M, Scardino P T. The appearance of prostate cancer on transrectal ultrasonography: correlation of imaging and pathological examinations. J Urol 1989; 142: 76–82

57. Terris M K, McNeal J E, Stamey T A. Detection of clinically significant prostate cancer by transrectal ultrasound-guided systematic biopsies. J Urol 1992; 148: 829–832

58. Flanigan R C, Catalona W J, Richie J P et al. Accuracy of digital rectal examination and transrectal ultrasonography in localizing prostate cancer. J Urol 1994; 152: 1506–1509

59. Hodge K K, McNeal J E, Stamey T A. Ultrasound guided transrectal core biopsies of the palpably abnormal prostate. J Urol 1989; 142: 66–70

60. Bazinet M, Meshref A W, Trudel C et al. Prospective evaluation of prostate specific antigen density and systematic biopsies for early detection of prostatic carcinoma. Urology 1994; 43: 44–51

61. Ravery V, Boccon-Gibod L A, Dauge-Geffroy M C et al. Systematic biopsies accurately predict extracapsular extension of prostate cancer and persistent/recurrent detectable PSA after radical prostatectomy. Urology 1994; 44: 371–376

62. Haggman M, Nybacka O, Nordin B, Busch C. Standardised in vitro mapping with multiple core biopsies of prostatectomy specimens: localisation and prediction of volume and grade. Br J Urol 1994; 74: 617–625

63. Lui P D, Terris M K, McNeal J E, Stamey T A. Indications for ultrasound guided transition zone biopsies in the detection of prostate cancer. J Urol 1995; 153: 1000–1003

64. Terris M K, Freiha F S, McNeal J E, Stamey T A. Efficacy of transrectal ultrasound for identification of clinically undetected prostate cancer. J Urol 1991; 146: 78–83

65. McNeal J E, Bostwick D G, Kindrachuk R A et al. Patterns of progression in prostate cancer. Lancet 1986; 1: 60–63

66. Breslow N, Chan C W, Dhom G et al. Latent carcinoma of prostate at autopsy in seven areas. Int J Cancer 1977; 20: 680–688

67. Franks L M. Latent carcinoma of the prostate. J Pathol Bacteriol 1954; 68: 603–616

68. Epstein J I, Carmichael M J, Partin A W, Walsh P C. Small high grade adenocarcinoma of the prostate in radical prostatectomy specimens performed for nonpalpable disease: pathogenetic and clinical implications. J Urol 1994; 151: 1587–1592

69. Cupp M R, Bostwick D G, Myers R P, Oesterling J E. The volume of prostate cancer in the biopsy specimen cannot reliably predict the quantity of cancer in the radical prostatectomy specimen on an individual basis. J Urol 1995; 153: 1543–1548

70. Stamey T A, Kabalin J N, McNeal J E et al. Prostate specific antigen in the diagnosis and treatment of adenocarcinoma of the prostate. II. Radical prostatectomy treated patients. J Urol 1989; 141: 1076–1083

71. Terris M K, McNeal J E, Stamey T A. Estimation of prostate cancer volume by transrectal ultrasound imaging. J Urol 1992; 147: 855–857

72. Dietrick D D, McNeal J E, Stamey T A. Core cancer length in ultrasound-guided systematic sextant biopsies: a preoperative evaluation of prostate cancer volume. Urology 1995; 45: 987–992

73. Terris M K, Haney D J, Johnston I M et al. Prediction of prostate cancer volume using PSA levels, transrectal prostatic ultrasound and systematic sextant biopsies. Urology 1995; 45: 75–80

74. Troncoso P, Babaian R J, Ro J Y et al. Prostatic intraepithelial neoplasia and invasive prostatic adenocarcinoma in cystoprostatectomy specimens. Urology 1989; 34 (suppl): 52–56

75. Bostwick D G. Prostatic intra-epithelial neoplasia (PIN): current concepts. J Cell Biochem 1992; 16H (suppl): 10–19

76. Webb J A W, Shanmuganathan K, McLean A. The complications of ultrasound guided transperineal prostate biopsy: a prospective study. Br J Urol 1993; 72: 775–777

77. Thompson P M, Pryor J P, Williams J P et al. The problem of infection after prostatic biopsy: the case for the transperineal approach. Br J Urol 1982; 54: 736–740

78. Ryan P G, Peeling W B. Perineal prostatic tumour seedling after 'Tru-Cut' needle biopsy: case report and review of the literature. Eur Urol 1990; 17: 189–192

79. Bastacky S S, Walsh P C, Epstein J I. Needle biopsy associated tumor tracking of adenocarcinoma of the prostate. J Urol 1991; 145: 1003–1007

80. Bostwick D G. Pathologic changes in the prostate following contemporary 18-gauge needle biopsy: no apparent risk of tumour seeding. J Urol Pathol 1994; 2: 203–211

81. Gaudin B, Epstein J I. Adenosis of the prostate. Am J Surg Pathol 1994; 18: 863–870

82. Bostwick D G, Qian J. Atypical adenomatous hyperplasia of the prostate. Relationship with carcinoma in 217 whole-mount radical prostatectomies. Am J Surg Pathol 1995; 19: 506–518

83. Epstein J I. Relationship of dysplasia to prostate carcinoma. Semin Urol 1990; 8: 2–8

84. McNeal J E, Villers A, Redwine E A et al. Microcarcinoma in the prostate: its association with duct-acinar dysplasia. Hum Pathol 1991; 22: 644–652

85. Brawer M K. Prostatic intraepithelial neoplasia: a premalignant lesion. Hum Pathol 1992; 23: 242–248

86. Srigley J R. Small-acinar patterns in the prostate gland with emphasis on atypical adenomatous hyperplasia and small acinar carcinoma. Semin Diagn Pathol 1988; 5: 254–272.

87. Epstein J I, Fynheer J. Acid mucin in the prostate. Can it differentiate adenosis from adenocarcinoma? Hum Pathol 1992; 23: 1321–1325

88. Bostwick D G, Srigley J, Grignon D et al. Atypical adenomatous hyperplasia of the prostate: morphologic criteria for its distinction from well-differentiated carcinoma. Hum Pathol 1993; 24: 819–832

89. Kramer C E, Epstein J I. Nucleoli in low-grade prostate adenocarcinoma and adenosis. Hum Pathol 1993; 24: 618–623

90. McNeal J E, Bostwick D G. Intraduct dysplasia: a pre-malignant lesion of the prostate. Hum Pathol 1986; 17: 64–71

91. Drago J R, Mostofi F K, Lee K. Introductory remarks and workshop summary. Urology 1989; 34 (suppl): 2–3

92. Parkinson M C. Preneoplastic lesions of the prostate. Histopathology 1995; 27: 301–311

93. Garnett J E, Oyasu R. Urologic evaluation of atypical prostatic hyperplasia. Urology 1989; 34 (suppl): 66–69

94. Markham C W. Prostatic intraepithelial neoplasia: detection and correlation with invasive cancer in fine-needle biopsy. Urology 1989; 34 (suppl): 57–61

95. Brawer M K, Bigler S A, Sohlberg O E et al. Significance of prostatic intraepithelial neoplasia on prostate needle biopsy. Urology 1991; 38 (suppl): 103–107

96. Weinstein M H, Epstein J I. Significance of high-grade prostatic intraepithelial neoplasia on needle biopsy. Hum Pathol 1993; 24: 624–629

97. Davidson D, Siroky M, Rudders R et al. Prostatic intraepithelial neoplasia is predictive of adenocarcinoma. Mod Pathol 1994; 7: 410 (abstr)

98. Stahl D, Keetch D, Smith D, Humphrey P H. Isolated prostatic intraepithelial neoplasia in needle biopsy as a marker for detection of adenocarcinom on re-biopsy. Mod Pathol 1994; 7: 479 (abstr)

99. Keetch D W, Humphrey P, Stahl D et al. Morphometric analysis and clinical followup of isolated prostatic intraepithelial neoplasia in needle biopsy of the prostate. J Urol 1995; 154: 347–351

100. Bostwick D G, Brawer M K. Prostatic intraepithelial neoplasia and early invasion in prostate cancer. Cancer 1987; 59: 788–794

101. Moore R A. The morphology of small prostatic carcinoma. J Urol 1935; 33: 224–234

102. Andrews G S. Latent carcinoma of the prostate. J Clin Pathol 1949; 2: 197–208

103. Liavag F. Atrophy and regeneration in the pathogenesis of prostatic carcinoma. Acta Pathol Microbiol Scand 1968; 73: 338–350

104. De Varaj L T, Bostwick D G. Atypical basal cell hyperplasia of the prostate. Immunophenotypic profile and proposed classification of basal cell proliferations. Am J Surg Pathol 1993; 17: 645–659

105. Grignon D J, Ro J Y, Srigley J R et al. Sclerosing adenosis of the prostate gland. A lesion showing myoepithelial differentiation. Am J Surg Pathol 1992; 16: 383–391

106. Jones E C, Young R H. The differential diagnosis of prostatic carcinoma. Am J Clin Pathol 1994; 101: 48–68

107. Malpica A, Ro J Y, Troncoso P et al. Nephrogenic adenoma of the prostatic urethra involving the prostate gland. Hum Pathol 1994; 25: 390–395

108. Gagucas R J, Brown R W, Wheeler T M. Verumontanum gland mucosal hyperplasia. Am J Surg Pathol 1995; 19: 30–36

109. Gikas P W, Del Buono E A, Epstein J I. Florid hyperplasia of mesonephric remnants involving prostate and periprostatic tissue. Possible confusion with adenocarcinoma. Am J Surg Pathol 1993; 17: 454–460

110. Epstein J I. Prostatic intraepithelial neoplasia. Adv Anat Pathol 1994; 1: 123–134

111. Ayala A G, Srigley J R, Ro J Y et al. Clear cell cribriform hyperplasia of prostate. Report of 10 cases. Am J Surg Pathol 1986; 10: 665–671

112. Epstein J I, Armas O A. Atypical basal cell hyperplasia of the prostate. Am J Surg Pathol 1992; 16: 1205–1214

113. Bostwick D G. Premalignant lesions of the prostate. Semin Diagn Pathol 1988; 5: 240–253

114. Mahadevia P S, Koss L G, Tar I J. Prostatic involvement in bladder cancer. Prostate mapping in 20 cystoprostatectomy specimens. Cancer 1986; 58: 2096–2102

19

Neurological and neurophysiological assessment
C. J. Fowler R. S. Kirby

Introduction

Symptomatic benign prostatic hyperplasia (BPH) is so prevalent that there is a tendency for urologists to assume that any lower urinary tract symptoms in any man over the age of 50 are likely to be the result of bladder outflow obstruction due to prostatic hypertrophy. The usual investigations that have already been discussed — including digital rectal examination (DRE), prostate-specific antigen (PSA), ultrasound determination of post-void residual urine and urinary flow rates — often do not distinguish between those male patients with uncomplicated BPH and those with neurological disease producing a similar clinical picture.

The neurological disorders most often implicated as causing bladder symptoms include neurodegenerative diseases such as multiple system atrophy (Shy–Drager syndrome), idiopathic Parkinson's disease and other conditions that affect the autonomic nervous system, such as the autonomic neuropathy of diabetes mellitus, pelvic nerve injury secondary to procedures such as abdominoperineal resection of the rectum, or lesions causing cauda equina damage. Furthermore, patients with upper motor neuron lesions due to spinal cord disease, or diseases affecting the cerebral hemispheres such as cerebrovascular accidents (CVA), may complain of bladder symptoms that may closely mimic those of BPH. Finally, it must be remembered that, as BPH is such a common condition it may well occur in men with established neurological disease, although the decision whether to operate on such patients is often difficult.

The differentiation between neuropathic involvement of the bladder and bladder outflow obstruction due to BPH is important, as surgical reduction of outflow resistance by transurethral resection of the prostate (TURP) is inappropriate when the disease is primarily neurological. Indeed, in circumstances such as multiple system atrophy or pelvic nerve injury following anteroposterior resection, where the distal sphincter mechanism is already denervated, surgery to the bladder neck and prostatic urethra is highly likely to cause postoperative urinary incontinence.

Focused neurological examination

In many situations the astute urologist can, after taking a clinical history and making a brief but focused clinical examination, tentatively diagnose neuropathic involvement of the bladder. In the past, neurological examination of the perineum was stressed as being important in recognizing neurological disease that was responsible for bladder dysfunction. In fact, cauda equina lesions, which may be detected by examining parts innervated by S2–S4, are relatively rare compared with the much more commonly occurring suprasacral spinal pathologies. The neural programmes that determine whether the bladder is in storage or voiding mode exist in centres in the dorsal tegmentum of the pons.[1] For these programmes to be effected there must be intact spinal connections between the sacral part of the spinal cord (which is the level of efferent and afferent neural connections to the lower urinary tract) and the pons. Because the innervation of the bladder arises from cord segments lower than those which innervate the lower limbs (Fig. 19.1) much can be learnt of spinal integrity by a neurological examination of the legs. Table 19.1 summarizes the sites of various lesions that can give rise to bladder dysfunction, together with the expected physical findings.

It is unusual to have a lesion between the pons and the sacral part of the cord giving rise to a neurogenic bladder that does not also produce signs of an upper motor neuron lesion in the lower limbs. This is undoubtedly the case in patients with multiple sclerosis (MS),[2] but it also appears to hold for most other instances of spinal pathology unless the lesion is small and intramedullary.

A predictable exception to the rule that spinal pathways for bladder function are unlikely to be

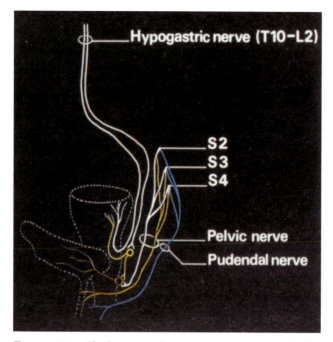

Figure 19.1. *The lower spinal segments innervating the bladder (parasympathetic) and pelvic floor (pudendal). The sympathetic innervation of the bladder neck, seminal vesicles and prostate comes from the higher (T10–L1) thoracolumbar levels.*

Table 19.1. *Neurological conditions that can produce bladder symptoms*

Nature/site of lesion	Physical signs
Spinal cord (tumour, vascular, MS, trauma)	Pathologically brisk knee and ankle jerks, extensor plantar responses
Cauda equina	Absent ankle jerks and possibly loss also of knee jerks; wasting of calf muscles and intrinsic foot muscles; perineal sensory loss; lax anal sphincter
Generalized peripheral neuropathy	Absent knee and ankle reflexes; impaired sensation in the feet
Multiple system atrophy	History of erectile failure; parkinsonian features, particularly bradykinesia, often poorly responding to L-dopa; postural hypotension; quiet voice or laryngeal stridor; cerebellar ataxia

damaged without also producing symptoms and signs in the legs might be expected from a conus or cauda equina lesion affecting only S2–S4. It seems, however, that even with such extreme caudal lesions there are usually neurological abnormalities in the lower limbs, and foot deformities may be present if the problem is a long-standing one.

The contribution of suprapontine pathology to neurogenic bladder dysfunction, with the exception of areas in the frontal lobes is poorly defined. Patients with frontal lobe incontinence usually have quite profound neuropsychological impairment, including a change of personality, but are often not indifferent to their incontinence.[3] Hydrocephalus can also cause bladder dysfunction in combination with unsteadiness of gait and dementia.[4]

The suggestion is sometimes made that a patient's peripheral neuropathy might be responsible for bladder dysfunction. Many forms of neuropathy are dependent on the length of the nerve fibres involved, the maximum deficit being evident in the longest fibres.[5] Because the nerve fibres to the bladder are comparatively short, there should usually be clinical evidence of extensive disease with loss of both knee and ankle jerks and sensory impairment to a level well above the level of the ankles for its innervation to have been affected as part of a generalized neuropathy. Even if the neuropathy is selective for small fibres (i.e. autonomic function, pain and temperature sensations), symptomatic bladder involvement occurs relatively late and only in patients with other profound neuropathic symptoms.

Blood pressure measurement

Every patient with BPH should have his blood pressure measured in both the standing and sitting (or ideally standing and lying) position. The most common abnormality is hypertension. It has been the authors' experience that approximately 30% of patients entering BPH studies are found to be hypertensive if a definition of hypertension is taken as a diastolic blood pressure greater than 90 mmHg. There has been some suggestion recently that there may be some concomitance of hypertension and BPH, the rationale behind this suggestion being overactivity of the sympathetic nervous system in men beyond middle age. Postural hypertension is even more important to detect before initiating therapy for BPH, especially in the era when alpha-blocking agents are more increasingly being used in the treatment of this condition. Pre-existing postural hypertension, such as that which commonly occurs with diabetic autonomic neuropathy, should preclude the use of alpha-blocking agents. In the absence of diabetes mellitus it may also be a sign of developing multiple system atrophy, which may be characterized by progressive autonomic failure. If a TURP is performed in the early stages of the disease, then the subsequent incontinence and impotence that are attributable to the neurological condition itself are often incorrectly ascribed to the operating urologist.

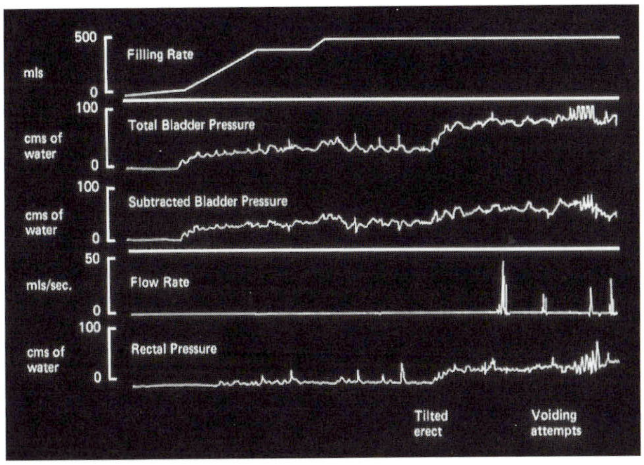

Urodynamics

The classic urodynamic appearances of bladder outflow obstruction due to BPH have been discussed in Chapter 16. Neurological disorders of the bladder, especially upper motor neuron lesions, usually cause a more profound form of detrusor hyperreflexia with phasic unstable contractions. In a severe cord lesion there may be loss of the voiding reflex. In lower motor neuron lesions an unstable filling pattern is still seen, but this is more often characterized by a slow progressive rise in bladder pressure during filling and, again, a loss of the normal voiding reflex (Fig. 19.2). In lower motor neuron lesions the bladder neck is often open at rest (Fig. 19.3) and voiding is achieved by abdominal straining, leaving a considerable post-micturition residue.

Pelvic floor neurophysiology

Electromyography

Electromyography (EMG) of the pelvic floor and sphincters has been performed with two distinct aims: EMG in the urodynamic suite has been used to examine sphincteric activity during bladder filling and voiding, while in the neurophysiology laboratory EMG has usually been performed to assess the integrity of innervation of the sphincter muscle. For the latter studies a needle electrode can be used, but for kinesiological studies various types of surface electrodes

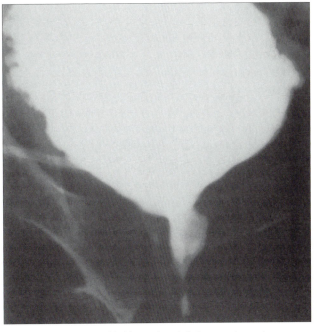

Figure 19.2. *Cystometrogram in a patient with a lower motor neuron lesion of the bladder. Note the loss of compliance during bladder filling and the loss of the normal voiding reflex.*

Figure 19.3. *An open bladder neck and slight stress incontinence seen in a male patient with a lower motor neuron lesion of the bladder.*

have been developed as alternatives to needles (see ref. 6 for review).

Sphincter EMG recorded during urodynamics

Studies of detrusor and sphincter activity show that there is continuous EMG activity in the sphincters and pelvic floor throughout bladder filling and that EMG silence of the urethral sphincter is the first recordable event in normally coordinated voiding. If there is a spinal lesion interrupting the bulbospinal pathways, this normal pattern of behaviour is lost and sphincter contraction occurs during detrusor contraction — the so-called detrusor–sphincter dyssynergia.[7] In suprapontine lesions, such as those following CVA, there may be uninhibited detrusor activity but the pattern of detrusor sphincter behaviour is normal.

Concentric needle electrode and single-fibre EMG recordings of the pelvic floor and urethral sphincter

The male subject lies in the left lateral position with knees and hips flexed and the needle is inserted percutaneously in the midline of the perineum and guided towards the apex of the prostate with the examiner's finger in the rectum. The audio output of the EMG machine is essential for finding the correct needle position. On inserting the needle electrode into the urethral sphincter there is a characteristic burst of activity recordable, which then fades to a resting interference pattern made up of three or four tonically firing units. Histochemical studies have shown that these muscles have type 1 fibre properties, suiting them to sustained contraction. These units fire continuously at all times, even during sleep and light general anaesthesia; the muscle becomes transiently electrically silent only at the onset of micturition.

Neuropathic units are of prolonged duration and polyphasic character and are readily distinguished from the less complex normal units found in control subjects (see ref. 6 for review).

Recognition of multiple system atrophy by sphincter EMG

The term multiple system atrophy (Shy–Drager syndrome) has been applied to a number of disease entities that have a common pathological expression of neuronal atrophy in a variety of overlapping combinations. Disturbances of continence and micturition invariably accompany other neurological changes in the Shy–Drager syndrome and may be the presenting symptom.[8]

Selective sole loss of the anterior horn cells in Onuf's nucleus occurs in multiple system atrophy, resulting in denervation of the striated muscle of both anal and urethral sphincters. Sakuta et al.[9] demonstrated the changes in the EMG of the anal sphincter in patients with multiple system atrophy and compared them with such findings in patients with motor neuron disease. Kirby et al.[10] examined motor units in the urethral sphincter and demonstrated marked prolongation and increased polyphasic potentials indicating chronic reinnervation. Eardley et al.[11] proposed that sphincter EMG should be used to differentiate between multiple system atrophy and idiopathic Parkinson's disease in patients with parkinsonism and bladder symptoms.

Cauda equina lesions and pelvic nerve injury

Like the pattern of denervation and reinnervation seen in the Shy–Drager syndrome, patients with either cauda equina lesions or pelvic nerve injury show neuropathic motor units from the external sphincter when an EMG needle is introduced. In these circumstances the demonstration of neuropathy affecting this muscle has obvious implications in terms of continence if the urologist is considering prostatic resection. In circumstances such as urinary retention following an abdominoperineal resection of the rectum when the prostate is suspected to be enlarged, transurethral resection will reduce outflow resistance at the bladder neck and in the prostatic urethra, but if the urethral sphincter has been denervated by the surgical process then there is a substantial risk of urinary incontinence. For this reason it is recommended that EMG should be performed on such patients before a decision to undertake a TURP is made.

Sacral reflexes and cortical evoked responses

Sacral reflexes are reflex contractions of the striated muscle structures in the pelvic floor that occur in response to stimulation of the perineal genital region. Methods for neurophysiological recordings of the bulbocavernosus reflex were described 30 years ago and although this reflex is easier to elicit in men than women, the intensity of stimulation needed to produce the reflex is very variable. Moreover, the presence or absence of a definite response does not always correlate with definite pathology. Cortical evoked potentials can be recorded following stimulation of the pudendal nerve and may be useful in selected cases, but it is unusual for this to be abnormal without an abnormality on clinical examination.[12]

Conclusions

Only a minority of patients presenting with BPH will require the sophisticated neurophysiological testing described above. However, all patients would benefit from a careful, focused neurological examination and recording of blood pressure in the standing and lying positions. If neurological disease is suspected, the authors recommend formal urodynamic studies and/or referral to a neurologist. Neurophysiological examination of the pelvic floor may be indicated in a few, a positive result confirming the presence of either neuropathic bladder dysfunction or denervation of the pelvic floor. Such a finding would have important implications in terms of the correct selection of treatment strategy.

References

1. de Groat W C. Central neural control of the lower urinary tract. In: Bock C, Whelan J (eds) Neurobiology of incontinence. Ciba Foundation Symposium 151. Chichester: Wiley, 1990: 27–56
2. Betts C D, D'Mellow M T, Fowler C J. Urinary symptoms and the neurological features of bladder dysfunction in multiple sclerosis. J Neurol Neurosurg Psychiatry 1993; 56: 245–250
3. Andrew J, Nathan P W. Lesions of the anterior frontal lobes and disturbances of micturition and defaecation. Brain 1964; 87: 233–262
4. Fisher C M. Hydrocephalus as a cause of disturbances of gait in the elderly. Neurology 1982; 32: 1358–1363
5. Sabin T. Classification of peripheral neuropathy: the long and short of it. Muscle Nerve 1986; 9: 711–719
6. Fowler C J. Pelvic floor neurophysiology. In: Osselton J (ed) Clinical neurophysiology. Oxford: Butterworth-Heinemann, 1995: 233–252
7. Blaivas J G, Sinha H P, Zayed A A H, Labib K B. Detrusor–external sphincter dysynergia. J Urol 1981; 125: 542–545
8. Beck R O, Betts C D, Fowler C J. Genito-urinary dysfunction in multiple system atrophy: clinical features and treatment in 62 cases. J Urol 1994; 151: 1336–1341
9. Sakuta M, Nakanishi T, Tohokura Y. Anal muscle electromyograms differ in amyotrophic lateral sclerosis and Shy–Drager syndrome. Neurology 1978; 28: 1289–1293
10. Kirby R S, Fowler G J, Gosling J, Bannister R. Urethro-vesical dysfunction in progressive autonomic failure with multiple system atrophy. J Neurol Neurosurg Psychiatry 1986; 49: 554–562
11. Eardley I, Quinn N P, Fowler C J. The value of urethral sphincter electromyography in the differential diagnosis of parkinsonism. Br J Urol 1989; 64: 360–362
12. Delodovici M L, Fowler C J. The clinical value of the pudendal somatosensory evoked potential is examined. Electroencephalogr Clin Neurophysiol 1995; in press

Medical Treatment

IV

Watchful waiting
F. A. Madsen R. C. Bruskewitz

20

Introduction

Benign prostatic hyperplasia (BPH) is a common problem of ageing men, affecting the majority of individuals aged 60 years and above. Today, the patient presenting with symptoms of BPH is offered a wide variety of treatment options, both medical and surgical, but before the physician and the patient make any decisions with respect to treatment, three basic issues have to be resolved, These include how bothered the patient is by his urinary symptoms, whether he desires any treatment for them, and whether it is safe to refrain from active treatment. For patients who do not find their symptoms sufficiently troublesome or who do not accept the morbidity or regular medication use associated with existing and surgical medical treatment modalities for BPH, watchful waiting might be the appropriate treatment strategy.

Watchful waiting (WW) is a strategy of management in which the patient is monitored by his physician but receives no active intervention for BPH. Although WW is the most common treatment strategy for patients with mild to moderate symptoms of BPH, relatively little is known about WW as a treatment option.

In this chapter WW is discussed as if it was an active treatment modality for BPH.

Indications

When transurethral resection of the prostate (TURP) was introduced more than 70 years ago, the mortality and morbidity rates associated with the procedure were high and the treatment was reserved for potentially life-threatening illness, such as haemorrhage, urinary retention, azotaemia or sepsis. These severe manifestations of BPH are still regarded as strong indications for surgery, but over the years there has been a gradual reduction in the mortality rate associated with TURP, from 5% in the 1930s[1] to 0.2% in 1989.[2] This progress, together with the emergence of new treatment

modalities such as less invasive approaches (laser prostatectomy, transurethral incision of the prostate, balloon dilatation) and medical therapy, has expanded immensely the indications for treatment.

Strong indications for treatment or WW

The clear-cut indications for *treatment* are relatively easy to define. Today, surgical treatment is recommended in BPH patients with (a) refractory urinary retention, who have failed at least one attempt of catheter removal with or without concomitant alpha-blockade, (b) recurrent urinary tract infections caused by bacterial prostatitis, in cases where the infection is resistant to medical therapy, (c) bladder stones, (d) renal insufficiency secondary to outlet obstruction or (e) severe gross haematuria leading to urinary tract clotting and retention or anaemia where possibilities other than BPH have been excluded.[3]

The strong indications for *no treatment* are not well defined, but currently it seems prudent to recommend a strategy of WW for patients with mild symptoms of BPH [roughly those with American Urological Association (AUA) Symptom Scores ≤ 7].[3]

Moderate indications for treatment or WW

The issue concerning whether patients with moderate manifestations of BPH should receive active treatment is controversial. It is crucial that these patients are informed about the benefits and harmful aspects of each treatment and are asked to share in the selection of treatment. Many patients, however, wish to have the physician's opinion on the best treatment options and in those cases it is appropriate for the physician to select the optimal treatment. To do so, attention should be focused on the clinical findings and optional tests that might predict a better outcome after certain treatment modalities. For WW these include (a) the patient's bother from urinary symptoms, (b) large post-void residual (PVR) urine measurements, and (c) uroflowmetry.

Bother

Two patients with the same level of urinary symptoms (same AUA Symptom Score) might be bothered by their urinary difficulties to different degrees. In a recently published study[4] (discussed later), comparing WW with TURP, it is concluded that patients who are substantially bothered by their symptoms have more to gain from TURP than WW. For men who find their symptoms less troublesome, WW is usually a safe alternative. One way of assessing how a given level of urinary symptoms affects the patient's quality of life is to use a bother score system such as the BPH Impact Index.[5] This index measures how much the patient's urinary problems affect various day-to-day activities.

Post-void residual

It is a common assumption that the amount of PVR urine predicts which men will improve after surgery. This assumption cannot be supported by currently available data, partly because it has not been exhaustively studied and partly because the volume of PVR correlates poorly with other signs and symptoms of prostatism. However, on the basis of data from the Department of Veteran Affairs (DVA) cooperative study,[4] it seems likely that higher residual urines may lead to a higher failure rate for WW. Currently, it is not possible to assign an exact volume at which intervention should be recommended.

Uroflowmetry

In the evaluation of BPH, uroflowmetry is often performed in an attempt to gain objective evidence of obstruction. The maximal urinary flow rate is considered to be the most useful flow variable and in some studies[6–8] appears to predict surgical outcome. There is good evidence[8,9] that patients with maximal urinary flow rates greater than 15 ml/s have a lower success rate following surgical treatment (TURP) than those with maximal flow rates less than 15 ml/s.

Conclusions

Moderate indications for WW include low bother score, high urinary flow rate and low PVR urine volume, but the decision on whether to treat should never be based on these measurements alone.

The indications for WW and therapeutic intervention are listed in Table 20.1.

Strategy

When the decision to follow a patient in a strategy of WW is made, it is important that the waiting period really is *watchful*. The patient's symptoms and clinical

Table 20.1. *Indications for therapeutic intervention vs watchful waiting in BPH*

Strength of indication	Strategy	
	Watchful waiting	Therapeutic intervention
Strong	Mild symptoms (AUA Score ≤ 7)	Recurrent urinary retention (more than a single episode)
		Recurrent urinary tract infections
		Recurrent gross haematuria
		Bladder stones
		Renal insufficiency due to BPH
Moderate	Moderate symptoms (AUA Score ≥ 8 and ≤ 19) but not bothersome (low BPH Impact Score)	Moderate to severe symptoms (AUA Score ≥ 8) and bothersome (high BPH Impact Score)
	Higher peak urinary flow rate (rate not specified)	High post-voiding residual and low peak urinary flow rate (volume and rate not specified)
	Low post-void urinary residual (volume not specified)	

course should be monitored, usually annually. Further research is required to determine if anything is gained, in terms of better outcome, when the patient is checked more (or less) often. The patient should receive information about medication that might make his symptoms worse, and given instructions on simple behavioural modifications, such as avoidance of coffee and alcohol after dinner. At each follow-up visit, a reassessment of symptoms (using the baseline symptom scoring instrument), a physical examination and routine laboratory testing (such as serum creatinine, urinalysis) should be performed and optional diagnostic procedures, such as uroflow and residual urine measurements, should be considered.

If the patient's symptoms progress or the bother from his urinary difficulties increases, it is appropriate to offer him other treatment options.

Studies of untreated BPH

Of primary consideration when evaluating studies on untreated BPH is that BPH is a heterogeneous disease, described in a number of ways. The definition of BPH, the estimates of outcome, the indications for treatment and the study design vary from one study to another and this makes comparison of different BPH studies difficult. The following is a description of some of the previous studies of untreated BPH.

Baltimore Longitudinal Study of Aging

An epidemiological study of great interest, providing information of the natural history of BPH, was published in 1991 by Arrighi:[10] this was the Baltimore Longitudinal Study of Aging. The study was established in 1958 and adult volunteers were enrolled, with a new participant recruited when another left the study. A total of 1371 men were enrolled. All patients completed a self-administered questionnaire and underwent a physical examination, including a digital rectal examination (DRE). The final analysis was based on 1057 men who did not have a history of prostatectomy or prostate cancer. The risk of eventual surgery for BPH was found to increase with increasing age. For men aged 50–59 years the 20-year probability for prostatectomy was 24% and for men aged 60 or older the risk was 39%. Change in prostate size (determined by DRE) and

obstructive symptoms, especially weak urinary stream and sensation of incomplete bladder emptying, were found to be predictive factors for subsequent prostatectomy.

The association between age and risk of prostatectomy, as found in this study, does not necessarily reflect a progression of BPH with age, in that historical prostatectomy rates may reflect different attitudes among urologists at different times.

Prospective study of patients with voiding symptoms

In 1969, Craigen et al.[11] published the results of a prospective study of 251 patients with voiding symptoms. The length of follow-up was 4–6 years. At baseline 39 patients had prostate cancer, 89 acute urinary retention and 123 patients had symptoms of prostatism. Of the 123 patients with prostatism, eight (6.5%) developed urinary retention and 48 (39%) underwent prostate surgery during the follow-up period.

Of the 67 patients who presented with symptoms of BPH and did not have surgery, 32 (48%) became symptom free in 4–6 years. There was no significant difference between the group of patients who underwent surgery and the group of patients who did not, with respect to age, baseline symptoms or general health.

This study can be criticized for a poor description of urinary symptoms and the method of selection of patients. Nevertheless, it suggests that patients with symptoms of BPH are much more likely to improve than to progress to acute urinary retention.

TURP waiting list

In 1993, Barham et al.[12] reported the results of a study evaluating 118 patients who were on a waiting list for TURP because of symptoms of BPH *and* the clinical finding of an enlarged prostate gland on rectal examination. The mean age was 70 years (55–89 years) and the mean period of time on the waiting list was 3 years (1–9 years). Eleven patients were excluded from the study because they either died, refused reassessment or underwent surgery at another location. A total of 107 patients were then reassessed. On the basis of symptoms, 70 patients (65%) reported no change, 13 (12%) had improved and 24 (22%) had deteriorated. A total of 29 patients (27%) were kept on the waiting list because of severe symptoms and reduced peak urinary flow rates (≤ 6.0 ml/s) but the remaining 78 patients were re-evaluated. Of these 51 (65%) were discharged from the waiting list because of mild or absent urinary symptoms, nine patients (12%) were kept under outpatient review because of mild symptoms but severe objective signs of obstruction (peak flow rates between 6 and 15 ml/s, and residual urine volumes ≥ 150 ml), and 18 (23%) were retained on the waiting list because of troublesome symptoms.

In summary, of the original 107 patients who were evaluated, 47 (44%) were kept on the waiting list, 51 (48%) were discharged and nine (8%) were kept under outpatient review.

This study shows the variability of BPH symptoms. The authors concluded that if the patients are reassured about the natural history of BPH and that their symptoms are caused by a benign disease, most of them will decide to avoid surgery. However, as is the case with the studies described previously, this study suffers from a lack of clear definition of symptoms and indications for surgery.

Prospective trial of TURP vs conservative management

In 1988, Kadow et al.[13] reported the results of a randomized, prospective trial comparing TURP with conservative management in 38 patients with bladder outlet obstruction. Twenty-one patients unaderwent TURP and 17 patients were followed in a strategy of WW. The patients were assessed urodynamically and asked about their urinary symptoms before treatment and 6 months after treatment.

After conservative therapy 56% of patients were rendered asymptomatic or improved, compared with 71% following TURP. The incidence of irritative urinary symptoms, such as nocturia and frequency, decreased significantly in both groups, as well as the number of patients with detrusor instability, where 79% showed reversion to stability following TURP compared with 50% following conservative management. The peak urinary flow rates improved from 8.5 to 19.0 ml/s in the TURP group and were little changed (from 9.8 to 11.2 ml/s) following conservative management.

This study concludes that TURP is superior to WW in terms of urinary flow improvement but it also confirms the findings of Craigen et al.[11] that in about one-half of the cases the natural course of untreated BPH is towards symptom improvement.

DVA cooperative study

The DVA cooperative study[4] was initiated in 1986 and has yielded a considerable amount of information about WW and TURP. The aim of this study was to compare WW with TURP in terms of efficacy and cost-effectiveness in patients with moderate symptoms of BPH. A total of 800 patients were screened at nine VA clinics. Excluded from the study were patients younger than 55 years, those who previously had undergone prostate surgery or who had prostate or bladder cancer, patients with residual urinary volumes exceeding 350 ml and those who had evidence of neurogenic bladder. A final total of 556 men with a median age of 65 years were included in the study and randomized to either surgery (280 patients) or WW (276 patients).

At baseline the patients were evaluated by a physical examination including a DRE, measurement of serum creatinine, urinalysis and measurements of residual urinary volume and peak urinary flow rate. The severity of symptoms was assessed by the Madsen Symptom Score and the degree to which the symptoms bothered the patients was assessed by a quality-of-life questionnaire. At baseline, there was no significant difference between the two groups with respect to all these parameters.

During follow-up, the peak urinary flow rates and the residual volumes were measured every 6 months and symptom/bother scores were obtained at 1, 2 and 3 years. All patients were told to avoid coffee and alcohol, and received information about medications that might make their symptoms worse. The primary outcome measure was treatment failure defined as the occurrence of any of the following events during follow-up: death; urinary retention; residual urine of more than 350 ml; developmemt of bladder calculus; new persistent incontinence; or a Madsen Symptom Score greater than 24 at one visit or of more than 21 in two consecutive visits.

Baseline and 3-year follow-up values are listed in Table 20.2. TURP was associated with a significantly higher improvement in peak urinary flow rates than WW, where the flow rates remained virtually

Table 20.2. *Baseline and 3-year follow-up values for patients in the DVA cooperative study*

Parameter	WW		TURP	
	Baseline	3-year follow-up	Baseline	3-year follow-up
Peak urinary flow rate (ml/s)*	12.3	12.7	11.6	17.8
Residual urine volume (ml)*	113	72	110	51
Symptom score (points)*	14.6	9.1	14.5	4.9
Bother from urinary difficulties (points†)*	48.0	57.6	46.4	75.7
Sexual performance (points†)	38.6	35.6	40.0	36.0
General well-being (points†)	71.3	71.4	73.2	76.2

*Changes on TURP significantly different ($p < 0.01$) from changes on WW. †Scale ranges from 0 (most impaired) to 100 (least impaired). (Adapted from ref. 4. with permission.)

unchanged over 3 years. The volume of residual urine decreased in both groups, but the improvement was most pronounced in the TURP group. With respect to symptoms and the perception of bother from urinary difficulties, both groups improved but, again, the improvement was greatest in the TURP group. There was no change in general well-being or sexual performance after either TURP or WW.

Treatment outcomes are presented in Table 20.3. There were significantly more treatment failures in the WW group (17%) than in the TURP group (8%). Three parameters associated with successful outcome for WW were high urinary flow rates, lower residual urine and less urinary bother, whereas high baseline bother was the only factor that predicted successful outcome after TURP.

The DVA cooperative study has demonstrated that TURP, across a broad range of outcomes, is more effective than WW. The more a man is bothered by his urinary symptoms, the more there is to gain from surgery. WW is a safe alternative to surgery for men who are less bothered by urinary difficulties. Eight out of ten patients followed in a strategy of WW will not experience treatment failure.

Treatment preference

As already mentioned, the patient should participate in the treatment decision to the extent that he desires, and physicians must accept that this decision might be based more on personal values than on scientific evidence. The more a patient is bothered by his urinary symptoms, the more likely it is that he will prefer a treatment with high efficacy and that he will view this intervention as

Table 20.3. *Treatment outcome for the DVA cooperative study at 3 years**

Outcome	WW (n=276)	TURP (n=280)
Treatment failures	47 (17)†	23 (8)
Deaths‡	10 (4)	13 (5)
Urinary retention	8 (3)	1 (0.3)
Residual urine > 350 ml	17 (6)	3 (1)
Renal azotaemia	1 (0.4)	4 (1)
High symptom score	13 (5)	1 (0.4)
Severe incontinence	4 (1)	4 (1)

*The average period of follow-up was 2.8 years. †Percentages in parentheses. ‡No genitourinary deaths occurred. (Adapted from ref. 4. with permission.)

successful. The patient's view on the relative disadvantages and benefits of each treatment option will help to determine his therapeutic preference.

Recently, the BPH Guideline Panel[3] performed a patient preference analysis in 53 patients with symptoms of BPH. On the basis of their AUA Symptom Score, the patients were categorized as having mild symptoms (12), moderate symptoms (26) and severe symptoms (15). The patients were given information about the benefits and disadvantages of four different treatment modalities (WW, alpha-blocker, TURP and balloon dilatation) and were then asked to select a personal treatment option. In the group of patients with mild symptoms, 80% preferred WW and 12% TURP; and in the group with moderate symptoms, 45% preferred WW and 18% TURP; and in the group with severe symptoms, 35% preferred WW and 55% TURP. The fact that almost one-half of the patients with moderate symptoms and one-third of the patients with severe symptoms decided against treatment clearly reflects that factors other than the severity of symptoms are important for the patient in the decision-making process. Such factors could be that he is not bothered sufficiently by his symptoms, or that he is not willing to accept the morbidity associated with the other treatment options.

Conclusions

When physicians evaluate treatment modalities for BPH, they often focus on certain outcomes, such as the improvement in symptom score and increase in urinary flow rates. These parameters are easy to measure and document scientifically. Naturally, the risk of side effects associated with the procedure is considered too, but many urologists are willing to accept a minor risk of even serious side effects (as the 1% risk of severe incontinence following TURP) if the chance of success (in terms of symptom improvement and uroflow improvement) following the treatment is high.

For the patient, however, the degree to which his symptoms bother him is of major importance and is what will determine his choice of treatment. Furthermore, the potential harm of certain approaches

is sufficient for many patients to make them decide against active or more aggressive therapy.

On the basis of the literature reviewed in this chapter, it is appropriate to recommend a strategy of WW for patients with mild symptoms of BPH (AUA Score ≤ 7). For patients with moderate symptoms, WW should be considered as a valid alternative to treatment, especially for patients who are not substantially bothered by their urinary difficulties.

Future research is required to determine the most appropriate way to follow untreated BPH patients and to answer such questions as whether it is necessary to monitor the renal function with serum creatinine, how often the patient should be examined, and how much PVR urine is too much.

References

1. Perrin P, Barnes R, Hadley H et al. Forty years of transurethral prostatic resections. J Urol 1976; 16: 757–758
2. Mebust W K, Holtgrewe H L, Cockett A T K et al. Immediate and postoperative complications. A cooperative study of 13 participating institutions evaluating 3,885 patients J Urol 1989; 141: 243
3. McConnell J D, Barry M J, Bruskewitz R C et al. Benign prostatic hyperplasia: diagnosis and treatment. Clinical practice guideline No 8. AHCPR publication No. 94-0582. Rockville: Agency for Health Care Policy and Research, Public Health Service, US Department of Health and Human Services, 1994.
4. Wasson J H, Reda D J, Bruskewitz R C et al. Comparison of transurethral surgery with watchful waiting for moderate symptoms of benign prostatic hyperplasia. N Engl J Med 1995; 332: 75–79
5. Barry M J, Fowler F J, O'Leary M P et al. Measuring disease-specific health status in men with benign prostatic hyperplasia. Med Care 1995; 33: AS145–AS155
6. Jensen K M E, Bruskewitz R C, Iversen P et al. Spontanous uroflowmetry in prostatism. Urology 1984; 24: 403–409
7. Jensen K M E, Jørgensen J B, Mogensen P. Urodynamics in prostatism I. Prognostic value of uroflowmetry. Scand J Urol Nephrol 1988; 22: 109–117
8. Abrams P H. Prostatism and prostatectomy: the value of urine flow rate measurement in the preoperative assessment for operation. J Urol 1977; 117: 70–71
9. Jensen K M E. Clinical evaluation of routine urodynamic investigations in prostatism. Neurourol Urodyn 1989; 8: 545–578
10. Arrighi H M, Metter E J, Guess H A et al. Natural history of benign prostatic hyperplasia and risk of prostatectomy. Urology 1991; 38: 4–8
11. Craigen A A, Hickling J B, Saunders C R et al. Natural history of prostatic obstruction. J R Coll Gen Pract 1969; 18: 226–232
12. Barham C P, Pocock R D, James E D. Who needs a prostatectomy? Review of a waiting list. Br J Urol 1993; 72: 314–317
13. Kadow C, Feneley R C L, Abrams P H. Prostatectomy or conservative management in the treatment of benign prostatic hypertrophy? Br J Urol 1988; 61: 432–434

21

The placebo effect in the treatment of benign prostatic hyperplasia

C. G. Roehrborn

The principal quality of a physician, as well as of a poet (for Apollo is the God of physics and poetry), is that of fine lying, or flattering the patient... And it is doubtless as well for the patient to be cured by the working of his imagination, or a reliance upon the promise of his doctor, as by repeated doses of physics.[1]

Is it ethical to use a placebo? The answer to this question will depend, I suggest, upon whether there is already available an orthodox treatment of proven or accepted value.
If there is such an orthodox treatment the question will hardly arise, for the doctor will wish to know whether a new treatment is more, or less, effective than the old, not that it is more effective than nothing.[2]

Placebo and placebo effect: definitions and theoretical considerations

It has long been recognized by practising physicians that procedures that offer patients reassurance or the expectation of help may lead to marked improvement in their clinical status. The Latin derived term 'placebo' originally appears in the Bible (*placebo domino in regione vivorum*, Psalm 116; 9), where it may be literally translated as 'I shall please'. This original meaning of 'please' is still found in the first medical definition of the term 'placebo' in *Hooper's Medical Dictionary* in the early 19th century: 'quality ascribed to any drug prescribed to please the patient rather than being useful'. The first article dedicated to the placebo effect did not appear until 1945: 'A note on placebo' by Pepper.[3] The potency of belief and expectation in effecting health is also underscored by such dramatic harmful effects as voodoo death, which in contrast can be referred to as a 'nocebo' ('I shall harm') effect.[4]

In a clinical context, placebo has come to denote a deceptive practice, a view that originates from the practice of singing vespers for pay. This negative connotation of placebo has come to dominate contemporary thinking, owing to the emergence of double-blind placebo-controlled drug studies, in which the differentiation of effects of the pharmacological action of a compound from other unspecified effects is a primary consideration. Placebo effects are so omnipresent that, if they are not controlled for in therapeutic studies, the findings are considered unreliable. Conditions in which placebo effects have been described include cough, mood changes, angina pectoris, headache, anxiety, hypertension, asthma, depression, lymphosarcoma, gastric motility, dermatitis, and pain from a variety of sources.[5]

A prevalent view of placebo is that its use is mandatory in clinical trials but unethical in clinical practice, a view that may be challenged on both counts.[5]

One of the most influential writers in the field of placebo research is Arthur K. Shapiro who offers the following definition:

> *A placebo is defined as any therapy or component of therapy that is deliberately used for its nonspecific, psychological, or psychophysiological effect, or that is used for its presumed specific effect, but is without specific activity for the conditions being treated. A placebo effect is defined as the psychological or psychophysiological effect produced by placebos.*[6]

Others have suggested definitions that differ from the one quoted above,[7] or have further elaborated on Shapiro's theory. Grünbaum developed a diagram to illustrate his definition of placebo (Fig. 21.1).[8] If a therapeutic theory recommends a therapy 't' for a condition, this treatment usually consists of a spectrum of factors, namely characteristic factors 'F' and incidental treatment factors 'C'. These incidental treatment factors may be known or unknown. The patient's life activities and functions are subdivided into two parts — the target disorder 'D', e.g. benign prostatic hyperplasia (BPH), and other aspects of the patient's life functions or health. The arrows in Fig. 21.1 illustrate the possible causations (effects). The characteristic

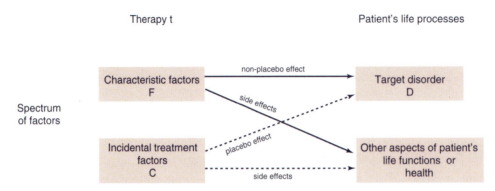

Figure 21.1. *Illustration of a therapeutic theory used to clarify the definition of 'placebo'. For further explanation, see text. (Adapted from ref. 8 with permission.)*

factors 'F' may have a positive or a negative effect on the target disorder (or may have no effect whatsoever). Similarly, the factors 'F' may have influences, good or bad, on other aspects of the patient's life, which are known as side effects. The incidental treatment factors 'C' may have side effects, but they may also affect the target disorder, which is referred to as a placebo effect.

If, for example the target disorder is BPH and the therapeutic theory the administration of alpha-blocking drugs by a physician who evaluates the patient at regular intervals, then the relaxation of the smooth muscle in the bladder neck and prostate has a positive effect on the symptoms of BPH (non-placebo effect), but the drug also causes side effects, namely a lowering of the blood pressure (positive) and asthenia (negative). An incidental treatment factor is the manner of dispensation of the drug by the physician: if he expresses his confidence in the medication, it may result in a positive placebo effect; if he is neutral or makes a comment such as 'We might try this for a while before we have to do something more serious', it may result in a negative placebo effect. Obviously, the frequent visits to the physician's office also have an impact on the patient's life functions by forcing him to set aside time for the visits (negative side effect of incidental treatment factors).

Brody[9] listed three possible reasons why a patient improves after a certain therapy is instituted:

1. The patient got better owing to the natural history of the condition in an organism with intact healing and recuperative powers.

2. The patient got better owing to the symbolic effect of the treatment, that is its impact on the patient's imagination, beliefs and/or emotions.

3. The patient got better owing to some specific or characteristic feature of the treatment that can be studied, isolated and predicted within the context of contemporary medical theory.

A positive placebo effect (no. 2 in the above list) is most likely to occur when three factors are present:[9]

1. The meaning of the illness experience for the patient is altered in a positive manner, given the patient's belief system and world view.

2. The patient is supported by a caring group.

3. The patient's sense of mastery or control over the illness is restored or enhanced.

This theory, emphasizing the importance of the patient's belief system and his or her expectations, highlights the cultural dimension of the placebo phenomenon and the importance of cross-cultural studies in placebo research.

White et al.[10] pointed out that there is no single placebo effect with a single mechanism and efficacy, but rather a multiplicity of effects with differential efficacy and mechanisms; these authors provide a list of placebogenic variables or determinants of a placebo response (Table 21.1). Turner et al.,[11] in a recent review of the importance of the placebo effect in pain treatment and research, listed similar factors influencing the placebo response. Among the patients' factors contributing to a high placebo response rate were

Table 22.1. *Biopsychosocial determinants of placebo response*

Cultural context
    Belief system
    Faith
Environmental milieu
Instruction
Suggestion
Preparation characteristics
Doctor–patient relationship
Patient's expectations and beliefs
Patient's personality
Psychological state
Symptom severity
Discomfort severity
Anxiety and stress
    Central evaluative processes
    Cognitive processes
Cognitive schema
Self-schema
Self-control
Expectancy
Outcome expectancy
Efficacy expectations
Operant behaviour
Symbolic processes
Imagination
Covert rehearsal
Emotions
Central nervous system influences upon physiology
    Immune system
    Stress mechanism
    Endogenous opiates
Classical conditioning
Spontaneous remissions

(From ref. 10 with permission.)

anticipation and expectations, a positive attitude toward provider and treatment, anxiety and compliance with the prescribed treatment. As an example of the latter, a randomized trial to evaluate the efficacy of a lipid-lowering drug in the therapy of coronary heart disease may be mentioned. Patients in the placebo arm were stratified by whether they took more or less than 80% of the placebo tablets.[12] Even after controlling for 40 known or suspected risk factors, the non-compliers had a 57% higher 5-year mortality rate than the compliant patients. Either the placebo lowered the rate of mortality, or patients' compliance was related to other characteristics associated with mortality that were not assessed in this study. Among the providers' factors they listed warmth, friendliness, interest, sympathy, empathy, prestige and, again, a positive attitude towards the patient and the treatment.

These considerations all address the issue of a 'placebo treatment' and the 'placebo effect' in the usually understood sense of a medical treatment with a drug. Placebo effects, however, are equally important to consider when the treatment consists of a procedure or surgical therapy. Instead of using an inactive preparation, a procedure or surgical intervention is performed that is similar in all respects to the active procedure or surgery but differs in that the key aspect of the procedure, which is believed to convey the main therapeutic benefit, is omitted. Such procedures are referred to as 'sham treatment' and the incidental causes or effects as 'sham effects'. Throughout this chapter, the term 'placebo/sham' is used to indicate the pertinence of the observation to both medical (drug) treatments and procedural (surgical) interventions.

Rationale for placebo/sham-controlled trials

The value of controlled clinical trials in the determination of the safety and effectiveness of a new intervention is largely undisputed. The US Food and Drug Administration (FDA) recognizes four types of comparative trials:

1. No treatment, which involves a comparison of the results in comparable concurrent groups of treated and untreated patients. This type of control is utilized when objective measurements of effectiveness are available and placebo effect or spontaneous improvement of the condition is negligible.
2. Placebo control, which involves a comparison of the results of a particular therapy with an inactive preparation or a sham procedure.
3. Active treatment control, which involves a comparison of the results with the new intervention with those with a treatment known to be effective.
4. Historical control, which involves comparison of the results with a new intervention with prior experience obtained in a comparable group of patients receiving no therapy or a known effective regimen.

The caveat listed in the first paragraph is of great relevance in BPH treatment trials. While better objective outcome measures are being developed and utilized, there is certainly a placebo effect and the natural history of the disease is such that spontaneous remissions are quite common. Thus, in clinical BPH research the only alternatives are placebo-/sham-controlled trials, or active treatment-controlled trials. Active control trials might substitute for placebo-controlled trials: (a) when there is reasonable certainty that a new treatment will be more effective than other agents known to be effective, (b) when the effectiveness of the new treatment is self-evident, or (c) where the nature of the therapy or procedure is such that it is not possible to blind the patients or the observers.[13] Whereas the first two arguments are rarely valid in BPH treatment trials, the third argument demands a closer look. Experience has shown that it is feasible to blind both patients and observers responsible for outcomes assessment regarding the randomization in a trial comparing balloon dilatation of the prostate with a sham procedure (cystoscopy).[14] As is discussed below, blinding is also possible in treatment trials using microwave-induced heat and other minimally invasive treatments. Whether true blinding could be achieved in a trial comparing transurethral resection of the prostate (TURP) with a sham procedure is more questionable because of the need for catheterization, and the bleeding, and the irrigation necessary following TURP. Despite the lack of any such trial, TURP is currently considered the gold standard of BPH treatments and, in fact, serves occasionally as an active treatment control for other invasive treatment modalities.

Despite the general acceptance of placebo/sham controls in medical research, others have warned against the 'continuing unethical use of placebo controls',[15] stating that in many cases the use of placebo control groups is in direct violation of the declaration of Helsinki.[16] The Declaration states that 'In any medical study every patient — including those of a control group, if any — should be assured of the best proven diagnostic and therapeutic method'.[16] Thus, Rothman and Michels argue, the use of a placebo is unethical whenever there is a proven therapy available, according to the Declaration of Helsinki. The two ethical counter-arguments that can be made are the notion that withholding of active treatment may not lead to any harm to the patient depending on the underlying condition and, second, that patients in fact give their informed consent, after being fully informed, to their participation in a placebo-/sham-controlled trial.

In the field of clinical BPH research, the American Urological Association (AUA), the FDA, and the World Health Organization (WHO) advocate rather strictly the use of placebo controls.

The AUA BPH Clinical Trials Subcommittee is currently preparing a blueprint for the design and reporting of clinical trials in BPH. It is noted that:

> BPH is a disease characterized by a somewhat unpredictable natural history. A significant minority of patients experience stabilization of symptoms or actual improvement. Moreover, improvements in symptoms and uroflow are seen in patients treated with placebo. This makes a randomized, placebo (or sham)-controlled design mandatory . . . New surgical technologies should be compared to standard surgical treatments, such as TURP or TUIP, utilizing a randomized design. For BPH medical therapies and minimally invasive technologies, efficacy relative to placebo or sham must be established. (Personal communication by John D. McConnell)

The document furthermore stipulates that patients have to be blinded towards the assigned treatment and that, preferentially, the treating physician also be blinded (double-blind).

The FDA has circulated a Draft Guidance for the Clinical Investigation of Hyperthermia Devices Used for the Treatment of BPH. This document stipulates that the study protocol should include a randomized active control, which best can be accomplished by a blinded, sham-treated control. The FDA specifically discusses the use of a watchful waiting control or historical controls, and expresses concern regarding both these suggestions: the watchful waiting control does not assess the placebo effect of repeated catheterization, which is part of the heat treatment, and the historical TURP control group might not be well matched, owing to different selection criteria and evaluation methodologies. However, the use of an active, randomized, concurrent TURP control group is recommended, to enhance further the evaluation of hyperthermia therapy. This draft guidance document has not yet been finalized, but it is widely used in the design of trials for hyperthermia devices or other minimally invasive treatment modalities [such as thermotherapy, transurethral needle ablation of the prostate (TUNA) or high-intensity focused ultrasound (HIFU)].

The International Consultation on BPH[17] has published, under the patronage of the WHO in 1991 and 1993, a consensus document that addresses the standardization of the evaluation of treatment modalities. The following recommendations were made: 'Technologies aiming to imitate the tissue ablative effect of TURP should be compared with TURP', while 'Technologies not claiming such . . . effect should be tested against a sham (placebo) treatment arm'; 'Pharmacological treatments for BPH should be compared with an appropriate control. The most appropriate control for pharmacological treatments is a placebo arm'. The recommendations of the 3rd Consultation, which met in 1995, will be almost identical to the one quoted above.

Despite the ethical concerns voiced by some, with regard to BPH treatment trials there appears to be unanimity between physicians, industry, the US Government (FDA) and the WHO regarding the mandatory use of placebo-/sham-control groups, at least in those trials considered pivotal for a new treatment.

Placebo effects in other fields of medicine

Blackwell et al.[18] chose the setting of a medical-school class to demonstrate the range of possible placebo effects. Fifty-six second-year medical student volunteers were conditioned to expect either stimulant or sedative effects but, in fact, all received placebo in either one or two blue or pink capsules without knowing that the number and colour of the capsules dispensed differed between the volunteers. Following the ingestion of the study medication, 30% of participants reported drug-associated changes, which were severe in some of the participants: two capsules produced more changes than one, and blue capsules were associated with more sedative effects than the pink capsules.

Physicians are powerful therapeutic agents, and their (placebo) influence can be felt to a greater or lesser degree at every consultation. In an unusual study, 200 patients with non-specific symptoms but no definite diagnosis were selected for one of four consultations — a positive consultation with therapy (thiamine hydrochloride 3 mg tablets) or without treatment, or a negative consultation with or without treatment.[19] In a positive consultation, the patient was given a firm diagnosis and told that he would be better in a few days: if no treatment was given, he was told he needed none; if treatment was given, he was told that the treatment would make him better, with certainty. In a negative consultation the doctor stated that he could not be sure about the diagnosis and that therefore no treatment was given (no treatment group), or that a treatment would be tried without assuring that it would help (treatment group). During the period to the follow-up visit, 64% of patients in the positive consultation group improved versus 39% in the negative consultation group ($p=0.001$); however, there was no significant difference between the treated (53%) and the untreated (50%) patients ($p=0.5$). In this example, the physician-related placebo effect was clearly stronger than the effect conveyed by the medication.

The largest body of literature regarding placebo effects exists in the area of pain treatment. Turner et al.[11] identified over 150 papers describing placebo effects in pain treatment and research. They found that placebo response rates vary greatly. Frequently, they were found to be higher than the widely accepted one-third placebo response rate based on the classic article by Beecher.[20] Placebos have time–effect curves, and peak, cumulative and carry-over effects similar to those of active medications. A certain placebo-responder personality could not be identified, and the roles of anxiety, expectations and learning were emphasized. The authors conclude that placebo effects plus natural history, and regression to the mean,[21] may result in high rates of good outcomes in pain treatment, that may be misattributed to specific treatment effects. The important role of the physician as administrator of the treatment for pain, be it active or placebo, was emphasized by Gracely et al.[22] Dental patients were told that they would receive either a placebo, a narcotic analgesic, or a narcotic antagonist, and that this treatment might increase, decrease, or have no effect on their pain. The physicians administering the drugs knew, however, that one group of patients would receive either placebo or the narcotic antagonist but not the narcotic analgesic (group A), while another group would receive either one of the three agents (group B). Thus, the two groups of placebo-treated patients in groups A and B differed only in the clinician's knowledge of the range of possible double-blind treatments, including the knowledge that patients in group A had no chance of receiving active pain medication; nevertheless, the placebo-treated patients in group B had significantly less pain than those in group A. This experiment shows clearly that analgesia depends not only on the action of the treatment administered, but also on the expectations of the patient and — most surprisingly — on those of the physician, who may influence the patient's response by a subtle behavioural change. This phenomenon of expectation and anticipation of analgesia must be taken into account when designing a crossover study, as patients' past experience of pain relief (i.e. during phase I of a crossover trial) may influence their subsequent (i.e. during phase II of a crossover trial) response to treatment.[23]

Surgical procedures may also have a very strong placebo effect, as described earlier by Beecher.[24] A most striking and classic example is the history of internal mammary artery ligation for the treatment of angina pectoris, which was popular in the first half of the 20th century as a means of increasing blood flow to the coronary circulation. Beecher analysed the early experience and divided the reports in to those written by 'enthusiasts' versus those of 'sceptics': the former group found complete relief of chest pain in 71/213 patients (38%); the latter in only 6/56 (10%).[24] Cobb et al.[25] and Diamond et al.[26] performed a double-blind study (the cardiologist was blinded as to the procedure performed by the cardiac surgeon) of internal mammary artery ligation versus a sham procedure, namely skin incision only, and published remarkably similar results: Cobb et al. reported a 63% significant improvement and 34% decrease in the use of nitroglycerine use in the ligation group versus a 56% improvement and 42% decrease in nitroglycerine use in the sham group; Diamond et al. reported a 100% improvement in both groups regarding exercise tolerance, nitroglycerine use and angina pain. During the year after surgery, 69% of patients reported over 50% improvement in pain in the ligation group versus 100% who experienced an over

50% improvement in the sham group. In a very recent review, Johnson[27] discussed the possible placebo effect of extracorporeal shock wave lithotripsy (ESWL) for gallstones. In a randomized trial comparing ESWL with open cholecystectomy, the symptomatic response was similar in both groups but, surprisingly, the symptomatic response in the ESWL group was identical whether or not the stones had actually been cleared. Thus, the symptomatic response might be triggered, at least in part, by a placebo effect.

Comparatively little is known about the placebo effects on healthy volunteers in clinical pharmacology trials. Rosenzweig et al.[23] reviewed adverse events reported during placebo administration in 109 double-blind placebo-controlled studies involving 1228 volunteers. The overall incidence of adverse events was 19%, and complaints were more frequent after repeated dosing (28%) and in elderly subjects (26%). The most frequent adverse events were headache (7%), drowsiness (5%) and asthenia (4%). The overall incidence and distribution of adverse events appeared also to depend on the nature of the active investigational drug in the young volunteers in single-dose studies. The highest incidence of all adverse events was noted when the active drug had a central nervous system effect (16.7%); the incidence was lower when the active drug had miscellaneous effects (16.2%) or a cardiovascular system effect (6.1%).

Natural history and watchful waiting versus placebo effect

The importance of placebo-/sham-controlled trials in BPH research is emphasized by the highly variable natural history of the disease, and the tendency towards spontaneous improvement and regression documented in several watchful waiting studies and — to a lesser degree — in longitudinal studies of the natural history of the disease. Whereas natural history studies refer to the longitudinal study of a cohort of men with signs and symptoms of BPH over time, without any kind of treatment intervention, the watchful waiting studies usually entail at least a yearly follow-up visit with a 'treating' physician. According to the discussion above, this consultation may have a profound impact on the 'natural history' of the disease process, depending on the attitude and behaviour of the physician. It is probably reasonable to expect that at the end of each visit the physician would tell the patient that 'he is doing well and does not need any (additional or active) treatment', a statement that carries with it a considerable placebo effect. Even in a natural history study, the members of the study population have to be seen, interviewed and examined at regular intervals, thus providing for the possibility of a placebo effect. Longitudinal natural history studies may provide, none the less, the best information about the 'background activity' of the disease process. Watchful waiting studies add at least one known and powerful placebo effect, and they carry with them the possibility of 'treatment failure' and conversion to a presumably more active treatment. Lastly, placebo-/sham-control groups add additional non-specific effects, thus their outcomes, theoretically, should be superior to those of watchful waiting and natural history studies.

Natural history of BPH

The most informative natural history study to date is the Olmsted County Study of Urinary Symptoms and Health Status among Men, which has provided much information about the prevalence and severity of urinary symptoms, bother, worry and embarrassment, quality of life due to symptoms, and the relationship between symptoms and other parameters such as flow rates, prostate volume and prostate-specific antigen (PSA).[28–34] Recently, 4-year follow-up data regarding the changes in symptoms, bother and prostate volume were presented. On the basis of transrectal ultrasonography (TRUS), the growth of the prostate in these men (40–79 years old) was estimated to be about 0.6 ml/year, or 6 ml per decade of life. However, prostate growth followed an exponential growth pattern, with a slope estimate of 0.4 ml/year for men aged 40–59 years at baseline and of 1.2 ml/year for those aged 60–79 years at baseline.[35] Of 904 men reporting none to mild symptoms [AUA Symptom Index (AUA-SI) 0–7 points] at baseline, 118 reported moderate to severe symptoms (AUA-SI >7 points) at 18 months, and 196 at 42 months follow-up.[36] However, 47 men who had developed moderate to severe symptoms at 18 months had none to mild symptoms at 42 months. Bother followed a pattern similar to the symptom frequency,

and the change in AUA-SI was strongly correlated to changes in bother ($r=0.64$; $p<0.001$). Overall there was a slight increase in AUA-SI over the 42 months of follow-up (mean=0.72; SD=4.33; $p<0.001$). These data indicate the measurable progression of lower urinary tract symptoms over time in up to 4 years of follow-up in a randomly chosen community-based cohort of men aged 40–79 years old, who had not sought advice or treatment for these symptoms prior to enrolment in the study. They do, however, also give an indication of the tendency towards spontaneous remission in symptoms that may be seen in a subset of patients.

Diokno et al.[37] have given estimates of the prevalence, incidence and remission of lower urinary tract symptoms in 803 community-dwelling men aged 60 years or older. The annual incidence of prostate surgery was 2.6 and 3.3% during years 1 and 2 of follow-up. The prevalence of at least one symptom was 35%, with annual incidence rates during years 1 and 2 of follow-up of 16.4 and 16.1%. Remission was also noted, in that 22.9% of those having severe symptoms at baseline were asymptomatic at follow-up. Table 21.2 details the changes in symptom severity from one survey to the next. The tendency for fluctuation and spontaneous remission of symptoms, as well as the regression to the mean, become evident from an analysis of these data.

Watchful waiting studies

In the absence of other longitudinal natural history studies, several watchful waiting studies are available for review. Most of these studies have significant shortcomings: inclusion and exclusion criteria are poorly defined, follow-up is loose, assessment instruments are either not defined or insufficient, and patient accounting is incomplete.

Five such studies, reported between 1919 and 1988 and totalling 456 patients, with follow-up ranging from 3 to 6 years,[38–42] were analysed for the Agency for Health Care Policy and Research (AHCPR) BPH Guidelines.[43] A change in symptom status was reported for all 456 patients, although none of the studies utilized a quantitative symptom-severity scale. Data on urinary flow rate and residual urine were available for 223 and 197 patients, respectively. The peak urinary flow rate deteriorated in 66% and improved in 20%. Residual

Table 21.2. *Changes in status of obstruction severity from one survey to the next*

Obstruction severity	Year	No. of patients	Severity in following year (percentage of patients)*			
			None	Mild	Moderate	Severe
None	Baseline	293	83.6	12.3	2.7	1.4
	Year 1	223	83.9	9.0	2.2	4.9
Mild	Baseline	88	18.2	55.7	11.4	14.8
	Year 1	84	33.3	52.4	8.3	6.0
Moderate	Baseline	38	7.9	31.6	26.3	34.2
	Year 1	27	3.7	33.3	22.2	40.7
Severe	Baseline	35	22.9	17.1	11.4	48.6
	Year 1	31	9.7	22.6	12.9	54.8

*Patients who underwent prostatectomy in the preceding year were excluded from the subsequent survey. (Adapted from ref. 37 with permission.)

urine increased (35%), decreased (37%) and remained unchanged (28%) in about the same number of all patients. The mean change in peak flow rate (in those patients for whom data are available) was 2.2 (from a mean of 9.0 to 11.2) ml/s or 24%, while the mean change in residual urine was +37 (from a mean of 115 to 152) ml or 32%. The data on symptom improvement were dichotomized (improved versus not improved). The probability of symptom improvement was then calculated using the confidence profile method (CPM) described by Eddy.[44] The mean probability of improvement in symptom severity was estimated to be 42.5% [90% confidence interval (CI) 30.8–54.8] — surprisingly similar to the probability of improvement noted in the placebo arms and in a carefully designed, prospective study discussed below (Fig. 21.2). It must, however, be recognized that, because of limitations of the dataset, the magnitude of the improvement cannot be estimated.

Recently, a randomized study with a 3-year follow-up was reported comparing watchful waiting with TURP in 556 men with symptoms of BPH[45] (Fig. 21.2). Inclusion criteria included a Madsen–Iversen symptom score between 10 and 20 points (0–27-point scale), thus limiting the informational value of the watchful waiting arm of the study to patients with moderate lower urinary tract symptoms. There were 47 treatment failures (defined as death, recurrent infection, residual urine volume over 350 ml, development of bladder calculus,

incontinence, a symptom score of 24 or higher, or a doubling of serum creatinine from baseline) in the watchful waiting arm (n=276) versus 23 in the surgery arm (n=280) over 3 years of follow-up (relative risk 0.48; 95% CI 0.3–0.77). Sixty-five (24%) men assigned to watchful waiting underwent surgery during follow-up, 20 of them for treatment failure. The majority of these men were classified as more bothered at baseline (Fig. 21.3). It should be noted that about 40% of patients in

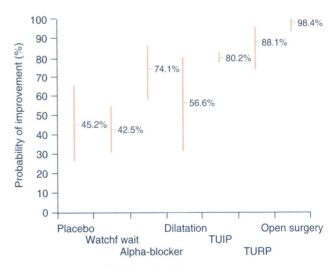

Figure 21.2. *Probability of achieving symptom improvement following various treatment interventions (Watchf wait, watchful waiting; TUIP, transurethral incision of the prostate; TURP, transurethral resection of the prostate). Mean probability and 90% confidence interval calculated with the confidence profile method (ref. 44) using hierarchical Bayes'. (Adapted from ref. 43.)*

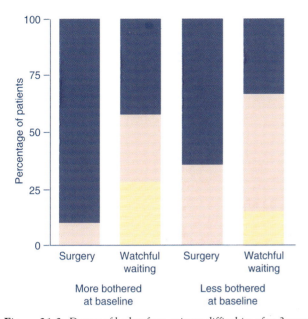

Figure 21.3. *Degree of bother from urinary difficulties after 3 years of follow-up (■, improved; ▨, worse, or no change; ▨, cross-over to surgery) among men with BPH managed with transurethral resection or watchful waiting, according to the degree of bother at baseline. A total of 148 men in the surgery group and 155 in the watchful waiting group were classified as more bothered by urinary difficulties at baseline (score > 55); 73 men in the surgery group and 97 in the watchful waiting group were classified as less bothered at baseline (score ≤ 55).*

this category experienced improvement in the degree of bother from urinary difficulties (Fig. 21. 3). The changes from baseline for the watchful waiting patients are shown in Table 21.3. It should be noted that the mean changes represented in almost all categories an improvement for those men who were followed in the assigned treatment arm (watchful waiting) over 3 years. The magnitude of the improvement, however, was less than that realized by surgery in almost all categories (*p* values in Table 21.3). Furthermore, this analysis excludes those men who were categorized as treatment failures, underwent surgery (crossover) or were lost to follow-up.

Placebo arms of controlled medical treatment trials for BPH

For the AHCPR BPH Guidelines, data on 1417 patients treated in 45 placebo arms of placebo-controlled trials were analysed.[43] Table 21.4 and Figure 21.2 allow a direct comparison between the watchful waiting and the placebo studies. For none of the examined parameters can a significant difference between the two treatment modalities be identified. However, several points merit discussion. As opposed to the long-term follow-up in the watchful waiting studies, the placebo studies are part of short- to mid-term medical treatment trials, ranging from 3 days to 52 weeks in duration (mean 13 weeks). In all these studies the patients are blinded as to the treatment arm and thus have, in most cases, at least a 50/50 (or better in case of 2:1 or 3:1 randomization) chance of receiving active drug. Dropping out of such studies because of failure does not have the same implications that it has in watchful waiting studies, where the patients willingly assume a conservative treatment approach knowing that it might fail (i.e. they might fail and go on to active treatment). In contrast, in some placebo-controlled studies a promise — either

Table 21.3. *Changes from baseline for men followed over 3 years in a watchful waiting protocol*

Outcome	Baseline (n=276)	Follow-up*	Mean change±SD	*p* value[†]
Symptom score (0–27)	14.6	9.1	−5.5±5.2	<0.001
Residual urine (ml)	113	72	−41±90	0.015
Peak flow rate (ml/s)	12.5	12.7	0.4±9.2	<0.001
Bother from urinary difficulties[‡]	46.3	57.6	9.6±29.7	<0.001
Sexual performance[‡]	42.5	35.6	−3.2±26.6	0.92
Activities of daily living[‡]	69.0	75.6	6.4±30.3	<0.001
General well being[‡]	71.2	71.4	0.1±28.3	0.217
Social activities[‡]	74.2	73.1	−1.7±23.5	0.945

*Only patients who were followed over 3 years, excluding crossovers, failures, etc. [†]For difference between treatment groups (surgery versus watchful waiting). [‡] On a scale from 0 (greatest impairment) to 100 (least impairment). (Adapted from ref. 45 with permission.)

Table 21.4. *Comparison of outcomes following watchful waiting and placebo treatment*

Outcomes	Watchful waiting	Placebo
Total number of patients in database	456	1417
Peak flow rate		
Probability of flow rate increase (%)	19.7	35.8
Probability of no change in flow rate (%)	14.2	41.1
Probability of flow rate decrease (%)	66.1	23.1
Mean pretreatment flow rate (ml/s)	9.0	9.1
Mean post-treatment flow rate (ml/s)	11.2	9.7
Difference (ml/s)	+2.2	+0.6
Percentage change in peak flow rate	+24.4	+6.6
Residual urine		
Probability of decrease in residual urine (%)	35.0	38.0
Probability of residual urine remaining unchanged (%)	28.0	26.1
Probability of increase in residual urine (%)	37.0	35.9
Mean pretreatment residual urine (ml)	115	87
Mean post-treatment residual urine (ml)	152	76
Difference (ml)	+37	−11
Percentage change in residual urine	+32.2	−12.6
Symptom improvement		
Probability of symptom improvement (%)	41.7	41.7
Probability of symptoms remaining unchanged (%)	25.8	53.5
Probability of symptom worsening (%)	32.4	4.7
Mean probability of symptom improvement* (%)	41.7	41.7
90% confidence interval for symptom improvement* (%)	30.8–54.8	26.3–65.1

*Calculated by confidence profile method (ref. 44) using hierarchical Bayes'.

tacit or overt — is made, stating that, following the conclusion of the trial, the patient would be eligible for either 'free' active treatment, or he would be 'moved up' on the surgical waiting list (this phenomenon is unique to those studies conducted in the UK). The inactive preparation given should, theoretically, add to the placebo effect and, thus improve the outcome above those noted for watchful waiting studies. The probability of a patient experiencing improvement, however, is estimated to be about 40% in the uncontrolled watchful waiting studies, the randomized watchful waiting versus TURP study, and the combined placebo arms. The changes in peak flow rate and residual urine are similar — and similarly minor — for these three groups as well (see Tables 21.3 and 21.4). Figure 21.4 shows a comparison of the percentage changes in peak flow rate and residual urine as well as the percentage of patients experiencing symptom

improvement between various treatment modalities. It becomes evident that a 40% rate of patients reporting improvement, and the minimal fluctuation of peak flow rate and residual urine, represent the 'placebo effect' background against which the more substantial changes in these parameters achieved by active treatment modalities must be seen.

With the advent of symptom-severity assessment tools or symptom scores, it is possible to describe quantitatively the response of patients treated by a variety of treatment interventions, including placebo and watchful waiting (see Chapter 42). Unfortunately, the different symptom-scoring instruments differ regarding their foot points (0 or different from 0), their scale and, occasionally, even their direction (increasing or decreasing severity of symptoms with increasing score). While, currently, the AUA-SI,[46–48] with its scale from 0 to 35 points, is the most widely utilized instrument, thus

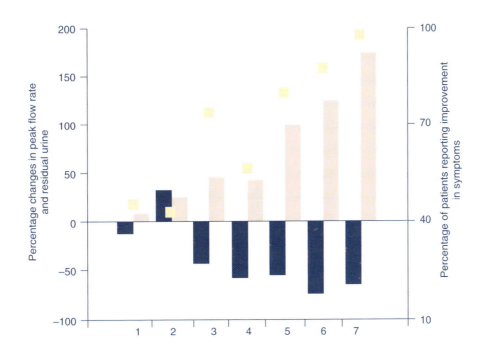

Figure 21.4. *Percentage changes in peak flow rate (■) and residual urine ( ), and percentage of patients reporting improvement in symptoms ( ) following various treatment interventions (1, placebo; 2, watchful waiting; 3, alpha-blocker; 4, dilatation; 5, transurethral incision of the prostate; 6, TURP; 7, open surgery). (Adapted from ref. 43 with permission.)*

facilitating direct comparisons between studies, in past years different scores with different scales were used. The only way to compare symptom improvement in different trials quantitatively in such cases is to rescale the individual scales to a 100% scale, and to express the changes as the drop in percentage symptom score from before to after treatment. Using this technique, seven placebo-controlled trials were reanalysed and compared with the most significant watchful waiting study[45] (Fig. 21.5). These seven trials enrolled between 11 and 267 subjects per arm, lasted from 4 to 24 weeks, and utilized an injectable steroid hormone (norprogesterone),[49] a prolactin inhibitor (bromocriptine),[50] an H_2-blocker (cimetidine),[51] an alpha-blocker (alfuzosin),[52] or candicin[53–55] as the 'active' drug. Each study is represented by its active and the placebo arm, side by side. Several points are noteworthy. The pretreatment symptom-severity score expressed as a percentage of the achievable score on a 100% scale ranges from 35 to almost 60%, and the drop in symptom severity from 7 to 33% for the placebo arms. Moreover, the pre- to post-treatment symptom-score range does not even overlap between some of the trials

listed, indicating that vastly different patient populations were treated. Specifically addressing the three placebo-controlled double-blind trials using candicin as the active drug, the drops in symptom score were 9, 15 and 33% (placebo), and 6, 26 and 22% (candicin). With the exception of the bromocriptine trial, the baseline symptom severity was reasonably similar between the placebo and the active treatment arm, and in all such cases the placebo response closely matched the active drug response. These observations allow several conclusions: (1) a strong placebo response is noted in medical treatment trials for BPH when quantitative symptom-severity scores are used; (2) the placebo response in medical treatment trials for BPH depends largely on the pretreatment characteristics of the treated cohort; (3) even when the baseline symptom severity is similar between two trials (A and B), the response of the placebo group in trial A matches more closely its actively treated cohort than the placebo group in trial B; (4) the latter fact indicates that factors other than the active drug or placebo are primarily responsible for the placebo effect. These factors may include patient selection criteria (solicitation,

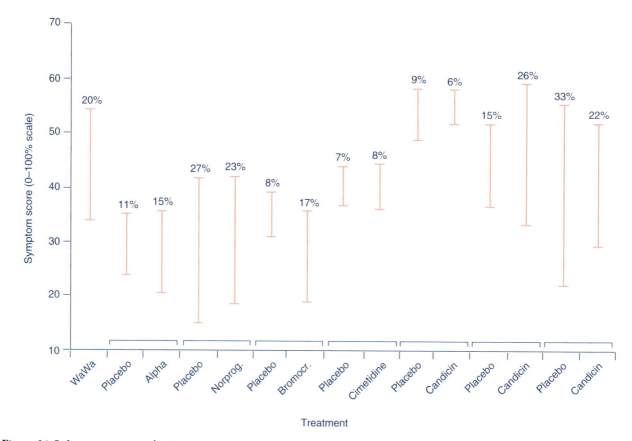

Figure 21.5. *Improvements noted using a quantitative symptom score in seven placebo-controlled trials and a watchful waiting (WaWa) study. Because of the different scales used, all scores were rescaled to a 100% scale and the reported changes were expressed as mean pretreatment and mean post-treatment percentage symptom scores. The percentage above the vertical bar indicates the change noted following treatment. Norprog, norprogesterone; bromocr, bromocriptine; alpha, alpha-blocker (alfuzosin).*

advertising), design and duration of study, incentives offered to patients (financial or otherwise), conduct and attitude of the treating physician or research coordinator (sympathetic versus unsympathetic, friendly versus unfriendly, positive versus negative), and other unrecognized factors. In fact, given the parallel changes in both treatment groups in most trials, the latter factors, which are provider factors, are more likely to be responsible than the previously mentioned patient factors.

It could be reasoned that placebo-treated patients enrolled with similar inclusion and exclusion criteria into clinical trials using the same class of active drugs might have a similar placebo response. A comparison of three alpha-1-receptor-blocker trials allows this hypothesis to be tested: 82 patients were treated with doxazosin versus placebo over 16 weeks,[56] 2064 patients with terazosin versus placebo over 52 weeks,[57] and 296

patients with tamsulosin versus placebo over 12 weeks.[58] In all three trials, a different symptom score was used: in the doxazosin trial, the scale ranged from 0 to 30 points, in the terazosin trials from 0 to 35 points (AUA-SI) and in the tamsulosin trial from 0 to 27 (Boyarsky score). In Figure 21.6 all scores are rescaled to a 100% scale and the pre- and post-treatment mean scores are expressed as a percentage of the 100% scale. Although the pretreatment symptom severity differs in the three trials, the placebo responses are very similar, ranging from 8.1 to 10.6% on the 100% scale, roughly half of the active drug cohort in each trial.

Improvements in peak urinary flow rates are also similar between these three drug trials, ranging from 0.4 to 0.8 ml/s in the three placebo groups, despite the fact that the baseline mean peak flow rates are rather different (Fig. 21.7). It should be noted that this improvement in peak flow rate is very similar to the

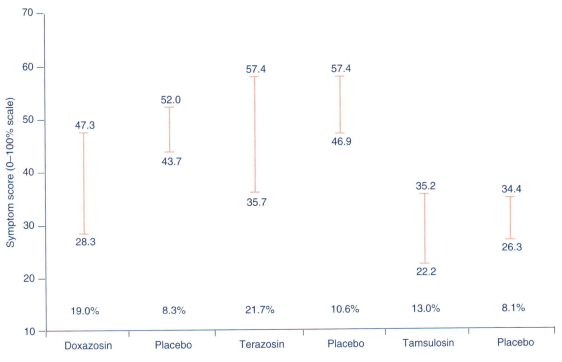

Figure 21.6. *Pre- and post-treatment mean symptom scores (upper and lower horizontal rules of vertical bar) rescaled to 100% for active drug- and placebo-treated cohorts in three randomized alpha-blocker trials (for details see text). The percentage at the bottom of the graph represents the improvement achieved.*

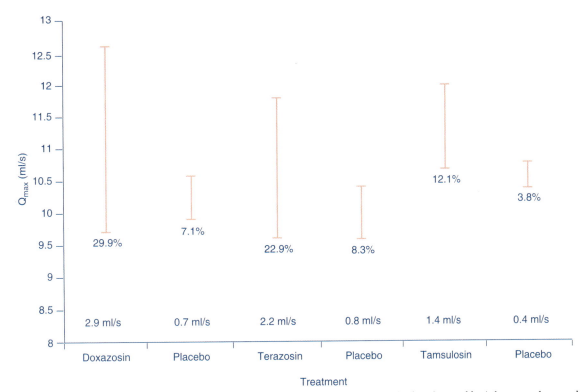

Figure 21.7. *Pre- and post-treatment mean peak flow rates (Q_{max}; lower and upper horizontal rules of vertical bar) for active drug- and placebo-treated cohorts in three randomized alpha-blocker trials (for details see text). The percentage below the vertical line indicates the percentage improvement in mean peak flow rate, while the ml/s value at the bottom of the graph represents the absolute mean improvement.*

mean changes noted in the combined placebo arm analysis (0.6 ml/s),[43] and the watchful waiting study (0.4 ml/s).[45] The percentage improvement calculated for the combined placebo arms (6.6%) falls also in the range of improvements seen in these three alpha-blocker trials (3.8–8.3%) (Fig. 21 7).

Sham arms of controlled device treatment trials for BPH

In recent years a multitude of minimally invasive device treatments for BPH have been developed and tested in randomized, sham-controlled, open, single or even double-blind trials. Although the majority of these trials compare various types of heat treatments (transrectal or transurethral hyperthermia or thermotherapy) with a sham treatment, one investigator compared balloon dilatation with 'sham' cystoscopy alone in a randomized, double-blind trial involving 33 men with BPH.[14] Blinding of the patients was effective in that an equal number of patients in each arm thought that they had undergone balloon dilatation. After 3 months, 40% of balloon-dilated patients noted marked improvement, while 27% noted no change; after cystoscopy, 63% had marked improvement and 12% no change. The changes in symptom score were significant at 3 months in both groups, whereas the peak urinary flow rate changes did not differ significantly from baseline in either group (Table 21.5). Most importantly, there was no difference in the symptom score or peak flow rate data at 3 months between the 'active' and the 'sham' treatment. This study is widely used to support the notion that balloon dilatation has no role in the treatment of BPH, and is not better than placebo/sham treatment.

Figures 21.8 and 21.9 analyse the outcomes of the balloon dilatation versus cystoscopy trial, one multicentre trial using transrectal or transurethral hyperthermia in comparison with a sham control,[59] and five transurethral microwave thermotherapy (TUMT) trials and their respective sham control arms.[60–63] The following observations can be made. The baseline or pretreatment mean symptom severity expressed as a percentage of total achievable severity (rescaled to 100%) differs from trial to trial. The mean improvements in symptom severity in the sham groups ranged from 5.2 to 15.6% (on a 100% scale), whereas the active thermotherapy-treated patients had improvements ranging from 27.0 to 37.8%, or in most cases twice the improvement of that of the sham control. The multicentre hyperthermia trial is the exception, in that the actively treated cohort has an improvement similar to that of the sham control, which is well within the range of the other sham-control trials. The changes in peak urinary flow rate follow a similar pattern (Fig. 21.9): with the exception of TUMT trials 2 and 4, the changes in peak flow rate are either very modest improvements or deteriorations (0.5 and 0.6 to 0.2 and 1.0 ml/s, respectively), whereas the active treatment arms report substantial improvements (with the exception of the hyperthermia trial). The changes noted in the sham arms (and the largely ineffective hyperthermia treatment arm) are very similar to those observed after alpha-blocker therapy (see Figs 21.6 and 21.7). Both thermotherapy trial 5 and the terazosin trial have similar entry criteria and baseline mean symptom severity. The improvements noted in the placebo and sham arms were 3.3 points (10.6%) and 2.6 points

Table 21.5. *Outcomes at 3 months following balloon dilatation or cystoscopy in a randomized, double-blind study*

Parameter	Procedure	Measurement		*p* value	
		Baseline	3 months	Baseline vs 3 months	Cystoscopy vs balloon dilatation at 3 months
Peak flow rate (ml/s)	Cystoscopy	10.5	12.9	n.s.	0.48
	Balloon dilatation	9.2	11.5	n.s.	
Symptom score	Cystoscopy	11.9	8.8	<0.01	0.33
	Balloon diltaation	12.4	7.5	<0.05	

(From ref. 14 with permission.)

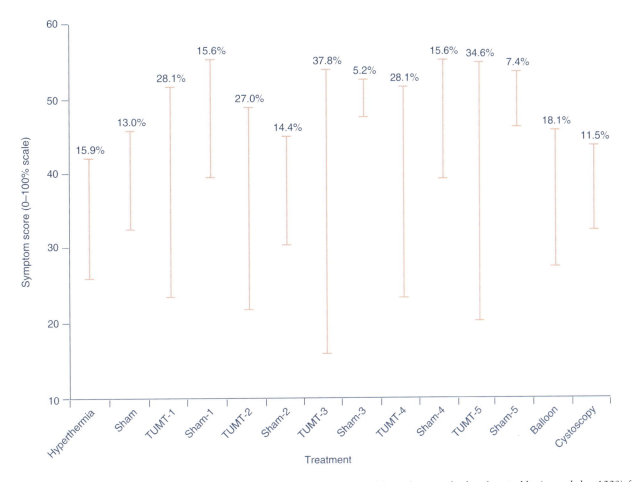

Figure 21.8. *Pre- and post-treatment (3 months) mean symptom scores (upper and lower horizontal rules of vertical bar) rescaled to 100% for active-treated and sham-treated patients in a multicentre hyperthermia trial, five transurethral microwave thermotherapy (TUMT) trials, and a balloon dilatation versus cystoscopy trial. The percentage improvement is noted above the horizontal rule.*

(6.4%), respectively, whereas in the active treatment arms the improvements were 7.6 points (21.7%) and 12.1 points (34.6%), respectively (see Fig. 42.7).

Placebo/sham effect and baseline symptom severity

An area of considerable interest is that of to what degree the placebo/sham effect depends on the baseline status of the patients. This could pertain to baseline symptom severity, baseline bother, quality of life, baseline flow rate, and all other imaginable parameters. Although very few investigators have thus far reported data stratified by baseline parameters, the results of a multicentre placebo-controlled 12-month alpha-blocker (terazosin) trial can be analysed.[57] Figure 21.10 shows

the absolute and percentage improvement in AUA symptom score for the placebo- and drug-treated patients stratified in six strata by symptom severity: whereas the active drug-treated cohort has almost twice the improvement within each stratum, the placebo-treated patients have improvements ranging from 1.6 points (4.6%) to 7.5 points (21.4%). The placebo improvements for the entire placebo cohort were 3.3 points (10.6%). A similar increase in the placebo effect with increasing baseline symptom severity has been reported for patients treated with finasteride in the phase III trials.[64] Data for minimally invasive treatment modalities have not been reported and thus it can only be speculated that the baseline symptom severity may also affect the sham effect seen in these trials. This

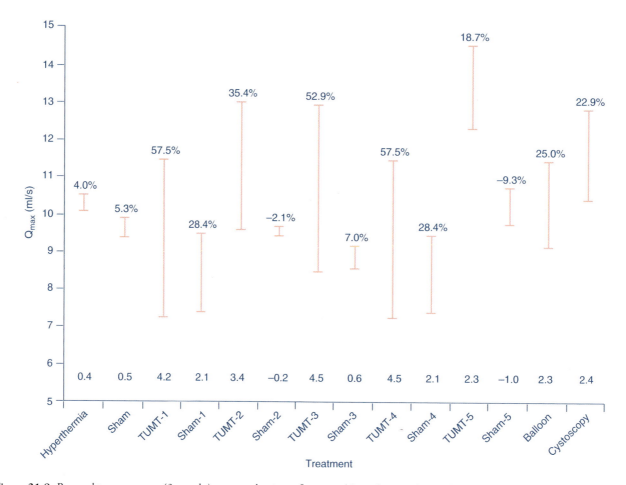

Figure 21.9. *Pre- and post-treatment (3 months) mean peak urinary flow rates (Q_{max}; lower and upper horizontal rules of vertical bar) for active-treated and sham-treated patients in a multicentre hyperthermia trial, five TUMT trials, and a balloon dilatation versus cystoscopy trial. The percentage changes are noted above the horizontal rules and the absolute improvement (or deterioration) (in ml/s) at the bottom of the graph.*

phenomenon may be attributable to increased expectations in patients with more severe baseline symptoms, or simply to a regression to the mean.

Relationship between placebo/sham effect and perception of improvement

Barry et al.[65] recently reported an important observation after assessing the relationship between changes in the AUA-SI and patients' global rating of improvement in over 1200 men treated in a medical treatment trial for BPH. They noted that a mean decrease in AUA-SI of 3.1 points was associated with a slight improvement; however, this relationship was strictly dependent on the baseline AUA-SI (Fig. 21.11). For patients to perceive a slight, moderate or marked improvement, increasing

drops in AUA-SI were required with increasing baseline symptom severity. In Figure 21.11 this relationship is illustrated graphically for slight, moderate and marked improvement. The symbols indicate the improvement in AUA-SI noted in the already mentioned alpha-blocker trial active drug and placebo arms.[57] It is evident that, for every symptom-severity stratum, the improvement in the placebo arm fell roughly on the 'slight' improvement line, which is the minimum improvement noticeable to patients: thus, for each baseline symptom severity level, patients treated with placebo would have a noticeable symptom improvement; however, the patients treated with active drug experienced, in all strata analysed, at least a 'moderate' improvement.

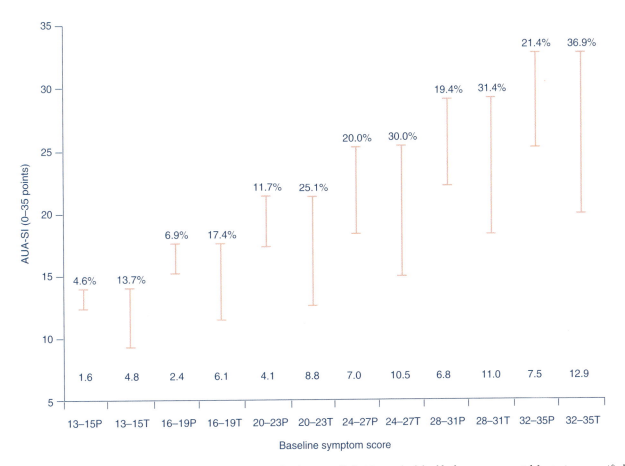

Figure 21.10. *Improvements in symptom score recorded in a placebo-controlled, 12-month alpha-blocker treatment trial for patients stratified in six baseline symptom-severity strata [along x-axis labelled as P (placebo) and T (terazosin treated)]. The percentage improvement (100% scale) and the absolute changes (at the bottom of the graph) are shown.*

Summary and conclusions

The data discussed demonstrate fairly convincingly that, in both medical and minimally invasive device treatment trials for BPH, a placebo/sham effect must be expected. This effect is surprisingly stable across different trials and different treatment modalities: about 40% of patients experience some unspecified degree of improvement, albeit marginal, in watchful waiting and placebo-/sham-control cohorts. Improvements in symptom severity scores range from 5 to 15% (about 2–5 points using the AUA-SI ranging from 0 to 35 points) for placebo-/sham-treated cohorts, whereas changes in peak urinary flow rate are, in general, more modest, ranging from actual deterioration to improvements of 1.0 ml/s, with few exceptions. The magnitude of this effect is similar to that seen in watchful waiting studies.

Of great importance is the observation that the magnitude of the improvement correlates directly with the baseline symptom severity. Patients' perceptions of improvement also correlate with baseline symptom severity and, in general, a greater drop in symptom score is associated with a global rating of a slight, moderate or marked improvement with increasing baseline symptom score. In the limited datasets available, the placebo effect for each symptom-severity stratum is of a magnitude associated with a global perception of slight improvement.

The statement that treatment for BPH is associated with a '40% placebo/sham effect' is clearly an inadequate oversimplification. More detailed and sophisticated analyses of responses in placebo-/sham-treated cohorts of men with BPH are needed to further our understanding of the complex relationship between

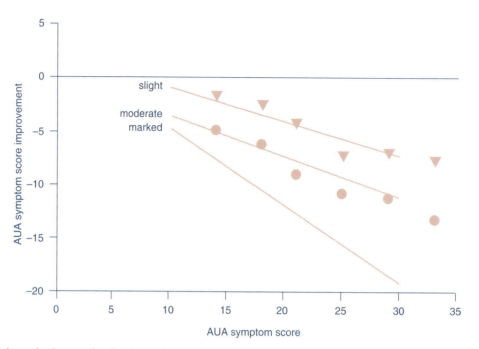

Figure 21.11. *Relationship between baseline (x-axis) symptom score and absolute changes in scores for subjects rating global improvement as slight, moderate or marked. The symbols (▼, placebo; ●, alpha-blocker) indicate the absolute drops in symptom scores from baseline for patients treated in a placebo-controlled, 12-month alpha-blocker treatment trial stratified in six strata by baseline symptom severity. (Adapted from ref. 65 with permission.)*

patients' expectations, baseline symptom severity, bother, quality of life, nature and invasiveness of the active treatment arm, and the responses noted with regard to symptom, bother, quality of life, and indirect outcomes such as urinary flow rates. Only once a matrix of these responses and their predictors has been established will we be able to judge newly developed treatments for BPH against the backdrop of their associated placebo/sham effects.

References

1. Shaw P. The reflector: representing human affairs, as they are; and may be improved. 1750. Cited in: Claridge G, Drugs and human behavior. London: 1970

2. Hill A B. Medical ethics and controlled trials. Br Med J 1963; 1: 1043–1049

3. Pepper O H P. A note on placebo. Ann J Pharm 1945; 117: 409–412

4. Kennedy W P. The nocebo reaction. Med Word 1961; 344: 203–205

5. White L, Tursky B, Schwartz G E. Placebo in perspective. In: White L, Tursky B, Schwartz G E (eds) Placebo. Theory, research, and mechanism. New York: Guilford Press, 1985: 3–6

6. Shapiro A K, Morris L A. The placebo effect in medical and psychological therapies. In: Garfield S L, Bergin A E (eds) Handbook of psychotherapy and behavior change. New York: Wiley, 1978: 371

7. Brody H. Placebos and the philosophy of medicine. Chicago: University of Chicago Press, 1977

8. Grünbaum A. Explication and implications of the placebo concept. In: White L, Tursky B, Schwartz G E (eds) Placebo. Theory, research, and mechanisms. New York: Guilford Press, 1985: 9–36

9. Brody H. Placebo effect: an examination of Grünbaum's definition. In: White L, Tursky B, Schwartz G E (eds) Placebo. Theory, research, and mechanisms. New York: Guilford Press, 1985: 37–58

10. White L, Tursky B, Schwartz G E. Proposed synthesis of placebo models. In: White L, Tursky B, Schwartz G E (eds) Placebo. Theory, research, and mechanisms. New York: Guilford Press, 1985: 431–448

11. Turner J A, Deyo R A, Loeser J D et al. The importance of placebo effects in pain treatment and research. JAMA 1994; 271: 1609–1614

12. Coronary Drug Project Research Group. Influence of adherence to treatment and response of cholesterol on mortality in the coronary drug project. N Engl J Med 1980; 303: 1038–1041

13. Finkel M J. Placebo controls are not always necessary. In: White L, Tursky B, Schwartz G E (eds) Placebo. Theory, research, and mechanisms. New York: Guilford Press, 1985: 419–428

14. Lepor H, Sypherd D, Machi G, Derus J. Randomized double-blind study comparing the effectiveness of balloon dilation of the prostate and cystoscopy for the treatment of symptomatic benign prostatic hyperplasia. J Urol 1992; 147: 639–644

15. Rothman K J, Michels K B. The continuing unethical use of placebo controls. N Engl J Med 1994; 331: 394–398

16. Declaration of Helsinki IV, World Medical Association, 41st World Medical Assembly HK September 1989. Placebo controls are not always necessary. In: Annas G J, Grodin M A, Schwartz G E (eds) The Nazi doctors and the Nuremberg Code: human rights in human experimentation. New York: Oxford University Press, 1992: 331–342

17. Cockett A T K, Aso Y, Denis L et al. Recommendations of the International Consensus Committee. In: Cockett A T K, Khoury S, Aso Y et al. (eds) The 2nd International Consultation on Benign Prostatic Hyperplasia (BPH). Jersey, Channel Islands: SCI, 1993: 553–564

18. Blackwell B, Bloomfield S S, Buncher C R. Demonstration to medical students of placebo responses and non-drug factors. Lancet 1972; 294: 1279–1282

19. Thomas K B. General practice consultations: is there any point in being positive? Br Med J 1987; 294: 1200–1202

20. Beecher H K. The powerful placebo. JAMA 1955; 159: 1602–1606

21. Whitney C W, Von Korff M. Regression to the mean in treated versus untreated chronic pain. Pain 1992; 50: 281–285

22. Gracely R H, Dubner R, Deeter W R, Wolskee P J. Clinicians' expectations influence placebo analgesia. Lancet 1985; 294: 43

23. Rosenzweig P, Brohier S, Zipfel A. The placebo effect in healthy volunteers: influence of experimental conditions on the adverse events profile during phase I studies. Clin Pharmacol Ther 1993; 54: 578–583

24. Beecher H K. Surgery as placebo. JAMA 1961; 176: 1102–1107

25. Cobb L A, Thomas G I, Dillard D H et al. An evaluation of internal-mammary-artery-ligation by a double-blind technic. N Engl J Med 1959; 260: 115–118

26. Diamond E G, Kittle C F, Crockett J E. Comparison of internal mammary ligation and sham operation for angina pectoris. Am J Cardiol 1960; 5: 483–486

27. Johnson A G. Surgery as placebo. Lancet 1994; 344: 1140–1142

28. Oesterling J E, Jacobsen S J, Chute C G et al. Serum prostate-specific antigen in a community-based population of healthy men. JAMA 1993; 270: 860–864

29. Guess H A, Chute C G, Garraway W M et al. Similar levels of urological symptoms have similar impact on Scottish and American men — although Scots report less symptoms. J Urol 1993; 150: 1701–1705

30. Jacobsen S J, Girman C J, Guess H A et al. Natural history of prostatism: factors associated with discordance between frequency and bother of urinary symptoms. Urology 1993; 42: 663–671

31. Chute C G, Panser L A, Girman C J et al. The prevalence of prostatism: a population-based survey of urinary symptoms. J Urol 1993; 150: 85–89

32. Oesterling J E, Girman C J, Panser L A et al. Correlation between urinary flow rate, voided volume, and patient age in a community-based population. Prog Clin Biol Res 1994; 386: 125–139

33. Girman C J, Epstein R S, Jacobsen S J et al. Natural history of prostatism: impact of urinary symptoms on quality of life in 2115 randomly selected community men. Urology 1994; 44: 825–831

34. Roberts R O, Jacobsen S J, Rhodes T et al. Cigarette smoking and prostatism: a biphasic association? Urology 1994; 43: 797–801

35. Rhodes T, Girman C J, Jacobsen S J et al. Longitudinal measures of prostate volume in a community-based sample: 3.5 year followup in the Olmsted County study of health status and urinary symptoms among men. J Urol 1995; 153: 301A

36. Jacobsen S J, Girman C J, Guess H A et al. Natural history of prostatism: four-year change in urinary symptom frequency and bother. J Urol 1995; 153: 300A

37. Diokno A C, Brown M B, Goldstein N, Herzog A R. Epidemiology of bladder emptying symptoms in elderly men. J Urol 1992; 148: 1817–1821

38. Clarke R. The prostate and the endocrines. 1919; : 254–271

39. Craigen A A, Hickling J B, Saunders C R, Carpenter R G. Natural history of prostatic obstruction. J R Coll Gen Pract 1969; 18: 226–232

40. Birkhoff J D, Wiederhorn A R, Hamilton M L, Zinsser H H. Natural history of benign prostatic hypertrophy and acute urinary retention. Urology 1976; 7: 48–52

41. Ball A J, Feneley R C, Abrams P H. The natural history of untreated 'prostatism'. Br J Urol 1981; 53: 613–616

42. Kadow C, Feneley R C, Abrams P H. Prostatectomy or conservative management in the treatment of benign prostatic hypertrophy? Br J Urol 1988; 61: 432–434

43. McConnell J D, Barry M J, Bruskewitz R C et al. Benign prostatic hyperplasia: diagnosis and treatment. Clinical Practice Guideline, Number 8. Rockville, Md: Agency for Health Care Policy and Research, Public Health Service, US Department of Health and Human Services, 1994

44. Eddy D M, Hasselblad V. FAST*PRO. Software for meta-analysis by the confidence profile method. San Diego: Academic Press/Harcourt Brace Jovanovich, 1992

45. Wasson J H, Reda D J, Bruskewitz R C et al. A comparison of transurethral surgery with watchful waiting for moderate symptoms of benign prostatic hyperplasia. The Veterans Affairs Cooperative Study Group on Transurethral Resection of the Prostate. N Engl J Med 1995; 332: 75–79

46. Barry M J, Fowler F J Jr, O'Leary M P et al. Correlation of the American Urological Association symptom index with self-administered versions of the Madsen–Iversen, Boyarsky and Maine Medical Assessment Program symptom indexes. Measurement Committee of the American Urological Association. J Urol 1992; 148: 1558–1563

47. Barry M J, Fowler F J Jr, O'Leary M P et al. The American Urological Association symptom index for benign prostatic hyperplasia. The Measurement Committee of the American Urological Association. J Urol 1992; 148: 1549–1557

48. O'Leary M P, Barry M J, Fowler F J Jr. Hard measures of subjective outcomes: validating symptom indexes in urology. J Urol 1992; 148: 1546–1548

49. Aubrey D A, Khosla T. The effect of 17-alpha-hydroxy-19-norprogesterone caproate (SH582) on benign prostatic hypertrophy. Br J Surg 1971; 58: 648–652

50. Van Poppel H, Boeckx G, Westelinck K J et al. The efficacy of bromocriptine in benign prostatic hypertrophy. A double-blind study. Br J Urol 1987; 60: 150–152

51. Lindner A, Ramon J, Brooks M E. Controlled study of cimetidine in the treatment of benign prostatic hypertrophy. Br J Urol 1990; 66: 55–57

52. Jardin A, Bensadoun H, Delauche-Cavallier M C, Attali P. Alfuzosin for treatment of benign prostatic hypertrophy. The BPH-ALF Group (see comments). Lancet 1991; 337: 1457–1461

53. Abrams P H. A double-blind trial of the effects of candicidin on patients with benign prostatic hypertrophy. Br J Urol 1977; 49: 67–71

54. Jensen K M, Madsen P O. Candicidin treatment of prostatism: a prospective double-blind placebo-controlled study. Urol Res 1983; 11: 7–10

55. Madsen P O, Dorflinger T, Frimodt-Moeller P C, Jensen K M. Candicidin in treatment of benign prostatic hypertrophy. J Urol 1984; 132: 1235–1238

56. Gillenwater J Y, Conn R L, Chrysant S G et al. Doxazosin for the treatment of benign prostatic hyperplasia in patients with mild to moderate essential hypertension: a double-blind, placebo-controlled, dose-response multicenter study. J Urol 1995; 154: 110–115

57. Roehrborn C G, Oesterling J E, Auerbach S et al. Effectiveness and safety of terazosin versus placebo in the treatment of men with symptomatic benign prostatic hyperplasia in the HYCAT study. 1995: :

58. Abrams P, Schulman C C, Vaage S, Stavanger. The efficacy and safety of 0.4 mg tamsulosin once daily in symptomatic BPH. J Urol 1995; 153: 274A

59. Abbou C C, Colombel M, Payan C et al. The efficacy of microwave induced hyperthermia in the treatment of BPH: the Paris public hospitals' experience. Prog Clin Biol Res 1994; 386: 449–453

60. Ogden C W, Reddy P, Johnson H et al. Sham versus transurethral microwave thermotherapy in patients with symptoms of benign prostatic bladder outflow obstruction. Lancet 1993; 341: 14–17

61. Blute M L, Tomera K M, Hellerstein D K et al. Transurethral microwave thermotherapy for management of benign prostatic hyperplasia: results of the United States Prostatron Cooperative Study (see comments). J Urol 1993; 150: 1591–1596

62. De la Rosette J J, de Wildt M J, Alivizatos G et al. Transurethral microwave thermotherapy (TUMT) in benign prostatic hyperplasia: placebo versus TUMT. Urology 1994; 44: 58–63

63. Bdesha A S, Bunce C J, Snell M E, Witherow R O. A sham controlled trial of transurethral microwave therapy with subsequent treatment of the control group. J Urol 1994; 152: 453–458

64. Gormley G J, Stoner E, Bruskewitz R C et al. The effect of finasteride in men with benign prostatic hyperplasia. The Finasteride Study Group (see comments). N Engl J Med 1992; 327: 1185–1191

65. Barry M J, Williford W O, Chang Y C et al. BPH-specific health status measures in clinical research: how much change in AUA Symptom Index and the BPH Impact Index is perceptible to patients? J Urol 1995; 154: 1770–1774.

22

Finasteride therapy for benign prostatic hyperplasia
J. D. McConnell

Introduction

Finasteride is a potent inhibitor of 5 alpha-reductase, the intracellular enzyme that converts testosterone to dihydrotestosterone (DHT). Clinical studies have shown this compound to be effective in reducing the volume of the prostate, so improving the obstructive component of benign prostatic hyperplasia (BPH). There are, however, limitations to the efficacy of finasteride, causing researchers to conclude that the importance of DHT in established BPH has been, to some extent, overestimated.

Dihydrotestosterone and BPH

The prostate gland is androgen dependent, requiring a source of testosterone for its growth, development, differentiation and function. The development of BPH clearly requires a combination of testicular androgens and ageing;[1–3] the role of the former is more probably permissive than causative. Evidence for this comes from the fact that men castrated before puberty do not develop BPH, and that genetic diseases that inhibit androgen production or action result in impaired or non-existent prostatic growth. In addition, studies on androgen withdrawal therapies have clearly shown regression of established BPH. The return of the prostate to a normal volume may be harder to achieve; even castration (medical or surgical) is not successful in this. Partial involution may be insufficient to relieve the obstructed bladder.

Within the prostate, testosterone is converted to DHT. Levels of this androgen are not elevated with age or in BPH, despite a decrease in plasma testosterone.[4] DHT preferentially binds to the androgen receptor in target cells and the formation of the DHT–androgen receptor complex is critical to the subsequent role of androgens in stimulating both normal and hyperplastic growth.[3] Downregulation of androgen-receptor levels after puberty has been noted in certain androgen-dependent tissues, so limiting further androgen-dependent growth. This does not appear to occur in the ageing prostate[3] or in BPH,[5,6] hence, androgen-dependent growth continues.[3]

5 Alpha-reductase

Two 5 alpha-reductase enzymes have been identified, each encoded by a separate gene.[7–9] The predominant enzyme in extraprostatic tissues (e.g. skin, liver) is type 1 5 alpha-reductase and is normally expressed in 5 alpha-reductase deficiency syndrome. Type 2 5 alpha-reductase is the major, if not only, form of the enzyme expressed in prostatic tissues, and is also expressed in extraprostatic tissues; it is absent in 5 alpha-reductase deficiency syndrome. In terms of sensitivity to finasteride, type 1 enzyme is poorly inhibited whereas type 2 is extremely sensitive.

The role of the type 1 form of the enzyme in normal and abnormal prostate growth is yet to be defined; trace levels of type 1 mRNA have been detected in normal prostates, although the protein itself has not been identified in BPH or prostatic cancer tissue.[10] Type 2 enzyme is critical to normal development of the prostate and hyperplastic growth later in life. Its location within the prostate is primarily the stroma.[11] Acinar epithelial cells uniformly lack type 2 protein, whereas some basal epithelial cells stain positively.

Individuals with a deficiency in 5 alpha-reductase were first observed in the 1960s. The condition was termed 'pseudovaginal perineoscrotal hypospadias' and involved a 46,XY karyotype, normally differentiated testes, male internal ducts and ambiguous genitalia. As adults, the prostate in these patients is non-palpable, despite otherwise normal virilization at puberty. Walsh et al.[12] and Imperato-McGinley et al.[13] described two groups of patients with this inherited form of male pseudohermaphroditism due to deficient DHT production. A genetic mutation in the type 2 isozyme gene was detected that resulted in defective or deficient 5 alpha-reductase enzyme activity.[14] At puberty in these patients, the increase in gonadotropins stimulates a significant rise in testosterone levels, which allows the production of external virilization. As type 1 5 alpha-reductase activity is normal, plasma DHT is detectable, suggesting that circulating DHT may have a true endocrine effect on androgen-dependent tissues. Adult men with this disorder have normal muscular development and male sexuality, and other organ systems function normally.

A rationale was developed for the treatment of BPH following the discovery of this rare genetic mutation. It was thought possible that an inhibitor of 5 alpha-reductase could reduce prostatic growth without affecting sexual function or breast growth, as seen with other androgen withdrawal therapies. In addition, as the enzyme's only activity is to convert testosterone to DHT, then total blockade of the enzyme should not lead to significant adverse effects.

Development of finasteride

A variety of 4-azosteroid 5 alpha-reductase inhibitors were synthesized that lacked affinity for the androgen receptor. N-(2-Methyl-2-propyl)-3-oxo-4-aza-5-alpha-androst-1-ene-17-beta-carboxamide (MK–906; finasteride; Proscar[TM]), one such compound, significantly decreased DHT levels in the hyperplastic canine prostate and also reduced the prostatic volume by up to 64%.[15] Further studies on finasteride showed that it is a potent, reversible inhibitor of type 2 5 alpha-reductase that can suppress plasma DHT levels (by approximately 80–90%) without affecting testosterone levels[16–19] — a fact that is critically important in terms of maintaining normal libido and sexual function. Intraprostatic testosterone levels are elevated, however, which may affect treatment efficacy. Uninhibited type 1 enzyme activity may explain the failure of finasteride to decrease serum and prostatic DHT levels to zero.[20]

Clinical development of finasteride

Clinical trials designed to determine the safety and efficacy of finasteride in men with BPH have been completed. A 6-month, placebo-controlled phase II study of finasteride in a limited number of patients with BPH resulted in a 30% decrease in prostatic size and a statistically significant improvement in urinary flow rate;[21] these results are comparable to those with other androgen withdrawal therapies. Although there was a trend towards symptom improvement, this effect of finasteride did not differ statistically from placebo. The limited numbers of patients in this trial do not permit an adequate assessment of clinical efficacy.

The safety and efficacy of finasteride has been assessed in two international multicentre, phase III trials.[7,22] These large-scale trials, in combination, treated 533 men with 5 mg finasteride for 12 months; an equal number were given placebo (Table 22.1). In the North American trial after 12 months of finasteride therapy, a 70% reduction in serum DHT and a 19% reduction in prostatic volume were recorded.[23] Maximal urinary flow rate improved by 1.6 ml/s in the finasteride group compared with 0.7 ml/s in the placebo group. Following the initial placebo run-in phase, there was a mean decrease in total symptom score of 2.6 in the finasteride treatment group. Results from the international study were similar (Table 22.1, Fig. 22.1).[7] Preliminary evidence that finasteride may reduce urodynamic obstruction in a subset of patients requires further study.[8,9,24]

A 3- and 4-year non-controlled extension of a subset of men was also conducted.[25] Analysis of patients maintained on therapy for 36 (n = 192) and 48 (n = 154) months in the North American trial, demonstrated maintenance of the effects on prostatic volume, urinary flow rate and symptom score (Table 22.1).[25,26] Whether the additional improvement seen in urinary flow and symptom score between months 12 and 48 represents ongoing improvement, as opposed to dropout of unresponsive patients, is not clear; maintenance of response for up to 5 years has been recorded in a smaller number of men.[27] The lack of a control group in the extension study, as well as the small growth rate of the prostate, prevents these data from being used as unequivocal proof that finasteride prevents further progression of BPH.

A 2-year, placebo-controlled Scandinavian finasteride study has recently been completed.[28] The objectives were to study whether placebo-induced improvements in men with symptomatic BPH could be maintained over a 2-year period, and to study the efficacy and safety of 2 years of therapy with finasteride. This multicentre study involved 707 men with moderate symptoms of BPH who were randomized into

Table 22.1. *Multicentre phase III trials of finasteride: summary of finasteride efficacy variables at month 12 of the controlled study, and months 36 and 48 of the extension*

	North American study			
	Controlled study, month 12		Extension, month 36	Extension, month 48
Change from baseline	Placebo (n = 299)	5 mg (n = 291)	5 mg[†] (n = 192)	5 mg (n = 154)
DHT (median; %)	3.2	−70.0***	−75**	NR[‡]
Prostate volume (median; %)	−3.0	−19.2***	−26.6**	−23.8
Maximum urinary flow (mean; ml/s)	0.7	1.6*	2.4**	+2.2
Total symptom score (mean)	−1.0	−2.6*	−3.6**	−3.6

	International study			
	(n = 254)	(n = 242)	(n = 105)	(n = 85)
DHT (median; %)	0.0	59.6***	NR	NR
Prostate volume (median; %)	−6.1	−26.0***	−27.1**	−29.4
Maximum urinary flow (mean; ml/s)	0.4	1.3*	2.3**	+2.6
Total symptom score (mean)	−2.6	−3.9*	−3.6**	−4.0

[†]All patients received finasteride 5 mg for 36 months. [‡]NR = not recorded. Asterisks indicate significant differences from placebo (*$p < 0.05$; ***$p < 0.01$) or baseline (**$p < 0.01$).

two groups, to receive finasteride (5 mg) or placebo. Symptoms were defined and quantified according to a previously defined symptom questionnaire.[29] Modified Boyarsky symptom scores for finasteride patients improved throughout the study, with the difference between the two groups reaching significance at 2 years ($p < 0.01$) (Table 22.2, Fig. 22.2). In the placebo group, there was an initial improvement in the symptom score but no change from baseline at 24 months. The maximum urinary flow rate decreased in the placebo group, but improved in the finasteride group, resulting in a between-group difference of 1.8 ml/s at 2 years

($p < 0.01$). Prostate volumes increased by 12% in the placebo group and decreased by 19% in the finasteride group ($p < 0.01$). Substantially fewer patients in the finasteride treated group than in the placebo group developed urinary retention during the study, 4 (1.1%) versus 15 (4.2%) ($P = 0.02$). In addition, a lower incidence of the need for prostate surgery was reported in the finasteride group, 0 versus 9 (2.5%) ($P \leq 0.01$). Finasteride was generally well tolerated throughout the study period. On the basis of the results of the study it was concluded that the improvements produced by finasteride in the treatment of BPH can be maintained

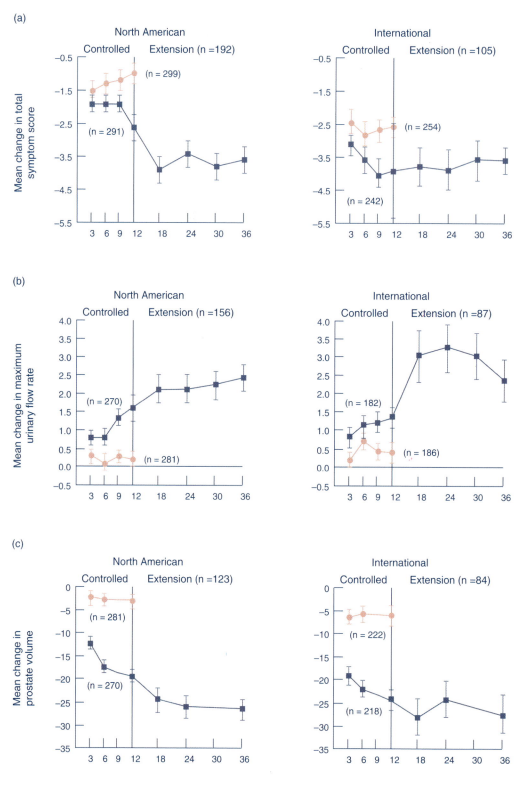

Figure 22.1. *Mean changes (± SE) from baseline in (a) total symptom score improvement, (b) maximum urinary flow rate and (c) prostate volume. (From ref. 25 with permission.)* ● *Placebo,* ■ *finasteride 5 mg.*

Table 22.2. *Results of the Scandinavian multicentre study of finasteride vs placebo in a total of 707 men: 2 year data*

Change from baseline	Placebo	Finasteride (5 mg)
Prostate volume (mean; %)	11.5 (n = 197)	−19.2*[†] (n = 197)
Maximum urinary flow (ml/s)	−0.3 (n = 309)	1.5*[†] (n = 308)
Total symptom score (units)	0.2 (n = 346)	−2.0*[†] (n = 347)

Asterisks indicate significant differences from placebo (*$p < 0.01$); daggers indicate significant differences within treatment ([†]$p < 0.01$).

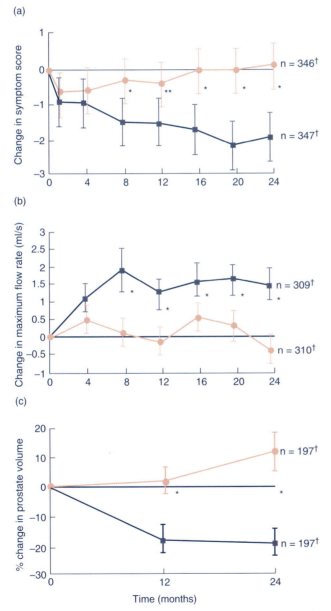

(a)

(b)

(c)

Figure 22.2. *Percentage changes in (a) total symptom scores, (b) maximum urinary flow rate and (c) prostate volume from baseline. Means ± 95% confidence interval. (From ref. 28 with permission.) Difference between treatment groups: * = $p ± 0.01$, ** = $p ± 0.05$.* —●— *Placebo,* —■—*Finasteride.* [†] *At 24 months.*

over a 2-year period, whereas no overall improvement — indeed, some deterioration — is seen with placebo.

Improvements in health-related quality of life have been demonstrated in men with BPH administered finasteride.[30,31] The side effects of this therapy also appear to be minimal: 3–4% of patients develop sexually related adverse effects, including abnormalities of ejaculate volume, libido and erectile function (Table 22.3). The rate of adverse effects does not appear to increase with time and does not result in large numbers of patients discontinuing therapy (Table 22.4). An unexpected (low) incidence of impotence was noted, despite the fact that serum testosterone levels are not affected significantly by finasteride. However sleep-related erections were not affected significantly by finasteride, compared with placebo, in a recent sleep laboratory study.[32]

Finasteride partially suppresses the expression of prostate-specific antigen (PSA). It remains to be seen whether this suppression will impact on prostate cancer detection or mortality rates, especially given the uncertain impact of routine PSA measurement on prostate cancer death rates in general. In men on finasteride, the cumulative distribution of serum PSA levels at baseline is nearly identical to the distribution of twice the serum PSA levels after 12 months of treatment.[33,34,35] In such circumstances, therefore, the upper PSA limit should be taken as 2 ng/ml (instead of the normal 4 ng/ml), in which case a PSA level of 3 ng/ml in a man on finasteride is just as elevated as a PSA of 6 ng/ml in a man not on finasteride. Finasteride reduces serum PSA with the same kinetics in men with high (4–10 ng/ml) vs low (<4 ng/ml) PSA levels.[36,37] However, finasteride also reduces serum PSA in men with known prostate cancer.[38,39] In some patients, ultimately diagnosed as having prostate cancer,

Table 22.3. *Finasteride-related adverse experiences*

	Controlled studies (12 months)		Open extension (5 mg)		
	5 mg (n = 543)	Placebo (n = 555)	Year 2 (n = 1325)	Year 3 (n = 1174)	Year 4 (n = 1036)
Decreased libido	3.3	1.6	2.4	1.6	1.5
Ejaculate volume decreased	2.6*	0.9	1.4	0.9	0.3
Impotence	3.7**	1.1	3.2	2.1	2.1
Orgasmic dysfunction	NR†	0.2	0.3	0.1	NR

†NR = not recorded. Asterisks indicate significant differences from placebo (*$p < 0.05$; **$p < 0.01$).

Table 22.4. *Primary reason why patients discontinued therapy with finasteride 5 mg**

	Double-blind		Year 2	Year 3	Year 4†
	5 mg (n = 547)	Placebo (n = 558)	5 mg (n = 1337)	5 mg (n = 1182)	5 mg (n = 1034)
Treatment failure	5.9	6.3	4.3	3.5	1.5
Sexual adverse experience	0.9	0.4	0.7	0.3	0.8
Prostate cancer	0.9	0.7	0.5	0.7	0.9
Death	–	–	0.7	1.2	0.9
Other clinical adverse events	3.5	4.5	2.3	1.2	1.2
Lost to follow-up	4.2	3.9	2.6	2.5	2.8
Total	15.4	15.8	11.1	9.4	8.1

* Values are percentages. † Rate of discontinuation due to drug-related adverse events over 4-year period was 2.6%.

the serum PSA did not increase in longitudinal follow-up.[34] Certainly, finasteride-induced suppression of the serum PSA does not appear to be a useful test to discriminate cancer from BPH.[39] Further study is needed to determine whether finasteride will suppress the expected rise in PSA in men who develop prostate cancer while on therapy.[22,40,41]

Conclusions

The benefit of finasteride over placebo in the treatment of BPH has been demonstrated in randomized, placebo-controlled trials. Approximately one-third to one-half of patients have clinically significant improvements, while modest benefits overall were seen in the study population. Uncontrolled studies suggest that the response to therapy may be sustained for up to 4 years, although it is yet to be determined whether the progression of BPH with time can be prevented. Given its minimal side effects, finasteride should be considered an acceptable treatment option for BPH. With regard to prostate cancer, patients should be informed of the effect finasteride has in lowering serum PSA levels and the potential impact this may have on the detection of prostate cancer.

References

1. Coffey D S, Berry S J, Ewing L L. An overview of current concepts in the study of benign prostatic hyperplasia. In: Rodgers C H (ed). Benign prostatic hyperplasia. Vol 2. Bethesda: National Institutes of Health, 1987

2. Walsh P C. Benign prostatic hyperplasia. In: Walsh P C, Gittes R F, Perlmutter A D, Stamey T A (eds). Campbell's urology, vol. 2, 5th ed. Baltimore: Saunders, 1985

3. Wilson J D. The pathogenesis of benign prostatic hyperplasia. Am J Med 1980; 68: 745–756

4. Walsh P C, Hutchins G M, Ewing L L. Tissue content of dihydrotestosterone in human prostatic hyperplasia is not supranormal. J Clin Invest 1983; 72: 1772–1777

5. Robel P, Eychenne B, Blondeau J P et al. Sex steroid receptors in normal and hyperplastic prostate. Prostate 1985; 6: 255–267

6. Barrack E R, Bujnovszky P, Walsh P C. Subcellular distribution of androgen receptors in human normal, benign hyperplastic, and malignant prostatic tissue: characterization of nuclear salt-resistant receptors. Cancer Res 1983; 43: 1107–1106

7. Finasteride Study Group. Finasteride (MK-906) in the treatment of benign prostatic hyperplasia. Prostate 1993; 22: 291–299

8. Kirby R S, Bryan J, Eardley I et al. Finasteride in the treatment of benign prostatic hyperplasia: a urodynamic evaluation. Br J Urol 1992; 70: 65–72

9. Tammela T L J, Kontturi M J. Urodynamic effects of finasteride in the treatment of bladder outlet obstruction due to benign prostatic hyperplasia. J Urol 1993; 149: 342–344

10. Silver R I, Wiley E L, Davis D L et al. Expression and regulation of steroid 5 α-reductase 2 in prostate disease. J Urol 1994a; 152: 433–437

11. Silver R I, Wiley E L, Thigpen A E et al. Cell type specific expression of steroid 5 α-reductase 2. J Urol 1994b; 152: 438–442

12. Walsh P C, Madden J D, Harrod M J et al. Familial incomplete male pseudohermaphroditism, Type 2: decreased dihydrotestosterone formation in pseudovaginal perineoscrotal hypospadias. New Engl J Med 1974; 291: 944–949

13. Imperato-McGinley J, Guerrero L, Gautier T, Peterson R E. Steroid 5 α-reductase deficiency in man: an inherited form of male pseudohermaphroditism. Science 1974; 186: 1213–1215

14. Thigpen A E, Davis D L, Milatovich A et al. Molecular genetics of steroid 5 α-reductase 2 deficiency. J Clin Invest 1992; 90: 799–809

15. Brooks J R, Berman C, Garnes D et al. Prostatic effects induced in dogs by chronic or acute oral administration of 5 α-reductase inhibitors. Prostate 1986; 9: 65–75

16. Rittmaster R S, Stoner E, Thompson D L et al. Effect of MK–906, a specific 5 α-reductase inhibitor, on serum androgens and androgen conjugates in normal men. J Androl 1989; 10: 259–262

17. Vermeulen A, Giagulli V A, Schepper P D et al. Hormonal effects of an orally active 4-azasteroid inhibitor or 5 α-reductase in humans. Prostate 1989; 14: 45–53

18. McConnell J D, Wilson J D, George F W et al. Finasteride, an inhibitor of 5 α-reductase, suppresses prostatic dihydrotestosterone in men with benign prostatic hyperplasia. J Clin Endocrinol Metab 1992; 74: 505–508

19. Norman R W, Coakes K E, Wright A S, Rittmaster R S. Androgen metabolism in men receiving finasteride before prostatectomy. J Urol 1993; 150: 1736–1739

20. Thigpen A E, Silver R I, Guileyardo J M et al. Tissue distribution and ontogeny of steroid 5 α-reductase isozyme expression. J Clin Invest 1993; 92: 903–910

21. Stoner E and the Finasteride Study Group. The clinical effects of a 5 α-reductase inhibitor, finasteride on benign prostatic hyperplasia. J Urol 1992; 147: 1298–1302

22. Gormley G J, Stoner E, Bruskewitz R C et al. The effect of finasteride in men with benign prostatic hyperplasia. New Engl J Med 1992; 327: 1185–1191

23. Jenkins E P, Andersson S, Imperato-McGinley J et al. Genetic and pharmacological evidence for more than one human steroid 5 α-reductase. J Clin Invest 1992; 89: 293–300

24. Kirby R S, Vale J, Bryan J et al. Long-term urodynamic effects of finasteride in benign prostatic hyperplasia: a pilot study. Eur Urol 1993; 24(1): 20–26

25. Stoner E and the Finasteride Study Group. Three year safety and efficacy data on the use of finasteride in the treatment of benign prostatic hyperplasia. Urology 1994; 43: 284–294

26. Lepor H, Stoner E. Long-term results of medical therapies for benign prostatic hyperplasia. Curr Opin Urol 1995; 5: 18–24

27. Geller J. Five year follow-up of patients with benign prostatic hyperplasia treated with finasteride. Eur Urol 1995; 21: 267-73

28. Anderson J T, Ekman P, Wolf H et al. Can finasteride reverse the progress of BPH? A two year placebo controlled study. Urology 1995; 46(5): 631–637

29. Bolognese J A, Kozloff R C, Kunik S C et al. Validation of a symptoms questionnaire for benign prostatic hyperplasia. Prostate 1992; 21: 247–254

30. Byrnes C A, Morton A S, Liss C L et al. Efficacy, tolerability and effect on health-related quality of life of finasteride compared to placebo in men with symptomatic benign prostatic hyperplasia: the community-based urology study of Proscar. Clin Ther 1995; 17(5): 956–969

31. Girman C J, Kolman C, Liss C L et al. Effects of finasteride on health-related quality of life in men with benign prostatic hyperplasia. (Submitted)

32. Cunningham G R, Hirshkowitz M. Inhibition of steroid 5 α-reductase with finasteride: sleep-related erections, potency, and libido in healthy men. J Clin Endocrin 1995; 80: 1–7

33. Stoner E, Guess H. Treatment of benign prostatic hyperplasia with 5 α-reductase inhibitors. Endocrinologist 1995; 5: 140–146

34. Stoner E and the Finasteride Study Group. Clinical experience of the detection of prostate cancer in patients with benign prostatic hyperplasia treated with finasteride. J Urol 1994; 151: 1296–1300

35. Guess H A, Heyse J F, Gormley G J. The effect of finasteride on prostate-specific antigen in men with benign prostatic hyperplasia. Prostate 1993; 22: 31–37

36. Waldstreicher P F, Tocker J C, Shown T E et al. The effects of finasteride on serum prostate specific antigen (PSA) in men with benign prostatic hyperplasia. J Urol 1995; 153: 396a

37. Guess H A, Gormley G J, Stoner E, Oesterling J E. The effect of finasteride on prostate-specific antigen: review of available data. J Urol; 155: 3–9

38. Andriole G, Lieber M, Smith J et al. Treatment with finasteride following radical prostatectomy for prostate cancer. Urology 1995;45(3): 491–497

39. Bach M A, Tucker P F, Malice M P et al. The effects of finasteride on serum prostate specific antigen in men with benign prostatic hyperplasia and prostate cancer. J Urol 1995; 153: 397a

40. Brawley O W, Thompson I M. Chemoprevention of prostate cancer. Urology 1994; 43: 594–599

41. Tsukamoto S, Akaza H, Imada S et al. Chemoprevention of rat prostate carcinogenesis by use of finasteride or Casodex. J Natl Cancer Inst 1995; 87: 842–844

Epristeride: a new 5 alpha-reductase inhibitor for the treatment of benign prostatic hyperplasia

C. R. Chapple Y. J. Lamb R. K. Knight M. A. Levy

23

Introduction

It is clear from clinical laboratory data that prostate growth exhibits dependence on androgens. Those individuals with genetic defects in the synthesis of androgens or defective androgen receptors have small underdeveloped prostates. Despite a reduction in the serum testosterone with ageing, intraprostatic androgen levels remain high. In contrast, castration of boys prior to puberty prevents the development of benign prostatic hyperplasia (BPH). It has been recognized for more than 100 years that castration or other forms of androgen ablation do also cause some prostatic regression even after development of the disease.

Testosterone production is ultimately controlled by the hypothalamic–pituitary–gonadal axis through the release of gonadotropin-releasing and luteinizing hormones. Although testosterone is the major circulating androgen, 90% of intraprostatic androgen is in the form of dihydrotestosterone (DHT), a 5 alpha-reduced metabolite. The binding of DHT to androgen receptors in the prostate is the critical element in the growth of this androgen-dependent tissue.

It is, therefore, clear that DHT is an essential element in prostate function and possibly in the development of BPH. The enzyme 5 alpha-reductase (type 2 isoenzyme is the predominant form in the prostate) controls the formation of DHT and is a significant therapeutic target. On this basis, the hypothesis has been advanced that inhibition of this enzyme could decrease intraprostatic DHT formation and reduce the size of the prostate. This decrease in prostate volume would reduce bladder outflow obstruction and thereby provide both objective and symptomatic improvement. A great deal of work has been carried out with the index compound for steroid 5 alpha-reductase inhibition, namely finasteride, and this is reviewed in Chapter 22.

Pharmacological actions of epristeride

Epristeride (SK&F 105657, 17-beta-[N-(1,1-dimethylethyl)aminocarbonyl] androsta-3,5-diene-3-carboxylic acid) has been shown to be a potent inhibitor of the steroid 5 alpha-reductase present in human hyperplastic prostate tissues.[1] Furthermore, studies in vitro using recombinant enzymes have shown that epristeride is a selective inhibitor of the type 2 isoform of human 5 alpha-reductase ($K_{i,app}$ = 0.7–2 nM) in comparison with the type 1 enzyme ($K_{i,app}$ = 400–450 nM).[3] It has also been shown to inhibit steroid 5 alpha-reductase activity in rat prostate ($K_{i,app}$ = 10–20 nM), rat epididymis ($K_{i,app}$ = 2–4 nM) and the prostate of the *Cynomolgus* monkey ($K_{i,app}$ <1 nM).[5–7]

Epristeride has also been shown to be an uncompetitive inhibitor against both testosterone and NADPH.[1,8] These results suggest that its inhibitory action results from a preferential association of epristeride to an enzyme binary complex containing NADP. As a uncompetitive inhibitor against testosterone, inhibition by epristeride cannot be overcome completely by an increase of testosterone concentration. By comparison, finasteride is a competitive inhibitor against testosterone as a result of an enzyme complex formed with NADPH.[1,8]

Studies in vitro have shown epristeride to have minimal inhibitory action against several alternative, mechanistically related enzymatic activities. In addition, the compound has been shown to have no detectable affinity for oestrogen, androgen, or other steroid hormone receptors.[3] It therefore provides a specific inhibition of the type 2 enzyme, which is the principal form of 5 alpha-reductase in the human prostate.

Oral administration of epristeride to rats at a dose of 25 mg/kg twice daily reduced the prostatic DHT content of intact animals to the same low level produced by surgical castration. However, unlike castration, treatment with epristeride was followed by an increase of prostatic testosterone of more than fivefold. The decrease of prostatic DHT coupled with increase of prostatic testosterone was specifically due to inhibition in vivo of the 5 alpha-reductase activity as these changes were not observed in rats that had been castrated and maintained with endogenous DHT. Treatment with epristeride was followed by inhibition of prostatic secretion and prostatic glandular cell proliferation and there was an increase of prostatic glandular cell death. However, these effects were less than those observed after surgical castration.

In humans, epristeride is well absorbed when given by mouth and maximal plasma levels are achieved 1.5–3 h after ingestion.[9] Plasma half-life is about 24 h and plasma clearance is low (approximately 0.33 ml/min/kg). Epristeride is 98.9% bound to plasma proteins and this is independent of concentration when present over therapeutic ranges. Steady-state conditions are achieved within one week.

Existing clinical studies of epristeride

Phase I studies

Phase I studies in young healthy males given a single oral dose of epristeride showed a decline of serum DHT concentration of over 50% in 86% of subjects at a median dose of epristeride of 0.25 mg/kg.[7] A dose of at least 0.25 mg/kg sustained serum DHT suppression consistently for more than 24 h.

Other phase I studies compared the effects on plasma DHT concentration of doses of epristeride varying from 0.4 to 160 mg daily and showed that, within this range, the drug was well tolerated and that the pharmacokinetics were similar in young and elderly men. When given at a dose of 0.4 mg daily, epristeride was less effective at suppressing serum DHT levels than higher doses of the drug,[10] and observations indicated that once-daily administration was adequate.

Phase II studies

Two double-blind placebo-controlled trials have been undertaken to measure serum and prostatic DHT levels in men pretreated with epristeride 10–14 days prior to planned transurethral prostatectomy (TURP).[11,12]

Study design

In one of these studies, conducted in the UK,[11] 60 male patients (mean age 66.9 years; range 50–83 years) were recruited for a study to assess the effect of epristeride on plasma and prostatic levels of DHT and testosterone in men with BPH. At the initial visit the presence and severity of symptoms from BPH were established by a full clinical history and physical examination, Madsen–Iversen symptom scores and peak urinary flow rates. BPH had produced symptoms in these patients sufficient to require TURP; patients were included in the study provided that they had no history of previous prostatic surgery, were not in acute or chronic urinary retention and did not have infected urine. Two other exclusion conditions were residual urinary bladder volume of over 250 ml and previous treatment with an alpha-receptor antagonist within the previous week. Fully informed written consent was obtained before entry into the study.

Patients were randomized into four groups to receive epristeride (2, 10 or 80 mg) or placebo by mouth once daily for 10 days prior to a scheduled TURP. Blood samples were taken before treatment was started, before the final dose of study medication and again 2 days after surgery; these were in order that routine biochemical and haematological parameters, as well as plasma epristeride levels, could be measured. Plasma testosterone and DHT levels were measured on days 1 and 10 of the study, immediately before the patient took his last dose of medication. A sample of blood was also taken at the time of induction of anaesthesia for measurement of plasma testosterone and DHT.

Tissue samples were obtained at TUR(P) and frozen to −70°C. These were then assayed for intraprostatic testosterone and DHT levels by selected ion-monitoring mass spectrometry/gas-liquid chromatography.

Effect of epristeride on prostatic DHT and testosterone (Table 23.1)

After 10 days treatment with placebo the mean level of DHT within the prostate was 3.21 ng/g. This was no different from mean prostatic DHT levels (3.21 ng/g) after 10 days' treatment (2 mg/day) with epristeride; however, as dosage of epristeride increased, mean levels of prostatic DHT were reduced to 2.13 ng/g following 10 days' treatment with 10 mg/day and to 0.85 ng/g with

Table 23.1. *Prostatic DHT and testosterone levels*

Epristeride dose (mg/day)	DHT (ng/g)	Testosterone (ng/g)
0 (placebo)	3.21	0.18
2	3.21	0.53
10	2.13	1.05
80	0.85	1.37

80 mg/day. The latter figure represented a reduction of 74% compared with placebo ($p<0.01$).

Mean levels of prostatic testosterone after treatment with placebo were 0.18 ng/g, increasing to 0.53 ng/g with 2 mg/day epristeride, and to 1.05 and 1.37 ng/g with epristeride doses of 10 and 80 mg/day, respectively. Epristeride at each treatment dose was associated with a statistically significant increase of prostatic testosterone compared with placebo ($p<0.05$). Furthermore, intraprostatic testosterone levels recorded in the 10 and 80 mg/day groups of patients were significantly higher than those in patients treated with epristeride at 2 mg/day ($p<0.05$). However, there was no significant difference in intraprostatic testosterone after 10 days' treatment with epristeride at either 10 or 80 mg/day.

Effect of epristeride on plasma DHT and testosterone (Table 23.2)

Treatment at all three doses was followed by a significant reduction of plasma DHT levels when compared with placebo ($p<0.001$). In the placebo group, there was no change of plasma DHT after 10 days of treatment (1.86 nmol/l). After 10 days of epristeride treatment at 2 mg/day, plasma DHT levels were reduced

from 1.77 to 0.88 nmol/l, which did not differ significantly from the fall of plasma DHT levels following the 10 mg/day dosage regimen (1.78–0.72 nmol/l). In addition, there was no significant difference between the reductions in plasma DHT with the 10 mg/day dose of epristeride and those after 80 mg/day (1.9–0.6 nmol/l) but the 80 mg/day regimen was significantly more effective at reducing plasma DHT than was 2 mg/day ($p<0.05$).

For plasma testosterone changes after 10 days' treatment, only the level observed in the 80 mg/day group was significantly greater than that observed with placebo ($p<0.05$).

Tolerability of epristeride

In this study most adverse events that were reported were self-limiting and there was no difference in the incidence of these events between groups treated with placebo or epristeride. Two men, both under treatment with 10 mg/day, were withdrawn because of gastrointestinal events, whereas urinary tract infection was reported as an adverse event in seven others; however, in all cases the investigators' assessment was that the adverse events were unrelated to treatment with epristeride.

Discussion

Similar observations on safety and efficacy were made in the smaller study conducted un the United States.[12]

Epristeride is a promising additional form of pharmacotherapy for BPH. It is effective in reducing levels of prostatic DHT, producing a 74% reduction in prostatic DHT on an 80 mg/day dose regimen, which is

Table 23.2. *Plasma DHT and testosterone levels*

Epristeride dose (mg/day)	DHT (nmol/l)		Testosterone (nmol/l)	
	Before treatment	At 10 days	Before treatment	At 10 days
0 (placebo)	1.86	1.86	12.72	12.89
2	1.77	0.88	10.56	13.17
10	1.78	0.72	11.23	13.58
80	1.90	0.60	11.53	15.10

very comparable to that seen with luteinizing hormone-releasing hormone (LHRH) analogues.[13] In these patients plasma testosterone levels remained within the normal range in all men.

Epristeride is the first uncompetitive inhibitor of the human type 2 steroid 5 alpha-reductase enzyme in clinical development. Epristeride does not bind to steroid hormone receptors. The uncompetitive mechanism of action of this agent is unlikely to be affected by an increase of intraprostatic testosterone during therapy. This may be an important distinguishing feature from finasteride, where there is a competitive inhibition versus testosterone. Inevitably, as a consequence of inhibition of the steroid 5 alpha-reductase enzyme there will be accumulation of testosterone in the prostate. The clinical relevance of this increase in intraprostatic testosterone remains unknown and investigation of this drug is currently the subject of clinical trials. Four large international phase III studies are in progress. The final results of three of these are expected later in 1996.

Preliminary work with tumour cell lines has shown that this agent can attenuate the growth rate of some androgen-responsive prostate cancers, in comparison to finasteride which appears to be inactive in this context.[14,15] This raises the possibility that an uncompetitive inhibitor such as epristeride may prove to be more effective in depleting DHT levels in prostate cancer cells.

References

1. Metcalf B W, Holt D A, Levy M A et al. Potent inhibition of human steroid 5α–reductase (ECI.3.30) by 3–androsten–3–carboxylic acids. Bioorg Chem 1989; 17: 372–376

2. Audet P R, Baine N H, Benincosa L J et al. Epristeride: a steroid 5α–reductase inhibitor, treatment for benign prostatic hyperplasia. Drugs Future 1994; 19: 646–650

3. Peeling W B, Lamb Y J, Levy M A. The effects of epristeride. In: Motta M, Serio M (eds) Sex hormones and antihormones in endocrine dependent pathology: basic and chemical aspects. Excerpta Medica International Congress series 1064. Amsterdam: Elsevier Science, 1994: 19–124

4. Levy M A, Brandt M, Sheedy K M et al. Epristeride as a selective and specific uncompetitive inhibitor of human steroid 5α–reductase isoform 2. J Steroid Biochem Molec Biol 1994; 48: 197–206

5. Holt D A, Levy M A, Oh H-J et al. Inhibition of steroid 5α–reductase by unsaturated 3-carboxysteroids. J Med Chem 1990; 33: 943–950

6. Levy M A, Metcalf B W, Brandt M et al. 3-phosphinic acid and 3-phosphonic acid steroids as inhibitors of steroid 5α–reductase. Species comparison and mechanistic studies. Bioorg Chem 1991; 19: 245–260

7. Audet P, Ilson B, Jorkasky D. Hormonal effects of SK&F 105657, a 5 alpha–reductase inhibitor in normal healthy male subjects. Presented at the International Society of Endocrinology, Nice, France, August 1992. Abstract #13.03.033, p. 446

8. Levy M A, Brandt M, Heys R et al. Inhibition of rat liver steroid 5α–reductase by 3-androstene-3-carboxylic acids. Mechanism of enzyme–inhibitor interaction. Biochemistry 1990; 29: 2815–2824

9. Chapelsky M C, Nichols A, Jorkasky D K et al. Pharmacokinetics and pharmacodynamics of SK&F 105657 in healthy elderly male subjects. Clin Pharmacol Ther 1992; 51: 154

10. Audet P, Nurcombe H, Lamb Y et al. Effects of multiple doses of epristeride, a steroid 5α–reductase inhibitor, on serum dihydro-testosterone (DHT) in older male subjects. Clin Pharmacol Ther 1993; 53: 231

11. Peeling W B, Abrams P, Ramsay J W A et al. Double–blind placebo controlled study to evaluate the pharmacodynamic effect of SK&F 105657 in patients with benign prostatic hypertrophy. Proc Tenth Congress Eur Assos Urol (Genoa) 1992; 240: 148

12. Johnsonbaugh R E, Cohen B R, McCormack E M et al. Effect of 14 days treatment with epristeride an uncompetitive 5 alpha reductase inhibitor on serum and prostatic testosterone (T) and dihydrotestosterone (DHT) in men with benign prostatic hyperplasia (BPH). J Urol 1993; 877: 432A

13. Forti G, Salerno R, Monetri G et al. Three-month treatment with a long-acting gonadotrophin-releasing hormone agonist of patients with benign prostatic hyperplasia: effects on tissue andogen concentrations, 5-alpha-reductase activity and andogen receptor content. J Endocrinol Metab 1989; 68: 461–468

14. Lamb J C, Levy M A, Johnson R K, Isaacs J T. Response of rat and human prostatic cancers to the novel 5α-reductase inhibitor, SK&F 105657. Prostate 1992; 21: 15–34

15. Brooks J R, Berman C, Ngyern H et al. Effect of castration, DES, flutamide, and the 5 alpha-reductase inhibitor, MK-906, on the growth of the Dunning rat prostatic carcinoma, R-3327. Prostate 1991; 18: 215–227

24

Other hormonal treatments

J. D. McConnell

Introduction

Benign prostatic hyperplasia (BPH) is an androgen-dependent process in which oestrogens may have a synergistic role and a variety of treatment strategies based on inhibition of androgen production/action in the prostate have been devised. The rationale for androgen withdrawal therapy for BPH is based on a number of scientific observations. A critical level of prostatic androgen is required to maintain the hyperplastic state and significant involution in the size of the prostate results from androgen withdrawal, leading to a reduction in outflow resistance and improvement in symptoms. In addition, men castrated prior to puberty do not develop BPH, and in patients with a variety of diseases affecting androgen production there is impaired or absent prostatic growth. The pathophysiology of BPH is multifactorial, however, as demonstrated by the observation that androgen withdrawal in humans does not return the hyperplastic prostate to a normal state.

The role of oestrogens in BPH is not as firmly established as that of androgens. In the dog model of BPH, produced by the synergistic action of oestrogens and androgens,[1,2] oestrogen is involved in the induction of the androgen receptor.[3] Oestrogen may, in fact, in the same way 'sensitize' the ageing dog prostate to the effects of androgen.[1] An abundance of high-affinity oestrogen receptors exists in the canine prostate and oestrogen treatment stimulates the stroma, leading to an increase in the total amount of collagen.[4,5]

Detailed reviews of the proposed role of oestrogens in the development of human BPH have been published.[6–8] Serum oestrogen levels increase with age in men, both in absolute terms and relative to testosterone levels; increased intraprostatic levels may also be noted in men with BPH.[7] Higher levels of oestradiol in the peripheral circulation have been observed in men with larger volumes of BPH.[9] The relatively low concentrations of classic high-affinity oestrogen receptor that are present in human BPH may,

in fact, be sufficient for biological activity.[10] Experimental studies in animal models using aromatase inhibitors have shown that decreases in intraprostatic oestrogen may lead to a reduction in oestrogen-induced stromal hyperplasia.

Normal sex hormone production

The control of androgen production in the testis is directly mediated by hypothalamic–pituitary hormones.[11] Gonadotropin-releasing hormone (GnRH) or luteinizing hormone-releasing hormone (LHRH) is secreted by neurons in the hypothalamus. This small peptide subsequently stimulates the release of both luteinizing hormone (LH) and follicle-stimulating hormones (FSH) in the anterior pituitary. LH secretion is regulated by the negative feedback action of androgens and oestrogens on the hypothalamus and pituitary.[11] On reaching the testes, LH interacts with specific high-affinity cell surface receptors in the plasma membrane of Leydig cells, activating the key biochemical events that lead to the synthesis of testosterone.

Testosterone acts directly in the brain, skeletal muscle and seminiferous epithelium, in stimulating the androgen-dependent process. In the prostate, however, testosterone is converted into dihydrotestosterone (DHT) by the action of the enzyme 5 alpha-reductase.[11] DHT is the principal androgen in the prostate, comprising 90% of total prostatic androgens, and is derived mainly from testicular androgens. Adrenal androgens make up 10% of total prostatic androgens, although the importance of this source in the pathophysiology of BPH is probably negligible. DHT has a higher affinity for the androgen receptor inside the cell and, as such, is considered to be a more 'potent' androgen; in addition the DHT–receptor complex may be more stable than the testosterone–receptor complex. By binding to specific DNA sites, the hormone–receptor complex increases transcription of androgen-dependent genes and hence protein production. Conversely, a decrease in protein production and tissue involution accompanies androgen withdrawal from androgen-sensitive tissues. Androgen withdrawal also leads to activation of specific genes involved in apoptosis (programmed cell death).[12]

Oestrogen can also be produced from testosterone in certain tissues (principally fat) that contain the enzyme aromatase. Prostatic oestrogen is formed mainly from the peripheral conversion of testosterone and subsequently reaches the prostate via the circulation.[13] The importance of intraprostatic aromatase activity is uncertain. As GnRH secretion is inhibited by oestrogen, androgen levels will rise secondarily in response to therapy that lowers peripheral oestrogen levels.

Normal levels of testosterone are required to maintain male sexual function, primarily libido; alteration in the synthesis or action of testosterone may therefore produce sexual dysfunction. Selective inhibition of DHT, however, should not result in altered libido or erectile function. The role of physiological levels of oestrogen in male sexual function, although unclear, is unlikely to be important.

The following is a review of various hormonal therapies available for the treatment of BPH. These are analysed in terms of rationale for use, efficacy and side effects.

Therapies based on androgen withdrawal

Androgen withdrawal therapies can be based on true anti-androgens, which block the action of testosterone and DHT at the receptor level, or those agents that impair androgen production (androgen ablation). Certain therapies may exhibit both activities (Table 24.1). Knowing the mechanism of action may be useful in determining potential side effects: for example, therapies that impair testosterone production are usually associated with sexual dysfunction.

Androgen ablation: surgical castration

It was noted as early as 1885 by White[14] that, of 200 men castrated as treatment of presumed BPH, 87% subsequently showed a decrease in prostatic size; approximately 50% of patients showed an improvement in clinical symptoms. In a series of 61 patients studied by Cabot in 1896, urinary retention ceased in 43% of

patients following castration and 83% showed overall improvement in symptoms.[15] In a recent study using transrectal ultrasound, Schroeder et al.[16] found an average decrease in prostate volume of 31% in five patients with BPH, four of whom had been castrated and one of whom had received a GnRH agonist. The limitations of anti-androgen therapy, however, were highlighted in 1940 by Huggins and Stevens:[17] in a study of three castrated BPH patients, significant epithelial atrophy did not occur until 90 days after androgen withdrawal; by contrast, there was negligible change in the stroma. Later studies confirmed that castration results in a reduction in the epithelial component of the prostate in men with prostate cancer.[18] Although the specific effects of androgen withdrawal on the stroma are inconclusive, it may be necessary to provide additional therapy aimed primarily at the stromal component in order to achieve maximal regression of BPH.

Androgen ablation: medical castration

Potent GnRH (LHRH) analogues can be used to block testicular androgen production. Their primary effect is desensitization of the GnRH receptor complex in the pituitary. The efficacy of GnRH analogues in men with uroflow obstruction due to BPH has been demonstrated in a number of clinical studies. Salerno et al.[19] showed reductions in prostatic DHT (90%) and in prostatic testosterone (75%) following 3 months of therapy with a long-acting GnRH analogue. Decreases in 5 alpha-reductase activity and nuclear androgen receptor levels may also result.[20] Thus, GnRH therapy may affect prostate growth, not only by lowering androgen levels but also by decreasing responsiveness to androgens.

An uncontrolled trial, involving nine patients with bladder outlet obstruction secondary to BPH, was conducted by Peters and Walsh to assess the effects of 6 months of therapy with nafarelin acetate.[21] Reductions in the level of testosterone to that recorded following castration resulted in decreased libido and impotence. Prostate size decreased by an average of 24.2%; a plateau was reached after 4 months of therapy. Within 6 months of cessation of treatment, however, all prostates returned essentially to their pretreatment sizes. Only one-third of patients showed a significant clinical improvement on the basis of maximum urinary flow rate and symptom assessment, despite the significant reduction in prostate

Table 24.1. *Mechanisms and side effects of androgen withdrawal therapies**

Agent	Mechanism	Side effects[†]
Androgen ablation/reduction		
GnRH agonists (e.g. nafarelin, leuprolide, buserelin)	Inhibit pituitary LH secretion; Decrease T and DHT	Hot flushes, loss of libido/impotence, gynaecomastia
5 alpha-reductase inhibitors (e.g. finasteride, epristeride)	Decrease DHT; no alteration in T or LH	3–4% incidence of sexual dysfunction[‡]
Anti-androgens		
Androgen-receptor antagonists (e.g. flutamide, Casodex™, zanoterone)	Androgen-receptor inhibition	Gynaecomastia/nipple tenderness; no significant incidence of impotence
Mixed mechanism of action		
Progestational agents (e.g. megestrol acetate, hydroxyprogesterone caproate, medrogestone, chlormadinone acetate, cyproterone acetate)	Inhibit pituitary LH secretion, variable decreases in T and DHT; variable androgen-receptor inhibition	Loss of libido/impotence, heat intolerance

*GnRH = gonadotropin-releasing hormone; LH = luteinizing hormone; T = testosterone; DHT = dihydrotestosterone. [†]Excluding gastrointestinal, haematological and central nervous system reactions. [‡]With finasteride.

volume. Epithelial and stromal volumes were reduced by 40 and 21%, respectively, based on morphometric analysis of biopsy specimens. Gabrilove et al.[22] showed a significant decrease in prostatic volume (58%) in patients treated with leuprolide for 6 months; urinary retention was alleviated in one patient. An approximate 30% decrease in prostate size was noted by Bosch et al.[23] following 12 weeks of therapy with buserelin; this was not associated with a concomitant improvement in urodynamic parameters. These results have been repeated in similar studies.[24–28]

Eri and Tveter recently published the results of a well-designed prospective placebo-controlled study of leuprolide.[29] Prostate volume decreased by 34.5% in the leuprolide group compared with 2.6% in the placebo group; there were also significant improvements in maximum urinary flow rate and symptoms. Clear, although modest, improvement in urodynamic parameters, such as detrusor pressure at maximal flow, were recorded in this study, in contrast to earlier studies. All patients had hot flushes and the majority of patients incurred loss of sexual function.[30] Additional possible side effects of medical castration include an effect on bone density in ageing men, which would limit the long-term safety of this approach. In patients with

significant medical co-morbidities and limited life span, however, androgen ablation may be of some value.

Although GnRH antagonists such as cetrorelix (SB-75) may produce a more rapid reduction in prostate size than the GnRH agonists discussed above,[31] their clinical advantage is unproven at this stage.

Androgen withdrawal side effects and cost constraints limit the use of GnRH therapy for BPH; cost per month may exceed US$400 compared with the US$30–50 for other BPH medical therapies that are commonly used. However, uncontrolled studies indicate that GnRH analogues may be beneficial in patients with urinary retention in whom the risks of surgery are very high.

Androgen-receptor antagonists

The non-steroidal anti-androgen flutamide competes with testosterone and DHT for androgen-receptor sites.[32] This compound, which requires metabolism to its active hydroxylated form, has no antigonadotropic or progestational activity and, consequently, plasma testosterone levels are not suppressed. To compensate for the androgen blockade, serum testosterone levels actually rise slightly, giving concerns about the effectiveness of flutamide monotherapy.

A number of studies have been conducted on flutamide therapy for BPH. Caine et al.[33] in a double-blind placebo-controlled study in 30 patients with BPH, noted a significant increase in urinary flow rate; residual urine volume and prostate size were unchanged. Symptom improvement was difficult to assess because, as in many other anti-androgen studies, response rates in the placebo-treated group were high. Nipple pain and gynaecomastia were experienced by seven of 15 patients treated with flutamide. The latter side effect appears to be related to unopposed oestrogen action in the breast; Bonard et al.[34] noted similar results.

The preliminary results of an ongoing multicentre trial on flutamide therapy for BPH have been reported by Stone et al.[35] Prostatic volume was significantly decreased in the treatment group after 3 months of therapy, with further regression in patients who continued therapy for longer than 6 months. Significant improvements were seen in maximum urinary flow rates and symptom scores in patients treated for 6 months. Breast pain or gynaecomastia were reported by 54% of flutamide-treated patients; gastrointestinal side effects were experienced by 49% of patients. Only one patient in the flutamide-treatment group experienced decrease in erectile function, suggesting that either the drug does not block the action of testosterone in the central nervous system (CNS), or that the perceived activity of androgens in the CNS should be re-examined.

A multicentre dose-ranging study on flutamide in 367 patients compared with BPH indicated no significant change in maximum urinary flow rate or symptom score compared with placebo after 6 months of therapy (unpublished observations). Reductions in prostate volume and serum prostate-specific antigen (PSA) levels were of the order of 20–30%, which are comparable to those seen with the 5 alpha-reductase inhibitor, finasteride. A significant number of patients experienced diarrhoea and breast tenderness and approximately one-third of patients withdrew from the study owing to side effects.

Bicalutamide (Casodex™), another non-steroidal androgen-receptor antagonist that has been studied with regard to BPH treatment, is structurally related to flutamide. Results of a double-blind placebo-controlled trial indicated a 26% reduction in prostate volume, but no statistically significant changes in maximum urinary

flow rate or detrusor pressure;[36] modest, but slightly significant, improvements were seen in symptom scores. Breast tenderness and enlargement occurred in 13 and nine patients, respectively, of a total of 14 treated. Five of these 14 patients experienced partial loss of sexual function, compared with none of 13 placebo patients.

Zanoterone, a steroidal androgen-receptor antagonist, has been evaluated in a phase II dose-ranging study.[37] A total of 463 men were randomized to receive zanoterone or placebo over a 6-month period. Significant increases in urinary flow rate compared with placebo were recorded after 3 months of therapy with zanoterone, 200 mg or 800 mg; at 6 months, the increase was significant only with the 200 mg dose. No statistically significant differences were seen in prostate volume reduction or symptom improvement between the two groups. Of the patients on active treatment, 18–32% withdrew from the study owing to breast pain or gynaecomastia.

Progestational agents

Progestational hormones decrease GnRH secretion, thus inhibiting the production of androgens; by blocking the androgen receptor they also inhibit the subsequent action of androgens in the prostate. A number of such agents have been clinically tested in men with BPH, with limited success. Geller et al.[38] showed regression of prostatic growth by hydroxyprogesterone caproate in an uncontrolled study. The importance of conducting placebo-controlled studies containing an adequate number of patients was shown in a subsequent study by Geller et al.[39] The efficacy of 20 weeks of therapy with megestrol acetate in 61 patients with BPH was studied in a double-blind placebo-controlled trial.[39] Subjective improvement occurred in 78 and 57% of the megestrol- and placebo-treated patients, respectively. Again, improvement in maximum urinary flow rates did not differ significantly in the two groups. Loss of libido occurred in 70% of patients in the active treatment group. Objective improvement on a similar scale has been reported following therapy with megestrol acetate,[40] hydroxyprogesterone[41] and medrogestone.[42] Impotence and antigonadotrophic side effects are common with this class of drugs.

Cyproterone acetate (CPA), a synthetic anti-androgen that acts primarily as an androgen-receptor inhibitor, also inhibits the release of gonadotropins from the pituitary. The efficacy of CPA treatment over a 15-month period was studied in an uncontrolled trial in 13 men with BPH.[43] Increases in urinary flow rate were recorded in nine patients, while voiding symptoms improved subjectively in 11. A decrease in epithelial cell height in eight of 11 patients evaluated was detected on the basis of needle biopsy of prostate tissue. Varying degrees of impotence were recorded in four patients, two of whom discontinued therapy for this reason. Bosch et al.[23] reported an approximate 30% decrease in prostatic size after 12 weeks of therapy with CPA or the GnRH agonist, buserelin. There were only slight clinical improvements, however, based on flow and pressure–flow studies. Improvement has been reported in other clinical studies, but proof of objective efficacy is lacking.[44,45]

Another progestational agent that is widely used in Japan for the treatment of BPH and prostate cancer is chlormadinone (CMA). Plasma androgen levels are reduced in most patients with BPH who are given CMA, but only modest improvements are seen in prostatic size reduction, urinary flow rate and symptom score.[46,47] In men with prostate cancer, serum testosterone levels were reduced to less than 1 ng/ml and prostate volume reduction was similar to that produced by flutamide.[48] The long acting form of CMA was compared with finasteride in a double-blind study in Japanese men with BPH. After 6 months of therapy, CMA (50 mg) was found to be as effective as finasteride in reducing prostate size (29 vs 22.2%), improving symptom score (8.2 vs 7.6) and improving maximum urinary flow rate (3.4 vs 2.2 ml/s); serum testosterone levels were lowered with both treatments. However, impotence was produced in 12.4 and 4.1% of patients treated with CMA and finasteride, respectively. Although CMA appears to be a moderately effective treatment for BPH, the significant risk of sexual dysfunction limits its tolerability.

Therapies based on oestrogen withdrawal

In comparison with androgens or other growth-stimulatory factors, the relative importance of oestrogens in the prostate is uncertain. Evidence suggests that oestrogens have a part in the development of BPH and preliminary clinical studies have been aimed at determining whether anti-oestrogen methods can be utilized clinically. Only aromatase inhibition, however, has been studied in detail.

Aromatase inhibition

Testolactone, an aromatase inhibitor, had a marginal effect on symptoms and uroflow in an uncontrolled study involving 13 patients with BPH.[8] A more potent inhibitor, atamestane (1-MEA) produced a significant decrease in plasma oestrone and oestradiol;[13,49] prostate volume and urinary flow were also affected beneficially. These results were not repeated in a US multicentre trial (Berlex Laboratories, personal communication). More recently, a European multicentre, placebo-controlled trial with atamestane in 160 patients with BPH resulted in reductions in mean oestradiol and oestrone levels of approximately 40 and 60%, respectively, in the active treatment group.[50] No difference between placebo and atamestane was found from the analysis of clinical parameters (symptom score, urinary flow rate and prostate size). Side effects in both groups were comparable. Testosterone concentration was increased by more than 40% and DHT by 30% in the atamestane treatment group. Such levels could stimulate epithelial cell activity, thus overriding any stromal cell regression; combination therapy with anti-androgens might therefore be considered in future clinical trials.

Conclusions

Although interesting possibilities exist for future study, there are no currently available hormone therapies, other than 5 alpha-reductase inhibitors, that fulfil the safety and efficacy criteria or those of cost effectiveness for the medical management of BPH.

References

1. Barrack E R, Berry S J. DNA synthesis in the canine prostate: effects of androgen and estrogen treatment. Prostate 1987; 10: 45–56
2. Walsh P C, Wilson J D. The induction of prostatic hypertrophy in the dog with androstanediol. J Clin Invest 1976; 57: 1093–1097
3. Moore R J, Gazak J M, Wilson J D. Regulation of cytoplasmic dihydrotestosterone binding in dog prostate by 17 beta-estradiol. J Clin Invest 1979; 63: 351–357
4. Berry S J. A study of spontaneous prostatic hyperplasia in the beagle (doctoral thesis). Baltimore, The Johns Hopkins University, 1984

5. Berry S J, Isaacs J T. Comparative aspects of prostatic growth and androgen metabolism with aging in the dog versus the rat. Endocrinology 1984; 114: 511–520

6. Henderson D, Habenicht U F, Nishino Y et al. Aromatase inhibitors and benign prostatic hyperplasia. J Biochem 1986; 25: 867–875

7. Henderson D, Habenicht U F, Nishino Y, El Etreby M F. Estrogens in benign prostatic hyperplasia: the basis for aromatase inhibitor therapy. Steroids 1987; 50: 219–233

8. Tunn U W, Schweikert H U. Aromatase inhibitors in the management of benign prostatic hyperplasia. New Dev Biosci 1989; 5: 139–149

9. Coffey D S, Walsh P C. Clinical and experimental studies of benign prostatic hyperplasia. Urol Clin North Am 1990; 17: 461–475

10. Berry S J, Coffey D S, Walsh P C. The development of human benign prostatic hyperplasia with age. J Urol 1984; 132: 474–479

11. Griffin J E, Wilson J D. Disorders of the testes and male reproductive tract. In: Wilson J D, Foster D W (eds) Williams textbook of endocrinology. Philadelphia: Saunders, 1985: 259

12. Isaacs J T. Control of cell proliferation and cell death in the normal and neoplastic prostate: a stem cell model. In: Rodgers C H, Coffey D S, Cunha G et al (eds) Benign prostatic hyperplasia, Vol. 2. NIH 87–2881. Washington DC: National Institutes of Health, US Department of Health and Human Services, 1987: 85–94

13. Etreby M F, Habenicht U F. The function and the role of aromatase inhibitors in the treatment of BPH. In: Benign prostatic hyperplasia. Wiley-Liss, 1994: 209–230

14. White J W. The results of double castration in hypertrophy of the prostate. Ann Surg 1895; 25: 1–59

15. Cabot A T. The question of castration for enlarged prostate. Ann Surg 1896; 26: 265–285

16. Schroeder F H, Westerhof M, Bosch R J, Kurth K H. Benign prostatic hyperplasia treated by castration or the LH–RH analogue buserelin: a report on 6 cases. Eur Urol 1986; 12: 318–321

17. Huggins C, Stevens R A. The effect of castration on benign hypertrophy of the prostate in man. J Urol 1940; 43: 705–714

18. Wendel E F, Brannen G E, Putong P B, Grayhack J T. The effect of orchiectomy and estrogens in benign prostatic hyperplasia. J Urol 1972; 108: 116–119

19. Salerno R, Moneti G, Forti G et al. Simultaneous determination of testosterone, dihydrotestosterone and 5α-androstan-3α-17ß-diol by isotopic dilution mass spectrometry in plasma and prostatic tissue of patients affected by benign prostatic hyperplasia: effects of a 3-month treatment with a GnRH analog. J Androl 1988; 9: 234

20. Forti G, Salerno R, Moneti G et al. Three months' treatment with a long acting gonadotropin releasing hormone agonist of patients with benign prostatic hyperplasia: effects of tissue androgen concentration, 5 alpha reductase activity and androgen receptor contents. J Clin Endocrinol 1989; 68: 461–468

21. Peters C A, Walsh P C. The effect of nafarelin acetate, a luteinizing-hormone-releasing hormone agonist, on benign prostatic hyperplasia. New Engl J Med 1987; 317: 599–604

22. Gabrilove J L, Levine A C, Kirschenbaum A, Droller M. Effect of long-acting gonadotropin-releasing hormone analog (leuprolide) therapy on prostatic size and symptoms in 15 men with benign prostatic hypertrophy. J Clin Endocrinol 1989; 69: 629–632

23. Bosch R J, Griffiths D J, Blom J H, Schroeder F H. Treatment of benign prostatic hyperplasia by androgen deprivation: effects on prostate size and urodynamic parameters. J Urol 1989; 141: 68–72

24. Bianchi S, Gravina G, Podestà A et al. Treatment of complicated benign prostatic hyperplasia with LHRH-analogues in aged patients. Int J Androl 1989; 12: 104–109

25. Keane P F, Timoney A G, Kiely E et al. Response of the benign hypertrophied prostate to treatment with an LHRH analogue. Br J Urol 1988; 62: 163–165

26. Lukkarinen O. Effect of LH–RH analogue in patients with benign prostatic hyperplasia. Urology 1991; 37: 92–94

27. Matzkin H, Chen J, Lewysohn O, Braf Z. Treatment of benign prostatic hypertrophy by a long-acting gonadotropin-releasing hormone analogue: 1-year experience. J Urol 1991; 145: 309–312

28. Schlegel P N, Brendler C B. Management of urinary retention due to benign prostatic hyperplasia using luteinizing hormone-releasing hormone agonist. Urology 1989; 34: 69–72

29. Eri L M, Tveter K J. A prospective, placebo-controlled study of the luteinizing hormone-releasing hormone agonist leuprolide as treatment for patients with benign prostatic hyperplasia. J Urol 1993; 150: 359–364

30. Eri L M, Tveter K J. Safety, side effects and patient acceptance of the luteinizing hormone releasing hormone agonist leuprolide in treatment of benign prostatic hyperplasia. J Urol 1994; 152: 448–452

31. Barcena D G, Buenfil M V, Gomez-Orta F et al. Responses to the antagonistic analog of LH-RH (SB-75, Cetrorelix) in patients with benign prostatic hyperplasia and prostatic cancer. Prostate 1994; 24: 84–92

32. Sufrin G, Coffey D S. Mechanism of action of a new nonsteroidal antiandrogen: flutamide. Invest Urol 1976; 13: 429–434

33. Caine M, Perlberg S, Gordon R. The treatment of benign prostatic hypertrophy with flutamide (SCH: 13521): a placebo-controlled study. J Urol 1975; 114: 564–568

34. Bonard M, de Almeida S, von Niederhäusern W. Placebo-controlled double-blind study in human benign obstructive prostatic hypertrophy with flutamide. Eur Urol 1976; 2: 24–28

35. Stone N N, Krongrad A, Chodak G W et al. A double blind randomized controlled study of the effect of flutamide in benign prostatic hypertrophy: clinical efficacy. Urol Res 1989; 17: 338

36. Eri L M, Tveter K J. A prospective placebo-controlled study of the antiandrogen Casodex as treatment for patients with benign prostatic hyperplasia. J Urol 1993; 150: 90–94

37. Berger B M, Naadimuthu A, Boddy A et al. The effect of zanoterone, a steroidal androgen receptor antagonist, in men with benign prostatic hyperplasia. The Zanoterone Study Group. J Urol 1995; 154: 1060–1064

38. Geller J, Bora R, Roberts T et al. Treatment of benign prostatic hypertrophy with hydroxyprogesterone caproate. JAMA 1965; 193: 115–122

39. Geller J, Nelson C G, Albert J D, Pratt C. Effect of megestrol acetate on uroflow rates in patients with benign prostatic hypertrophy: a double-blind study. Urology 1979; 5: 467

40. Donkervoort T, Sterling A M, van Ness J et al. Megestrol acetate in treatment of benign prostatic hyperplasia. Urology 1975; 6: 580

41. Brooks M E, Braf Z F. Effect of 17-α-hydroxyprogesterone 17-n-caproate on urine flow. Urology 1981; 17: 488–491

42. Paulson D F, Kane R D. Medrogestone: a prospective study in the pharmacological management of benign prostatic hyperplasia. J Urol 1975; 113: 811–815

43. Scott W W, Wade J C. Medical treatment of benign nodular prostatic hyperplasia with cyproterone acetate. J Urol 1969; 101: 81–85

44. Cocimano V, Marino G, Surleti D et al. Il ciproterone acetato nella iperplasia prostatica benigna. Minerva Urol Nefrol 1989; 41: 275–276

45. Geller J, Fishman J, Cantor T L. Effect of cyproterone acetate on clinical endocrine and pathological features of benign prostatic hypertrophy. J Biochem 1975; 6: 837–843

46. Moriyama M, Akiyama T, Yamamoto T et al. Studies on therapeutic effects and adverse effects of chlormadinone acetate for patients with benign prostatic hypertrophy. Nishinihon J Urol 1991; 53: 563–571

47. Shida K. Clinical effects of allylestrenol on benign prostatic hypertrophy by double-blind method. Acta Urol Jpn 1986; 32: 625–648

48. Akaza H, Usami M, Kotaka T et al. A randomized phase II trial of flutamide vs chlormadinone acetate in previously untreated advanced prostatic cancer. Jpn J Clin Oncol 1993; 23: 178–185

49. Etreby M F. Atamestane: an aromatse inhibitor for the treatment of benign prostatic hyperplasia. A short review. J Biochem 1993; 44: 565–572

50. Gingell J C, Knönagel H, Kurth K H et al. Placebo controlled double-blind study to test the efficacy of the aromatase inhibitor atamestane in patients with benign prostatic hyperplasia not requiring operation. J Urol 1995; 154: 309–401

Rationale for alpha-1 blockade in BPH

The rationale for alpha-1 blockade in benign prostatic hyperplasia (BPH) is based upon the following observations and assumptions: the tension of prostatic smooth muscle is mediated by the alpha-1-adrenoceptor (alpha-1-AR); the tension of prostate smooth muscle in males with BPH contributes to bladder outlet obstruction; and the severity of bladder outlet obstruction is related to prostatic smooth muscle tension.

Raz et al.[1] were the first investigators to study the physiology and pharmacology of prostatic smooth muscle. Isometric tension studies demonstrated that the rat prostate contracts in the presence of noradrenaline (norepinephrine), an adrenergic agonist. Caine and associates subsequently demonstrated that the human prostate adenoma and capsule also contracts in the presence of noradrenaline.[2] Caine et al.[3] recognized the therapeutic implications of pharmacologically altering the tension of prostatic smooth muscle in males with clinical BPH. Lepor et al.[4] reported isometric tension studies demonstrating that human BPH tissues challenged with alpha-1-adrenergic agonists elicit a potent contractile response whereas alpha-2 and muscarinic agonists elicit a weak contractile response. Antagonist dissociation[5,6] and in vivo[7] studies have provided further evidence that the contractile properties of the human prostate adenoma are mediated by alpha-1-AR. Radioligand receptor-binding studies have shown that the human prostate contains a relative abundance of alpha-1-AR[8–10] and that alpha-1-AR is associated exclusively with the stromal elements of the prostate.[9] Comparative binding and functional studies of lower genitourinary tissues have demonstrated that alpha-1-ARs are sparse in the bladder body and abundant in the bladder base and prostate.[11] On the basis of the aforementioned physiological and pharmacological observations, alpha-1-adrenergic blockers should decrease the resistance along the prostatic urethra by relaxing the smooth muscle component of the prostate. Theoretically, selective alpha-1-adrenergic antagonists are ideally suited for the treatment of the dynamic component of bladder outlet obstruction since the resistance along the bladder outlet can be selectively reduced without impairing detrusor contraction.

Bartsch et al.[12] reported in 1979 that BPH is predominantly a stromal proliferative process. Shapiro et al.[13] subsequently reported that the development of clinical BPH is related to the cellular content of the prostate. This conclusion was based upon the observation that the stromal epithelial ratio was significantly greater in males with symptomatic BPH relative to asymptomatic BPH.

Shapiro et al.[14,15] recently developed a technique for quantifying the cellular elements of the prostate. Double immunoenzymatic staining and colour-assisted image analysis on 26 prostatic biopsy specimens obtained from males with clinical BPH revealed that the mean area densities of smooth muscle, connective tissue, epithelium and glandular lumen in these biopsy specimens were $39 \pm 3\%$, $38 \pm 3\%$, $12 \pm 1\%$ and $11 \pm 1\%$, respectively.[16] These morphometric studies confirmed Bartsch's observation that BPH is primarily stromal (smooth muscle and connective tissue) hyperplasia,[12] and that a significant component of the prostatic enlargement is due to smooth muscle proliferation.

The proposed mechanism for the efficacy of selective alpha-1-blockade in BPH is via relaxation of prostatic smooth muscle. It therefore follows that the magnitude of the clinical response to selective alpha-1-blockade in BPH should be related directly to the proportion of the hyperplasia that is smooth muscle. Shapiro et al.[16] reported the relationship between the percentage area density of prostatic smooth muscle and the clinical response to terazosin, a selective long-acting alpha-1-blocker. Prostatic biopsy specimens were obtained from 26 males with clinical BPH prior to initiating terazosin therapy. The dose of terazosin was titrated to 5 mg provided that serious adverse events were not observed. The percentage area density of smooth muscle in the biopsy specimens was quantified using double immunoenzymatic staining and colour-assisted computer image analysis: a direct relationship between the increase in peak urinary flow rate (Q_{max}) and the percentage area density of smooth muscle was observed. The direct relationship between the area density of prostatic smooth muscle and improvement in Q_{max} strongly supports the hypothesis that the development of bladder outlet obstruction is mediated by prostatic smooth muscle tension.

Although bladder outlet obstruction in the ageing male population is often mediated by prostatic smooth muscle proliferation, there is increasing evidence that the severity of urinary symptoms is not exclusively the result of bladder outlet obstruction. The correlation between symptom severity captured by the American Urological Association (AUA) symptom index and Q_{max} is weak.[17] Unlike Q_{max}, the density of prostatic smooth muscle is not directly correlated with symptom severity.[16] These observations suggest that urinary symptoms in the ageing male are probably multifactorial. It is also conceivable that symptom improvement in males with prostatism is achieved via non-prostate smooth muscle events mediated by the alpha-1-AR.

The alpha-blockers administered in the BPH studies can be subgrouped according to receptor subtype selectivity and duration of serum elimination half-lives. Phenoxybenzamine, a non-selective alpha-blocker, antagonizes alpha-1- and alpha-2-AR. The drugs that are selective for only the alpha-1-AR include prazosin, alfuzosin, indoramin, terazosin, doxazosin and tamsulosin (YM617). The primary advantage of the selective alpha-1-antagonists is that the incidence and severity of adverse events are significantly less than the non-selective alpha-blockers. Terazosin represents the alpha-blocker that has been most extensively studied in BPH. The advantages of selective long-acting (once-a-day) alpha-blockers are related to compliance and tolerance. The most common adverse events associated with selective alpha-1-blockers include dizziness, light-headedness and asthenia. The administration of a once-a-day formulation at bedtime appears to reduce the incidence and severity of these adverse events.

Lepor has critically analysed and summarized the reported clinical experiences with alpha-blockers.[18–20] Randomized double-blind placebo-controlled studies have consistently demonstrated that selective alpha-1-blockers are safe and effective for the treatment of BPH. Improvements in symptom scores and urinary flow rates have consistently been statistically and clinically significant. The response to alpha-1-blockers is dose dependent. The efficacy and toxicity of the different alpha-1-blockers appear comparable. Terazosin is the most widely prescribed alpha-1-blocker, its published literature related to BPH being the most extensive.

Terazosin

Terazosin is a highly selective and potent inhibitor of prostatic alpha-1-AR.[21] Isometric tension studies have shown that terazosin inhibits phenylephrine-mediated prostate smooth contraction via alpha-1-blockade.[4] As the half-life of terazosin is approximately 8 h, the drug is effective as a once-a-day dose. Lepor et al. reported one of the first open-label experiences with terazosin in males with BPH in 1990.[22] This preliminary and uncontrolled study reported mean improvements in Q_{max} and in obstructive and irritative Boyarsky symptom scores of 42, 63 and 35%, respectively. Qualitatively, 67% of subjects exhibited a favourable clinical response.

Lepor et al.[23] reported the results of a phase III multicentre, double-blind, parallel group, randomized placebo-controlled study of once-a-day administration of terazosin to patients with symptomatic BPH. A total of 285 patients entered the double-blind treatment receiving either placebo or 2, 5 or 10 mg terazosin once daily. Statistically significant decreases from baseline obstructive, irritative and total symptom scores were observed for all terazosin treatment groups (Table 25.1). The 10 mg terazosin treatment group also exhibited significantly greater decreases in mean irritative and total symptom scores relative to the placebo group. The 5 and 10 mg terazosin treatment groups exhibited a significantly greater mean decrease in obstructive scores relative to the placebo group. The level of improvements in the symptom scores was dose dependent. The percentages of patients experiencing a greater than 30% improvement in the total symptom scores for the

Table 25.1. *Effectiveness of terazosin (TRZ)*

Outcome measures	Treatment	Assessment Baseline	Assessment 12 weeks	%Δ*	p value[†]
Symptom score‡	Placebo	9.7	7.4	−23.5	< 0.001
	TRZ (10 mg)	10.1	5.5	−45.1	
Q_{max} (ml/s)	Placebo	10.1	10.2	+10.4	0.009
	TRZ (10 mg)	8.8	12.2	+34.0	

*Values correspond to means of changes from baseline in each man and therefore cannot be derived from baseline and 12 weeks' results. [†]Comparison between mean %Δ placebo vs TRZ. ‡Boyarsky symptom score.

placebo and the 2, 5 and 10 mg treatment groups were 40, 51, 57 and 69%, respectively (Fig. 25.1). The percentage of patients experiencing greater than 30% improvement in total symptom score in the 10 mg treatment groups was significantly greater than the placebo group.

A statistically significant improvement from baseline was observed in the peak and mean urinary flow rates for all treatment groups (Table 25.1) The 10 mg treatment group exhibited a significantly greater increase from baseline in peak and mean urinary flow rates relative to the placebo group. The changes in Q_{max} were also dose dependent. The percentages of patients experiencing a greater than 30% increase in Q_{max} in the placebo and the 2, 5 and 10 mg treatment groups were 26, 40, 35 and 52%, respectively (Fig. 25.1). A significantly greater proportion of patients in the 10 mg terazosin treatment group exhibited a greater than 30% improvement in Q_{max} compared with the placebo group.

Overall, the adverse events in the four treatment groups were minor and reversible. Although a higher incidence of asthenia, flu syndrome and dizziness were observed in the terazosin treatment groups, the differences from placebo were not statistically significant when tested using Fisher's exact test. There was a significantly greater incidence of postural hypotension in the 5 mg terazosin group than in the placebo group. One patient in the 10 mg treatment group developed syncope at the 5 mg dose of terazosin. The incidence of syncope in the 10 mg treatment group was one out of 79 (1.3%). The incidence of syncope for all terazosin-treated patients was less than 0.5%.

An effort was made to identify clinical or urodynamic factors that predict response to terazosin therapy. The relationships between percentage change in total symptom score and Q_{max} vs baseline age, prostate size, Q_{max}, mean urinary flow rate, post-void residual and total symptom score were examined. No significant association was observed between treatment effect and baseline factors when tested using an analysis of covariance model with terms for baseline factor, treatment groups and their interaction.

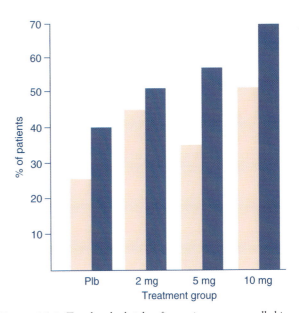

Figure 25.1. *Two hundred eighty-five patients were enrolled into a randomized double-blind study comparing placebo (Plb) and 2, 5 and 10 mg terazosin once daily. Percentages of patients experiencing greater than 30% improvement in total symptom scores (■) and peak urinary flow rates (□) are shown.*

Di Silverio[24] recently reported a multicentre, randomized, placebo-controlled, double-blind study in Italy evaluating the safety and efficacy of terazosin in patients with BPH: 137 patients were randomly assigned to receive a daily dose of either placebo or 2, 5 or 10 mg terazosin for 8 weeks. The mean percentage change in Q_{max} for the placebo and for the 2, 5 and 10 mg terazosin groups was 16.6, 32.5, 39.4 and 32.2%, respectively. The differences between the placebo and treatment groups were comparable to those in Lepor's (US) study.[23] Symptom improvement was evaluated using the Boyarsky symptom score. The mean percentage change in obstructive symptom score for the placebo, and for the 2, 5 and 10 mg terazosin groups was 57.6, 62.1, 60.1 and 68.5%, respectively. The author did not present data for changes in irritative or total symptom scores. The differences between the changes in Q_{max} and obstructive symptom score in the placebo and treatment groups were not statistically significant because of the relatively small sample size and the excessive effect of placebo on the symptom score. The safety of terazosin was unequivocally confirmed: only one serious event (urinary retention) was reported throughout the study and the changes in blood pressure in the predominantly normotensive population were small.

Lloyd et al.[25] in the UK recently reported a multicentre, randomized, placebo-controlled trial evaluating terazosin for BPH: 86 patients were randomized to receive a daily dose of placebo or 2, 5 or 10 mg terazosin for 8 weeks. The mean change in Q_{max} for the placebo and the 2, 5 and 10 mg terazosin groups was 45.5, 22.8, 33.7 and 39.5%, respectively. The differences between the placebo and active treatment groups were not statistically significant because of the unexplained exceedingly high placebo response: the effect of placebo on Q_{max} is typically less than 20%. The change in Q_{max} for the active treatment groups was dose dependent. Although symptoms were evaluated using the Boyarsky symptom score, the authors did not report the total symptom scores. The mean percentage change in obstructive symptom score in the placebo and 2, 5 and 10 mg groups was 22.4, 51.1, 49.0 and 57.1%, respectively. The mean percentage change in the irritative symptom score in the placebo and 2, 5 and 10 mg drug groups was 17.1, 10.8, 26.9 and 25.3%, respectively. The differences between placebo and the

active treatment groups were not statistically significant because of the small sample size. The percentage changes in obstructive and irritative symptom scores are compared in the British and US studies. Treatment was discontinued in only four randomized patients because of adverse events. The severe adverse events felt to be 'probably' related to terazosin were one episode of syncope and one episode of peripheral oedema. One patient each in the placebo group and in the 2 and 5 mg drug groups, and two patients in the 10 mg group, reported dizziness.

Overall, the three multicentre, randomized, placebo-controlled studies support the safety and efficacy of terazosin for the treatment of BPH. The only discrepancies in the three trials are the exceedingly high placebo effects reported for Q_{max} in the British study and the obstructive symptom score in the Italian study. The changes in Q_{max} and symptom scores appear to be dose dependent, and doses of up to 10 mg were well tolerated. In the author's opinion, the dose should be titrated to at least 10 mg, unless adverse events develop.

Long-term studies

Because BPH is a chronic and potentially progressive condition, any form of medical management for BPH must achieve durable clinical responses in order to assume a meaningful role in the treatment of this disease. Between December 1989 and December 1991, 494 men with clinical BPH were enrolled at 23 medical centres into a long-term open-label study evaluating the safety and efficacy of terazosin.[26] Patients diagnosed as having symptomatic BPH but lacking absolute indications for surgical intervention were eligible. Initially, the study protocol was designed to follow patients undergoing terazosin administration for a maximum of 2 years, but the duration of follow-up was subsequently extended to 4 years. Terazosin was started at 1 mg/day and titrated upward at monthly intervals, according to the investigators' discretion, to a maximum dose of 20 mg/day. The primary efficacy variables were peak urinary flow rate and total Boyarsky symptom score. The study visits were conducted at 1-month intervals up to 3 months, at 3-month intervals up to 24 months and at 6-month intervals thereafter. Duration of follow-up ranged from 3 to 42 months. Of the 494 patients, 213 (43.1%) withdrew prematurely — 55 (11%) owing to therapeutic failure, 96 (19%) owing to adverse events and 62 (13%) for administrative reasons. The duration of the study was extended to 4 years after some patients had completed 2 years of treatment. Specifically, 102 patients (21%) of 494 patients had completed the study protocol according to the original 2-year protocol and were, therefore, not included among premature withdrawals.

At all follow-up visits, the mean peak urinary flow rates were significantly higher than baseline values (Fig. 25.2). The baseline Q_{max} was 10.0 ml/s. From 3 to 42 months, the improvements in Q_{max} ranged from 2.3 to 4.0 ml/s above baseline. Between months 3 and 42, at least a 30% improvement in Q_{max} from baseline was observed in 40–59% of patients. The level of improvement in Q_{max} is comparable to that achieved in double-blind and open-label studies evaluating terazosin for BPH.

At all follow-up intervals, the mean Boyarsky symptom scores were significantly lower than at baseline; this was true of obstructive, irritative and total scores (Fig. 25.3). At baseline, the mean total score for the overall population was 10.5, with a mean obstructive score of 6.2 and a mean irritative score of 4.3. From 3 months onward, improvements ranged from 4.0 to 5.4. Between months 3 and 42, at least a 30% improvement in total symptom score from baseline was observed in 62.4–77.1% of the patients.

The most common adverse events resulting in discontinuation from the long-term study were dizziness (6.7%), asthenia (3.8%) and somnolence (2.0%). The proportion of adverse events that were treatment related is unknown as the study design did not include a parallel placebo group.

The mean changes from baseline for systolic and diastolic blood pressures for normotensive patients ranged between 1 and 4 mmHg. The mean changes from baseline for systolic and diastolic blood pressures for patients hypertensive at baseline ranged from 10 to 15 mmHg. Thus, terazosin lowered blood pressure in patients with BPH primarily when it was a desirable clinical outcome. The drug had no clinically significant effect on the blood pressure of normotensive patients.

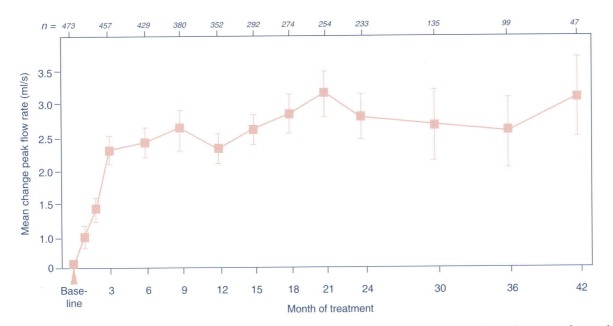

Figure 25.2. *Mean change in peak flow rate between baseline and 42 months in terazosin-treated patients. The n values across the top of the graph indicate the number of patients available at each time interval. All data points were significantly different from baseline at the p ≤0.05 level.*

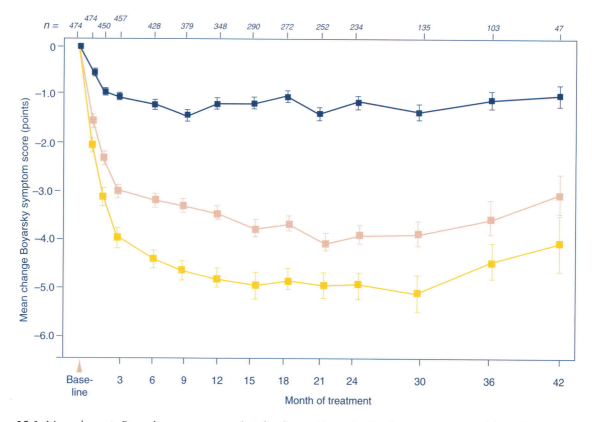

Figure 25.3. *Mean change in Boyarsky symptom scores from baseline to 42 months. Baseline scores were 10.5 for total scores (■), 6.2 for obstructive scores (■) and 4.3 for irritative scores (■). The n values across the top of the graph indicate the number of patients available at each time interval. All changes were significant at the p≤0.05 level.*

The terazosin experience provides the longest available follow-up observations on the safety and efficacy of alpha-1-blockers for the treatment of BPH. These data, and those of any long-term open-label study, must be interpreted with caution since non-responders are unlikely to remain on long-term drug therapy when an agent has failed to produce the desired effect. Although the data are encouraging, the efficacy and safety of terazosin need to be studied for even longer periods. The findings of the 42-month study confirm previously reported observations related to the efficacy, safety and tolerability of terazosin in the treatment of BPH.

Alpha-blockade: the future

Minneman and associates recently characterized two pharmacological subtypes of alpha-1-AR based upon differential binding affinities to the antagonists 5-methylurapidil (5-MU) and WB4101, and by differential sensitivity to the non-competitive antagonist chloroethylclonidine (CEC).[27,28] The alpha-

1A-AR exhibited relatively high affinity for WB4101 and 5-MU and was CEC sensitive. The alpha-1B-AR exhibited relatively low affinity for WB4101 and 5-MU and was CEC sensitive. The predominant subtype in the rat vas deferens and hippocampus was the alpha-1A-AR whereas in the rat liver and spleen it was of the alpha-1B-AR subtype. Lepor et al.[29,30] were the first investigators to characterize pharmacological subtypes in the human prostate. The ratio of high- to low-affinity WB4101 and 5-MU binding sites in the human prostate was 1.8:1 and 1.6:1, respectively. CEC inactivated 44% of the prostatic alpha-1-AR. These binding studies indicated that both alpha-1A- and alpha-1B-binding sites are present in the human prostate, the alpha-1A being the dominant binding site.

Recently, several investigators have characterized and cloned distinct cDNAs encoding for three distinct subtypes of the alpha-1-AR. The alpha-1-AR subtypes were initially cloned from rat, hamster and bovine tissues.[31–33] Investigators at Synaptic Pharmaceutical cloned these alpha-1-AR subtypes from human tissue.[34–36]

These alpha-1-AR cDNAs were transfected into LM (TK-) or CHO cells, and the membrane preparations were assayed for the ability to bind [^{3}H]prazosin. Competitive binding studies were performed using non-subtype-selective antagonists (albanoquil, alfuzosin, doxazosin, prazosin and terazosin) and subtype-selective alpha-1-AR antagonists (5-MU, niguldepine, indoramin, SK & F 104856 and SNAP 1069). The selective alpha-1-AR antagonists exhibited varying levels of selectivity for the different alpha-1-AR subtypes. The binding properties of the pharmacological alpha-1-AR described by Minneman were similar to the binding properties of the cloned alpha-1c-AR. Similarly, the binding properties of the pharmacological alpha-1B-AR was similar to the binding properties of the cloned alpha-1b-AR. A tissue expressing the cloned alpha-1a has yet to be identified. Based upon these relationships, several investigators have suggested altering the nomenclature so that the cloned alpha-1c-AR is redefined as the alpha-1a-AR.

The relationships between the binding affinities of alpha-antagonists for the three expressed alpha-1-ARs and the affinity of these antagonists for inhibiting phenylephrine-mediated contraction of human prostatic tissue strips were examined recently.[37] The correlation between the pK_i of the alpha-1a- vs the alpha-1b-AR and the pA_2 were weak, whereas a direct relationship existed ($r=0.94$) for the relationship between the pK_i of the alpha-1c-AR and the pA_2 values. These comparative binding and functional studies provide the most compelling evidence that the tension of human prostatic smooth muscle is mediated by the alpha-1c-AR. Lepor et al.[38] using quantitative image analysis and autoradiography, recently reported that the alpha-1a-AR is the predominant receptor in the prostate, and that the stromal alpha-1-ARs are exclusively the alpha-1a-AR subtype. These studies are consistent with the observation of Price et al.[39] that 70% of the total alpha-1-AR mRNA encodes for the alpha-1c-AR. Recently, the cloned alpha-1-AR subtypes have been reclassified in order to coincide with the pharmacological subtypes of the alpha-1-AR. The previously described alpha-1c-AR has been renamed the alpha-1a. Thus, it is the alpha-1a-AR that mediates the tension of prostate smooth muscle.

One of the limitations of drug therapy is the development of untoward adverse experiences. These adverse experiences are the result of undesirable effects of drugs on non-target tissues also expressing the receptor. Advances in drug development are often achieved by identifying compounds that exhibit tissue selectivity. The development of tissue-selective antagonists often minimizes or eliminates side effects. The development of tissue-selective alpha-adrenergic antagonists has already had an effect on the medical management of BPH. Phenoxybenzamine, a non-selective alpha blocker, was shown by Caine et al.[3] in 1975 to be highly effective for the treatment of BPH. The primary limitation of phenoxybenzamine was the incidence and severity of adverse experiences. Berthelson and Pettinger[40] reported in 1977 the existence of two different subtypes of the alpha-receptor (alpha-1 vs alpha-2). Binding and functional studies demonstrated that the prostate smooth muscle tension is mediated by the alpha-1-AR. Prazosin and other selective alpha-1-blockers were shown to achieve the same level of effectiveness as phenoxybenzamine with fewer adverse events. The development of tissue-selective alpha-AR antagonists significantly improved the tolerance of alpha-blockers and led to the eventual widespread acceptance of this therapeutic approach for the management of BPH.

The alpha-1-AR subtype mediating prostate smooth muscle tension is unequivocally the alpha-1a-AR (previously defined as the alpha-1c-AR). The ultimate role of alpha-1-AR subtype-selective antagonists will depend upon the alpha-1-AR subtype mediating efficacy, blood-pressure changes and adverse experiences. At present, the alpha-1-AR subtype mediating these events is not known. It is conceivable that factors other than prostate smooth muscle may mediate the therapeutic benefit of alpha-1-blockers. There is a great deal of interest among the pharmaceutical industry in developing alpha-1 subtype-selective (prostate-selective) blockers. Several highly selective alpha-1a drugs have already been synthesized. The impact of alpha-1a-selective antagonists in the treatment of BPH will be defined by future randomized double-blind trials evaluating these new and promising agents.

References

1. Raz S, Ziegler M, Caine M. Pharmacologic receptors in the prostate. Br J Urol 1973; 45: 663–667

2. Caine M, Raz S, Ziegler M. Adrenergic and cholinergic receptors in the human prostate, prostatic capsule and bladder neck. Br J Urol 1975; 27: 193–202,

3. Caine M, Pfau A, Perlberg S. The use of alpha adrenergic blockers in benign prostatic obstruction. Br J Urol 1976; 48: 255–263

4. Lepor H, Gup D I, Baumann M, Shapiro E. Laboratory assessment of terazosin and alpha1 blockade in prostatic hyperplasia. Urology 1988; 32(suppl): 21–26

5. Hieble J P, Boyce A J, Canine M. Comparison of the alpha adrenoceptor characteristics in human and canine prostate. Fed Proc 1986; 45: 2609–2614

6. Hieble J P, Caine M, Zalaznik E. In vitro characterization of the alpha-adrenoceptors in human prostate. Eur J Pharmacol 1985; 107: 111–117

7. Breslin D, Fields D W, Chou T C et al. Medical management of benign prostatic hyperplasia: a canine model comparing the in vivo efficacy of alpha$_1$ adrenergic antagonists in the prostate. J Urol 1993; 149: 395–399

8. Gup D I, Shapiro E, Baumann M, Lepor H. Autonomic receptors in asymptomatic and symptomatic BPH. J Urol 1990; 143: 179–185

9. Kobayashi S, Tang R, Shapiro E, Lepor H. Characterization of human alpha$_1$ adrenoceptor binding sites using radioligand receptor binding on slide-mounted tissue sections. J Urol 1993; 150: 2002–2006.

10. Lepor H, Shapiro E. Characterization of the alpha$_1$ adrenergic receptor in human benign prostatic hyperplasia. J Urol 1984; 132: 1226–1229

11. Lepor H, Shapiro E. Alpha$_1$ adrenergic receptors in the lower genitourinary tissues: insight into development and function. J Urol 1987; 138: 979–983

12. Bartsch G, Muller H R, Oberholzer M, Rohr H P. Light microscopic stereological analysis of the normal human prostate and of benign prostatic hyperplasia. J Urol 1979; 122: 487–491

13. Shapiro E, Becich M J, Lepor H. The relative proportion of stromal and epithelia hyperplasia is related to the development of clinical BPH. J Urol 1992; 147: 1293–1297

14. Shapiro E, Hartanto V, Lepor H. Quantifying the smooth muscle content of the prostate using double-immunoenzymatic staining and color assisted image analysis. J Urol 1992; 147: 1167–1170

15. Shapiro E, Hartanto V, Lepor H. Anti-desmin vs. anti-actin for quantifying the area density of prostate smooth muscle. Prostate 1992; 20: 259–268

16. Shapiro E, Hartanto V, Lepor H. The response to alpha blockade in benign prostatic hyperplasia is related to the percent area density of prostate smooth muscle. Prostate 1992; 21: 297–307

17. Barry M J, Cockett A T K, Holtgrewe H L et al. Relationship of symptoms of prostatism to commonly used physiological and anatomical measures of the severity of benign prostatic hyperplasia. J Urol 1993; 150: 351–358

18. Lepor H. The role of alpha blockade in the treatment of BPH. In: Lepor H, Lawson R K (eds) Prostatic diseases. Philadelphia: Saunders, 1993: 170–182

19. Lepor H. The treatment of BPH with alpha$_1$ blocker. Curr Opin Urol 1994; 4: 16–21

20. Lepor H. Alpha blockade for the treatment of BPH. Urol Clin North Am, in press

21. Lepor H, Baumann M, Shapiro E. The alpha adrenoceptor binding properties of terazosin in the human prostate and canine brain. J Urol 1988; 140: 664

22. Lepor H, Knapp-Maloney G, Sunshine H. A dose titration study evaluating terazosin: a selective once-a-day alpha$_1$ blocker for the treatment of symptomatic BPH. J Urol 1990; 144: 1393–1398

23. Lepor H, Auerbach S, Puras-Baez A et al. A randomized multicenter placebo controlled study of the efficacy and safety of terazosin in the treatment of benign prostatic hyperplasia. J Urol 1992; 148: 1467–1474

24. Di Silverio F. Use of terazosin in the medical treatment of benign prostatic hyperplasia: experience in Italy. Br J Urol 1992; 70: 22–26

25. Lloyd S N, Buckley J F, Chilton C P et al. Terazosin in the treatment of benign prostatic hyperplasia: a multicentre placebo-controlled trial. Br J Urol 1992; 70: 22–26

26. Lepor H. Long-term safety and effectiveness of terazosin for the treatment of BPH. Urology, in press

27. Hahn C, Able P W, Minneman K P. Heterogeneity of alpha$_1$ adrenergic receptors revealed by chlorethylclonidine. Mol Pharmacol 1987; 32: 505–510

28. Minneman K P, Hahn C, Able P W. Comparison of alpha$_1$ adrenergic receptor subtypes distinguished by chlorethylclonidine and WB-4101. Mol Pharmacol 1988; 33: 509–514

29. Lepor H, Tang R, Meretyk S, Shapiro E. Alpha$_1$ adrenoceptors subtypes in the human prostate. J Urol 1993; 149: 640–642

30. Lepor H, Tang R, Shapiro E. The alpha adrenoceptor subtype mediating the tension of human prostatic smooth muscle. Prostate 1993; 22: 301–307

31. Cotecchia S, Schwinn D A, Randall R R et al. Molecular cloning and expression of the cDNA for the hamster alpha$_1$ adrenergic receptor. Proc Natl Acad Sci USA 1988; 85: 7159–7163

32. Lomasney J W, Cotecchia S, Lorenz W et al. Molecular cloning and expression of the cDNA for the alpha$_{1c}$ adrenergic receptor. J Biol Chem 1991; 266: 6365–6369

33. Schwinn D A, Lomasney J W, Lorenz W et al. Molecular cloning and expression of the cDNA for a novel alpha$_1$ adrenergic receptor subtype. J Biol Chem 1990; 265: 8183–8189

34. Bruno J F, Whittaker J, Song J, Berelowitz M. Molecular cloning and sequencing of a cDNA encoding a human alpha$_{1a}$ adrenergic receptor. Biochem Biophys Res Commun 1991; 179: 1485–1490

35. Hirasawa A K, Horie T, Tanaka K et al. Cloning, functional expression and tissue distribution of human cDNA for the alpha$_{1c}$ adrenergic receptor. Biochem Biophys Res Commun 1993; 195: 902–909

36. Ramarao C S, Denker J M, Perez D M et al. Genomic organization and expression of the human alpha$_{1B}$ adrenergic receptor. J Biol Chem 1992; 267: 21936–21945

37. Forray C, Bard J A, Wetzel J M et al. The alpha$_1$ adrenergic receptor that mediates smooth muscle contraction in human prostate has the pharmacologic properties of a cloned human alpha$_{1C}$ subtype. Pharmacology 1994; 45: 703–709

38. Lepor H, Tang R, Shapiro E et al. Location of the alpha$_{1c}$ adrenoceptor subtypes in the human prostate. J Urol 1994; 151: 381A

39. Price D T, Schwinn D A, Lomasney L F et al. Identification, quantification, and localization of mRNA for three distinct alpha$_1$ adrenergic receptor subtypes in human prostate. J Urol 1993; 150: 546–515

40. Berthelson S, Pettinger W A. A functional basis for the classification of alpha adrenergic receptor. Life Sci 1977; 21: 595–606

26

Doxazosin in the treatment of obstruction of the lower urinary tract

R. S. Kirby

Introduction

The treatment with alpha-1-adrenoceptor antagonists of the benign prostatic hyperplasia (BPH) symptom complex associated with obstruction of the lower urinary tract has evolved substantially from the pioneering work of Caine with phenoxybenzamine. Initially, only two types of alpha-adrenoceptor (alpha-1 and alpha-2) were identified. Phenoxybenzamine, an antagonist at both alpha-adrenoceptors, was classified as a non-selective alpha-adrenoceptor antagonist. Subsequently, the prime determinant of periurethral smooth muscle tone was found to be the alpha-1-adrenoceptor, which led to the clinical evaluation of the first alpha-1-selective antagonist, prazosin, in an attempt to improve the side-effect profile of phenoxybenzamine. Understanding has increased further, to an extent where three major subtypes of the alpha-1-adrenoceptor have been identified; namely alpha-1A, alpha-1B and alpha-1D. The evolution of the nomenclature, which has been confusing and has undergone change over the last few years, is described in a review by Bylund et al.[1]

As a class, alpha-1-adrenoceptor antagonists have been shown to be safe and effective in the treatment of obstruction-related lower urinary tract symptoms.[2] Both obstructive and irritative symptoms are improved, and there are changes in urinary flow and residual volume consistent with a reduction in urethral resistance. Prazosin has been used in this context for several years, but its therapeutic potential has been limited owing to the dosing regimen and the side effects associated with the rapidity of onset of action. Doxazosin, a selective alpha-1-adrenoceptor antagonist, was developed to overcome these shortcomings. It has similar affinity at all three alpha-1 subtypes and, therefore, can be considered to have a balanced pharmacological profile.[3] In addition, doxazosin can be distinguished from prazosin on the basis of physiochemical differences, which result in a more gradual onset of action and an extended plasma half-life (22 h), consistent with utility as a once-a-day agent (Fig. 26.1).[4,5] Doxazosin has had a wide exposure in BPH and hypertensive patients, and also in the high proportion of patients with concomitant disease.[6]

This chapter reviews the currently available data with doxazosin, and considers whether the balanced action of doxazosin on all alpha-1-adrenoceptors translates into clinical advantages for patient, primary-care physician and urologist, alike.

Alpha-1-adrenoceptor heterogeneity

To understand the clinical profile of doxazosin it is necessary to consider briefly the pathophysiological roles of alpha-1-adrenoceptor subtypes. A comprehensive review of the literature is not within the scope of this chapter, but the salient features are summarized below.

The best correlation between the prostatic contractile response and any subtype is with the alpha-1A-adrenoceptor subtype.[7–9] This correlation is not absolute, and a contribution from other subtypes to the maintenance of periurethral stromal tone cannot be ruled out. However, in an attempt to circumvent side effects and increase efficacy, targeting the alpha-1A-

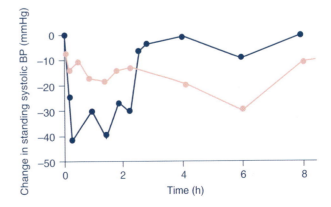

Figure 26.1. *Onset of action of doxazosin (●; mean dose 0.95 mg i.v.) and prazosin (●; mean dose 1 mg i.v.): effect on standing systolic blood pressure. (From ref. 4 with permission.)*

adrenoceptor would represent a logical starting point. The disadvantages and advantages of such a strategy are discussed in more detail later. Whereas with regard to the prostate there is some level of consensus, the roles of the subtypes in other organs and physiological processes, and in the underlying aetiology of disease progression, are more equivocal.

Safety and efficacy of doxazosin in BPH treatment

Short-term efficacy

To date, seven double-blind placebo-controlled clinical studies of doxazosin in patients with BPH have been completed, and five of these are now reported in the literature.[10–14] Patients enrolled in the studies have been men aged between 50 and 80 years with clinical evidence of BPH and maximum flow rates below 15 ml/s. In general, patients receiving treatment with other alpha-1-adrenoceptor antagonists, and patients with urinary tract infections or other serious illnesses, were excluded from these studies. A wash-out phase of at least 1 week was followed by a double-blind treatment period of between 1 and 6 months. Patients were randomized either to doxazosin (at an initial dose of 1 mg/day and increased sequentially according to protocol) or to placebo. Both normotensive and hypertensive patients were included in these studies.

Treatment with doxazosin increased both maximum and average urinary flow rates in almost all studies. The changes achieved statistical significance compared with placebo in the majority of patients. The usual effective dose was 4 mg/day, although additional benefits in some patients were seen with doses up to 8 mg/day. Doxazosin also produced a consistently reduced residual urine volume, albeit small and variable, compared with placebo.

BPH-associated symptoms were also improved to a statistically significant extent in the majority of studies. Irrespective of the different symptom scores used in these studies, consistently greater responses were recorded in patients treated with doxazosin than in those given placebo. A retrospective study has demonstrated that doxazosin produced a greater than 30% reduction in the American Urological Association (AUA) symptom score in almost two-thirds of patients, and that the degree of symptom bothersomeness was also significantly improved.

The beneficial effects of doxazosin on symptoms and uroflow are seen within the first few weeks of treatment, often before doxazosin has been titrated to the optimum dose (Fig. 26.2). This has important clinical implications, in that patients may be encouraged to continue to comply with treatment if they experience an early improvement in symptoms.

Long-term efficacy

The longest double-blind study with doxazosin currently available was conducted by Holme et al.,[13] with a duration of 29 weeks. This trial demonstrated that

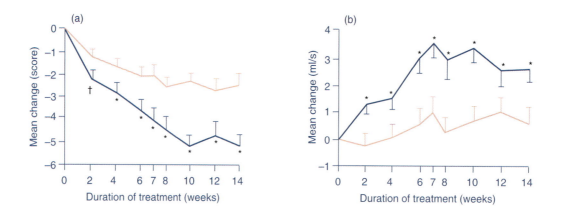

Figure 26.2. *Effect of doxazosin (blue line) vs placebo (pink line) on (a) symptom score and (b) peak uroflow. Asterisks indicate significant differences from placebo (*p < 0.005); dagger indicates significant difference from baseline (†p < 0.05). (From ref. 12 with permission.)*

efficacy was maintained throughout the period. The long-term efficacy of doxazosin is also currently being evaluated in an open extension study of patients who completed three initial double-blind trials.[15] A total of 450 men (86%) have chosen to participate in these open-phase studies. Currently, data are available for up to 48 months of BPH treatment with doxazosin. Results indicate that patients have experienced significant, sustained increases in maximum flow rate from baseline (Fig. 26.3) and

sustained, significant improvements in total, obstructive and irritative symptom scores (Fig. 26.4).

Safety profile

The clinical database for doxazosin in the treatment of hypertension extends to more than 2 billion patient days. Data are now emerging from studies of doxazosin in BPH to suggest that the compound is equally well tolerated in patients with this condition and,

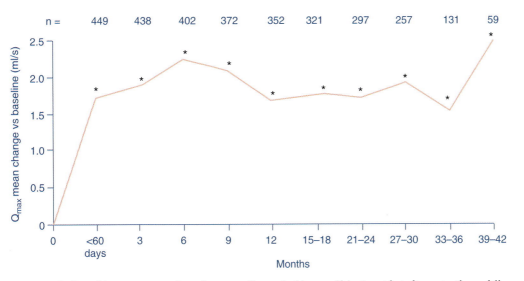

Figure 26.3. *Sustained effect of doxazosin on peak uroflow over 42 months (data on file). Asterisks indicate significant differences from baseline (*p = 0.001).*

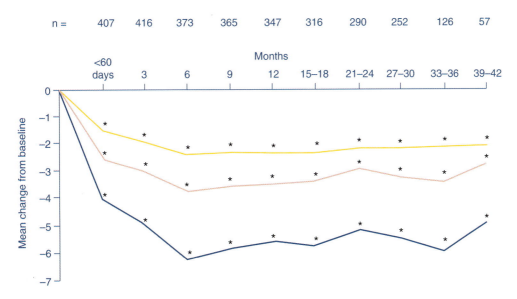

Figure 26.4. *Sustained effect of doxazosin on obstructive (——), irritative (——) and total symptom scores (——) over 42 months (data on file). Asterisks indicate significant differences from baseline (*p = 0.0001).*

intriguingly, perhaps is even better tolerated in normotensive than in hypertensive patients. In the seven studies that have been completed so far, overall, 46% of doxazosin-treated patients reported at least one adverse event compared with 38% of placebo-treated patients (representing an overall 8% increase in side effects over placebo). The most commonly reported adverse events in both groups were dizziness, vertigo, headache and fatigue; cardiovascular events such as postural hypotension were infrequent. The majority of adverse events were mild and did not require discontinuation of treatment.

Doxazosin is also well tolerated over time: adverse events reported during the long-term, open extension study were similar to those occurring during the initial double-blind studies. Again, the most frequently reported adverse events were dizziness, headache and fatigue. The incidence of adverse events with doxazosin did not increase over time. In fact, a reverse Kaplan–Meier plot of patient withdrawals from therapy during long-term treatment illustrates a levelling-off of discontinuations after the first few months. Approximately half of those patients who discontinued therapy with doxazosin owing to adverse events did so within the first 9 months of therapy (Fig. 26.5).

Treatment of the whole patient
Effects on blood pressure control
The involvement of alpha-1-adrenoceptor subtypes in cardiovascular control is of prime importance in normotensive and hypertensive patients. Not surprisingly, as blood pressure regulation is the algebraic sum of many cardiac and vascular processes, the 'blood pressure subtype' of the alpha-1-adrenoceptor has not been identified. Although there may be differential distributions within the vasculature, all three alpha-1 subtypes are ubiquitous.[16,17] On this basis, it could be assumed that cardiovascular homeostasis depends on all three subtypes, and effective blood pressure control will be achieved only with a balanced alpha-1-adrenoceptor antagonist. Equally, a prostate-selective antagonist may be incapable of providing effective blood pressure control in BPH patients with associated hypertension.

It is well documented that the effects of alpha-1-adrenoceptor antagonists are highly dependent on the haemodynamic baseline. Doxazosin lowers blood pressure when sympathetic drive is high, for example in hypertension. In contrast, doxazosin has less effect on resistance vessel tone in normotensive patients, and clinically insignificant changes in blood pressure are observed (Fig. 26.6).[18,19] Interestingly, there is no effect

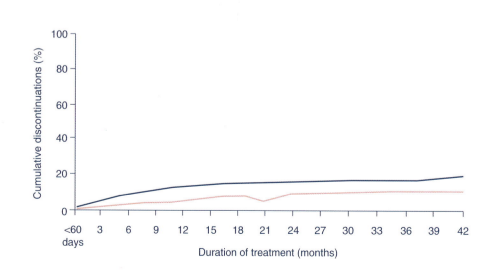

Figure 26.5. *Reverse Kaplan–Meier plot of discontinuations from long-term doxazosin therapy because of adverse events (upper curve) or inadequate clinical response (lower curve) (data on file).*

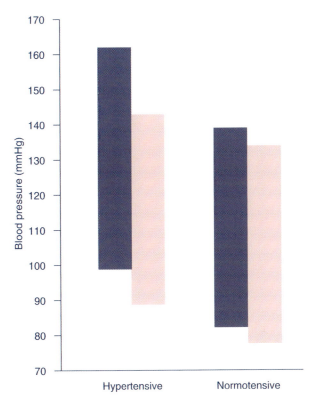

Figure 26.6. *Effect of doxazosin ( ) on the blood pressure of hypertensive and normotensive BPH patients (■, baseline). (From ref. 19 with permission.)*

has identified several in vitro loci that could account for the clinical observations. Increases in LDL-receptor activity and lipoprotein lipase activity, and decreases in intracellular LDL synthesis and cholesterol absorption, have been observed in the presence of these drugs. No one alpha-1-adrenoceptor subtype has been linked to these effects. Indeed, studies of doxazosin metabolites indicate that a component of the drug's actions may arise from a direct action on signal transduction, independent of the alpha-1-adrenoceptor.[23]

In the context of cardiovascular risk factors, catecholamines are involved in smooth muscle proliferation in the vasculature via an alpha-1-adrenoceptor mechanism.[24,25] Alpha-1-adrenoceptor-antagonist attenuation of a proliferative vascular response could have important implications in the prevention of hypertension, coronary heart disease (CHD) and atherosclerosis.

Doxazosin has also been shown to have a favourable effect on other cardiovascular risk factors, including increased fibrinolysis, inhibition of platelet aggregation, attenuation of the adverse haemodynamic and haemostatic effects of smoking, and regression of left ventricular hypertrophy.[20,21]

Extensive studies of almost 5000 hypertensive patients in general practice show a beneficial effect of doxazosin in significantly reducing CHD.[26] On the basis of the Framingham Study equation,[27] an approximate 20% reduction in CHD incidence would be predicted to result from these changes in CHD risk factors. Thus, the beneficial effects of doxazosin on cardiovascular risk further support the use of a balanced agent in the treatment of the BPH patient as a whole.

on the haemodynamic baseline, irrespective of whether BPH patients are physiologically normotensive or are stabilized on antihypertensive therapy.[18]

Cardiovascular risk factors

Many of the risk factors for hypertension are common to congestive heart failure and atherosclerosis.[20] Particularly relevant are an aberrant lipid profile and insulin resistance/glucose intolerance. The effects of doxazosin compared with other quinazolines and other antihypertensive agents have been extensively reviewed by Pool.[20,21] Clearly, doxazosin offers a number of benefits in this respect. In the Treatment of Mild Hypertension Study (TOMHS),[22] doxazosin, in contrast to other antihypertensive agents, produced sustained reductions over a 48-month period in total and low-density-lipoprotein (LDL) cholesterol and triglycerides, and increases in high-density-lipoprotein (HDL) cholesterol and HDL:total cholesterol ratios.

Although understanding of the effect of alpha-blockers on serum lipid profile is incomplete, Pool[20,21]

Sexual function

Although specific studies in male erectile dysfunction have not been carried out, there is good evidence that doxazosin has a positive effect on impotent males. In the 4-year TOMHS study,[22] a much-reduced incidence of erectile dysfunction was reported in the doxazosin group compared with placebo (Fig. 26.7). In contrast, other antihypertensive agents (e.g. beta-blockers, diuretics) appeared to increase the incidence. In the placebo group, 50% of males recording erectile dysfunction at the start of the study underwent spontaneous 'remission' during the trial. By comparison,

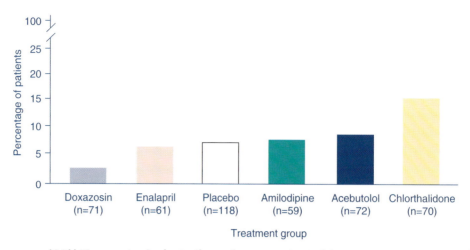

Figure 26.7. *Treatment of Mild Hypertension Study: incidence of men reporting inability to maintain an erection. (From ref. 22 with permission.)*

in the doxazosin groups all males returned to normal potency. This positive effect is consistent with the well-documented role of alpha-1-adrenoceptors in the control of corpus cavernosal tone[28] and the clinical benefit observed with intracavernosal injection of alpha-1-adrenoceptor antagonists.

Urogenital tract

When considering the urogenital tract it is important to remember the potential contribution from extraprostatic actions to the overall clinical profile of BPH.[28] There is no direct correlation between flow rates and urethral resistance and the observed improvement in symptoms. Furthermore, it should be remembered that patients generally present because of symptoms and bothersomeness, not because of a reduced urinary flow. Thus, the extraprostatic actions that have been observed with doxazosin on the bladder,[28] spinal cord[29] and efferent pathways[30] may be just as important as changes induced in periurethral stromal tone.

Conclusions

Doxazosin has a balanced pharmacological action at all three subtypes of the alpha-1-adrenoceptor, which is reflected clinically in a beneficial effect on the whole patient. At the level of the prostate, the action of doxazosin on the alpha-1A-adrenoceptor subtype undoubtedly accounts for the significant changes in

urinary flow rates and voiding pressure, secondary to changes in urethral resistance. The prostatic action, and the extraprostatic effects of doxazosin on the bladder, bladder neck and higher centres, account for the significant changes in symptoms and bothersomeness.

Doxazosin produces clinically important blood pressure reductions in hypertensive BPH patients. It is likely that an action on all three adrenoceptor subtypes is required to produce this profile. In subjects with physiological or drug-controlled normotension, only minor, clinically insignificant changes in blood pressure are observed.

Doxazosin appears to have a beneficial effect on several risk factors (e.g. lipid profile, glucose metabolism) associated with hypertension, CHD and atherosclerosis. The alpha-1-adrenoceptor subtype involved has not been identified, and there may be a contribution from receptor-independent events.

In addition to these pharmacological actions, the physiochemical properties of the drug offer considerable advantages. In particular, doxazosin, compared with other alpha-1-adrenoceptor antagonists, has a long plasma half-life consistent with once-daily dosing. The associated gradual onset of action also underpins the reduced propensity for side effects. Importantly, the pharmacokinetics are unchanged in the elderly and in renal failure.

Doxazosin is extremely well tolerated in both old and young patients. Most adverse events are mild or moderate in severity and do not require discontinuation of therapy. There is no evidence of a deleterious impact on sexual function — in fact, there is evidence of a positive effective of doxazosin on erectile dysfunction.

Overall, the balanced action of doxazosin on all alpha-1-adrenoceptor subtypes is associated with a highly desirable clinical profile for the BPH patient. Any advantages arising from a genuinely prostate-selective antagonist will ultimately have to be weighed against the deficits of such therapy in the treatment of the whole patient.

References

1. Bylund B D, Eikenberg D C, Hieble J P et al. International Union of Pharmacology nomenclature of adrenoceptors. Pharmacol Rev 1994; 46: 121–136

2. Eri L M, Tveter K J. Alpha-blockade in the treatment of symptomatic benign prostatic hyperplasia. J Urol 1995; 154: 923–934

3. Kenny B A, Naylor A M, Carter A J et al. Effect of alpha$_1$ adrenoceptor antagonists on prostatic pressure and blood pressure in the anesthetized dog. Urology 1994; 44: 52–57

4. Elliot H L, Meredith P A, Sumner D J et al. A pharmacodynamic and pharmacokinetic assessment of a new alpha-adrenoceptor antagonist, doxazosin (UK-33274) in normotensive subjects. Br J Clin Pharmacol 1982; 13: 699–703

5. Young R A, Brogden R N. Doxazosin: a review of its pharmacodynamic and pharmacokinetic properties and therapeutic efficacy in mild to moderate hypertension. Drugs 1988; 35: 535–541

6. Boyle P, Napalkov P. The epidemiology of benign prostatic hyperplasia and observations on concomitant hypertension. Scand J Urol Nephrol 1995; 168: 7–12

7. Forray C, Chiu G, Wetzel J M et al. Effects of novel alpha1-C adrenergic receptor antagonists on the contraction of human prostate smooth muscle. J Urol 1994; 151: 267A (abstr 159)

8. Goetz A S, Lutz M W, Rimele T J, Saussy D L Jr. Characterization of alpha1 adrenoceptor subtypes in human and canine prostate membranes. J Pharmacol Exp Ther 1994; 271: 1228–1233

9. Ford A P D W, Arredondo N F, Blue D R Jr et al. Do alpha1-A (alpha1-C)-adrenoceptors (AR) mediate prostatic smooth muscle contraction in man? Studies with a novel, selective alpha1-A-AR antagonist, RS 17053. Br J Pharmacol 1996; in press

10. Chapple C R, Carter P, Christmas T J et al. A three month double-blind study of doxazosin as treatment for benign prostatic bladder outlet obstruction. Br J Urol 1994; 74: 50–56

11. Gillenwater J Y, Conn R L, Chrysant S G et al. Doxazosin for the treatment of benign prostatic hyperplasia in patients with mild to moderate essential hypertension: a double-blind, placebo-controlled, dose-response multicenter study. J Urol 1995; 154: 110–115

12. Fawzy A, Braun K, Lewis G P et al. Doxazosin in the treatment of benign prostatic hyperplasia in normotensive patients: a multicenter study. J Urol 1995; 154: 105–110

13. Holme J B, Christensen M M, Rasmussen P C et al. 29 weeks doxazosin treatment in patients with symptomatic benign prostatic hyperplasia. Scand J Urol Nephrol 1994; 28: 77–82

14. Christensen M M, Holme J B, Rasmussen P C et al. Doxazosin treatment in patients with prostatic obstruction. A double-blind placebo-controlled study. Scand J Urol Nephrol 1993; 27: 39–44

15. Lepor H. Long-term efficacy and safety of doxazosin for the treatment of benign prostatic hyperplasia. J Urol 1995; 153:273A (abstr 180)

16. Bylund D B, Regan J W, Faber J E et al. Vascular α-adrenoceptors: from the gene to the human. Can J Physiol Pharmacol 1995; 73: 533–543

17. Hoffman B B, Hu Z-H. Regulation of responses mediated by alpha1-adrenergic receptors in smooth muscle cultures. Pharmacol Commun 1995; 6: 1–3

18. Kaplan S A, Meade-D'Alisera P, Quinones S, Soldo K A. Doxazosin in physiologically and pharmacologically normotensive men with benign prostatic hyperplasia. Urol 1995; 46: 512–517

19. Kirby R. Doxazosin in benign prostatic hyperplasia: effects on blood pressure and urinary flow in normotensive and hypertensive men. Urology 1995; 46: 182–186

20. Pool J L. Effects of doxazosin on coronary heart disease risk factors in the hypertensive patients. Br J Clin Pract Symp Suppl 1994; 74: 8–12

21. Pool J L. Effects of doxazosin on serum lipids. A review of the clinical data and molecular basis for altered lipid metabolism. Am Heart J 1991; 121: 251–260

22. Neaton J D, Grimm R H, Prineas R J et al. Treatment of Mild Hypertension Study: final results. JAMA 1993; 270: 713–724

23. Chait A, Gilmore M, Kawamura M. Inhibition of low density lipoprotein oxidation in vitro by the 6- and 7- hydroxy metabolites of doxazosin, an alpha1-adrenergic antihypertensive agent. Am J Hypertens 1994; 7: 159–164

24. Jackson C L, Schwartz S M. Pharmacology of smooth muscle cell replication. Hypertension 1992; 20: 713–736

25. Hu Z-H, Shi X-Y, Okazaki M, Hoffman B B. Angiotensin II induces transcription and expression of α_1-adrenergic receptors in vascular smooth muscle. Am J Physiol 1995; 268: H1006–1014

26. Langdon C G, Packard R S. Doxazosin in hypertension: results of a general practice study in 4809 patients. Br J Clin Pract 1994; 48: 293–298

27. Levy D, Wilson P W F, Anderson K M, Castelli W P. Stratifying patients at risk from coronary heart disease; new insights from the Framingham Heart Study. Am Heart J 1990; 119: 71–77

28. Andersson K-E. Pharmacology of lower urinary tract smooth muscles and penile erectile tissues. Pharmacol Rev 1993; 45: 253–308

29. Ishizuka O, Persson K, Mattiasson A et al. Micturition in conscious rats with and without outlet obstruction: role of spinal α_1 adrenoceptors. Br J Pharmacol 1996; in press

30. Ramage A G, Wyllie M G. Effects of doxazosin and terazosin on inferior mesenteric nerve activity, spontaneous bladder contraction and blood pressure in anaesthetised cats. Br J Pharmacol 1994; 112: 526P

27

Alfuzosin

A. Jardin

Introduction

Alfuzosin, a quinazoline derivative, acts as a selective antagonist of alpha-1-adrenoceptor-mediated contraction of bladder neck, proximal urethral and prostatic smooth muscle. Bladder outlet resistance resulting from benign prostatic hyperplasia (BPH) is consequently reduced. Alfuzosin has been authorized in France since 1989, and now in numerous European countries, for the treatment of symptomatic BPH.

Pharmacological profile of alfuzosin at alpha-1-adrenoceptor subtypes

Alpha-1-adrenoceptors have recently been shown to comprise a family of distinct subtypes. In addition to the native alpha-1-adrenoceptors, which have been subdivided into two pharmacologically different subtypes, namely alpha-1A and alpha-1B, three pharmacologically and structurally distinct members of the alpha-1-adrenoceptor subfamily (which have been termed alpha-1b, alpha-1c and alpha-1d) have been identified by molecular cloning techniques (for review see ref. 1).

In permanent HeLa cell lines stably transfected with either the hamster smooth muscle alpha-1b-adrenoceptor, the bovine brain alpha-1c-adrenoceptor or the rat cerebral cortex alpha-1d-adrenoceptor, Faure et al.[2] have shown that [3H]prazosin-binding to these various alpha-1-adrenoceptor preparations is potently inhibited by alfuzosin as well as by terazosin or parazosin (Table 27.1). Comparable results are reported by Forray et al.[3] on membrane preparations from LM (tk−) cells stably transfected with the cloned human alpha-1-adrenoceptor subtype genes, since neither alfuzosin, terazosin or prazosin show significant differences in their potencies to inhibit [3H]prazosin-binding to the three alpha-1-adrenoceptor subtypes. In contrast, WB-4101 and 5-methylurapidil display a higher affinity for the cloned bovine brain or human hippocampus alpha-1c-adrenoceptor subtype (Table 27.1).[3]

Table 27.1. *Affinity of alfuzosin for the various alpha-1-adrenoceptor subtypes expressed in cDNA stably transfected cell lines*

Compound	pK_i*		
	Hamster smooth muscle (alpha-1b)	Bovine brain (alpha-1c)	Rat cerebral cortex (alpha-1d)
Alfuzosin	8.93	8.42	8.58
Terazosin	9.16	8.53	8.74
Prazosin	10.18	9.73	9.71
WB-4101	8.43	10.09	9.37
5-Methylurapidil	7.21	8.89	7.75

*The concentration of each drug that inhibited specific [3H]prazosin-binding by 50% (IC_{50}) is used to calculate K_i values. The potencies of the drugs is expressed by the negative logarithms of their K_i values (pK_i). (Data from ref. 2.)

Affinity of alfuzosin for alpha-adrenoceptors in the human prostate

The cranial region of the human prostatic adenoma possesses high-affinity [3H]prazosin-binding sites.[4,5] These sites display the pharmacological characteristics of alpha-1-adrenoceptors. As shown in Table 27.2, [3H]prazosin-binding is potently displaced by alfuzosin and phentolamine, with IC_{50} values in the low nanomolar range, whereas the alpha-2-adrenoceptor antagonists, idazoxan and yohimbine, or the beta-adrenoceptor antagonist, propranolol, affect [3H]prazosin-binding only with IC_{50} values in the micromolar range. Thus, alfuzosin shows high affinity for alpha-1-adrenoceptors in the human prostate which may represent the pharmacological target in BPH. In support of this view, it has been reported that alfuzosin-displaceable [125I]HEAT (iodo-4-hydroxyphenyl-ethyl-aminomethyl-tetralone)-binding sites, which have the pharmacological characteristics of alpha-1-adrenoceptors, are exclusively associated with muscular stroma of the prostate and are globally elevated in sections from

Table 27.2. *Affinity of alfuzosin for alpha-1-adrenoceptor in cranial human prostatic adenoma labelled with [³H]prazosin*

Compound	IC$_{50}$*(µM)
Alfuzosin	0.035 ± 0.008
Phentolamine	0.018 ± 0.001
Idazoxan	3.5 ± 1.0
Yohimbine	6.0 ± 2.0
Propranolol	37 ± 9

*IC$_{50}$ values represent drug concentrations producing 50% inhibition of specific [³H]prazosin binding. (Data from refs 4 and 5.)

prostatic adenomas compared with non-hypertrophic tissue.[6]

As far as alpha-1-adrenoceptor subtypes are concerned, Faure et al.[7] have shown that the human prostate expresses, at the level of the apex, base, periurethra and lateral lobe, mRNA transcripts corresponding to alpha-1b-, alpha-1c- and alpha-1d-adrenoceptors. In addition, these authors have shown that a reconstituted partial sequence (349 amino acids) of the human prostatic alpha-1c-adrenoceptor shares 94% identity with the bovine brain alpha-1c-adrenoceptor, and that this receptor represents the predominant alpha-1-adrenoceptor subtype in this tissue.

Effects of alfuzosin on elevated urethral and blood pressure

Inhibition of urethral responses to stimulation of hypogastic sympathetic nerves in the cat can be considered to represent an animal model of the dynamic sympathetic constriction of urethral smooth muscle, which is regarded as a contributory factor in the obstructive disorders that characterize BPH. On the other hand, inhibition in alpha-1-adrenoceptor antagonists of blood pressure in spontaneously hypertensive rats is accepted as a model to assess antihypertensive drugs acting at receptors physiologically stimulated by an increased sympathetic tone. Thus, a relationship between the ability of alfuzosin to inhibit sympathetically mediated increases in urethral tone in the cat and to act on sympathetically mediated hypertension in the spontaneously hypertensive rat can be considered as a relevant way to

evaluate the therapeutic margin in BPH with respect to unwanted vascular effects (such as orthostatic hypotension).

Studies conducted in the anaesthetized cat and in conscious spontaneously hypertensive rats confirm the alpha-1-antagonist properties of alfuzosin. The compound produces a dose-related as well as a complete (Figs 27.1, 27.2) and prolonged (Fig. 27.2) inhibition of the rise in urethral pressure resulting from post-ganglionic stimulation of hypogastric sympathetic nerves in the cat. As shown in Table 27.3, the decrease by alfuzosin of the urethral resistance induced by hypogastric nerve stimulation in the cat occurs at doses 11 times lower than those that reduce blood pressure in the spontaneously hypertensive rat.[8]

Functional selectivity of alfuzosin for the lower urinary tract

The affinity of alfuzosin for alpha-1-adrenoceptors in the human prostate, on the one hand, and the predominant presence of alpha-1c-adrenoceptors in the

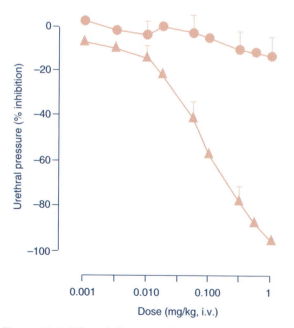

Figure 27.1. *Effect of alfuzosin (▲) compared with vehicle control (●) on an increase in urethral pressure in the anaesthetized cat. Doses of alfuzosin correspond to cumulative i.v. bolus administration of the drug. Increased urethral pressure was elicited by electrical stimulation of sympathetic hypogastric nerves. (From ref. 5 with permission.)*

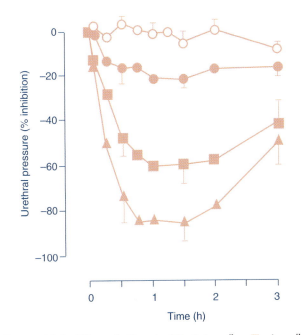

Figure 27.2. *Effect of alfuzosin (● , 0.1 mg/kg; ■ , 1 mg/kg; ▲ , 3 mg/kg) or vehicle control (○) on an increase in urethral pressure in the anaesthetized cat. Doses of alfuzosin correspond to cumulative i.v. bolus administration of the drug. Increased urethral pressure was elicited by electrical stimulation of sympathetic hypogastric nerves. (From ref. 5 with permission.)*

Table 27.3. *Effects of alfuzosin on urethral pressure (UP) in the cat and on mean arterial blood pressure (AP) in the spontaneously hypertensive rat*

Compound	UP [ID$_{50}$ (mg/kg,i.d.)]*	AP [ID$_{20}$ (mg/kg,p.o.)]*	Uroselectivity ratio (AP/UP)
Alfuzosin	0.36	4.0	11
Terazosin	0.12	0.42	3.5
Prazosin	0.12	0.13	1

*Values are doses of each compound producing a 50% reduction in urethral pressure (UP$_{50}$) in anaesthetized cats and 20% reduction in blood pressure (UP$_{20}$) in spontaneously hypertensive rats. (Data from ref. 8.)

human prostate, on the other hand, suggest that alfuzosin may exert its pharmacological properties in this particular tissue through the blockade of the alpha-1c-adrenoceptor subtype. In support of this view it has been shown that the alpha-1-adrenoceptor that mediates smooth muscle contraction induced by phenylephrine in the human prostate has the

pharmacological properties of the cloned human alpha-1c-adrenoceptor subtype.[3]

The hypothesis that a selective antagonist of the alpha-1c-adrenoceptor (alpha-1A-adrenoceptor under the recently proposed nomenclature)[9] might represent an effective agent for the treatment of BPH, with reduced systemic cardiovascular side effects, has been advanced by several investigators.[3,7] Selectivity for the alpha-1c-adrenoceptor subtype may, however, contribute only in part to the functional selectivity of an alpha-1-adrenoceptor blocker for the lower urinary tract, and further investigations to determine whether the alpha-1c-adrenergic receptor subtype present in the prostate differs from the functional subtype which controls vascular tone may be essential.

In this context, although alfuzosin does not show selectivity for any particular alpha-1-adrenoceptor subtype in animal models, the compound displays functional selectivity at the levels of the lower urinary tract. A pharmacokinetic property of alfuzosin leading to a preferential distribution at the level of the urethral or prostatic tissue may contribute to its uroselectivity.

In conclusion, alfuzosin is a potent and selective alpha-1-adrenoceptor antagonist that displays functional uroselectivity in animal models. These pharmacological properties support the rationale for expecting alfuzosin to alleviate the dynamic component of urinary obstruction attributable to sympathetic tone in BPH.

Pharmacokinetic properties

The pharmacokinetics of alfuzosin are linear and non-saturable. Absorption of oral alfuzosin is relatively rapid, with a maximum plasma concentration occurring after a mean of 1.5 h. Its bioavailability is 64%, with a negligible effect of concomitant administration of food on its absorption. Alfuzosin is approximately 90% protein bound in plasma. Its mean plasma elimination half-life is 4.8 h. Alfuzosin is extensively metabolized by the liver and the metabolites are inactive. Its main route of elimination is faecal. Because of the above pharmacokinetic profile, it has to be administered three times daily. The usual recommended dosage is 2.5 mg three times a day, i.e. 7.5 mg/day. This daily dose can be increased to 10 mg/day with a ratio of the AUC (area under curve) obtained corresponding to the ratio of the dosage.[10] Recently, a slow-release (SR) formulation has been developed in order to improve compliance with the treatment by reducing the number of daily doses from three to two. The relative bioavailability of this new formulation is 15% lower than the immediate-release (IR) formulation of alfuzosin. The time to reach the peak is longer, approximately 3 h instead of 1.5 h, confirming that the absorption is delayed, as well as its apparent elimination half-life, which is 8 h. The usual recommended daily dose is 5 mg twice daily, i.e. 10 mg/day; this higher daily dosage compares with the usual daily dose of 7.5 mg for the IR formulation, compensating for the relative loss of bioavailability.

Oral bioavailability is increased in the elderly: thus, a reduced initial dose is recommended. The overall pharmacokinetic profile of alfuzosin is not significantly changed in patients with renal insufficiency, in contrast to what is observed in patients with hepatic insufficiency, where dosage modifications appear to be necessary.

Pharmacodynamic effects in humans

Urodynamic effects

Intravenous alfuzosin significantly reduced high urethral pressure of neurological origin which is partly responsible for the voiding symptoms. In 163 patients with symptomatic neurogenic bladder disease (NBD) and a mean maximal urethral pressure of 108 cmH$_2$O included in a randomized, double-blind placebo-controlled study assessing the effect of a single i.v. injection of alfuzosin (0.5, 1 or 2 mg) or placebo, alfuzosin significantly and dose-dependently decreased urethral pressure with a mean decrease of 44% for the 2 mg dose.[11] A single i.v. test dose of 5 mg alfuzosin had previously been used to determine which patients with spinal cord injury (n=21) were likely to benefit from alfuzosin therapy. Response was assessed in terms of change in micturition, residual urine and posterior urethral pressure and diameter.[12] Furthermore, in a placebo-controlled study conducted in 66 patients with NBD, this decrease was maintained with oral alfuzosin for 12 weeks and associated with a significant improvement of voiding symptoms (–45%) and residual urine volume (–39%) compared with placebo.[13] This

effect appears to be in direct correlation with the alpha-1-adrenoceptor-antagonist effects of alfuzosin.

In patients with BPH, orally administered IR alfuzosin significantly and dose-dependently increased urinary flow rates from the first dose. At 90 min after a single alfuzosin dose, peak flow rate (PFR) was significantly increased by 23 and 34% with 1.25 and 2.5 mg, respectively, compared with placebo in 93 patients with initial PFR values of less than 15 ml/s. In patients with PFR values of less than 10 ml/s (n=47), mean increases in PFR with 1.25 or 2.5 mg alfuzosin, or placebo, were even greater — 26, 55 and 17%, respectively.[14] Similar results were observed with SR alfuzosin. At 180 min after a single SR alfuzosin dose, PFR was significantly increased by 29 and 36% with 3 and 5 mg doses, compared with placebo (+17%) in elderly patients (≥ 65 years) with initial PFR values of less than 15 ml/s.[15]

The 30% increase in flow rates, which is the rate of improvement expected with alpha-1-blocker therapy in patients with BPH, is maintained after multiple dose administration of alfuzosin (IR and SR formulations) (Tables 27.4, 27.5). Furthermore, this is of the same order of magnitude as that of prazosin,[16,17] with no statistical intertreatment differences. In those patients with an increase in PFR of at least 25% (i.e. 45–50% of patients) the mean increase is approximately 5 ml/s.

Residual urine volume is a parameter related to the decrease in urinary flow resistance but also to the bladder contractility. Furthermore, it shows wide intra-individual variability between serial examinations.[18] However, alfuzosin has been shown to decrease significantly the volume of residual urine, by 38% after 6 months of treatment compared with 9% in placebo recipients.[19] A few more complex urodynamic assessments have been carried out. In a 3-month, double-blind placebo-controlled study performed in 31 patients with urodynamically proven bladder outflow obstruction treated with alfuzosin (9 or 12 mg/day), there was a significant increase in the volume that produced a strong desire to void, which reflected the increase of bladder capacity.[20] A pressure–flow placebo-controlled study carried out in 32 patients with BPH treated with alfuzosin (7.5 mg/day for 4 and 8 weeks) showed that alfuzosin significantly decreases detrusor pressure compared with placebo (opening pressure, –48%; pressure at maximum flow, –42%; maximum pressure, –41%).[21]

Table 27.4. *Summary of the main placebo-controlled trials with alfuzosin in BPH*

Reference	No. of patients	Inclusion criteria	Dosage (mg/day)	Duration of treatment (months)	Results[†] (percentage increase or decrease)		
Jardin et al. (1991)[19]	518	Boyarsky ≥ 6	7.5–10	6	Symptoms PFR RUV	(P) –32 (P) –11 (P) –9	(A) –42* (A) –11.5 (A) –39
Carbin et al. (1994)[37]	30	PFR < 12 ml/s	7.5	2	Symptoms RUV	(P) –39 (P) –2	(A) –48 (A) –56*
Hansen et al. (1994)[22]	205	Madsen–Iversen > 6 PRF ≤ 10 ml/s	7.5	3	Symptoms PFR RUV	(P) –14 (P) +14 (P) +7	(A) –29* (A) +45* (A) –40
Schulman et al.[‡] (in press)[38]	160	Boyarsky > 10 PFR ≤ 12.5 ml/s	7.5	1	Symptoms PFR RUV	(P) –26 (P) +23 (P) –28	(A) –38 (A) +43* (A) –44*
Delmas et al. (1994)[32]	198	Irritative symptoms PFR ≤ 12 ml/s	(SR)[§] 10	1	Symptoms PFR	(P) –18 (P) +13	(A) –24 (A) +30
Algebi (unpublished data)	390	Irritative symptoms PFR ≤ 15 ml/s	(SR) 10	3	Symptoms PFR RUV	(P) –17 (P) +14 (P) –23	(A) –30* (A) +29* (A) –29*

*Intergroup comparison: $p < 0.05$. [†]A, alfuzosin; P placebo; PFR, peak flow rate; RUV, residual urine volume. [‡]Cross-over design. [§]SR, slow release

Table 27.5. *Peak flow rate (PFR) increases after SR alfuzosin 5 mg bid treatment for 3 months (unpublished data)*

Parameter	Treatment		p^*
	SR alfuzosin (5 mg bid)	Placebo	
Whole population (n)	176	176	
Baseline PFR (ml/s)	10.4	10.1	
Variation vs baseline			
1 month	+ 2.0	+.0.8	
2 months	+ 2.2	+ 1.1	
3 months	+ 2.4	+ 1.1	0.006
Percentage change at 3 months	+ 29	+ 14	
Percentage of responders at 3 months			
> 25% increase	45	31	0.008
> 50% increase	42	25	
Patients with initial PFR < 10 ml/s (n)	67	85	
Baseline PFR (ml/s)	7.6	7.8	
Variation vs baseline: 3 months	+ 3.2	+ 1.3	0.006
Percentage change at 3 months	+ 45	+ 21	
Percentage of responders at 3 months			
> 25% increase	55	38	0.04
> 50% increase	55	29	

*Intergroup comparison; intent to treat analysis.

From the above findings, it can be concluded that the urodynamic effect of alfuzosin is characterized by a decrease in urethral pressure of about 45%, an increase in flow rates in patients with BPH of 30% and a beneficial effect on bladder capacity and pressure.

Haemodynamic effects

The haemodynamic safety profile of single i.v. injections of alfuzosin was very satisfactory for all three dose levels and maximum changes in blood pressure measurements were comparable to those seen with the placebo (Fig. 27.3). This could be due to the high degree of functional uroselectivity, as described above with regard to animal experiments.

At dosages used for BPH treatment, alfuzosin has minor effects on blood pressure, owing to its previously mentioned functional uroselectivity. After single oral doses of alfuzosin [1.25 mg (n=31) and 2.5 mg (n = 31)] administered to patients with BPH, heart rate increased (by 5 beats/min) in the 2.5 mg recipients; asymptomatic hypotension occurred in five patients who received 2.5 mg, and in two patients who received 1.25 mg

alfuzosin. No such changes occurred in placebo recipients. However, mean supine and standing systolic and diastolic blood pressures were not significantly changed by alfuzosin compared with placebo (n=31).[14] This was confirmed in the single-dose study performed with the SR formulation of alfuzosin in elderly patients (mean age 70 years) considered as being at risk.[15] Mild symptomatic and asymptomatic orthostatic hypotension occurred in one and seven patients, respectively, of 117 patients who received SR alfuzosin. In medium-term treatment (3–6 months), minimal changes in blood pressure may be observed. A small but significant decrease in diastolic blood pressure compared with baseline, of 3 mmHg in the alfuzosin (7.5 mg/day) group versus 0 mmHg in the placebo group, was observed after 3 months in the study performed by Hansen et al.[22] The effect on blood pressure in a 3-month placebo-controlled study performed in 390 patients with BPH (unpublished data) is shown in Figure 27.4.

The decreases in standing blood pressure observed in volunteers after the administration of IR alfuzosin (5 mg bid) were compared with those of prazosin (1 mg bid).[23]

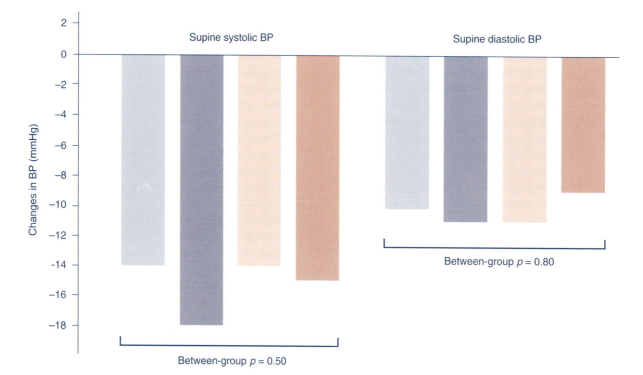

Figure 27.3. *Maximum changes in blood pressure (BP) from baseline following a single i.v. injection of alfuzosin of 0.5 (■), 1 (□) or 2 (■) mg in comparison with placebo (■).*

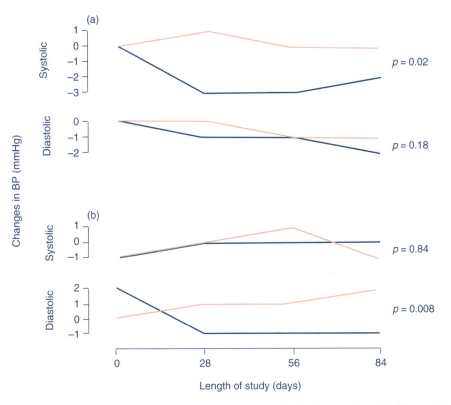

Figure 27.4. *Systolic and diastolic blood pressure (BP) in a 3-month study of placebo (———) vs SR alfuzosin 10 mg/day (———) in 390 patients with BPH: (a) changes from baseline in supine BP; (b) changes in upright minus supine BP. (Unpublished data.)*

They were of a lesser order of magnitude with alfuzosin than with prazosin, the latter inducing a significant decrease in both standing systolic (-22 cmH_2O) and diastolic blood pressure compared with placebo in acute administration, these results confirming the lower-grade effect on blood pressure of alfuzosin than of prazosin, as shown in animal experiments.

Therapeutic potential

More than 15 000 patients suffering from BPH have been included in European clinical studies assessing the efficacy and/or safety of alfuzosin, or the improvement in quality of life after administration of alfuzosin. Most of the studies assessed the IR formulation of alfuzosin (7.5–10 mg dose given in three divided doses) which is registered in almost all Western European countries for the treatment of symptomatic BPH. Its SR formulation (SR alfuzosin, 5 mg bid) is registered or under registration in most of these countries for the same indication.

Clinical efficacy

Jardin et al.[19] reported the efficacy of alfuzosin in a large multicentre placebo-controlled study of 518 patients with symptoms of BPH who received alfuzosin 7.5 or 10 mg/day, or placebo, for 6 months. Patients were evaluated using Boyarksky's symptom-scoring system, urinary flow rates and post-voided residual urine volume. Obstructive and irritative symptoms, assessed according to the Boyarsky scale, improved significantly in the alfuzosin group compared with the placebo group ($p=0.004$). Fewer patients in the alfuzosin group than in the placebo group dropped out due to lack of efficacy (6.8 vs 14.6%, $p=0.0004$) and the prevalence of spontaneous acute urine retention was lower in the alfuzosin group (0.4 vs 2.6%, $p=0.04$). By 6 months, mean urinary flow rates had increased ($p<0.05$) and residual volume had decreased ($p<0.017$) in the alfuzosin group, although the two groups were broadly similar with respect to increase in PFR. Clinical improvement with alfuzosin was apparent after 6 weeks and could be maintained for up to 30 months, as observed in non-comparative extensions of the original 6-month study[19,24,25] (Fig. 27.5).

The symptomatic improvement following alfuzosin treatment was analysed by pooling the data of 983 patients included in six randomized double-blind studies (three placebo-controlled studies, two comparative studies versus prazosin and an extract of the plant *Serenoa repens*, and one study versus prazosin and placebo). The results of the meta-analysis showed that 68, 59 and 73% of patients who received alfuzosin had at least a 25% improvement of their total, irritative and obstructive scores, respectively (Table 27.6) and a 50% improvement of these scores was obtained by 37, 29 and 50% of patients, respectively. These results were highly significant compared with placebo ($p<0.001$). These improvements were maintained at the same levels at the 3- and 6-month endpoints (Fig. 27.6). Alfuzosin was at least as effective as prazosin and significantly better than *Serenoa repens*. Of the placebo recipients, 55% had a 25% improvement in the total score at 6 weeks and this figure did not tend to decrease with time.[26] Interestingly,

in a 3-month placebo-controlled study with the SR formulation of alfuzosin (5 mg bid; unpublished data), symptoms were assessed according to both the Boyarsky and International Prostate Symptom Score (I-PSS) scoring systems. Following 3 months of treatment with alfuzosin, patients reported a clinically relevant and statistically significant improvement in their urinary symptoms in both scoring systems that was similar to that from the above-mentioned meta-analysis (Table 27.7). This clinical efficacy was observed from the first month. Furthermore, a good correlation between the two scores was demonstrated, with an excellent correlation in 54% of patients, a fair correlation in 30% of patients and a discordance between the two scores in only 16% of patients.

Quality of life is now becoming accepted as an important criterion in the evaluation of treatments for BPH.[27] Results from a study involving over 7000 outpatients treated with alfuzosin for 3 months showed quality-of-life scores to improve by 44% and to correlate significantly with symptom scores.[28] These results are

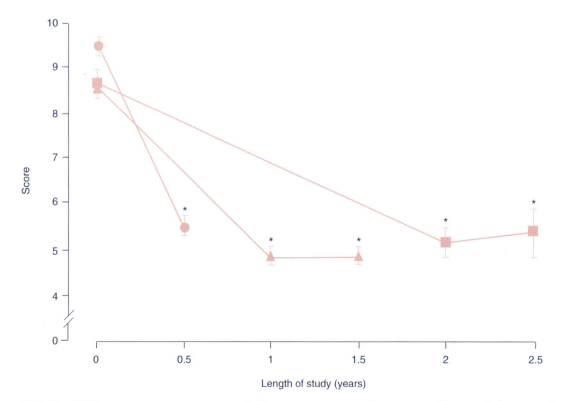

Figure 27.5. *Total BPH symptom score improvement with alfuzosin: maintenance of symptomatic efficacy in the long term. Part 1: 6-month placebo-controlled study (●; n=251); part 2: 1-year open extension (▲; n=131); part 3: 1-year (additional) open extension (■; n=50). *p < 0.05 vs baseline. (Data from refs 19, 24 and 25 with permission.)*

Table 27.6. *Results of meta-analysis of placebo-controlled studies: symptomatic improvement at week 6 endpoint*

Score improvement	Percentage of patients improved		p*
	Alfuzosin	Placebo	
Total score			
≥ 25%	68	55	< 0.001
≥ 50%	37	23	
Irritative score			
≥ 25%	59	48	0.003
≥ 50%	29	24	
Obstructive score			
≥ 25%	73	60	< 0.001
≥ 50%	50	36	

*Intergroup comparison: chi-square (Ridit scores)

supported by those of a study conducted by Martelli et al.[29] in which 3 months' treatment with alfuzosin had a positive impact on quality of life, especially on activity index, in patients with moderate or severe prostatism (n = 498).

Clinical improvement is associated with an increase in flow rates and decrease in residual urine volume, as mentioned above. Overall, alfuzosin has brought about a consequent symptomatic improvement in patients suffering from moderately symptomatic BPH (i.e. a 25% improvement in two-thirds of treated patients and a 50% improvement in one-third), with a favourable impact on quality of life. The increase in flow rates is 30%, which is that expected with alpha-1-blocker therapy,[30] and residual urine volume may be decreased by 40%. The relief is prompt and can be maintained over 2 years.

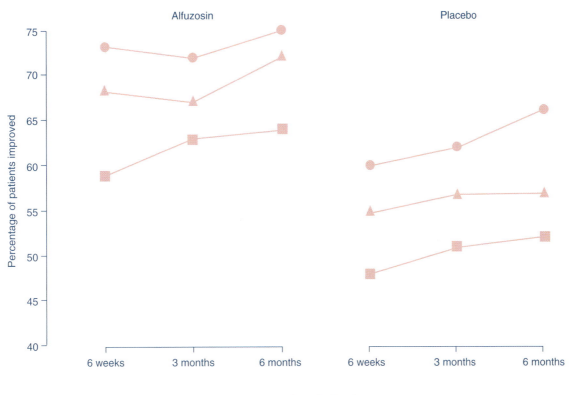

Figure 27.6. *Maintenance in the long term (up to 6 months) of at least 25% improvement in BPH symptoms (circles, obstructive scores; squares, irritative scores; triangular, total scores) in patients given alfuzosin or placebo.*

Table 27.7. *Symptomatic improvement according to the Boyarsky and I-PSS scoring systems with SR alfuzosin 5 mg bid administered for 3 months*

| | Treatment | | |
| | Alfuzosin | Placebo | |
Score	(10 mg/day; n = 194)	(n = 196)	p*
Boyarsky total score			
Initial[†]	9.9 (2.9)	10.3 (2.7)	
Absolute variation[†]	–3.1 (3.4)	–1.8 (3.1)	< 0.001
Percentage of patients with ≥ 25% improvement			
Total score	59	41	< 0.001
Irritative subscore	51	32	< 0.001
Obstructive subscore	69	48	< 0.001
I-PSS score			
Initial[†]	15.0 (5.3)	15.9 (5.4)	
Absolute variation[†]	–5.0 (6.1)	–3.4 (5.3)	0.007
Percentage of patients with ≥ 25% improvement			
I-PSS	64	48	0.004
Quality of life index	59	44	0.001

*Intergroup comparison. [†]Mean (±SD).

Tolerance

Oral alfuzosin (7.5–10 mg/day) has been generally well tolerated in clinical studies of up to 30 months' duration.[19,23,24] The overall incidence of adverse effects with alfuzosin appears to be similar to that seen with placebo, and the incidence of vasodilatation-related adverse effects with alfuzosin appears to be lower than that with prazosin. Reported adverse effects with alfuzosin are usually transitory: the majority occur within the first 4 weeks of treatment, resolve spontaneously after drug withdrawal and are largely related to its alpha-1-adrenoceptor-blocking properties. Furthermore, the SR formulation of alfuzosin is at least as well tolerated as the IR formulation.

In the 6-month placebo-controlled study,[19] the overall incidence of adverse events was similar in alfuzosin-treated patients (36%) and in placebo recipients (36%), with a similar rate of drop-out for adverse events (10 and 9%, respectively). In addition, the number of patients reporting at least one vasodilatation-related adverse effect also was similar in alfuzosin and placebo recipients (11 and 10%, respectively). Adverse effects occurring with an incidence of 1% or more in patients with BPH receiving alfuzosin include vasodilatation-related adverse effects such as dizziness and vertigo, headache, postural hypotension, drowsiness and malaise; tachycardia; gastrointestinal disorders such as diarrhoea, nausea and vomiting; dermatological conditions (skin rash); ischaemic heart disorders (chest pain); and other miscellaneous effects including dry mouth and asthenia. As a group, vasodilatation-related adverse effects occur most commonly, with dizziness having the highest overall incidence. A low incidence of impotence with alfuzosin compared with placebo may reflect the beneficial effect of alpha-adrenoceptor antagonists in this condition (Table 27.8).

Alfuzosin appeared to be well tolerated in the long term. In the first 1-year extension of the previous study, 6% of the 131 patients experienced an adverse effect that may have been related to alfuzosin during a total of 12–18 months of therapy: the overall incidence of vasodilatation-related adverse effects was 5.3%.[24] There were no withdrawals from treatment because of adverse events in this study, or in the further extension up to 24–30 months among 50 patients.[25] These results are of particular interest because BPH patients are likely to require long-term treatment.

In support of these data, results of a non-comparative, non-blinded, multicentre post-marketing general-practice survey involving over 5000 evaluable patients with BPH, who received alfuzosin 2.5 mg tid for

Table 27.8. *Adverse effects reported by patients with BPH during 6 months' treatment with alfuzosin (7.5–10 mg/day; n = 251) or placebo (n = 267)*

Adverse effect	Percentage alfuzosin recipients	Percentage placebo recipients
Vasodilatory		
Dizziness	7.2	5.2
Headache	6.4	4.9
Postural hypotension	1.9	1.2
Drowsiness	1.6	< 1
Tachycardia	1.6	< 1
Other		
Skin rash	4.4	5.2
Dry mouth	4.4	2.6
Diarrhoea	2.8	< 1
Nausea	2.4	< 1
Vomiting	1.6	1.9
Asthenia	2.0	3.8
Chest pain	2.0	< 1
Hypertension	1.6	2.3
Bad taste in mouth	< 1	3.4
Impotence	< 1	2.3

(Data from ref. 19.)

3 months, showed that two-thirds of patient withdrawals because of adverse effects (5.3%) were caused by vasodilatation-related adverse effects (vertigo, dizziness, postural hypotension and malaise). Two-thirds of the adverse effects leading to withdrawal occurred during the first week of treatment;[31] however, in fewer than 0.2% of withdrawals this occurred after the first dose. Hypotension-related adverse effects were more common in the elderly and in patients receiving concomitant alpha-adrenoceptor antagonists, diuretics, beta-adrenoceptor antagonists and calcium-channel antagonists. Alfuzosin may be better tolerated than prazosin in terms of vasodilatation-related adverse effects in patients with BPH. In the two available comparative studies,[16,17] vasodilatation-related adverse effects (dizziness, headache and malaise) occurred more frequently with prazosin than with alfuzosin (Table 27.9) in patients with BPH. These findings are clinically important, as the use of other alpha-adrenoceptor antagonists, including prazosin, has been limited by adverse effects such as first-dose postural hypotension and syncope. They also underline the consequences of the more powerful effect on standing blood pressure observed with prazosin than with alfuzosin.[23]

No significant laboratory abnormalities have been reported with alfuzosin. In particular, no tendency towards changes in blood counts, electrolyte levels or liver and renal function, has been observed either in the short term or the long term. The new SR formulation of alfuzosin is well tolerated even in patients over 75 years of age. In particular, there is a low incidence of vasodilatation-type adverse events. Only one case of transient and mild dizziness was observed among 98 BPH patients who received SR alfuzosin (5 mg bid) for 1 month; no worsening of concomitant cardiovascular

Table 27.9. *Comparative safety of alfuzosin and prazosin*

Adverse effect	Treatment		
	Alfuzosin (n = 84)	Prazosin (n = 91)	Placebo (n = 31)
Dizziness/vertigo	6 (7.1)	11 (12)	3 (9.7)
Malaise/syncope	1 (1.2)	5 (5.5)	2 (6.5)
Headache	3 (3.6)	8 (8.8)	1 (3.2)

Values are numbers of patients, with percentages in parentheses. (Data from refs 16 and 17.)

disorders was reported in those 37 of 98 patients who also suffered from hypertension and/or coronary heart disease.[32] Similarly, in the 3-month placebo-controlled study conducted in 390 BPH patients of whom 189 received SR alfuzosin 10 mg/day (unpublished data), a low incidence of dizziness and malaise/syncope was observed. It is worth noting that, except for the first 5 mg tablet given in the evening, the full dose (10 mg/day) was administered the next day without any titration. Apart from the intrinsic functional uroselectivity of alfuzosin, the low incidence of vasodilatation-type adverse events observed with the new formulation of alfuzosin could be related to its pharmacokinetic properties, i.e. delayed peak plasma concentrations owing to prolongation of the rate of release of the active drug.

Dosage and administration

The recommended oral daily dose of alfuzosin for the symptomatic treatment of BPH is 7.5–10 mg in three divided doses. Although alfuzosin has not been shown to be responsible for a first-dose effect, the first tablet should be taken at bedtime. No titration is necessary, the full dose being administered the next day. However, as elderly patients and patients with hypertension (whether or not receiving antihypertensive drugs) have an increased sensitivity to vasodilatation, the recommended initial daily dose in these patients is 2.5 mg twice daily. The dosage may subsequently increase progressively to 10 mg/day, depending on clinical response and tolerance. The dose of SR alfuzosin is 5 mg twice daily. Alfuzosin is contraindicated in patients with a history of postural hypotension and in those concurrently receiving an alpha-1-adrenoceptor antagonist. In patients receiving treatment for coronary heart disease, alfuzosin should be withdrawn if angina reappears or worsens. In addition, it is recommended that alfuzosin be withdrawn prior to general anaesthesia in an effort to minimize potential blood-pressure instability. Dosage modifications appear to be necessary in patients with hepatic insufficiency.

Place of alfuzosin in therapy

Although it is unlikely that a pharmacological agent would abolish both the mechanical and dynamic components of BPH as effectively as surgery, the pharmacological approaches to the symptomatic treatment of BPH have attracted increasing interest over recent years. The alternative to the use of agents that reduce the size of the prostate, and thus the mechanical component of obstruction (the most useful clinical class being 5 alpha-reductase inhibitors such as finasteride), are agents that reduce the tone of the prostatic smooth muscle (hence the dynamic component), such as alfuzosin.[33] The 5 alpha-reductase inhibitors that prevent the conversion of testosterone to 5-alpha-dihydrotestosterone can reduce the size of the prostate, but it may take months for finasteride to have such an effect.[34] In the overall study population the magnitude of benefit is modest.[35] The potential advantage of the association of alfuzosin with 5 alpha-reductase inhibitors has to be demonstrated.

The clinical advantage of alfuzosin over 5-alpha-adrenoceptors antagonists lies in the fact that it selectively antagonizes contraction mediated by alpha-1-adrenoceptros in the genitourinary tract rather than by receptors in the vasculature. Therefore, as mentioned above, alfuzosin may be effective in BPH at doses that produce minimal vasodilatation-related adverse effects, especially postural hypotension and syncope. The perceived advantage of alfuzosin therapy could be offset in clinical practice by its thrice-daily administration, as the midday intake might not be compatible with the normal daily routine. The SR formulation of alfuzosin overcomes this drawback and probably improves compliance, as previously shown by Greenberg,[36] who, in a literature review of patient compliance with medication dosing, reported that once-a-day and twice-a-day regimens were associated with better compliance (73 and 70%, respectively) than were thrice-daily regimens (52%).

Despite some gaps in our knowledge, such as the predictive criteria of those patients with BPH who are likely to respond to alpha-blockers and, of course, to alfuzosin, it appears that this compound is a first-line and safe agent in patients with uncomplicated but symptomatic BPH.

References

1. Bylund D B, Eikenberg D C, Hieble J P et al. IV International Union of Pharmacology nomenclature of adrenoceptors. Pharmacol Rev 1994; 46: 121–136

2. Faure C, Pimoule C, Arbilla S et al. Expression of α_1-adrenoceptor subtypes in rat tissues: implications for α_1-adrenoceptor classification. Eur J Pharmacol (Mol Pharmacol) 1994; 268: 141–149

3. Forray C, Bard J A, Wetzel J M et al. The α_1-adrenergic receptor that mediates smooth muscle contraction in human prostate has the pharmacological properties of the cloned α_{1C} subtype. Mol Pharmacol 1994; 45: 703–708

4. Pimoule C, Shoemaker H, Jardin A, Langer S Z. Identification and characterization of high affinity [^{3}H]-prazosin binding to the α-adrenoceptor in the human prostatic adenoma. Fundam Clin Pharmacol 1988; 3: 446

5. Lefevre-Borg F, O'Connor S E, Shoemaker H et al. Alfuzosin, a selective α_1-adrenoceptor antagonist in the lower urinary tract. Br J Pharmacol 1993; 109: 1282–1289

6. Benavides J, Peny B, Scatton B. Autoradiographic distribution of alfuzosin sensitive α_1-adrenoceptors in normal and hyperplasic human prostate. Bok S A Madrid, Editions, 1991: 384

7. Faure C, Pimoule C, Vallencien G et al. Identification of α_1-adrenoceptor subtypes present in the human prostate. Life Sci 1994; 54: 1595–1605

8. Lefevre-Borg F, Lechaire J, O'Connor S E. In vivo uroselectivity of alfuzosin compared to prazosin and terazosin. Br J Pharmacol 1992; 106: 84P

9. Ford A P D W, Williams T J, Blue D R, Clarke D E. α_1-Adrenoceptor classification: sharpening Occam's razor. Trends Pharmacol Sci 1994; 15: 167–169

10. Crome P, Wyawardhana P, Ankier S I et al. Alfuzosin: a comparison of the steady state pharmacokinetics of two dosages in middle-aged and elderly male volunteers. Drugs Invest 1993; 6: 156–161

11. Delauche-Cavallier M C, Costa P, Robain R et al. Efficacy and tolerability of 3 doses of intravenous alfuzosin in neurogenic bladder disease. Neurol Urodyn 1993; 12: abstr 24 B

12. Cramer P, Neveux E, Regnier F et al. Bladder-neck opening test in spinal cord injury patients using a new I.V. alpha-blocking agent, alfuzosin. Paraplegia 1989; 27: 119–124

13. Delauche-Cavallier M C, Richard M, Buzelin J M et al. Alpha-blocker therapy with alfuzosin in neurogenic bladder disease. Neurol Urodyn 1993; 12: abst 24 A

14. Teillac P, Delauche-Cavallier M C, Attali P et al. Urinary flow assessment after a single oral administration of alfuzosin, a new alpha blocker, in patients with benign prostatic hypertrophy. Br J Urol 1992; 70: 58–64

15. Costa P, Geffriaud C, Delauche-Cavallier M C et al. Effect of a single dose of alfuzosin SR on flow rate in elderly patients with symptomatic benign prostatic hyperplasia (BPH). Proc XIth Congr Eur Assoc Urol 13–16 July 1994, Berlin: abstr 44. Switzerland, Karger, 1994

16. Buzelin J M, Hebert M, Blondin P et al. Alpha-blocking treatment with alfuzosin in symptomatic benign prostatic hyperplasia: comparative study with prazozin. Br J Urol 1993; 72: 922–927

17. Stephenson T P, Jensen R D and the Pranalf Group. A placebo-controlled study of the efficacy and tolerability of alfuzosin and prazosin for the treatment of benign prostatic hypertrophy (BPH). Proc XIth Congr Eur Assoc Urol 13–16 July 1994, Berlin: abstr 48. Switzerland, Karger, 1994

18. Birsch N C, Hurst G, Doyle P T. Serial residual urine volumes in men with prostatic hypertrophy. Br J Urol 1988; 62: 571–575

19. Jardin A, Bensadoun H, Delauche-Cavallier M C et al. Alfuzosin for treatment of benign prostatic hypertrophy. Lancet 1991; 337: 1457–1461

20. Ramsay J W A, Scott G I, Whitfield H N. A double-blind controlled trial of a new α_1 blocking drug in the treatment of bladder outflow obstruction. Br J Urol 1985; 57: 657–659

21. Martorana G, Gilberti C, Pacella M et al. Urodynamic effects of alfuzosin on outlet obstruction of benign prostatic hyperplasia. Proc XIth Congr Eur Assoc Urol 13–16 July 1994, Berlin: abstr 42. Switzerland, Karger, 1994

22. Hansen B J, Nordling J, Mensik H J A et al. Alfuzosin in the treatment of benign prostatic hyperplasia: effects on symptom scores, urinary flow-rates and residual volume. A multicentre, double-blind placebo-controlled trial. Scand J Urol Nephrol 1994; (suppl 157): 169–176

23. Scott M G, Deering A H, McMahon M T et al. Haemodynamic and pharmacokinetic evaluation of alfuzosin in man. A dose-ranging study and comparison with prazosin. Eur J Clin Pharmacol 1989; 37: 53–58

24. Jardin A, Bensadoun H, Delauche-Cavallier M C et al. Long term treatment of benign prostatic hypertrophy with alfuzosin: a 12–18 month assessment. Br J Urol 1993; 72: 615–620

25. Jardin A, Bensadoun H, Delauche-Cavallier M C et al. Long term treatment of benign prostatic hyperplasia with alfuzosin: a 24–30 month survey. Br J Urol 1994; 74: 579–584

26. Jardin A, Delauche-Cavallier M C, Mathieu G et al. Symptomatic improvement in benign prostatic hyperplasia after alpha$_1$ blocker therapy with alfuzosin (metaanalysis). J Urol 1994; 151(suppl): abstr 165

27. Fowler F J, Barry M J. Quality of life assessment for evaluating benign prostatic hyperplasia treatments. Eur Urol 1993; 24(suppl 1): 24–27

28. Luckacs B, McCarthy C, Grange J C and the QOL BPH Study Group in General Practice. Long term quality of life in patients with benign prostatic hypertrophy: preliminary results of a cohort survey of 7,093 patients treated with alpha-1 adrenergic blocker, alfuzosin. Eur Urol 1993; 24(suppl 1): 34–40

29. Martelli A, Pacificio P, Casadei G and the Italien Alfuzosin Co-operative Group. Effect of alfuzosin on quality of life in benign prostatic hyperplasia patients: preliminary results. Eur Urol 1993; 24(suppl S1): 28–33

30. Lepor H. Non-operative management of benign hyperplasia. J Urol 1989; 141: 1283–1289

31. Conort P, Chaumet-Riffaud A E, McCarthy C et al. Safety of 3 months therapy with the alpha-blocker alfuzosin in 6 278 patients with benign prostatic hypertrophy (BPH). Ann Meet AUA, Washington, 1992. J Urol 1992; 147(suppl): 436A

32. Delmas V, Coulange C, Caille P et al. A placebo-controlled double blind study of sustained release alfuzosin in benign prostatic hyperplasia. Proc XIth Congr Assoc Urol 13–16 July 1994, Berlin: abstr 47. Swizerland, Karger, 1994

33. Wilde M J, Fitton A, McTavish D. Alfuzosin: a review of its pharmacodynamic and pharmacokinetic properties and therapeutic potential in benign prostatic hyperplasia. Drugs 1993; 45: 410–429

34. Garmley G J, Staner E, Bruskewitz R C et al. The effect of finasteride in men with benign prostatic hyperplasia. N Engl J Med 1992; 327: 1185–1191

35. McConnell J, Akakura K, Bartsch G et al. Hormonal treatment of benign prostatic hyperplasia. In: Cockett A T K et al (eds) Proc 2nd Int Consultation on benign prostate hyperplasia, 27–30 June. Paris, 1993: 417–441

36. Greenberg R N. Overview of patient compliance with medication dosing: a literature review. Clin Ther 1986; 6: 592–599

37. Carbin B E, Bauer P, Friskand M, Moyse D. Efficacy of alfuzosin (an α_1-adrenoceptor blocking drug) in benign hyperplasia of the prostate. Scand J Urol Nephrol 1991;(suppl 138): 73–75

38. Schulman C C, De Sy W, Valendris M et al. Belgian multicentre clinical study of alfuzosin, a selective alpha 1-blocker, in the treatment of benign prostatic hyperplasia. Acta Urol Belg, in press

28

Tamsulosin
C. C. Schulman

Introduction

Introduction to alpha-1-blockers

Alpha-blockers were originally developed for the treatment of hypertension. By blockade of postsynaptic alpha-1-adrenoceptors in the blood vessels, these agents cause vasodilatation. As a consequence, the peripheral vascular resistance and blood pressure are reduced. Examples of alpha-1-blockers that have been evaluated and/or are still used for hypertension are prazosin, doxazosin, alfuzosin and terazosin.

In 1976, Caine and colleagues proposed a hypothesis for the use of alpha-blockers in bladder outlet obstruction due to benign prostatic hyperplasia (BPH).[1] By antagonizing the effect of noradrenaline, the neurotransmitter of the sympathetic nervous system, at the alpha-1-adrenoceptor, the alpha-blockers reduce smooth muscle cell tone in the bladder neck, prostatic urethra, prostate capsule and prostatic adenoma (stroma) and, consequently, reduce the dynamic component of bladder outlet obstruction.[1-4] Thus, the short-acting alpha-1-blockers prazosin and alfuzosin and the long-acting alpha-1-blockers doxazosin and terazosin are effective in hypertension and in patients with functional symptoms of BPH.[2-3] They improve symptoms and urinary flow rate and a favourable clinical response is achieved in about 70% of patients.[2-3] The adverse events most commonly associated with alpha-1-blockers include dizziness, headache, asthenia, palpitation/tachycardia, postural hypotension and syncope. These side effects may be related to the blood-pressure-lowering effect. In order to reduce, in particular, the occurrence of postural hypotension and syncope, therapy is started with a low dose, gradually titrating to an optimal therapeutic dose.

Introduction to alpha-1c-adrenoceptor subtype selectivity

Since the late 1980s it has been clear that there are several subtypes of the alpha-1-adrenoceptor. However, there is some confusion concerning alpha-1-adrenoceptor subtype terminology. This is due to the fact that different subtypes were identified with pharmacological and molecular biological techniques while it was not clear how these different subtypes were related to each other.

With pharmacological techniques, two subtypes were discernable — alpha-1A and alpha-1B.[5-7] With molecular biological studies, however, it was possible to clone and express three subtypes — alpha-1b, alpha-1c and alpha-1d (also termed alpha-1a/d).[5-7] Recently it has been accepted that the cloned alpha-1b-adrenoceptor encodes for the pharmacological alpha-1B-adrenoceptor and that the cloned alpha-1c-adrenoceptor encodes for the pharmacological alpha-1A-adrenoceptor.[7-9] The new accepted classification is presented in Table 28.1.[7,53]

Table 28.1. *Pharmacologically and molecular biologically identified alpha-1-adrenoceptor subtypes and accepted classification*

Old classification		New (accepted) classification	
Pharmacological terminology	Molecular biological terminology	Pharmacological terminology	Molecular biological terminology
alpha-1A	alpha-1c	alpha-1A	alpha-1a
alpha-1B	alpha-1b	alpha-1B	alpha-1b
	alpha-1d or alpha-1a/d	alpha-1D	alpha-1d

(From refs. 7 and 23)

As the distribution and functionality of the alpha-1-adrenoceptor subtypes differ between human tissues,[10–11] it may be that the subtype responsible for prostatic smooth muscle contraction differs from that involved in blood pressure regulation and side effects associated with alpha-1-blockers. Several studies have demonstrated that in the human prostate the pharmacological alpha-1A-adrenoceptor[12,13] or the cloned alpha-1c-adrenoceptor[8,9,14–17] is predominantly present (about 70% of all alpha-1-adrenoceptors) and functional. So far, research has done little to determine which alpha-1-adrenoceptor is present in blood vessels and/or is responsible for smooth muscle contraction in the blood vessels and, consequently, for blood pressure regulation in humans. One recent study has demonstrated, however, that in large human arteries such as the internal iliac artery the alpha-1B-adrenoceptor subtype is probably responsible for vasoconstriction.[18] The authors conclude that 'an alpha-1-adrenoceptor antagonist with low affinity for the alpha-1B-adrenoceptor may attain a therapeutic response to bladder outlet obstruction with fewer side effects'. This has to be confirmed by further research.

The above data suggest that, in the treatment of BPH, an alpha-1-blocker with higher selectivity for the alpha-1c than for the alpha-1B-adrenoceptor subtype would maintain the therapeutic efficacy without a blood-pressure-lowering effect and side effects related to vasodilatation. This may result in a better benefit–risk ratio.[2,3,8,9,11,16–18]

Introduction to tamsulosin

Tamsulosin hydrochloride (YM-617) is a new, alpha-1c-subtype-selective, long-acting alpha-1-blocker specifically developed for the treatment of the functional symptoms of BPH by Yamanouchi Pharmaceutical Co., Ltd in Japan. It has been formulated into a long-acting modified release formulation.

The chemical structure of tamsulosin, a methoxybenzenesulfonamide, differs from that of other alpha-1-blockers such as alfuzosin, terazosin and doxazosin which are quinazoline derivatives (Fig. 28.1). This may have consequences for drug–receptor interaction.

Alpha-1c-subtype-selective alpha-1-blocker

Tamsulosin is a very potent, competitive and selective alpha-1-adrenoceptor antagonist that displays much higher affinity for alpha-1- than for alpha-2-adrenoceptors.[19] Furthermore, tamsulosin is an optically

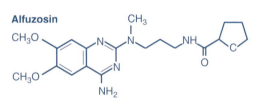

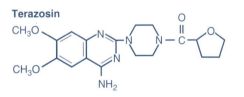

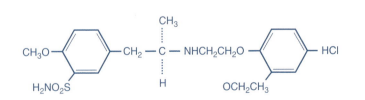

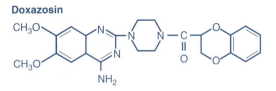

Figure 28.1. *Chemical structures of tamsulosin, alfuzosin, terazosin and doxazosin.*

$R(-)$ isomer that is about 100 times more potent at the alpha-1-adrenoceptors in the lower urinary tract than is the (+) isomer.[20,21] Tamsulosin displays higher selectivity for the alpha-1c-adrenoceptor than for the alpha-1B-adrenoceptor subtype.[22-29] (See also the section on safety of tamsulosin below.) This may result in a better risk–benefit ratio of tamsulosin compared with other alpha-1-blockers.

Long-acting alpha-1-blocker

Tamsulosin hydrochloride is available as modified release capsules. In European, elderly BPH patients, the elimination half-life of tamsulosin (0.4 mg once daily) is 13 h.[30] This long half-life supports the classification of tamsulosin as a long-acting alpha-1-blocker and the once daily dosage.[2,3]

In Japan, tamsulosin is available for prescription under the tradename Harnal® with a recommended dosage of 0.2 mg once daily. In Europe, 0.4 mg tamsulosin (modified release formulation) once daily has been evaluated in phase II and III clinical trials and will be marketed by Yamanouchi Europe (tradenames Omnic®, Flomax®) and/or by Boehringer Ingelheim (tradenames Alna®, Josir®, Mapelor®, Pradif®, Flomax®). This chapter focuses mainly on the clinical experience with 0.4 mg tamsulosin once daily in Europe.

Clinical efficacy and safety in phase II studies in Japan and Europe

Phase II clinical studies have been performed with tamsulosin once daily in Japan and Europe. In all clinical studies, tamsulosin was recommended to be administered after breakfast.

Japanese phase II study

A randomized, double-blind, placebo-controlled, parallel-group, phase II dose–effect study was performed in 270 Japanese BPH patients, using 0.1, 0.2 and 0.4 mg tamsulosin once daily for 4 weeks, after a 2-week placebo run-in period.[31]

The maximum urinary flow rate (Q_{max}) for the placebo, 0.2 mg and 0.4 mg groups improved by 1.4 ml/s (15%), 4.0 ml/s (44%) and 3.6 ml/s (35%), respectively. With respect to average urinary flow rate (Q_{ave}), there were statistically significant differences between 0.2 and

0.4 mg tamsulosin once daily (increase 26 and 41%, respectively) and placebo (decrease 4%). In addition, overall symptomatic improvement was similar in the 0.2 mg and the 0.4 mg dosing groups and significantly better in comparison with placebo. Approximately 80% of patients reported that their condition had (slightly, moderately or markedly) improved. The Boyarsky symptom score (nine questions, each to be graded on a scale from 0 to 3; total score range 0–27 points)[32] was used to assess the effect on symptoms. Each symptom was considered to be improved when the score was decreased by more than one grade/point. Compared with baseline values, the 0.4 mg dose significantly improved all obstructive and irritative symptoms, with the exception of daytime frequency.

Finally, tamsulosin was very well tolerated. Neither orthostatic hypotension nor a decrease in blood pressure was observed.

In conclusion, both 0.2 and 0.4 mg tamsulosin once daily are effective and well-tolerated dosages in the treatment of Japanese patients with symptomatic BPH.

European phase II study

A randomized, double-blind, placebo-controlled, parallel-group, phase II dose–effect study in 169 patients with symptomatic BPH comparing dosages of 0.2, 0.4 and 0.6 mg tamsulosin once daily with placebo was conducted in Europe.[30] After a 3-week placebo run-in period, 126 men with a Q_{max} of less than 15 ml/s, a voided volume of more than 100 ml and urethral resistance (P_{det}/Q^2_{max}) of 0.5 or more were randomized to one of the four treatment groups. Double-blind therapy lasted for 4 weeks. The main aim of the study was to establish the optimum dosage for phase III studies, based on the effects during free flow and pressure–flow studies and on symptoms. A modified Boyarsky symptom score, which evaluated eight symptoms to be rated on a scale from 0 to 5 (total symptom score range 0–40 points), was used. The effects on these efficacy parameters are presented in Table 28.2.

Both 0.4 and 0.6 mg tamsulosin once daily gave a statistically significant ($p<0.05$) increase in mean Q_{max} during free flow studies relative to placebo. The improvements in mean Q_{max} were 2.2 ml/s (+22.6%) with 0.4 mg and 1.8 ml/s (+20.2%) with 0.6 mg; the mean Q_{max} decreased slightly with placebo (–0.1 ml/s or –0.9%). Furthermore, detrusor pressure at Q_{max} ($P_{det}Q_{max}$)

Table 28.2. *Effect of placebo or 0.2, 0.4 or 0.6 mg tamsulosin once daily on mean free flow Q_{max}, mean $P_{det}Q_{max}$ and mean total symptom score*

| | | Tamsulosin | | |
Parameter	Placebo (n=23–26)	0.2 mg (n=25–34)	0.4 mg (n=23–28)	0.6 mg (n=21–30)
Q_{max} (ml/s)				
Baseline	10.9	9.6	9.8	9.1
4 weeks	10.9	10.7	12.1	10.9
Change (%)	–0.1 (–0.9%)	1.2 (+12.6%)	2.2 (+22.6%)*	1.8 (+20.2%)*
$P_{det}Q_{max}$ (cmH$_2$O)				
Baseline	88.4	84.2	93.6	90.7
4 weeks	87.2	74.7	67.8	75.7
Change (%)	4.9 (+5.7%)	–11.2 (–13.2%)	–26.6 (–28.2%)	–18.0 (–18.9%)
Total symptom score (points)				
Baseline	16.7	16.9	14.9	15.8
4 weeks	13.5	13.6	10.2	10.9
Change (%)	–2.9 (–17.7%)	–3.4 (–20.1%)	–4.1 (–28.7%)	–4.4 (–28.2%)

The number of patients that could be evaluated for pressure–flow results was smaller than the number of patients evaluated for free flow Q_{max} and total symptom score effects. Furthermore, the baseline and 4 weeks of treatment values are based on different numbers of patients; this explains why the change is not always exactly identical to the subtraction of the baseline and 4 weeks of treatment value. Asterisks indicate statistically significant difference from placebo (*$p<0.05$; ANOVA with multiple comparison test).

decreased to the greatest extent with 0.4 mg tamsulosin (decrease 26.6 cmH$_2$O or –28.2% compared with increase of 4.9 cmH$_2$O or +5.7% with placebo).

The decrease in mean total symptom score was comparable for the 0.4 mg dose (4.1 points or –28.7%) and the 0.6 mg dose (4.4 points or –28.2%). Although the decreases with these two dosages of tamsulosin were greater than with placebo (2.9 points or –17.7%), the improvements did not differ significantly from placebo.

The efficacy results showed optimum improvement with 0.4 mg tamsulosin once daily. The safety profile of this dosage was also good. Furthermore, the changes in blood pressure both during the first 8 h after administration of the first dose and after 4 weeks of therapy were comparable for placebo and 0.4 mg tamsulosin once daily and did not differ statistically significantly from each other. The 0.4 mg tamsulosin once daily dosage was therefore evaluated further in phase III clinical trials in Europe.

Clinical efficacy and safety in phase III studies in Europe

Four phase III studies evaluating the efficacy and safety of 0.4 mg tamsulosin once daily in patients with functional symptoms of BPH were initiated in Europe. Two studies were placebo-controlled studies, one was a comparative study against alfuzosin and one study assessed the long-term efficacy and safety.

Clinical efficacy in phase III studies in Europe

The major efficacy parameters in the phase III studies were total Boyarsky symptom score[32] and Q_{max} assessed during free flow studies.

With regard to improvement in symptoms, the percentage of total symptom score responders (i.e. patients with a decrease of 25% or more) and the effects on obstructive, irritative and individual symptom scores were also evaluated. For the improvement in objective parameters, the percentage of Q_{max} responders (i.e. patients with an increase of at least 30% or 3 ml/s increase) was also considered.

Tamsulosin versus placebo

Two multinational, multicentre, double-blind, randomized, placebo-controlled studies with 0.4 mg tamsulosin once daily have been performed in Europe. In each study more than 300 patients with functional symptoms of BPH (i.e. total Boyarsky symptom score greater than 6), Q_{max} 4–12 ml/s and voided volume of 120 ml or more were enrolled into a 2-week placebo run-in period after which they were randomized to 12 weeks of treatment with placebo or tamsulosin (ratio 1:2). Most of the efficacy assessments as discussed above took place at baseline and after 4, 8 and 12 weeks of therapy. Furthermore, an intention-to-treat endpoint analysis was performed in order not to exclude patients prematurely terminating the double-blind treatment period. As the inclusion/exclusion criteria, study design and assessments were the same for both studies, a meta-analysis of the two studies that involved 193 placebo and 381 tamsulosin patients was carried out.[54] The results of this meta-analysis are discussed for efficacy comparisons between tamsulosin and placebo at the endpoint. For the effects of both therapies over time, the results of one study with 98 placebo and 198 tamsulosin patients[33,34] are presented (see below). The effects over time in the other study were comparable. The results of the meta-analysis are in line with those of the individual placebo-controlled studies.

Symptoms. Tamsulosin reduced the mean total Boyarsky symptom score by 3.3 points (−35%) at the endpoint compared with baseline. Although there was a considerable placebo effect (decrease 2.4 points or −26%), the improvement in mean total symptom score with tamsulosin was statistically significantly ($p=0.002$) greater than with placebo (Fig. 28.2). Tamsulosin had a statistically significant beneficial effect on both irritative ($p=0.017$) and obstructive ($p=0.008$) symptom scores. For individual symptoms, tamsulosin improved the mean symptom scores for urgency, hesitancy and intermittency statistically significantly more than placebo, while a trend for a better effect of tamsulosin on daytime frequency ($p=0.084$) and impairment of size and force or urinary stream ($p=0.075$) was found.

A decrease in total symptom score of 25% or more has been proposed as a clinically significant response.[35,36] At the endpoint, significantly ($p<0.001$) more patients achieved a clinically significant response with tamsulosin (66%) than with placebo (49%).

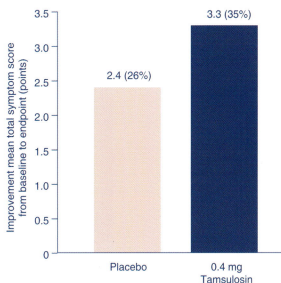

Figure 28.2. *Improvement in mean total Boyarsky symptom score with placebo (■; n=190) or 0.4 mg tamsulosin once daily (■; n=374) in the meta-analysis.[54] The baseline total symptom score was 9.4 points in both groups. Improvement with tamsulosin differs significantly from that with placebo (p=0.002; ANOVA with components for study centre and treatment.).*

Maximum urinary flow rate (Q_{max}). In addition to improving symptoms, tamsulosin also improved mean Q_{max} by 1.6 ml/s (+16%). Although there was again a considerable placebo effect of 0.6 ml/s (6%), the increase with tamsulosin was statistically significantly ($p=0.002$) greater than with placebo (Fig. 28.3).

Not only did tamsulosin improve mean Q_{max} but the percentage of patients achieving an increase in Q_{max} of 30% or more was also significantly ($p=0.003$) greater with tamsulosin (32%) than with placebo (20%). In addition, the percentage of patients who achieved an increase in Q_{max} of 3 ml/s or more was 29 and 20% for tamsulosin and placebo, respectively ($p=0.018$). Both an increase in Q_{max} of at least 30% and one of at least 3 ml/s have been proposed as clinically significant responses.[36]

Tamsulosin versus alfuzosin

A comparative phase III study between 0.4 mg tamsulosin once daily and 2.5 mg alfuzosin twice to thrice daily has been conducted in Europe.[30] The inclusion/exclusion criteria, study design and assessments were similar to those used in the placebo-controlled studies. A total of 282 patients were enrolled in a 2-week placebo run-in period, after which 256

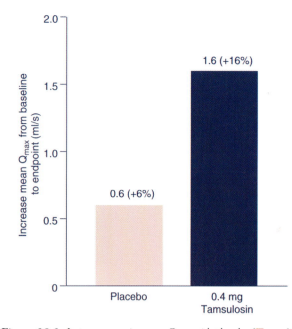

Figure 28.3. *Improvement in mean Q$_{max}$ with placebo (▆; n=185) or 0.4 mg tamsulosin once daily (▇; n=364) in the meta-analysis.[54] The baseline Q$_{max}$ was 10.1 ml/s (placebo) and 10.2 ml/s (tamsulosin). Increase with tamsulosin differs significantly from that with placebo (p=0.002; ANOVA with components for study centre and treatment).*

patients were randomized to 12 weeks of double-blind treatment with alfuzosin (n=124) or tamsulosin (n=132). For tamsulosin, only one dosage (0.4 mg once daily) was used during the entire 12 weeks. Patients randomized to alfuzosin started with 2.5 mg twice daily for 2 weeks; then the dosage was increased to 2.5 mg thrice daily for the last 10 weeks of double-blind treatment. Efficacy parameters were measured at baseline and after 2, 6 and 12 weeks of therapy.

The results of this study showed that tamsulosin 0.4 mg once daily is as effective as 2.5 mg alfuzosin thrice daily with regard to improvement of both total Boyarsky symptom score and Q$_{max}$. However, this is achieved with a once-daily dosage of tamsulosin and without dose titration. Lack of dose titration and once-daily administration are convenient aspects for patients and, therefore, may improve compliance, especially during long-term treatment.

The mean total symptom score was statistically significantly reduced from baseline to endpoint with both products — by 3.8 points (–38.8%) with alfuzosin and by 4.1 points (–39.8%) with tamsulosin. The

percentage of total symptom score responders was also comparable — 69% with alfuzosin and 68% with tamsulosin.

Both treatments increased mean Q$_{max}$ by 1.6 ml/s (+16%). The percentage of patients with a clinically significant increase in Q$_{max}$ was also quite similar — 34% with alfuzosin and 35% with tamsulosin.

Clinical efficacy of tamsulosin: onset of action and maximum effect

Tamsulosin 0.4 mg once daily has a fast onset of action. *Symptoms.* In the placebo-controlled studies, the first assessment of the effect on total Boyarsky symptom score took place after 4 weeks of therapy. By this time, there already was a statistically significantly greater reduction in total symptom score with 0.4 mg tamsulosin once daily than with placebo (*p*<0.001).[33,34] In the alfuzosin comparative study, a statistically significant reduction in total symptom score compared with baseline was already apparent at the first measurement after 2 weeks of tamsulosin treatment when about 50% of the maximum effect was reached.[30] In both studies, the maximum effect of tamsulosin seemed to be present after about 12 weeks of therapy. At that time a plateau in total Boyarsky symptom score of about 6 points was attained with both alfuzosin and tamsulosin (Fig. 28.4).

Tamsulosin has been evaluated also in phase III clinical studies in the USA. In these studies, the American Urological Association (AUA) symptom score[37] was assessed first after 1 week of double-blind treatment. Preliminary results demonstrate that at that time 0.4 mg tamsulosin once daily had already improved total symptom score statistically significantly compared with placebo.[38]

Maximum urinary flow rate (Q$_{max}$). In the European phase III studies, the first assessment of Q$_{max}$ changes from baseline was after 4 weeks of tamsulosin treatment in the placebo-controlled studies and after 2 weeks in the alfuzosin comparative study. Compared with placebo, the increase in Q$_{max}$ was statistically significant (*p*=0.027) and maximal (about 12 ml/s) at the first measurement after 4 weeks of tamsulosin treatment. There was no further increase in Q$_{max}$ after that time. In the alfuzosin comparative study, the increase was statistically significant compared with baseline and

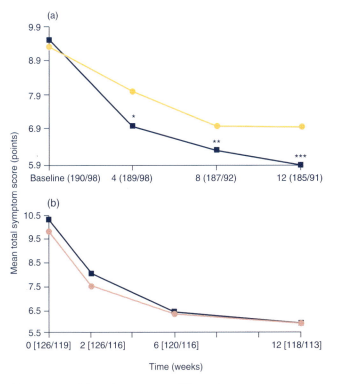

Figure 28.4. *Mean decrease in total Boyarsky symptom score over time in (a) a placebo-controlled study and (b) in the alfuzosin comparative study:* ■, *tamsulosin;* ●, *placebo;* ●, *alfuzosin. Values in parentheses are numbers of patients on tamsulosin/placebo; values in square brackets are numbers of patients on tamsulosin/alfuzosin. Asterisks indicate significant difference from placebo (*p<0.001; **p<0.016; ***p=0.004; ANOVA with components for study centre and treatment).*

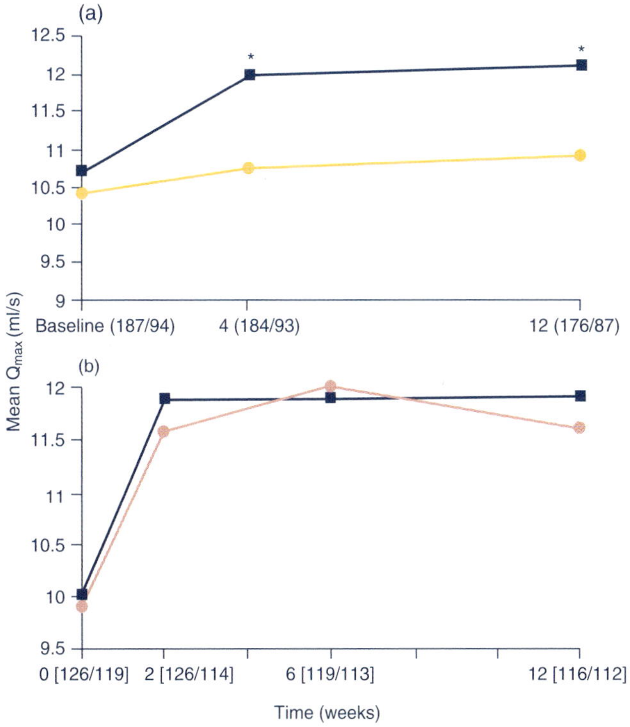

Figure 28.5. *Mean increase in Q_{max} over time in (a) a placebo-controlled study and (b) in the alfuzosin comparative study:* ■, *tamsulosin;* ●, *placebo;* ●, *alfuzosin. Values in parentheses are numbers of patients on tamsulosin/placebo; values in square brackets are numbers of patients on tamsulosin/alfuzosin. Asterisks indicate significant difference from placebo (*p=0.027; ANOVA with components for study centre and treatment).*

maximal (about 12 ml/s) at the first measurement after 2 weeks of tamsulosin treatment (Fig. 28.5).

Q_{max} after a single dose of 0.4 mg tamsulosin. In an open, early phase II study in 13 elderly BPH patients, Q_{max} was assessed for 8 h after the first dose of 0.4 mg tamsulosin and again for 8 h following 8 days of treatment with 0.4 mg tamsulosin once daily.[30] It appeared that mean Q_{max} was already statistically significantly increased by 4.2 ml/s (+53%) from baseline after 8 h following the single-dose administration with no further improvement after multiple doses of tamsulosin. The increase in mean Q_{max} in this study (4.2 ml/s) was greater than that in the phase II and III studies with 0.4 mg tamsulosin once daily (2.2 and 1.6 ml/s, respectively). This may partly be explained by the lower baseline Q_{max} value of 7.9 ml/s, because the mean Q_{max} attained after 8 h was 12.1 ml/s which is comparable to that achieved in the phase II and phase III studies (see Table 28.2 and Fig. 28.5).

The preliminary results of the placebo-controlled phase III studies in the USA also demonstrate that the effect of tamsulosin on mean Q_{max} is maximal after the first dose.[38]

Conclusion. Tamsulosin 0.4 mg once daily has a fast onset of action. Mean Q_{max} is already maximally increased to about 12 ml/s after the first dose of 0.4 mg, with no further improvement thereafter. Although a statistically significant improvement in mean total symptom score in comparison with placebo can already be seen after 1 week of therapy with tamsulosin, total symptom score is continuously reduced further to about 6 points (on the Boyarsky symptom score) after 12 weeks of treatment.

Clinical efficacy of tamsulosin: during long-term treatment

A long-term phase III efficacy and safety study with 0.4 mg tamsulosin once daily is ongoing in Europe. All patients who completed the two placebo-controlled studies, whether they had been randomized to tamsulosin or to placebo, could be enrolled in the long-term study to receive open-label tamsulosin treatment. In an interim analysis, 355 patients with functional symptoms of BPH were treated with tamsulosin for up to 60 weeks.[55] A total of 279 patients (79%) took the medication for approximately 1 year (48 weeks) and 184 patients (52%) for 60 weeks.

Figure 28.6 shows that the favourable effect on both mean total symptom score and mean Q_{max}, as achieved after 12 weeks of tamsulosin treatment in the placebo-controlled studies, is maintained during long-term therapy. The maximum mean total Boyarsky symptom score of about 6 points is reached after 12–14 weeks of medication and is maintained thereafter. The maximum mean Q_{max} of about 12 ml/s is achieved at the first assessment after 4 weeks of treatment and is also maintained thereafter. Furthermore, the percentage of total symptom score responders and Q_{max} responders remained constant over time (Fig. 28.7).

Clinical safety in phase III studies in Europe

Tamsulosin 0.4 mg once daily was well tolerated in the phase III studies in Europe. The most important safety parameters analysed were adverse events and vital signs (blood pressure and pulse rate).

Adverse events

In the meta-analysis of the two placebo-controlled studies, a total of 25 patients (6.6% of 381) in the tamsulosin and 15 patients (7.8% of 193) in the placebo group discontinued the study.[54] Discontinuation because of adverse events occurred in 17 patients (4.5%) treated with tamsulosin and in seven patients (3.6%) treated with placebo. The incidence of serious adverse events was also comparable for tamsulosin and placebo (2.4 and 3.6%, respectively) (Table 28.3).

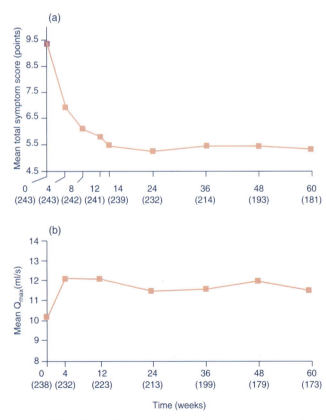

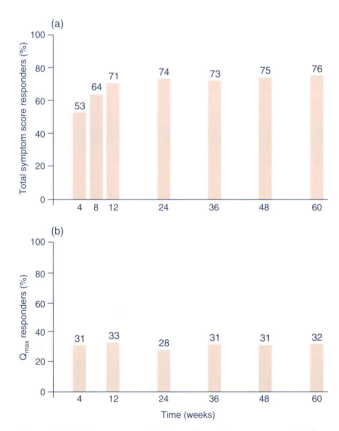

Figure 28.6. *Effect of long-term open-label treatment with tamsulosin on (a) mean total Boyarsky symptom score and (b) mean Q_{max} over time.[55] Values in parentheses are numbers of patients.*

Figure 28.7. *Percentage of (a) total symptom score responders (decrease ≥25%) and (b) Q_{max} responders (increase ≥30%) during long-term treatment with tamsulosin.[55]*

Table 28.3. *Adverse events in the European phase III placebo-controlled studies*

	Tamsulosin (n=381)	Placebo (n=193)
Adverse events possibly or probably related	50 (13)	24 (12)
Discontinuations due to adverse events	17 (4.5)	7 (3.6)
Serious adverse events	9 (2.4)	7 (3.6)

Values are numbers of patients, with percentages in parentheses.

In the meta-analysis, the percentage of patients with at least one adverse event was comparable for patients who received 0.4 mg tamsulosin once daily or placebo (36 and 32% respectively; *p*=0.290).[54] The most common adverse events (i.e. those that occurred in at least 3% of patients within a treatment group) were abnormal ejaculation (4.5%), dizziness (3.4%) and infection (3.1%) in the tamsulosin group and dizziness (3.1%) and flu syndrome (2.6%) in the placebo group. There were no statistically significant differences between tamsulosin and placebo for these adverse events in the individual placebo-controlled studies.

When a causal relationship with study medication, defined as adverse events possibly or probably related to study medication according to the investigator, was taken into account, the incidence of adverse events was also comparable for tamsulosin- and placebo-treated patients (Table 28.3: 13 and 12%, respectively; *p*=0.802).[54] The only adverse event for tamsulosin occurring in at least 3% of patients that was considered to have a causal relationship to study medication was abnormal ejaculation. The incidences of impotence and decreased libido were comparable for tamsulosin and placebo. Figure 28.8 shows all adverse events classified as possibly or probably related to medication occurring in at least three patients on tamsulosin (0.8%) or placebo (1.6%).

As mentioned earlier, adverse events commonly associated with alpha-1-blockers include dizziness, headache, palpitation/tachycardia, postural hypotension and syncope; these are possibly related to vasodilatation. Furthermore, asthenia, nasal congestion/rhinitis and flu syndrome (reported with terazosin)[36] are commonly attributed to therapy with alpha-1-blockers. Table 28.4 shows that the incidence of adverse events possibly related to vasodilatation with tamsulosin is comparable to that with placebo. The same is true for the occurrence of asthenia, nasal congestion/rhinitis and flu syndrome (Table 28.5).

It is particularly noteworthy that none of the patients treated with 0.4 mg tamsulosin once daily in the placebo-controlled studies reported (symptoms of) postural hypotension. Syncope occurred in one patient on tamsulosin; however, this was not considered by the investigator to be related to the medication.

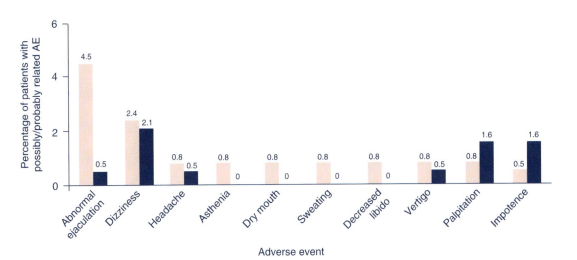

Figure 28.8. *Percentage of patients with adverse events (AE) possibly or probably related to medication, occurring in at least three patients with tamsulosin ( ) or placebo ( ) in the meta-analysis.*

Table 28.4. *Incidence of adverse events believed to be related to vasodilatation in patients who received placebo (n=193) or tamsulosin (n=381)*

Adverse event (AE)	All AEs reported		AEs possibly/probably related	
	Placebo	Tamsulosin	Placebo	Tamsulosin
Dizziness	6 (3.1)	13 (3.4)	4 (2.1)	9 (2.4)
Headache	4 (2.1)	8 (2.1)	1 (0.5)	3 (0.8)
Tachycardia/palpitation	3 (1.6)	5 (1.3)	3 (1.6)	3 (0.8)
Postural hypotension	1 (0.5)	0	1 (0.5)	0
Syncope	1 (0.5)	1 (0.3)	1 (0.5)	0
Total	15 (7.8)	27 (7.1)	10 (5.2)	15 (3.9)

Values are numbers of patients, with percentages in parentheses. However, the total number (%) concerns the total numbers of events and not the total numbers of patients experiencing adverse events possibly related to vasodilatation, as one patient may report more than one of these events simultaneously.

Table 28.5. *Incidence of asthenia, nasal congestion and flu syndrome in patients who received placebo (n=193) or tamsulosin (n=381)*

Adverse event (AE)	All AEs reported		AEs possibly/probably related	
	Placebo	Tamsulosin	Placebo	Tamsulosin
Asthenia	2 (1.0)	4 (1.0%)	0	3 (0.8)
Nasal congestion/rhinitis	1 (0.5)	1 (0.3)	0	0
Flu syndrome	5 (2.6)	6 (1.6)	0	0

Values are numbers of patients, with percentages in parentheses.

Blood pressure

In the meta-analysis of the two placebo-controlled studies there were no statistically significant differences between 0.4 mg tamsulosin once daily and placebo, with respect to the change in mean supine and standing blood pressure at endpoint relative to baseline values (Table 28.6).[54] The only exception was the standing diastolic blood pressure, which was reduced to a statistically significantly greater extent with tamsulosin than with placebo. The reduction was, however, small (2.5 mmHg) and was not considered to be of clinical relevance. This lack of effect on blood pressure was achieved despite about 20% of patients being treated with antihypertensive medication [i.e. beta-blockers, diuretics, angiotensin-converting-enzyme (ACE) inhibitors and calcium antagonists]. In addition, pulse rate was not significantly changed by tamsulosin.

The negligible effect of 0.4 mg tamsulosin once daily on blood pressure was also demonstrated in the alfuzosin comparative trial. Tamsulosin had statistically significantly less effect on blood pressure than 2.5 mg

alfuzosin thrice daily, with the exception of standing systolic blood pressure, for which the difference approached statistical significance (Fig. 28.9).

In conclusion, 0.4 mg tamsulosin once daily has no significant effect on supine or standing blood pressure and pulse rate in comparison with placebo. Furthermore, 2.5 mg alfuzosin thrice daily gives significantly greater blood pressure reductions than 0.4 mg tamsulosin once daily.

Interactions

Clinical drug interactions. Tamsulosin has been administered concomitantly with several antihypertensive drugs (the beta-blocker atenolol, the ACE inhibitor enalapril and the calcium antagonist nifedipine) in patients with essential hypertension.[30,56,57] There was no pharmacodynamic interaction between tamsulosin and any of the antihypertensive agents, i.e. there were no clinically important additional blood pressure reductions during concomitant therapy with tamsulosin than during treatment with the antihypertensive agent alone.

Table 28.6. *Change in mean systolic and diastolic blood pressure (SBP/DBP) and pulse rate at endpoint compared with baseline[†] values, with placebo or tamsulosin in the meta-analysis[54]*

Vital sign	Placebo (n=189)[‡]	Tamsulosin (n=373)[§]
Change in mean supine SBP/DBP (mmHg)	–3.5/–0.9	–3.1/–1.6
Change in mean standing SBP/DBP (mmHg)	–1.7/–0.4	–3.3/–2.5*
Change in mean supine pulse rate (beats/min)	–0.7	–0.4
Change in mean standing pulse rate (beats/min)	–0.3	+0.2

[†]Baseline supine SBP/DBP, 144.3/85.4 mmHg for placebo and 143.1/85.4 mmHg for tamsulosin; baseline standing SBP/DBP, 142.9/86.4 mmHg for placebo and 141.8/86.8 mmHg for tamsulosin. [‡]n=188 for pulse rate. [§]n=372 for pulse rate. Asterisk indicates statistically significant difference between tamsulosin and placebo (*$p=0.018$; ANOVA with components for study centre and treatment).

In addition, there were no clinically significant interactions between tamsulosin and the loop diuretic frusemide (furosemide), digoxin or the H_2-receptor blocking agent cimetidine in healthy male volunteers.[30]

Long-term safety

The good safety profile of 0.4 mg tamsulosin once daily during short-term therapy (12 weeks) in the placebo-controlled studies was maintained during long-term open-label tamsulosin medication in the follow-up study (Table 28.7).[55] In this study, 279 patients received tamsulosin for 48 weeks and 184 patients for 60 weeks.

Tamsulosin treatment was stopped in 73 patients (21% of 355) of whom 27 patients (8%) discontinued the follow-up study because of adverse events. Twenty-five patients (7%) experienced a total of 33 serious adverse events of which only three (9%) were, according to the investigator, possibly or probably related to tamsulosin treatment.

A total of 19% of patients experienced adverse events possibly or probably related to study medication

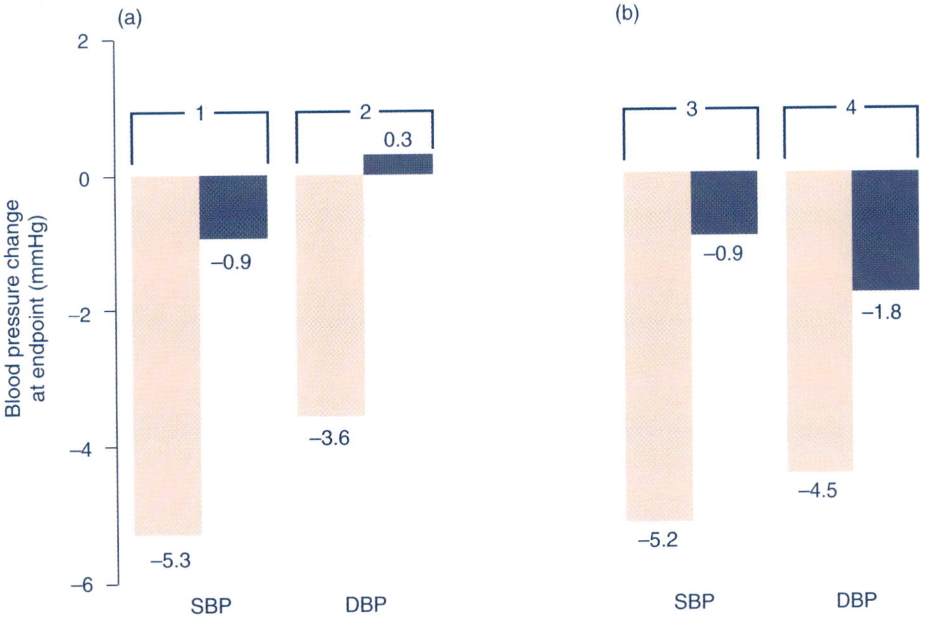

Figure 28.9. *Effect of alfuzosin (; n=118–120) or tamsulosin (■; n=127) on (a) supine and (b) standing systolic (SBP) and diastolic (DBP) blood pressure: mean change from baseline to endpoint. 1: $p=0.019$; 2: $p=0.002$; 3: $p=0.057$; 4: $p=0.044$. ANOVA with components for study centre and treatment. (From ref. 30.)*

Table 28.7. *Adverse events during long-term treatment (up to 60 weeks) with 0.4 mg tamsulosin once daily in 355 patients with functional symptoms of BPH*

	Tamsulosin (n=355)
Adverse events possibly or probably related to treatment	68 (19)
Discontinuations due to adverse events	27 (8)
Serious adverse events	25 (7)

(From ref. 30.)

during treatment for up to 60 weeks. Dizziness (4.8%) and abnormal ejaculation (3.9%) were the most common adverse events with a causal relationship to the medication (occurring in at least 3% of patients).

Safety of tamsulosin in relation to pharmacology

No requirement for dose titration and/or bedtime dosing. Several procedures have been recommended for alpha-1-blockers in order to reduce the risk of the first-dose effect and adverse events related possibly to vasodilatation. Treatment with most alpha-1-blockers (especially prazosin, terazosin and doxazosin), therefore, starts with a low dose, which then has to be carefully titrated to an optimal, therapeutic BPH dose.[2–4,36,39–40] Another method has been administration of the drug at bedtime;[2,3,41] however, it should be noted that nocturia (once or twice a night) may remain a problem in patients with symptomatic BPH despite treatment. Patients who take the dose of a long-acting alpha-1-blocker at bedtime have maximum plasma concentrations during the night and are susceptible to dizziness, (symptoms of) postural hypotension and syncope when they go to the lavatory at night.[41]

The good safety profile of 0.4 mg tamsulosin once daily in comparison with placebo, as shown by the low incidence of vasodilatory adverse events and the negligible effect on blood pressure, is achieved without dose titration or bedtime dosing. The 0.4 mg dose is administered, from the onset of therapy, after breakfast.

Safety in relation to alpha-1-adrenoceptor subtype selectivity. As discussed above, a good cardiovascular safety profile may also be due to a higher selectivity of tamsulosin for the alpha-1-adrenoceptor subtype predominantly present and functional in the human prostate (i.e. the alpha-1c-adrenoceptor) than in the human blood vessels (i.e. the alpha-1B-adrenoceptor).[2,3,8,9,11,16–18]

Whereas none of the currently available alpha-1-blockers (prazosin, alfuzosin, terazosin and doxazosin) is selective for any of the alpha-1-adrenoceptor subtypes,[8,9,22,24,25,28,29,42] in contrast, pharmacological studies have shown that tamsulosin is selective for the alpha-1A-adrenoceptor[22,23,29] and molecular biological studies have demonstrated that tamsulosin is also selective for the alpha-1c-adrenoceptor.[24–29] Tamsulosin is about 7–38 times more selective for the alpha-1c- than for the alpha-1b-adrenoceptor.[20,24] Consequently, tamsulosin is selective for the alpha-1-adrenoceptor subtype predominantly present and functional in the human prostate and displays less affinity for the alpha-1-adrenoceptor subtype that may be responsible for smooth muscle contraction in large human blood vessels (i.e. the alpha-1B-adrenoceptor). This is in line with the fact that tamsulosin is 12 times more selective for alpha-1-adrenoceptors in the human prostate than for those in the human aorta.[43]

Discussion and conclusion

Dosage and administration of tamsulosin

The recommended dosage of tamsulosin (modified release formulation) is 0.4 mg once daily after breakfast. This dosage can be administered right from the start of therapy without dose titration.

Therapeutic potential of tamsulosin

Consistent results have been achieved in European phase III clinical studies. Mean total Boyarsky symptom score is reduced by about 3.5–4 points (35–40%), from a mean score of about 9.5 points at baseline to 6 points after therapy. Mean Q_{max} is increased by about 1.6 ml/s (+16%), from about 10 ml/s at baseline to 11.5–12 ml/s during treatment with tamsulosin. The percentage of patients who achieve a clinically significant response is more than 65% for symptoms and more than 30% for Q_{max}. The effect on Q_{max} is present and maximum after the first dose of 0.4 mg tamsulosin. For total symptom score, a significant effect compared with placebo is already evident at the first measurement after 1 week of treatment in clinical trials, with continuing improvement up to 3 months. The improvement in both symptoms and Q_{max} is maintained during long-term administration. Furthermore, the efficacy of 0.4 mg tamsulosin is comparable to that of other alpha-1-blockers, such as alfuzosin (2.5 mg tid).

A mean Q_{max} of about 11.5–12 ml/s was also reached after 3 months of therapy with other alpha-1-blockers such as terazosin in a phase III placebo-controlled study[36] and after 12 months of therapy with the 5 alpha-reductase inhibitor finasteride in two phase III studies.[44,45] This observation suggests that, perhaps, it may not be possible to increase mean Q_{max} much above 12 ml/s with pharmacological therapy. This is supported by the fact that studies on the natural history of BPH have indicated that there is a mean decrease in Q_{max} of approximately 0.2 ml/s per year[46–48] and that, for a mixed group of symptomatic and asymptomatic men aged 65 years with a voided volume of 250 ml, the Q_{max} is about 14 ml/s.[47,48] Therefore, a Q_{max} of 12 ml/s may be physiological for men aged 65 years with a voided volume of 250 ml; these were the means for age and voided volume in the phase III studies with tamsulosin. This theory may also explain why the effect of pharmacological therapy on Q_{max} is modest (increase 1.5–2 ml/s) in comparison with transurethral resection of the prostate (TURP) (increase 8–9 ml/s or ±100%).[49] It has also been demonstrated that TURP in general substantially reduces symptom scores by about 80–85%.[49] This improvement is much greater than can be achieved with pharmacological therapy which, on average, gives a reduction in total symptom score of 35–40%.

One explanation for the difference in efficacy might be that the patient populations assessed in the TURP and pharmacological studies were not the same. This explanation is supported by the results of a study by Fowler and colleagues.[50] TURP was effective only in those patients with moderate to severe symptoms preoperatively. The reduction in symptom score compared with baseline was 29% in patients with moderate symptoms preoperatively and 52% in patients with severe symptoms preoperatively. TURP was not effective in patients with mild symptoms. Thus, in patients with moderate symptoms, the degree of symptomatic improvement after TURP, which is an important efficacy parameter from a patient's perspective, does not appear to differ greatly from results achieved with drug therapy, e.g. with tamsulosin.

Tamsulosin tolerance

The incidence of adverse events with 0.4 mg tamsulosin once daily is comparable to that with placebo in placebo-controlled studies. The adverse events had a causal relationship to medication in 13% of tamsulosin and in 12% of placebo patients ($p=0.802$). Adverse events possibly related to vasodilatation, such as dizziness, headache, palpitation/tachycardia, postural hypotension and syncope, and asthenia and nasal congestion/rhinitis which are adverse events commonly associated with alpha-1-blockers, occurred at a comparable incidence in tamsulosin- and placebo-treated patients.

Tamsulosin has no negative impact on sexual function, with the possible exception of abnormal ejaculation. Abnormal ejaculation was the only adverse event with a causal relationship to medication which occurred in at least 3% of tamsulosin patients and was reported more frequently with tamsulosin than with placebo. Abnormal (retrograde) ejaculation has also been attributed to other alpha-1-blockers and may be related to the pharmacological action, e.g. relaxation of smooth muscle in the bladder neck and prostatic urethra.[51,52] The incidences of impotence and decreased libido were comparable for tamsulosin and placebo.

Impairment of sexual function (i.e. impotence, decreased libido and ejaculation disorder) occurs more frequently with the 5 alpha-reductase inhibitor finasteride (there is a causal relationship in about 3% of patients) than with placebo.[44,45] Sexual dysfunction is also a common problem in TURP patients. This is especially true for retrograde ejaculation, which occurs in about 68% of TURP patients.[49,52]

There is no statistically significant difference between tamsulosin and placebo with respect to the effect on blood pressure. The only exception is the decrease in standing diastolic blood pressure which is reduced statistically significantly more with tamsulosin. This reduction is, however, small (2.5 mmHg) and is not of clinical significance. Compared with tamsulosin, alfuzosin decreases the blood pressure to a statistically significantly greater extent.

Benefit–risk ratio of tamsulosin

Tamsulosin hydrochloride (modified release formulation) will be available as 0.4 mg capsules in Europe. The recommended dosage is 0.4 mg once daily after breakfast. This can be administered right from the start of therapy without dose titration. In this dosage, tamsulosin has been shown to be effective in the (long-term) treatment of patients with functional symptoms of BPH, with regard to improvement of both symptoms and urinary flow rate. Its efficacy is comparable to that of other alpha-1-blockers, such as alfuzosin (2.5 mg tid). The incidence of adverse events is comparable to that with placebo in placebo-controlled studies. This is particularly the case for adverse events possibly related to vasodilatation, such as dizziness, headache, palpitation/tachycardia, postural hypotension and syncope. In addition, there is no clinically significant difference between tamsulosin and placebo with respect to the effect on blood pressure. In contrast, alfuzosin decreases the blood pressure to a statistically significantly greater extent than tamsulosin. The latter may be due to the fact that alfuzosin (and other alpha-1-blockers such as prazosin, terazosin and doxazosin) are not selective for any of the alpha-1-adrenoceptor subtypes. Tamsulosin, however, has higher affinity for the alpha-1-adrenoceptor subtype present and functional in the human prostate (i.e. the cloned alpha-1c- subtype). This may explain the good benefit–risk ratio of 0.4 mg tamsulosin once daily in patients with functional symptoms of BPH.

Acknowledgements

The author is very greatful to Bianca P. W. Meesen and Ruud G. L. van Tol, Yamanouchi Europe, for the worthwhile collaboration.

References

1. Caine M, Pfau A, Perlberg S. The use of alpha-adrenergic blockers in benign prostatic obstruction. Br J Urol 1976; 48: 255–263

2. Lepor H. Medical therapy for benign prostatic hyperplasia. Urology 1993; 42: 483–501

3. Lepor H. The treatment of benign prostatic hyperplasia with alpha$_1$ blockers. Curr Opin Urol 1994; 4: 16–21

4. Monda J M, Oesterling J E. Medical treatment of benign prostatic hyperplasia: 5α-reductase inhibitors and α-adrenergic antagonists. Mayo Clin Proc 1993; 68: 670–679

5. Minneman K P, Esbenshade T A. α1-Adrenergic receptor subtypes. Ann Rev Pharmacol Toxicol 1994; 34: 117–133

6. Bylund D B, Eikenberg D C, Hieble J P et al. IV. International Union of Pharmacology nomenclature of adrenoceptors. Pharmacol Rev 1994; 46: 121–136

7. Ford A P D W, Williams T J, Blue D R, Clarke D E. α$_1$-Adrenoceptor classification: sharpening Occam's razor. Trends Pharmacol Sci 1994; 15: 167–170

8. Faure C, Pimoule C, Vallancien G et al. Identification of α$_1$-adrenoceptor subtypes present in the human prostate. Life Sci 1994; 54: 1595–1605

9. Forray C, Bard J A, Wetzel J M et al. The α$_1$-adrenergic receptor that mediates smooth muscle contraction in human prostate has the pharmacological properties of the cloned human α$_{1C}$ subtype. Mol Pharmacol 1994; 45: 703–708

10. Price D T, Lefkowitz R J, Caron M G et al. Localization of mRNA for three distinct alpha1-adrenergic receptor subtypes in human tissue: implications for human alpha-adrenergic physiology. Mol Pharmacol 1994; 45: 171–175

11. Yamada S, Tanaka C, Kimura R, Kawabe K. Alpha$_1$-Adrenoceptors in human prostate: characterization and binding characteristics of alpha$_1$-antagonists. Life Sci 1994; 54: 1845–1854

12. Miranda H F, Ramirez H, Castillo O et al. α1A-Adrenergic receptors in the isolated human prostate. Pharmacol Commun 1994; 4: 181–188

13. Lepor H, Tang R, Meretyk S, Shapiro E. Alpha$_1$ adrenoceptor subtypes in the human prostate. J Urol 1993; 149: 640–642

14. Price D T, Schwinn D A, Lomasney J W et al. Identification, quantification, and localization of mRNA for three distinct alpha$_1$ adrenergic receptor subtypes in human prostate. J Urol 1993; 150: 546–551

15. Schalken J A, Van Stratum P, Smit F et al. Differential expression of alpha1-adrenergic receptor subtypes in BPH determined by reverse transcriptase PCR (polymerase chain reaction). Proc 23rd Congr Société Internationale d'Urologie, Sydney, 18–22 September 1994: 253 (abstr 648)

16. Lepor H, Tang R, Shapiro E. The alpha-adrenoceptor subtype mediating the tension of human prostatic smooth muscle. Prostate 1993; 22: 301–307

17. Chapple C R, Burt R P, Andersson P O et al. Alpha$_1$-adrenoceptor subtypes in the human prostate. Br J Urol 1994; 74: 585–589

18. Hatano A, Takahashi H, Tamaki M et al. Pharmacological evidence of distinct α$_1$-adrenoceptor subtypes mediating the contraction of human prostatic urethra and peripheral artery. Br J Pharmacol 1994; 113: 723–728

19. Honda K, Nakagawa C, Terai M. Further studies on (±)-YM-12617, a potent and selective α$_1$-adrenoceptor antagonist and its individual optical enantiomers. Naunyn-Schmiedebergs Arch Pharmacol 1987; 336: 295–302

20. Honda K, Nakagawa C. Alpha-1 adrenoceptor antagonist effects of the optical isomers of YM-12617 in rabbit lower urinary tract and prostate. J Pharmacol Exp Ther 1986; 239: 512–516

21. Yamada S, Ashizawa N, Ushijima H et al. Alpha-1 adrenoceptors in human prostate: characterization and alteration in benign prostatic hypertrophy. J Pharmacol Exp Ther 1987; 242: 326–330

22. Michel M C, Büscher R, Kerker J et al. α$_1$-Adrenoceptor subtype affinities of drugs for the treatment of prostatic hypertrophy. Evidence for heterogeneity of chloroethylclonidine-resistant rat renal α$_1$-adrenoceptors. Naunyn-Schmiedebergs Arch Pharmacol 1993; 348: 385–395

23. Chapple C R, Couldwell C J, Noble A J, Chess-Williams R. The in-vitro α$_1$ adrenoceptor mediated effects of tamsulosin on the human prostate. Proc 23rd Congr Société Internationale d'Urologie, Sydney, 18–22 September 1994: 210 (abstr 487)

24. Michel M C, Insel P A. Comparison of cloned and pharmacologically defined rat tissue α$_1$-adrenoceptor subtypes. Naunyn-Schmiedebergs Arch Pharmacol 1994; 350: 136–142

25. Michel M C, Grübbel B, Möllhoff S et al. α_1-Adrenoceptor affinities of drugs for the treatment of benign prostatic hyperplasia in human prostate, rat tissues and at cloned subtypes. Proc 23rd Congr Societé Internationale d'Urologie, Sydney, 18–22 September 1994: 254 (abstr 649)

26. Han C, Hollinger S, Theroux T L et al. ^{3}H-Tamsulosin binding to cloned α_1-adrenergic receptor subtypes stably expressed in human embryonic kidney 293 cells: antagonist potencies and sensitivity to inactivation by alkylating agents. Pharmacol Commun, 1995; 5: 117–126

27. Minneman K P, Han C, Hollinger S. Binding of ^{3}H-tamsulosin to α_1-adrenergic receptor (AR) subtypes. Proc 23rd Congr Societé Internationale d'Urologie, Sydney, 18–22 September 1994: 262 (abstr 680)

28. Schwinn D, Wilson K, Page S et al. Tamsulosin is selective for cloned α_{1C}-AR and $\alpha_{1A/D}$ subtypes. Proc 23rd Congr Societé Internationale d'Urologie, Sydney, 18–22 September 1994: 261 (abstr 678)

29. Testa R, Poggessi E, Taddei C et al. REC 15/2739, a new α_1-antagonist selective for the lower urinary tract: in vitro studies. Neurol Urodyn 1994; 13: 473–474 (abstr 84B)

30. Data on file, Yamanouchi Europe.

31. Kawabe K, Ueno A, Takimoto Y et al. Use of an α_1-blocker, YM617, in the treatment of benign prostatic hypertrophy. J Urol 1990; 144: 908–911

32. Boyarsky S, Jones G, Paulson D F, Prout G R. A new look at bladder neck obstruction by the food and drug administration regulators: guide lines for investigation of benign prostatic hypertrophy. Trans Am Assoc Genitourin Surg 1977; 68: 29–31

33. Abrams P, Schulman C C, Vaage S for the European Tamsulosin Study Group. The efficacy and safety of 0.4 mg tamsulosin once daily in symptomatic BPH. J Urol 1995; 153(suppl): 274A (abstr 123)

34. Abrams P, Schulman C C, Vaage S and the European Tamsulosin Study Group. Tamsulosin, a selective α_{1C}-adrenoceptor antagonist: a randomized, controlled trial in patients with benign 'obstruction' (symptomatic BPH). Br J Urol 1995; 76: 325–336

35. Aso Y, Boccon-Gibod L, Da Silva F C et al. Subjective response, objective response, impact on quality of life. In: Cockett A T K, Aso Y, Denis L, Khoury S (eds) Proceedings of the International Consultation on Benign Prostatic Hyperplasia (BPH), Paris, 26–27 June. SCI, 1991: 85–90

36. Lepor H, Auerbach S, Puras-Baez A et al. A randomized, placebo-controlled multicenter study of the efficacy and safety of terazosin in the treatment of BPH. J Urol 1992; 148: 1467–1474

37. Barry M J, Fowler F J, O'Leary M P et al. The American Urological Association symptom index for benign prostatic hyperplasia. J Urol 1992; 148:1549–1557

38. Lepor H for the Tamsulosin Investigator Group. Clinical evaluation of tamsulosin, a prostate selective alpha-1c antagonist Urol 1995; 153(suppl): 274A (abstr 182)

39. Wilde M I, Fitton A, Sorkin E M. Terazosin. A review of its pharmacodynamic and pharmacokinetic properties, and therapeutic potential in benign prostatic hyperplasia. Drugs Aging 1993; 3: 258–277

40. Janknegt R A, Chapple C R for the Doxazosin Study Groups. Efficacy and safety of the alpha-1 blockers doxazosin in the treatment of benign prostatic hyperplasia. Analysis of 5 studies. Eur Urol 1993; 24: 319–326

41. Kaplan S A, Soldo K A, Olsson C A. Effect of dosing regimen on efficacy and safety of doxazosin in normotensive men with symptomatic prostatism: a pilot study. Urology 1994; 44: 348–352

42. Faure C, Pimoule C, Arbilla S et al. Expression of α_1-adrenoceptor subtypes in rat tissues: implications for α_1-adrenoceptor classification. Eur J Pharmacol (Mol Pharmacol) 1994; 268: 141–149

43. Yamada S, Suzuki M, Tanaka C et al. Comparative study on α_1-adrenoceptor antagonist binding in human prostate and aorta. Clin Exp Pharmacol Physiol 1994; 21: 405–411

44. Gormley G J, Stoner E, Bruskewitz R C et al. The effect of finasteride in men with benign prostatic hyperplasia. N Engl J Med 1992; 327: 1185–1191

45. Finasteride Study Group. Finasteride (MK-906) in the treatment of benign prostatic hyperplasia. Prostate 1993; 22: 291–299

46. Drach G W, Layton T N, Binard W J. Male peak urinary flow rate: relationship to volume voided and age. J Urol 1979; 122: 210–214

47. Girman C J, Panser L A, Chute C G et al. Natural history of prostatism: urinary flow rates in a community-based study. J Urol 1993; 150: 887–892

48. Oesterling J E, Girman C J, Panser L A et al. Correlation between urinary flow rate, voided volume, and patient age in a community-based population. In: Kurth K, Newling D W W (eds) Benign prostatic hyperplasia. Recent progress in clinical research and practice. EORTC Genitourinary Group Monograph 12. New York: Wiley-Liss, 1994: 125–139

49. Brendler C, Schlegel P, Dowd J et al. Surgical treatment for benign prostatic hyperplasia. Cancer 1992; 70(suppl 1): 371–373

50. Fowler F J, Wennberg J E, Timothy R P et al. Symptom status and quality of life following prostatectomy. JAMA 1988; 259: 3018–3022

51. Kedia K R, Persky L. Effect of phenoxybenzamine (dibenzyline) on sexual function in man. Urology 1981; 18: 620–622

52. McConnell J D, Barry M J, Bruskewitz R C et al. Benign prostatic hyperplasia: diagnosis and treatment. Clinical practice guideline no. 8. Agency for Health Care Policy and Research (AHCPR) Publication no. 94-0582. Rockville: US Department of Health and Human Services, 1994: 99–103

53. Hieble J P, Bylund D B, Clarke D E et al. International Union of Pharmacology.x. Recommendation of nomenclature of α_1-adrenoceptors: consensus update. Pharmacol Rev 1995; 47(2): 267–270

54. Chapple C R, Wyndaele J J, Nordlung J et al. Tamsulosin, the first prostate-selective α_{1A}-adrenoceptor antagonist: a meta-analysis of two randomized, placebo-controlled, multicentre studies in patients with benign prostatic obstruction (symptomatic BPH). Eur Urol 1996; in press

55. Schulman C C, Denis L, Jonas U et al. Tamsulosin, the first prostate-selective α_{1A}-adrenoceptor antagonist: an interim analysis of a multinational, multicentre, open-label study assesssing the long-term efficacy and safety in patients with benign prostatic obstruction (symptomatic BPH). Eur Uol 1996; in press

56. Starkey L P, Trenga C, Miyazawa Y, Ito Y. Lack of clinical interaction effects between tamsulosin and enalapril. Clin Pharmacol Ther 1995; 57(2): 166 (abstr PII–11)

57. Starkey L P, Yasukawa K, Trenga C, Miyazawa Y, Ito Y. Study of possible pharmacodynamic interaction between tamsulosin and nifedipine in subjects with essential hypertension. J Clin Pharmacol 1994; 34(10): 1019 (abstr 45)

29

Combination therapies for benign prostatic hyperplasia

R. S. Kirby H. Lepor

Introduction

The use of medical therapies for bladder outflow obstruction due to benign prostatic hyperplasia (BPH) is growing rapidly worldwide; over one million individuals are, for example, receiving finasteride and probably as many taking an alpha-blocker for the symptoms of this disorder. As noted in previous chapters, the tolerability of these medications has been confirmed in many studies, but their efficacy still falls below that of transurethral resection of the prostate (TURP). Moreover, medical therapies are not always effective in every patient. These observations have provided the stimulus to evaluate a number of different combination therapies in patients with symptomatic BPH.

Theoretical considerations

The two major classes of pharmacological agent utilized in BPH are the alpha-1-adrenoceptor selective blockers and the 5 alpha-reductase inhibitors. In addition, aromatase inhibitors and anti-oestrogens, theoretically at least, may have some clinical value. BPH is characterized by proliferation of both stroma and epithelium in the transition zone of the prostate, but as Bartsch and subsequently Shapiro et al. have shown, the predominant tissue type is stroma.[1,2] It is predominantly the smooth muscle component of stroma at which alpha-blockers are directed. By contrast, 5 alpha-reductase inhibitors are mainly active against the epithelial cells. Androgen deprivation results in apoptosis of epithelial cells and pronounced glandular involution (Fig. 29.1). However, both 5 alpha-reductase enzymes and androgen receptors have been shown to be present in prostatic stromal cells and it is possible that some part of the 30% or so prostatic shrinkage that follows androgen deprivation may be the result of atrophy of stromal components of the gland. Smooth muscle cells of the prostate also possess oestrogen receptors, providing the rationale for anti-oestrogen and aromatase inhibitor therapy in BPH.

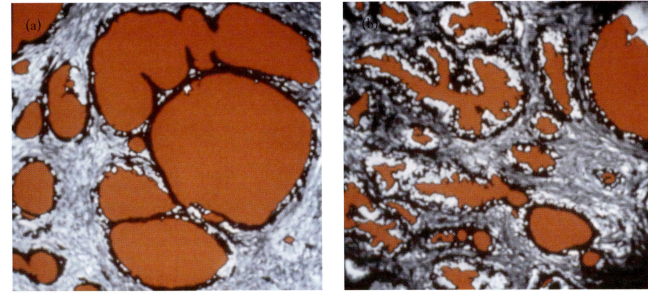

Figure 29.1. (a) Image analysis of a section of the prostate from a patient with BPH. This shows a predominant glandular hyperplasia with large acini. (b) Image analysis of a section of the prostate from a patient following 9 months of treatment with finasteride, showing glandular involution.

Efficacy of monotherapy

A recent meta-analysis of nearly 30 randomized, controlled trials of alpha-1 selective blockers in BPH suggested that a 14% fall in symptom score and 1.5 ml/s improvement in maximum uroflow could be expected with these agents (although, admittedly, maximum dosage had not always been achieved in many of these studies).[3] Finasteride, the 5 alpha-reductase inhibitor with which most experience has been gained, has been demonstrated to produce a 2.7-point fall in symptom score and 1.6 ml/s enhancement in uroflow at 1 year.[4] Open label studies have confirmed durability of response beyond 36 months, with a mean symptom score reduction of 3.6 points and a uroflow enhancement of 3.6 ml/s.[5] By contrast, a recent multicentre study of the aromatase inhibitor atamestane, tested in a randomized, controlled study of 160 patients, showed no greater efficacy than placebo and poor tolerability.[6] The reported effects of the most commonly used alpha-blockers and 5 alpha-reductase inhibitor are summarized in Tables 29.1 and 29.2.

The current question, therefore, is whether the combination of an alpha-1-adrenoceptor blocker and a therapy directed towards reducing the androgenic stimulation of the prostate will produce an additive efficacy with acceptable tolerability. This hypothesis is currently being tested both in single-arm pilot studies and in a number of multicentre randomized, controlled trials. The data available to date are reviewed below.

Combination therapy: a pilot study

At the time of writing there is only one published study evaluating combination therapy for BPH. Lepor and Machi reported a pilot study evaluating the safety and efficacy of the combination of terazosin and flutamide for the treatment of BPH.[7] Flutamide was administered because, at the time of patient enrolment, the 5 alpha-reductase inhibitor finasteride was not commercially available.

A total of 29 men with symptomatic BPH signed informed consent forms to participate in this open-label study evaluating the relative efficacy of terazosin versus terazosin and flutamide for the treatment of BPH. The exclusion parameters were patients aged less than 50

years or more than 80 years, insulin-dependent diabetes, symptomatic coronary artery disease, neurological disorders (cerebrovascular accident, Parkinson's disease and multiple sclerosis), urinary tract infections, urethral stricture disease, previous prostatectomy, orthostatic hypotension, creatinine level more than 2 mg/dl, total Boyarsky symptom score less than 7, peak urinary flow rate less than 4 ml/s or more than 15 ml/s, and post-void residual greater than 300 ml. Prostatic ultrasonography was performed on all patients prior to enrolment in the study using the 7 MHz Bruel and Kjaer transrectal transducer. The volume of the prostate was determined by ultrasound, and any suspicious hypoechoic foci were biopsied.

Terazosin was administered at bedtime throughout this study. The dose of terazosin was titrated in all patients to 5 mg, provided that significant adverse drug-related events did not develop. The dose titration proceeded as follows: 1 mg on days 1–3; 2 mg on days 4–14; 5 mg on days 15–183 (6 months). Flutamide was administered between days 30 and 183. The initial dosage of flutamide was 250 mg three times daily. The dosages of terazosin and flutamide were reduced if significant adverse events developed.

The efficacy parameters included changes in Boyarsky symptom scores and peak urinary flow rates. The patients also assessed their symptomatic improvement as marked, moderate, slight, none or worse. The efficacy parameters were evaluated at 1 month and 6 months (or at the time of early withdrawal from the study). The difference between Boyarsky symptom scores and peak urinary flow rates at baseline and 1 month represented the efficacy of terazosin alone. The difference between these outcome parameters at 1 month and 6 months, or at the time of early withdrawal from the study, represented the efficacy following the addition of flutamide. The efficacy of combination therapy was not evaluated for subjects receiving flutamide for less than 3 months.

The serum prostate-specific antigen (PSA) levels and prostate volumes were measured at 6 months or at the time of early withdrawal from the study. Complete blood counts and biochemistry parameters were evaluated at baseline, 2 months and 6 months. Two patients ultimately required a reduction of the dose level of terazosin to 2 mg. The effects of terazosin on the

Table 29.1. *Reported effects of the most commonly used alpha-blockers*

Alpha-blocker	Series	Patients (n)	Treatment duration (weeks)	Increase in max flow (ml/s)†	Increase in mean flow (ml/s)†	Fall in subtracted detrusor pressure (cmH₂O)	Reduction in symptom score†	Residual volume (ml)	No. of drop-outs‡
Phenoxybenzamine	Caine[8]	50	2	6.2 (87.5)	3.18 (81.9)	ND	NS	ND	1 (CVA)
	Brooks[9]	28	4	0.9 (14)	ND	ND	NS	NS	–
	Abrams[10]	61	4	3.1 (43)	ND	ND	–2	NS	3
Alfusozin	Ramsey[11]	31	13	0	NS	ND	Frequency*	NS	–
	Jardin[12]	518	24	3.1 (43)§	0.9 (13.6)	ND	(42)	–33 (–38)	70/92 (NS)
	Teillac[13]	93	Single dose	2.6 (34.3)	1.25*	ND	ND	ND	0
	Hanson[14]	205	12	2 (22)	(38.5)*	ND	(29)	20	5/12
Doxazosin	Christensen[15]	100	9	1.5 (23)	1.2 (26)	ND	(67)	–15 (15)	1/3
	Chapple[16]	135	12	2.6 (29)	1.0 (22.7)	4.6	(51)	ND	5/4
	Fawzy[17]	100	16	2.9	1.4	ND	(39)	–	7/1
Indoramin	Stott[18]	40	4	2.6 (39)	1.8 (25.3)	ND	Nocturia*	*	–
	Iacovou[19]	30	8	10.0 (11.8)	ND	ND	*	ND	3
	Chow[20]	139	8	4.9	ND	ND	*	ND	9 (6.5)
Prazosin	Martorana[21]	18	2	6.9 (96.8)	2.2 (47.8)	ND	NS	NS	0
	Hedlund[22]	20	4	2.0 (40.8)	1.1 (42.3)	7	NS	–53 (–5.3)	0
	Kirby[23]	80	4	4.8 (58.5)	ND	3	*	ND	0
	Chapple[24]	58	12	3.2 (34)	ND	17.7	–	–	5/3 (NS)
Terazosin	Dunzendorfer[25]	15	–	1.8 (30.5)	2.0 (47)	2	(48)	ND	0
	Lepor[26]	45	144	3.6 (42)	3.9 (48)	ND	(35) irr (63) obs	ND	5
	Fabricius[27]	57	24	4.2	2.7	ND	(68)	–52 (–56)	0
Tamsulosin	Kawabe[28]	270	4	3.6 (34.6)	2.0 (41)	ND	ND	–9	ND
	Abrams[29]	313	12	1.4 (13.1)	0.8 (15.4)	ND	(36)* (43)* obs	–20	3/8

†Percentages in parentheses; ‡dropouts due to adverse reaction or lack of efficacy (drug/placebo); §peak flow < 10 ml/s.
Asterisks indicate significant differences between groups. CVA, cerebrovascular accident; irr, irritative; ND, not done; NS, not significant; obs, obstructive. For more information, see text.

Table 29.2. *Reported effects of the most commonly used 5 alpha-reductase inhibitor, finasteride*

Series	Patients enrolled (n)	Treatment duration (weeks)	Increase in max flow (ml/s)*	Reduction of symptom score*	Prostatic shrinkage*	No. of dropouts[†]
Gormley[4]	892	52	1.6 (22)	2.7 (21)	11.9 (–19)	40/37
Finasteride Study Group[30]	750	52	1.7 (11.8)	3.3 (12.1)	12.3 (–22)	15/12
Andersen[31]	707	104	1.5 (11.7)	2.0 (11.4)	19.2 (–19)	66/64

*Percentages in parentheses;[†]dropouts due to adverse reaction or lack of efficacy (drug/placebo).

Boyarksy symptom scores, peak urinary flow rate and voided volume following 1 month of treatment are presented in Table 29.3. The mean peak urinary flow rate improved by 38%. The mean total, obstructive and irritative symptom scores improved by 56, 67 and 42%, respectively. The changes in all efficacy parameters from baseline were statistically significant. The patients' objective assessment of their symptomatic improvement was as follows: marked improvement, 41%; moderate improvement, 38%; and slight improvement, 21%. The only adverse event occurring with an incidence greater than 5% was nasal congestion.

A total of 29 patients entered the 5-month combination treatment period. Of these 29 subjects, two were lost to follow-up; 14 patients were withdrawn early owing to adverse events associated with flutamide. The efficacy of combination therapy was based on 24 patients who received any combined dosage of terazosin and flutamide for at least 3 months. Of these 24 patients, 16 (67%) required a reduction of flutamide dosage. The final daily dosage of flutamide for the 24

evaluable patients was 750 mg (n=8), 500 mg (n=3) and 250 mg (n=13).

The efficacy of terazosin versus combination therapy was compared for the 24 patients receiving terazosin and flutamide for at least 3 months (Table 29.4). The peak urinary flow rate, voided volume and symptom scores did not differ significantly between these two groups. Of the 24 patients, six (25%) exhibited moderate improvement following the addition of flutamide.

The adverse events related to flutamide were problematic. The most significant adverse event was breast tenderness. Decreased libido, diarrhoea, increased liver function tests and impotence also occurred in more than 5% of the subjects.

The adequacy of the dosage and duration of flutamide therapy to achieve maximal reduction of prostate volume and serum PSA was evaluated. Overall, the prostate volume and PSA decreased by 25 and 52%, respectively, following combination therapy. Serum testosterone increased by 48% following combination therapy.

Table 29.3. *Effects of terazosin* on peak flow rate and Boyarsky symptom score after 1 month of treatment*

Parameter	Baseline	Terazosin	Change (%)	p value
Max flow (ml/s)	9.3 (±0.6)	12.8 (±0.9)	38	< 0.0001
Symptom score	11.2 (±0.6)	4.9 (±0.4)	56	< 0.0001

*Dose titrated to 5 mg/day unless adverse drug-related events occurred.

Table 29.4. *Effects of terazosin* versus combination therapy (terazosin + flutamide[†]) on peak flow rate and Boyarsky symptom score*

Parameter	Terazosin	Combination	Difference (%)	p value
Max flow (ml/s)	12.7 (±1.0)	11.9 (±0.8)	–6	0.423
Symptom score	4.9 (±0.4)	4.5 (±0.6)	–8	0.382

*As in Table 29.3; [†]final daily dosage for 24 patients was 750 mg (n=8), 500 mg (n=3) or 250 mg (n=13).

The comparison of terazosin versus combination therapy assumed that the maximal clinical response following terazosin therapy occurred within 5 months of flutamide treatment. Lepor et al.[32] have previously reported that the changes in peak urinary flow rate and Boyarsky total symptom score following 2 months of terazosin treatment (5 mg/day) were 42 and 47%, respectively. The changes in these outcome parameters following 1 month of terazosin treatment in the present study were equivalent to the outcome analysis reported following 2 months of terazosin therapy. A multicentre randomized placebo-controlled study has demonstrated that maximal clinical response occurs following 2 weeks of terazosin dose adjustment.[26] Reduction of prostate volume following androgen suppression plateaus between 4 and 6 months. Although the combination treatment period in the present study was scheduled for 5 months, the majority of patients developed significant adverse events related to flutamide, which required dosage reduction and/or early withdrawal. The minimum effective dose of flutamide in BPH has not been determined. The mean reduction of prostate volume following combination treatment in these 24 evaluable subjects was 25%. The reported reduction of prostate volume in males with symptomatic BPH following the administration of gonadotropin-releasing hormone analogues and finasteride for 6 months was 24 and 27%, respectively.[4,33] Therefore, the evaluable patients in the combination treatment group exhibited the maximal reduction of prostate volume expected following androgen suppression. Thus, the study was appropriately designed to determine the relative efficacy of terazosin versus combination therapy for BPH.

This combination study did not identify any statistically significant therapeutic advantages for combination therapy relative to terazosin monotherapy. Combination therapy was associated with a 20% improvement in obstructive symptom scores relative to terazosin monotherapy. Twenty-five per cent of the subjects exhibited moderate symptomatic improvement following the addition of flutamide. The differences in the outcome parameters between terazosin versus combination therapy were not statistically significant, but this lack of statistical significance may be related to the very small sample size. The present study was not designed to compare the relative efficacy of terazosin

versus flutamide for the treatment of BPH. Therefore, conclusions regarding the relative efficacy of these treatment alternatives cannot be extrapolated from the clinical database.

Randomized controlled studies of combination therapy in BPH

Four studies are currently evaluating this concept. The Veteran Affairs (VA) cooperative study in the USA has compared terazosin and finasteride with terazosin or finasteride as monotherapy with placebo in a four-arm study of 1200 patients over 12 months. In Europe, the PREDICT study has a similar design but employs doxazosin rather than terazosin as the alpha-1-adrenoceptor blocker. In the UK, finasteride and indoramine have been evaluated as combination therapy whereas, in France, alfuzosin is the alpha-blocker that has been evaluated in this context.

At the time of writing, only the VA cooperative study has been completed but the results are not available, although publication of the full data is currently pending. As more data emerge, we should be able to judge more precisely the true efficacy of the combination of prostatic shrinkage and relaxation of the smooth muscle within the gland, and to evaluate whether this novel approach to BPH management lives up to its theoretical promise.

References

1. Bartsch G, Muller H, Boerholzer M, Rohr H. Light microscopic stereological analysis of the normal human prostate and benign prostatic hyperplasia. J Urol 1979; 122: 487–491

2. Shapiro E, Hartanto V, Beicich M, Lepor H. The relative proportions of stromal and epithelial hyperplasia is related to the development of symptomatic BPH. J Urol 1992; 147: 1293–1295

3. Eri L, Tveter K. Alpha-blockade in the treatment of symptomatic benign prostatic hyperplasia. J Urol 1995; 154: 923–934

4. Gormley G, Stoner E, Bruskewitz R, et al. The effect of finasteride in men with benign prostatic hyperplasia. N Engl J Med 1992; 327: 1185–1191

5. Stoner E, Members of the Finasteride Study Group. Three-year safety and efficacy data on the use of finasteride in the treatment of benign prostatic hyperplasia. Urology 1994; 43 (3): 284–294

6. Gingell J, Knonagel H, Kurth K, Tunn U, and the Schering 90.062 study group. Placebo controlled double-blind study to test the efficacy of the aromatase inhibitor atamestane in patients with benign prostatic hyperplasia not requiring operation. J Urol 1995; 154: 399–401

7. Lepor H, Machi G. The relative efficacy of terazosin versus terazosin and flutamide for the treatment of symptomatic BPH. Prostate 1992; 20: 89–95

8. Caine M, Perlnerg S, Meretyk S. A placebo-controlled double-blind study of the effect of phenoxybenzamine in benign prostatic obstruction. Br J Urol 1978; 50: 551–554

9. Brooks ME, Sidi AA, Hanani Y, Braf Z. Ineffectiveness of phenoxybenzamine in treatment of benign prostatic hypertrophy. A controlled study. Urology 1983; 21: 474–478

10. Abrams P, Shah P, Stone A, Choa R. Bladder outflow obstruction treated with phenoxybenzamine. Br J Urol 1982; 54: 527–530

11. Ramsay J, Scott GI, Whitfield HN. A double-blind controlled trial of a new alpha-1 blocking drug in the treatment of bladder outflow obstruction. Br J Urol 1985; 57: 657–659

12. Jardin A, Bensadoun H, Delauche-Cavalier MC, Attali P. Alfuzosin for treatment of benign prostatic hypertrophy. Lancet 1991; 337: 1457–1461

13. Teillac P, DeLauche-Cavalier M, Attali P, DUALF Group. Urinary flow rates in patients with benign prostatic hyperthrophy following treatment with alfuzosin. Br J Urol 1992; 70: 58–64

14. Hansen B, Nordling J, Mensink H, Walter S, Meyhoff H, ALFECH study group. Alfuzosin in the treatment of benign prostatic hyperplasia: effects on symptom scores, urinary flow rates and residual volume. A multicentre, double-blind, placebo-controlled trial. Scand J Urol Nephrol 1993; Suppl 157: 169–176

15. Christensen MM, Holme JB, Rasmussen PC, et al. Doxazosin treatment in patients with prostatic obstruction. A double-blind placebo-controlled study. Scan J Urol Nephrol 1993; 27: 39–44

16. Chapple C, Christmas T, Milroy E, Abrams P, Kirby R. A three month placebo-controlled study of doxazosin on prostatic outflow obstruction. J Urol 1992; 147: 366A

17. Fawzy A, Braun K, Lewis GP, et al. Doxazosin in the treatment of benign prostatic hyperplasia in normotensive patients: a multicenter study. J Urol 1995; 154: 105–110

18. Stott MA, Abrams PH. Indoramin in the treatment of prostatic bladder outflow obstruction. Br J Urol 1991; 67: 499–501

19. Iacovou JW, Dunn M. Indoramin - an effective new drug in the management of bladder outflow obstruction. Br J Urol 1987; 60: 526–528

20. Chow W, Hahn D, Sandhu D, et al. Multicentre controlled trial of indoramin in the symptomatic relief of benign prostatic hypertrophy. Br J Urol 1990; 65: 36–38

21. Martorana G, Giberti C, Damonte P. The effect of prazosin in benign prostatic hypertrophy: A placebo-controlled double-blind study. IRCS Med Sci 1984; 12: 11–12

22. Hedlund H, Andersson KE, Ek A. Effects of prazosin in patients with benign prostatic obstruction. J Urol 1983; 130: 275–278

23. Kirby R, Coppinger S, Corcoran M, Chapple C, Flannigan M, Milroy E. Prazosin in the treatment of prostatic obstruction. A placebo controlled study. Br J Urol 1987; 60: 136–142

24. Chapple CR, Christmas TJ, Milroy EJG. A twelve-week placebo controlled study of prazosin in the treatment of prostatic obstruction. Urol Int 1990; 45 (suppl 1): 47–55

25. Dunzendorfer U. Clinical experience: symptomatic management of BPH with terazosin. Urology 1988; 32: 27–31

26. Lepor H, Auerbach S, Puras-Baez A, et al. A randomised, placebo-controlled multicentre study of the efficacy and safety of terazosin in the treatment of benign prostatic hyperplasia. J Urol 1992; 148: 1467–1474

27. Fabricius PG, Weizert P, Dunzendorfer U, Mac Hannaford J, Maurath C. Efficacy of once-a-day terazosin in benign prostatic hyperplasia: A randomized placebo controlled clinical trial. Prostate 1990; 3 (suppl): 85–93

28. Kawabe K, Ueno A, Takimoto Y, Aso Y, Kato H. Use of an alpha-1 blocker, YM617, in the treatment of benign prostatic hypertrophy. J Urol 1990; 144: 908–912

29. Abrams P, Schulman C, Vaage S, European Tamsulosin Study Group. Tamsulosin, a selective alpha1c-adrenoceptor antagonist: a randomised, controlled trial in patients with benign prostatic obstruction (symptomatic BPH). Br J Urol 1995; 76: 325–326

30. Finasteride Study Group. Finasteride (MK-906) in the treatment of benign prostatic hyperplasia. Prostate 1993; 22: 291–299

31. Andersen J, Ekman P, Wolf H, et al. Can finasteride reverse the process of benign prostatic hyperplasia? A two-year placebo-controlled study. Urology 1995; 46: 631–637

32. Lepor H, Knapp-Maloney G, Sunshine H. A dose titration study evaluating terazosin, a selective, once-a-day alpha-1 blocker for the treatment of symptomatic benign prostatic hyperplasia. J Urol 1990; 144: 1393–1398

33. Peters CA, Walsh PC. The effect of nafarelin acetate, a luteinizing hormone releasing hormone agonist, on benign prostatic hyperplasia. N Eng J Med 1987; 317: 599–604

30

Phytotherapeutic agents
J. M. Fitzpatrick T. H. Lynch

Introduction

The increased interest in the management of symptomatic benign prostatic hyperplasia (BPH) has stimulated research into the aetiology, pathogenesis and diagnosis of the condition, in addition to critical evaluation of current therapies. Because the aetiology of BPH has been studied so carefully, and because the relationship between this and the development of bladder outlet obstruction is being defined, new pharmacological options in the management of BPH have been developed. At present, these are aimed at either reducing prostatic size or decreasing outflow resistance, but as our knowledge grows it is likely that there will be an increased possibility of the development of drugs that will be able to target closer to genetic influences within the nucleus. At present, most drugs are aimed at the more simplistic rationales stated above, but it is important to note that these drugs, such as 5 alpha-reductase inhibitors and alpha-blockers, have very specific rationales for use in symptomatic BPH.

The ultimate aim of all drugs that are introduced as a therapy for symptomatic BPH is that they improve symptoms and peak flow rate and that this will effectively decrease the requirement for transurethral resection of the prostate (TURP). In addition to these hopes of the efficacy of the drug, the aim that it be safe is also considered to be of the greatest importance. The balance between safety and efficacy is the rate-limiting factor associated with any drug.

Most patients with BPH in the developed world present to their doctors because their symptoms are bothering them rather than because of one of the serious complications of the condition, such as chronic retention or uraemia. It is, therefore, seen as a legitimate aim to find a drug that will cause a considerable improvement in symptoms. The secondary gain of a huge increase in peak flow rate or a decrease in residual urine would therefore be seen by many as being of lesser importance. Nevertheless, there must be some statistically significant improvement in objective indices in order that the drug can be differentiated from a placebo. In addition to this, as stated above, for a drug to be introduced it should be a requirement that the rationale for the use of such an agent should be known, or at least should be potentially related to one of the aetiological mechanisms of BPH.

As a result of the wish on the part of urologists and pharmaceutical companies to have a complete knowledge of the safety and efficacy of the various products, they have all been submitted to the most rigorous of clinical trials. This is very helpful and it allows the urologist the opportunity of seeing not only how well a drug works but also in which patients it will be of particular value. The therapeutic trials should be placebo-controlled, randomized and performed in several centres. In addition, the trials should ideally be evaluated by an outside observer. The 5 alpha-reductase inhibitors and alpha-adrenergic blockers have been tested carefully, but the phytotherapeutic agents, in the majority of cases, have not. There are exceptions to this and these are outlined in this chapter. There is strong evidence that there has been a dramatic change, and that phytotherapeutic agents are increasingly being submitted to clinical trials. This is, of course, a very satisfactory eventuality that will, it is hoped, continue. It is only from this approach that the universal acceptance of such agents in urological practice can be guaranteed.

There are drawbacks, however, in clinical trials. For example, different patients may be bothered more by different symptoms, and in many cases one patient will be able to endure symptoms of a severity that other patients will find intolerable. There is a fluctuation in the symptoms of BPH in the same patient, which must also be taken into account when results are being interpreted. These facts are further complicated by the profound placebo effect associated with any treatment. Furthermore, as pain is not usually a main symptom of BPH, there will be a variability as to when patients will present to their doctor, with many presenting very late. The placebo effect has been evaluated carefully by Schulze et al.[1] who collected all the data from the placebo arms of many drug trials in symptomatic BPH, and carried out a meta-analysis on these. They found that there was a marked spontaneous improvement of symptoms in the placebo groups, which occurred as early as 3–6 months and which lasted in some patients for as long as 2 years. The percentage of patients in whom such a placebo effect was demonstrable at 2 years was less than at 6 or 12 months, but it was still a large number. It is quite clear that these observations can also be criticized, in that placebo groups are present in drug trials only to be compared with treatment groups. It is as valid to lump all of the *treatment* groups together and compare them with nothing as it is to lump all of the *placebo* groups together and compare them with nothing. However, this work is an important pointer, and the placebo effect must be kept in mind when interpreting the results of any trial.

Natural therapy of BPH

The medical management of BPH other than with hormones or alpha-blockers continues to be of interest, and the possibility that there might be a 'natural' treatment for BPH is a very attractive one. If an agent has a natural ingredient with low side effects that is of value to patients, this would be a valuable contribution to the therapeutic options for treating this condition. Many such natural agents have been introduced and they are divided into four groups:[2,3]

1. Phytotherapeutic agents.
2. Cholesterol-lowering agents.
3. Amino acid complexes.
4. Organ extracts.

This is somewhat arbitrary division, with considerable crossover between the groups, particularly in the case of the phytotherapeutic and cholesterol-lowing agents. It is preferable, therefore, to group these two together and apply the term phytotherapeutic agents to both of them.

Phytotherapeutic agents

It may seem unlikely to some readers that taking plant extracts could ever be considered to be an appropriate therapy for symptomatic BPH. Nevertheless, they have been used since ancient times, and are immensely popular today throughout the world, but particularly in Europe. One publication suggested that the 16 most popular phytotherapeutic agents had a total sale value in Germany in 1986 of 131 million Deutschmarks.[4] Subsequent publications have not suggested that there has been a decrease in expenditure.[5] These agents have not been introduced with any clear rationale behind them, apart from the fact that they are natural compounds, but is fair to say that they have achieved patient satisfaction and so have been received with growing popularity by physicians and patients alike. This popularity has been maintained by the ease with which they can be purchased and also by the absence of any particular side effects.

The most frequently used plant extracts used are as follows:

1. The bark of *Pygeum africanum*.
2. Pollen extract.
3. The leaves of the trembling poplar.
4. The root of *Hypoxis rooperi*.
5. The seeds of *Cucurbita pepo*.
6. The fruit of *Serenoa repens* (*Sabal serrulata*).
7. The roots of *Echinacea purpura*.

These attractive names are often subsumed into the more pragmatic and marketable trade names. Many so-called cholesterol-lowering agents are also in use, and the best known of these are beta-sitosterol and mepartricin.

Contents of phytotherapeutic agents

Although a hidden natural ingredient may well be present, it has not definitely been found. It is more likely that one of the known ingredients has an unsuspected mode of action, and this is an area that is undergoing considerable study. What is certain is that most of the plant extracts contain (a) free fatty acids, (b) free fatty alcohols and (c) triterpenes and sterols (the most frequently found being sitosterol, tocopherol, campesterol, stigmasterol, lupenone and lipoxin). Exactly which of these is the most likely to be affecting the prostate is not certain, but each one has its own individual champion. It is also unclear which, if any, of these compounds is absorbed through the intestinal mucosa, but the specific radioisotope-labelled studies that would be required to establish this have not been performed.

Mode of action

Many different possible methods of action have been proposed for the different plant extracts. A rather large number of these have not yet been scientifically substantiated and are therefore just suggested as possible modes of action. It is interesting to note that an increasing number of studies are being performed in order to define accurately the action of various compounds, and it is to be hoped that the required answers will soon be achieved.

One of the problems with these studies is that, although they are excellently performed with considerable scientific expertise in the laboratory, the link between their action on the culture medium or cell line and the therapeutic action in the human body has not been made. Although the various compounds have been shown to have some effect on experimental animals or tissue culture, it is sometimes not clear whether the concentrations used have a definite clinical relevance. Because these are naturally occurring compounds present in the human diet, it is essential that their absorption into the human body and subsequent concentration in the target organ be defined by radiolabelled particles. Several possible modes of action have been suggested, as follows:

1. Anti-oestrogenic effect.
2. Anti-androgenic effect.
3. Decrease in sex hormone-binding globulin.
4. Inhibition of prostate-derived cell lines.
5. Inhibition of basic fibroblast growth factor (bFGF) and epidermal growth factor (EGF)-induced proliferation of 3T3 fibroblasts.
6. General inhibition of bFGF.
7. Interference with the metabolism of prostaglandin.
8. Overall anti-inflammatory effect.
9. Decrease of outflow resistance.
10. Reduction of prostatic size.

The following is a more detailed review of how the plant extracts may effect the prostate.

Cholesterol-lowering effect

The prostate contains cholesterol, and this is also present in its secretions. Hyperplastic tissue from the prostate contains twice as much cholesterol as non-hyperplastic tissue. This link has suggested that any agent that would lower the level of cholesterol in the prostate would also inhibit its growth, and that this would lead to a decrease in prostatic size with relief of symptoms of BPH.

Many plant extracts contain sitosterol, a compound that resembles cholesterol. Sitosterols are thought to be poorly absorbed and to have a cholesterol-lowering action because they bind cholesterol in the intestine. About 10 g sitosterols are required daily to lower the plasma cholesterol by 10–20%, and most of the phytotherapeutic agents contain only about 10 mg per tablet. In addition, about 200 mg sitosterol are consumed in an ordinary daily diet.[6]

Previously, polyene-macrolide antifungal antibiotics such as nystatin, amphotericin B and candicidin have been used to treat symptomatic BPH. Experimental studies have shown that these compounds do reduce prostatic cholesterol concentrations. As none of these drugs is absorbed from the bowel, it is very likely that they act by inhibiting cholesterol absorption.

Hormonal effects

Hormonal effects have also been claimed for some of the plant extracts. *Serenoa repens* is thought to have an anti-androgenic effect localized to the prostate. It is felt that it does this by being a multisite inhibitor of androgenic action, competing with dihydrotestosterone at androgen receptor level.[7]

A number of in vitro studies have also suggested some other possible hormonal actions — inhibition of [³H]methol-tremolone, inhibition of 5 alpha-reductase and partial inhibition of 3-alpha-oxidoreductase.[8] The inhibition of [³H]methol-tremolone effects targets as specific as the androgen receptor, because it is thought to be highly specific for androgen receptors at low concentrations. It has also been suggested by di Silverio and colleagues that *S. repens* causes a 50% reduction in conversion of testosterone to dihydrotestosterone. It has also been demonstrated in vitro that it has an anti-oestrogenic effect. Further studies have shown an anti-androgenic effect in vitro on the prostate cell lines LNCaP and PC3.[9]

A possible hormonal action has been a recurring theme in the in vitro work assessing modes of action of phytotherapeutic agents, but not all studies agree with this or accept it as a possibility. The work quoted above suggests a definite inhibition of 5 alpha-reductase, but a further investigation assessed a number of phytotherapeutic agents such as *Radix urtica*, *Hypoxis rooperi* and *S. repens* against finasteride for the activity.[10] None of these plant extracts was found in clinical or laboratory studies to have any demonstrable 5 alpha-reductase activity when compared with finasteride.

In addition, where a hormonal action or more specifically a 5 alpha-reductase inhibitory action is claimed, the expectation would be that there would be a reduction in the size of the prostate and a decrease in the level of prostate-specific antigen (PSA) in the blood. In the clinical trials with finasteride a roughly 29% reduction in prostate size and a 50% decrease in PSA after 6 months have been reported; these effects have not yet been reported as having taken place in any of the clinical studies with phytotherapeutic agents.

Action on bladder muscle

One of the other possibilities that has been raised is that there is a direct action on bladder muscle. This theory has been extensively studied in a series of experiments performed recently. In a model of partial bladder outlet obstruction in the rabbit,[11] the bladder muscle can be stimulated in a number of ways. The first method involves field stimulation, which sets up a pathway of events: there is a neurogenic release of transmitter, which then activate receptors and the receptors activate actin and myosin, which are the contractile mechanisms. The next method is bethanechol stimulation, which activates the receptors directly; finally, stimulation with KCl activates the contractile apparatus directly.

In a series of elegant experiments using this model,[12] it was found that the contractile responses to field stimulation, bethanechol and KCl were significantly greater in animals treated with *Pygeum africanum* than in controls. It was therefore shown that *P. africanum* protected the bladder against the severity of contractile abnormalities caused by partial bladder outlet obstruction, but the absolute cause was not certain. It was felt that it possibly protected the status of the contractile apparatus and the level of muscarinic receptors by being a membrane stabilizer, but further studies would be required to confirm this.

The doses used in these experiments were rather higher than would be used in the therapeutic situation in humans, but this is a study that shows a definite action on the bladder, albeit at the higher dose.

Effects on fibroblasts

It has also been shown that *P. africanum* has an in vitro effect on basal growth of fibroblasts.[13] This is a slight inhibitory effect, but *P africanum* has a much greater inhibitory effect on cell proliferation inducted by bFGF, and also a lesser inhibitory effect on cell proliferation induced by EGF. In obstruction models, there has been shown to be an increase in bFGF and a decrease in transforming growth factor-beta (TGFβ).

Histological effects

In a histological study into the effect of *Sabel serrulata* (= *Serenoa repens*) it has been shown that in patients receiving a placebo preparation there was oedema and mucoid degeneration of the periglandular stroma as stromal nodules. The authors also described the presence of intraglandular congestion and congestive periglandular prostatitis. There was a marked reduction in all of these findings in patients treated with *Sabal serrulata*.[14]

Effects of pollen extract

There have been extensive studies into the mode of action of pollen extract.[15] A standardized extract of rye pollen was tested in vitro and its effect on the synthesis of prostaglandin and leukotrienes was evaluated. Prostaglandins and leukotrienes are derived from arachidonic acid; this was labelled and its conversion to these compounds was assessed in the microsomes of the seminal vesicles of the ram. Pollen extracts have two fractions — water soluble and fat soluble. The water-soluble fraction had no effect, but the fat-soluble extract showed an anticongestive and anti-inflammatory effect. These results were somewhat equivocal, but pointed in the direction of an inhibition of prostaglandin and leukotriene synthesis.

Further studies have been performed in order to test with pollen extract the in vitro influence of phytotheraphy on 5 alpha-reductase and on 3-alpha- and 3-beta-hydroxysteroid oxidoreductase. These complicated and extensive studies failed to show conclusively that pollen extract inhibited these enzymes.[16]

Experiments have also been performed into the effect of pollen extract on the regulation of prostate cell growth. These demonstrated that pollen extract exerted a powerful mitogenic inhibition of the proliferation of fibroblasts and epithelial cells. An effect on EGF concentration was proposed as the likely cause of this, but the authors did not demonstrate a difference between control and experimental groups.[17]

Clinical evaluation

As has been stated above, the main problem associated with BPH as far as the patient is concerned is its symptomatology rather than its complications, which occur relatively infrequently. The aim of phytotherapeutic agents in this condition is mainly to relieve symptoms, and the fact that there is a low incidence of side effects is also important. It is mainly in this area that marketing advances have been made. The beneficial effects of these agents in the management of BPH have been evaluated in numerous studies and these have shown a symptomatic improvement of between 60 and 80%. In most cases, this observation has been made on a global scale rather than on a recognized symptom index. Clearly, this has meant that scientific evaluation of the results of the studies falls somewhat short of what would be considered ideal.

Objective evidence of efficacy is also required for these studies in order to outrule an essentially placebo effect. The fluctuation of symptoms has been alluded to above,[18,19] although most studies would suggest a gradual progression of symptoms over a long-term follow-up. This makes it a requirement that at the very least, a peak urinary flow rate should be measured. In addition, many of the previously performed studies are open-label, non-randomized, non-placebo-controlled, and do not attempt an objective evaluation of results.

Trials should be of adequate duration, with carefully stated inclusion and exclusion criteria. There has, however, been a gradual change in emphasis in trials using phytotherapeutic agents, leading to a greater scientific value of their results.

Pollen extract (Cernilton®) was given in one study to 26 patients who were compared with 24 patients who received placebo in a 6-month study. The Boyarsky symptom score was used, but each symptom was assessed individually. All symptoms were affected by both treatment and placebo, with statistical significance being apparent in only the feeling of incomplete bladder emptying. The peak flow rate changed from 11.8 to 12.1 ml/s in placebo patients and from 10.3 to 10.5 ml/s in treated patients, but these differences did not differ significantly.[20]

In a further study using Serenoa repens (Permixon®), 33 patients were randomized to the treatment group, and 37 to the placebo group. Subjective and objective observations were made at 2, 4, 8 and 12 weeks, looking at symptoms, flow rate and residual urine; no definite symptom score was used. A questionnaire was sent to patients at 6 months, and symptoms were found to have improved globally. The flow rate (not stated to have been either peak or mean) increased from 6.5 to 8.5 ml/s in both placebo and treatment groups.[21] This slightly uncritical study was hampered by the fact that many of the recently standardized criteria for assessment of results were not then available.

Sabal serrulata (Serenoa repens) has been evaluated in two large open-label studies. In the first of these,[22] 305 patients were evaluated at 3 months, when it was found that the International Prostate Symptom Score (I-PSS) had decreased from 19.0 to 12.4, and the peak urinary flow rate had improved from 9.8 to 12.2 ml/s. There was a considerable standard deviation to the mean values, and no change in prostate volume or PSA was seen. In the second study using the same agent,[23] 435 patients were evaluable. There was a fairly high drop-out rate (22.6%), mainly due to lack of efficacy, the requirement on the part of the patient to have a prostatectomy or the fact that the patient was lost to follow-up. In the remaining patients, a mean improvement in peak flow rate of 6.1 ml/s was noted.

Two further trials were performed in order to evaluate S. repens. In the first of these,[24] a major double-blind, placebo-controlled randomized trial, a total of 238 patients were evaluable. The results at 3 months were presented, which is rather a fairly short time in which to assess the effects of a particular treatment. Symptomatic improvement was significantly greater in the treated group and peak flow increased from 11.0 to 12.2 ml/s in the placebo group compared with an increase from 10.4 to 13.2 ml/s in the treated group. These were very satisfactory results, but a much longer follow-up period would have been helpful.

In a further placebo-controlled study of S. repens, interesting results were also obtained.[25] This study had a 30-day single-blind placebo run-in period, and only the 'non-responders' continued in the study. There were 176 non-responders with, by the authors' definition of non-response, a less than 30% improvement in peak urinary flow rate. These were then randomized to double-blind oral treatment, with S. repens (Permixon®) and followed up for 30 days. It is disappointing that the endpoint of a well-constructed trial was so short, and also that, of the 271 patients entered into it, only 176 preceded to the second phase; it is understandable that the majority of patients would not respond to placebo, but regrettable that as many as 39 patients dropped out of the trial. The results were very impressive, with the peak urinary flow rate increasing from 11.7 to 15.3 ml/s in the treated group, as opposed to from 12.4 to 13.5 ml/s in the controls.

A further interesting study has evaluated the effect of beta-sitosterol in patients with symptomatic BPH. Historically, this compound was not found to be particularly helpful in this condition; a study in 1986 evaluated its effect on patients, and used internationally recognized objective methods of evaluating patient response at the end of a 6-month period.[26] This was a double-blind placebo-based trial, which showed no difference between control and treatment groups relating to peak flow rates, residual urine volumes and pressure–flow studies.[26]

Interest in this compound has been rekindled by a more recent study performed in 1995 in Germany. A randomized, double-blind, placebo-controlled multicentre study was performed on 200 patients with symptomatic BPH. The primary endpoint of the study was the difference in modified Boyarsky symptom score between the groups at 6 months. There were secondary endpoints

also — I-PSS, peak urinary flow rate and prostatic volume.[27]

The modified Boyarsky score decreased from 14.9 to 12.2 in the placebo group and from 15.0 to 7.7 in the treatment group at 6 months. The I-PSS decreased from 15.1 to 12.8 in the placebo group and from 14.9 to 7.5 in the treatment group. The changes in the peak urinary flow rate were even more impressive — from 10.2 to 11.4 ml/s in the placebo group and from 9.9 to 15.2 ml/s in the treatment group. These excellent results, which it is hoped will be reproduced in other countries, are very encouraging and of considerable interest.

Other studies are currently being completed or prepared, with considerable care as to the trial designs: these are comparing Pygeum africanum with placebo, mepartricin with placebo and Serenoa repens with finasteride.

Amino acid complexes and organ extracts

Amino acid complexes such as Balometan® and Paraprostin® have been used widely, especially in the Far East, but have not been subjected to careful scientific evaluation. The impression is, therefore, that the use of most amino acid complexes is empirical, with no obvious rationale, and there is no evidence that they have any action other than a placebo effect. It is to be hoped that trials will be performed and that attempts will be made to find out how these agents work.

Organ extracts, such as extract of prostate, have also been used widely — once again, particularly in the Far East — but the reason why they should be used has not been clearly defined. It has been suggested that they may have a general effect on the lower urinary tract, which is proposed to include an improvement in detrusor contractility and a decreased sphincter tone. Unfortunately, the potential side effects from the use of these compounds in humans may prevent urologists from considering their use.

Conclusions

The continued enthusiastic use by many urologists of phytotherapeutic agents has shown that many consider that there is a place for their use in symptomatic BPH.

Equally, there is a continued wish on the part of urologists that studies be performed that will demonstrate a clearly defined mode of action and a rationale for their use. It is clear that some compounds have a 'clinical utility' that precludes, in the minds of many, the need for scientific evidence of their efficacy. The trend, however, is against this, and there is a gratifying increase in the number of scientific trials and scientific attempts at assessing the mode of action of the various compounds. None of them has been shown to decrease outflow obstruction on pressure–flow studies, nor has any brought about a significant decrease in prostatic size or PSA level. On the other side of the argument, there is evidence of an effect on symptom score and peak urinary flow rate. More studies will be required to confirm these findings, and to convince others of the efficacy of phytotherapeutic agents.

References

1. Schulze H, Berges R, Paschold K et al. Neue Konservative Therapieausaetze bei der benignen Prostatahyperplasie. Urologe [A] 1982; 31: 8–13

2. Fitzpatrick J M, Dreikorn K, Khoury S et al. The medical management of BPH with agents other than hormones or alpha-blockers. In: Cockett A T K, Khoury Y, Aso Y et al. (eds) Proceedings of the 2nd International Consultation on Benign Prostatic Hyperplasia (BPH), Jersey, Channel Islands. Scientific Communication International, 1993: 443–450

3. Fitzpatrick J M, Lynch T H. Phytotherapeutic agents in the management of symptomatic benign prostatic hyperplasia. Urol Clin North Am 1996; 22: 407–412

4. Dreikorn K, Richter R, Schoenhoefer P S. Konservative, Nicht-Hormonell Behaundlung der Benignen Prostatahyperplasie. Urologe [A] 1990; 29: 8–16

5. Dreikorn K, Schoenhoefer P S. Stellenwert von Phytotherapeutika bei der Behandlung der benignen Prostatahyperplasie (BPH). Urologe [A] 1995; 34: 119–129

6. Dreikorn K, Richter R. Nonhormonal treatment of benign prostatic hyperplasia. In: Ackermann R, Schroder F H (eds) Prostatic hyperplasia: etiology, surgical, and conservative management. Berlin: Walter de Gruyter, 1989: 109–121

7. Sultan C, Terraza C, Devillier C et al. Inhibition of androgen metabolism and binding by a liposterolic extract of Serenoa repens B in human foreskin fibroblasts. J Steroid Biochem 1984; 20: 515–520

8. Di Silverio F, D'Eramo G, Lubrano C et al. Evidence that Serenoa repens extract displays an antioestrogenic activity in prostatic tissue of benign prostatic hypertrophy patients. Eur Urol 1992; 21: 309–314

9. Petrangeli E, Di Silverio F. Antiandrogenic activity of Serenoa repens in LNCaP lines (unpublished data).

10. Rhodes L, Primica R, Berman C et al. Comparison of finasteride (Proscar®), a 5-alpha reductase inhibitor, and various commercial plant extracts in in-vitro and in-vivo 5-alpha reductase inhibition. Prostate 1993; 22: 43–51

11. Malkowicz S B, Wein A J, Whitmore K et al. Acute biochemical and functional alterations in the partially obstructed rabbit urinary bladder. J Urol 1986; 136: 1324–1329

12. Levin R M, Riffaud J-P, Habib M et al. Effect of Tadenan® oral therapy on rabbit bladder hypertrophy following partial outlet obstruction (unpublished data).

13. Paubert-Braquet M, Monboisse J C, Servent-Saez N et al. Inhibition of bFGF and EGF-induced proliferation of 3T3 fibroblasts by extract of Pygeum africanum (Tadenan®). Biomed Pharmacother 1994; 48(suppl 1): 435–475

14. Helpap B, Oehler U, Weisser H et al. Morphology of benign prostatic hyperplasia after treatment with Sabal Extract IDS 89 or placebo. J Urol Pathol 1995; in press

15. Loschen G, Ebeling L. Inhibition of the arachidonic acid metabolism by an extract from rye pollen. In: Vahlensieck W, Rutischauser G (eds) Benign prostatic diseases. Stuttgart: Georg Thieme Verlag, 1992: 65–72

16. Tunn S, Krieg M. Alterations in the intraprostatic hormonal metabolism by the pollen extract Cernilton®. In: Vahlensieck W, Rutishauser G (eds) Benign prostatic diseases. Stuttgart: Georg Thieme Verlag, 1992: 109–114

17. Habib F K, Ross M, Buck A C et al. In vitro evaluation of the pollen extract Cernilton® T-60 in the regulation of prostate cell growth. Br J Urol 1990; 66: 393–397

18. Ball A J, Feneley R C, Abrams P H. The natural history of untreated prostatism. Br J Urol 1982; 54: 527–530

19. Jacobsen S J, Girman C J, Guess H A et al. Natural history of prostatism; four-year change in urinary symptom frequency and bother. J Urol 1995; 153: 300A

20. Buck A C, Cox R, Rees R W M et al. Treatment of outflow tract obstruction due to benign prostatic hyperplasia with the pollen extract Cernilton®. Br J Urol 1990; 66: 398–404

21. Reece Smith H, Memon A, Smart C J et al. The value of Permixon® in benign prostatic hypertrophy. Br J Urol 1986; 58: 3–40

22. Braeckman J. The extract of Serenoa repens in the treatment of benign prostatic hyperplasia: a multicenter open study. Curr Ther Res 1994; 55: 776–785

23. Bach D, Ebeling L. Long-term drug treatment of benign prostatic hyperplasia — results of a prospective 3-year study using Sabal Extract IDS 89. Urologe [B] 1995; in press

24. Braeckman J, Denis L, De Leval J et al. A double-blind, placebo-controlled study of the plant extract Serenoa repens in the treatment of benign hyperplasia of the prostate (unpublished data).

25. Descotes J L, Rambeaud J J, Deschaseaux P, Faure G. Placebo-controlled evaluation of the efficacy and tolerability of Permixon® in benign prostatic hyperplasia after exclusion of placebo responders. Clin Drug Invest 1995; 9: 291–297

26. Kadow C, Abrams P H. A double-blind trial of the known effect of beta-sitosteryl glucoside (WA 184) in the treatment of benign prostatic hyperplasia. Eur Urol 1986; 12: 187–189

27. Berges R R, Windeler J, Trampisch H J, Senge I. Randomised, placebo-controlled, double-blind clinical trial of beta-sitosterol in patients with benign prostatic hyperplasia. Lancet 1995; 345: 1529–1532

Surgical/Interventional Options

V

Historical background

Surgical treatment for benign prostatic hyperplasia (BPH) was introduced over a century ago with the first description of a planned open enucleation of the prostate by Bellfield and McGill of Leeds, UK,[1] and later by Fuller at the New York Hospital.[2] Since the report by Freyer in 1900,[3] his name has been attached — perhaps incorrectly — to this particular approach, while the retropubic approach was first described and popularized by Millin in 1945.[4,5]

Credit for the first transurethral operation to relieve bladder outlet obstruction is given to Ambroise Paré (16th century), who used a curette and a sharpened hollow sound to shear off urethral strictures. The method was improved by other French surgeons, namely Mercier, Civiale and D'Etoilles, in 1830. According to Nesbit,[6] three concepts contributed to the development of modern transurethral resection. These were, first, the development of the incandescent lamp by Edison (1879); second, the development of high-frequency electrical current that could cut through tissue, discovered by Hertz (1888) and DeForest (1908); and third, the development of a fenestrated tube by Hugh Hampton Young in 1909, allowing the engagement and shearing off of tissue in the fenestrations. After Stern, in 1926, had introduced a tungsten wire loop that could be used to resect tissue, McCarthy brought all these concepts together by introducing the direct-vision resectoscope, with a foroblique lens built by Reinholdt Wappler and a wire loop for resection and cauterization of prostate tissue. Further improvements were the development of the fibreoptic lighting system together with the Hopkins wide-angle lens, in the 1970s, and the constant-flow low-pressure resectoscope, described by Iglesias in 1975.[7] The current use of video equipment allows the surgeon to work by looking at a television monitor instead of having to look through the lens, a further improvement in surgical technique.

An even less invasive surgical treatment for BPH, that is not associated with any actual removal of tissue — namely, transurethral incision of the prostate (TUIP) — is by no means a new procedure. Edwards et al.[8] give credit to Bottini (1897), and Hedlund and Ek[9] credit Guthrie (1834). The first modern description comes from Keitzer et al.,[10] who used the method for the treatment of bladder neck contracture. The first significant series of patients was published in 1973 by Orandi,[11] who popularized the method in the USA. To date, however, the technique has not found as widespread an acceptance as it deserves, when comparing the results obtained with those of other interventions.

Indication and patient selection

Actual incidence rates for TUIP are not available, but it probably can safely be assumed that the number of TUIPs done in the USA and in other developed countries is only a fraction of the number of transurethral resection of the prostate (TURP) operations done. Whereas in 1962 TURPs constituted over 50% of all major surgical interventions performed by American urologists, this number had dropped to 38% by 1986.[12] Although the number of TURPs performed on Medicare patients declined from an all-time peak of 258 000 in 1987 to 168 000 in 1993 — a 34% reduction — it remains second only to cataract surgery on the list of Medicare's most costly surgical procedures.

Both the number of prostatectomies performed, as well as the relative number of patients treated by TURP versus open surgery (OPSU), vary greatly from country to country (Table 31.1), probably reflecting surgeons' preferences rather than actual differences in disease prevalence and case mix.

According to the recently released Agency for Health Care Policy and Research (AHCPR) Guidelines for the diagnosis and treatment of BPH,[13] as well as the 2nd International Consultation on BPH,[14] there are a few indications for the treatment of men with BPH that make a surgical approach, rather than any of the other available treatment options, mandatory. These are:

Table 31.1. *Incidence (number/year) of prostatectomies per 1000 men aged 55 years or older and choice of surgical treatment in various countries*

Country	Prostatectomies (no./year)		Procedure chosen (as percentage of total)	
	1988	1990	TURP	OPSU
United States	15	13	97	3
France	14	13	69	31
Belgium	12	14	83	17
Sweden*	11	11	99	1
Denmark[†]	10	12	97	3
Japan	7	9	70	30
United Kingdom[‡]	–	7	92	8

*1988 data. [†]Approx. 66% of prostatectomies by general surgeons. [‡]Approx. 33% of prostatectomies by general surgeons; data for England only.
(From ref. 162 with permission.)

1. Refractory urinary retention (after at least one attempt to remove the catheter).
2. Recurrent urinary tract infections due to BPH.
3. Recurrent gross haematuria due to BPH.
4. Renal insufficiency due to BPH.
5. Bladder stones due to BPH.
6. Large bladder diverticula due to BPH.

However, at least in the USA, the vast majority of patients (at least until recently) have undergone surgical treatment either exclusively for symptom relief or for symptoms of prostatism in combination with other indications (Table 31.2).[15]

The differential indications for the various surgical treatment alternatives are also, with few exceptions, not clearly defined. The 2nd International Consultation on BPH[16] considered those patients with symptoms and/or signs secondary to prostate obstruction with acceptable surgical and anaesthetic risk factors to be candidates for TUIP, TURP or OPSU. TUIP, however, was recommended only if the weight of the prostate was estimated to be less than 30 g and if no median lobe was present. This recommendation is based on the fact that most studies reporting outcomes following TUIP excluded, a priori, patients with either a large median lobe or an estimated prostate weight of more than 30 g. Thus, although this recommendation intuitively seems reasonable, it is not based on a controlled clinical trial. Of 3885 TURPs retrospectively reviewed by Mebust et al.,[15] 35% produced 10 g tissue or less, 65% produced

20 g tissue or less, and 80% produced 30 g tissue or less (mean weight 22 g). Thus, even when listed criteria are applied, the majority of patients currently undergoing TURP could also be treated by TUIP. TURP was recommended if the resectionist believed that the procedure could be completed in less than 60 min. Beyond these recommendations, patients with large bladder stones not amenable to electrohydraulic

Table 31.2. *Indications for prostatectomy alone and in combination, in 3885 patients*

Indications for surgery	Patients	
	No.	%
Symptoms of prostatism	3522	90.7
Significant residual urine	1336	34.4
Urinary retention, acute	1053	27.1
Recurrent urinary tract infection	479	12.3
Haematuria	465	12.0
Altered urodynamic function	385	9.9
Renal insufficiency	176	4.5
Bladder stones	116	3.0
Symptoms of prostatism only	1145	29.5
Prostatism and residual urine	577	14.9
Prostatism and acute retention	372	9.6
Prostatism and acute retention and residual urine	217	5.6

(From ref. 15 with permission.)

lithotripsy (EHL) and the need for surgical removal of large bladder diverticula are probably best served by open enucleation using the suprapubic transvesical route.

Anaesthetic considerations

Open surgical enucleation of the prostate either by the supra- or retropubic routes is most commonly performed under general anaesthesia. Spinal or epidural anaesthesia was used in 79% of all TURP procedures in a national survey published in 1989,[12] and in 78% in a cooperative study of 13 institutions in 3885 patients.[15] McGowan and Smith,[17] as well as Nielson et al.,[18] found no significant differences between regional and general anaesthesia in terms of blood loss, complications and perioperative mortality. TURP under local anaesthesia had been reported as early as 1977.[19] More recently, Sinha et al.[20] and Birch et al.[21] presented a series of 100 men each, who underwent TURP under local anaesthesia supplemented with intravenous sedation. The latter group found that those with prostates estimated to be of less than 40 g resectable weight were suitable candidates. The average weight of tissue resected in this series, however, was only 11 g, compared with the average weight of 22 g reported by Mebust et al.[15]

Four studies describing TUIP performed under local anaesthesia have been published, of which three are non-randomized studies carried out entirely on high-risk patients.[22–24] Recently, Hugosson et al.[25] reported the results of 30 TUIPs performed under local anaesthesia as an outpatient procedure. None of the prostates was estimated to exceed 30 g resectable weight. Anaesthesia was achieved by instillation of lidocaine gel into the urethra and injection of local anaesthetic into the area of the bladder neck. All but one of the 30 patients tolerated the procedure well, without discomfort.

Apart from medical considerations (see Delayed Mortality, p. 367), the current climate of health-care economics will certainly encourage physicians to seek alternative ways of reducing costs of surgical procedures. The use of local as opposed to general anaesthesia, and the continuing attempts to shorten hospitalization time by the use of local anaesthesia and other measures, can be expected to continue in the foreseeable future.

Surgical technique

Transurethral incision of the prostate (Fig. 31.1)

A transurethral incision of the prostate and the bladder neck is fundamentally a fairly simple procedure. A wide range of knives have been developed and, recently, free beam and contact lasers have also been utilized. The incision(s) is (are) made from inside the bladder neck down to the verumontanum and should be deep enough to penetrate the prostate tissue down to and through the prostate capsule. In fact, the presence of fat tissue at the bottom of the incision indicates that the incision is of the correct depth. Following such an appropriately placed incision, the bladder neck usually springs apart. Despite the aggressiveness of the incision, complications such as injuries to adjacent organs (rectal injury) are very rarely encountered.

Several variations of the TUIP procedure have been introduced. Traditionally, a single incision at the 6 o'clock position is performed; alternatively, bilateral incisions are performed at the 5 and 7 o'clock positions. However, authors have reported on single or multiple incisions at a variety of locations all around the circumference of the bladder neck.[26]

Transurethral resection of the prostate (Fig. 31.2)

The TURP procedure has been described in detail by Nesbit,[6,27] Mebust[28] and others. After calibration of the urethra to a size accommodating easily the outer diameter of the resectoscope sheath, if necessary aided by a meatotomy, the bladder, bladder neck and prostatic urethra, as well as the external sphincter, are inspected. It is imperative that the resectionist maintains throughout the entire procedure a three-dimensional image of the anatomical relationships between the trigone, the ureteral orifices, the bladder neck, the lateral and median lobe of the prostate (if present), the verumontanum and, in particular, the external sphincter muscle.

Various techniques have been suggested for systematic removal of the adenomatous tissue. They all are based on the principle that the resection should be done step by step. Most techniques described suggest resection of the ventral tissue between 3 and 9 o'clock first, so that the anterior tissue will drop down, allowing the surgeon to resect from the top downwards rather

(a)   (b)

(c)

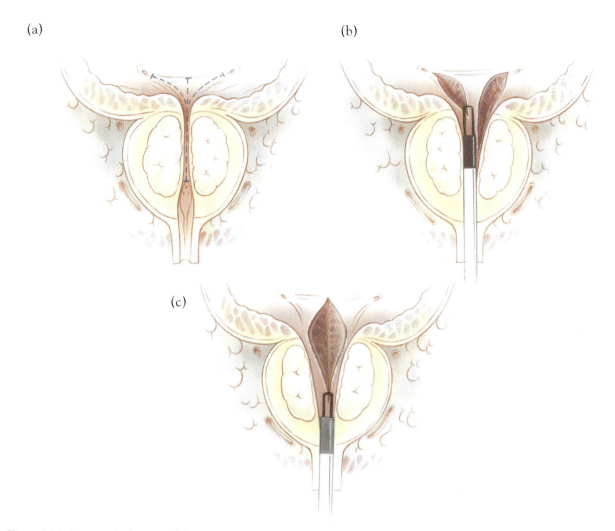

Figure 31.1. *Transurethral incision of the prostate.*

than from the floor upwards. As bleeding is the resectionist's nemesis, leading to loss of visual field and disorientation, it is imperative that resection and haemostasis should both be completed in one area of the fossa before the next area is tackled. The classic description of the transurethral resection has been given by Nesbit.[6,27,29] The Nesbit surgical technique has three stages. First (Fig. 31.2a), the fibres at the bladder neck and those of the immediately adjacent prostatic adenoma are resected with short, full-thickness bites circumferentially around the bladder neck. This process may be started at the 12 o'clock position and then carried out on either side until, finally, the bladder neck tissue between 5 and 7 o'clock is resected in this manner. Thereafter, the adenoma is resected in

quadrants (Fig. 31.2b). The resectoscope is placed in front of the verumontanum and the resection started at the 12 o'clock position, so that the lateral lobe tissue can fall into the middle of the prostatic fossa. The upper or ventral quadrants on both the right and left side are resected first down to the fibres of the surgical capsule. The fibres of the surgical capsule can be identified by a number of hallmarks: for example, the yellowish, nodular tissue of adenoma changes to the white glistening surface of the compressed peripheral zone of the prostate or surgical capsule. Once the resection has been carried out in the lower quadrants, another important hallmark allows the surgeon to identify when the surgical capsule is reached — namely, the presence of prostatic calculi, which are located between the

(a)

(b)

(c)

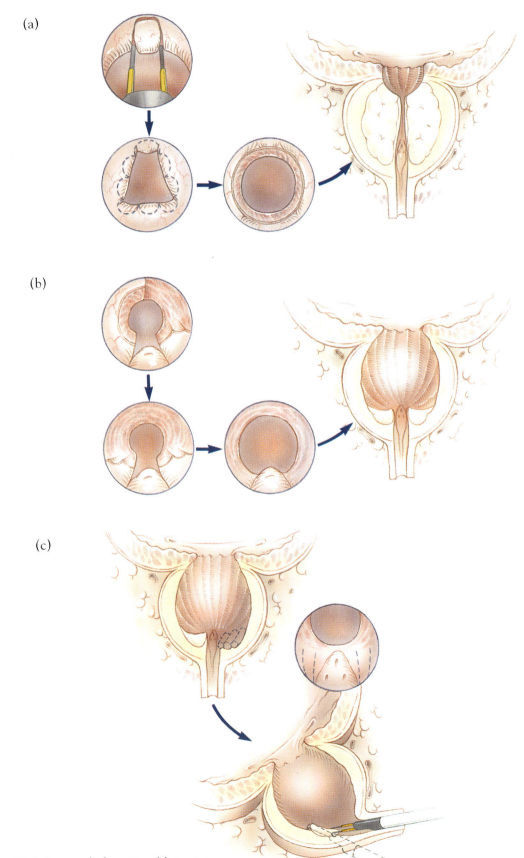

Figure 31.2. *Transurethral resection of the prostate.*

transition zone (i.e. the adenomatous part of the gland) and the compressed peripheral zone. The use of transrectal ultrasonography, now widespread, has shown that, in fact, these calcifications allow a clear separation of the transition zone from the peripheral zone. Once all four quadrants have been resected down to the surgical capsule, at the third stage (Fig. 31.2c) the adenomatous tissue surrounding the verumontanum is resected last. This tissue is located proximal to the external sphincter mechanism and, as the prostatic fossa is a biconcave cavity, a sweeping motion is used, so that the loop is moved from a lateral to a medial direction as it approaches the sphincter. From experience with radical prostatectomy, it is well known to most urologists that the verumontanum is, in fact, located in the middle of the prostate rather than at its extreme distal end. It should, therefore, not be surprising that adenomatous tissue can be safely resected lateral and even distal to the verumontanum without jeopardizing the sphincter mechanism.

Following the completion of the resection, with all adenomatous tissue removed down to the level of the surgical capsule circumferentially, an incision of the bladder neck may be performed, as recommended by Kulb et al.,[30] to prevent the formation of a bladder neck contracture, particularly in those with a small prostate.

A multitude of modifications have been suggested to improve TURP.[31] Among them are the introduction of the constant-flow resectoscope, which allows continuous resection, clearer vision and low-pressure conditions within the prostatic fossa, with decreased fluid absorption and shortened surgical time.[7] Other authors have recommended placement of a suprapubic tube to allow continuous irrigation without the use of the Iglesias instruments.

Following complete resection of the prostate by the preferred technique, great care must be taken to achieve perfect haemostasis within the prostatic fossa and, particularly, around the bladder neck, where small bleeding arterial vessels ('bleeders') are often noted. Whereas it is virtually impossible to control venous sinus bleeding with the resectoscope loop, all arterial bleeders can be easily controlled thus. After evacuation of any remaining prostate chips with the Ellik evacuator, further inspection is necessary, as the vigorous evacuation of chips often causes more bleeding. The

catheter of choice is a 24 Fr, three-way Foley that allows for either intermittent or constant irrigation, usually with normal saline solution. The balloon of the catheter is inflated with a variable amount of fluid. It is not recommended that the balloon should be inflated in the prostatic fossa; rather, the balloon should be inflated with gentle traction at the bladder neck to approximately 30 ml. Some authors recommend that a significant amount of traction should be exerted for up to a full day following the procedure, whereas others argue that this might increase the risk of bladder neck contractures. If meticulous haemostasis in the prostatic fossa is obtained, the remaining bleeding (usually from venous sinuses) will readily stop with the ensuing contraction of the capsule, and will not require continuous traction. The intermittent or continuous irrigation is stopped once the urine is clear. On the first or second postoperative day, the catheter may be removed. Whereas in the past, concomitant vasectomy has been recommended to prevent postoperative epididymitis, it has recently been shown that vasectomy is not effective for this purpose and it is, therefore, no longer recommended.[15]

Suprapubic prostatectomy (Fig. 31.3)

The open suprapubic or transvesical prostatectomy was the first method applied to the removal of the adenomatous gland, and may still be the most frequently performed type of open surgery. Although initially it was done as a blind procedure with a small suprapubic incision, it is now performed under direct vision, allowing control of bleeding and prevention of bladder neck contracture.

The patient is placed supine on the operating table in a slight Trendelenburg position, with the table broken so as to extend the lumbar spine for better access to the pelvis. A Foley catheter is placed in the bladder on the sterile field and the bladder is distended with saline or antibiotic solution and the catheter clamped. Either a vertical midline incision or a Pfannenstiel incision may be used to enter the extraperitoneal perivesical space. A self-holding retractor facilitates exposure of the bladder, which may be opened in either a vertical or transverse fashion (Fig. 31.3a). Two lateral and one caudally placed midline self-retaining retractor

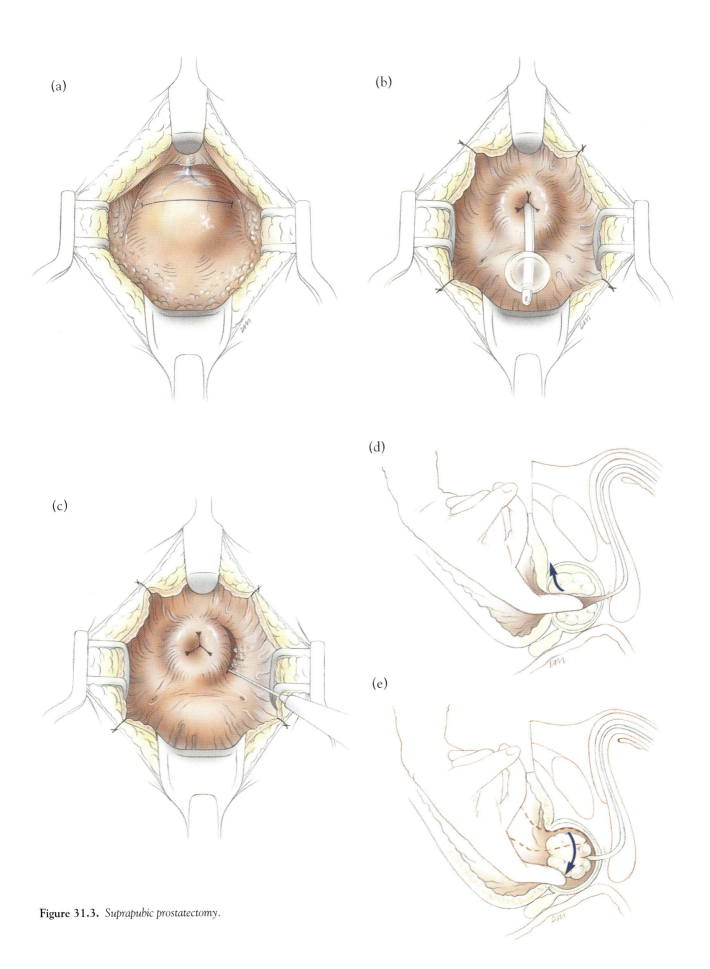

(a)

(b)

(c)

(d)

(e)

Figure 31.3. *Suprapubic prostatectomy.*

(f)

(h)

(g)

(i)

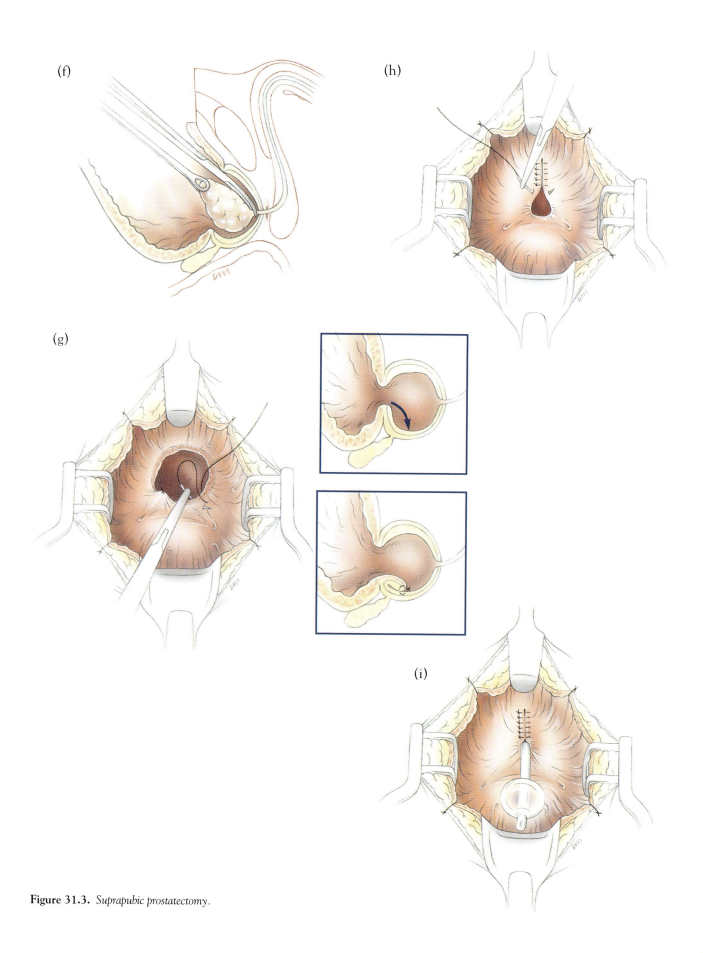

Figure 31.3. *Suprapubic prostatectomy.*

blades are inserted in the bladder to facilitate exposure. At this time, the internal urethral meatus or bladder neck is clearly identified (31.3b). The catheter is now removed and, using electrocautery, the mucosa over the prostate around the bladder neck is incised circumferentially with a radius of about 1 cm from the centre of the urethra (31.3c). Care is taken to avoid cautery too close to the ureteral orifices. This procedure is complicated if there is a large intravesical lobe present. It is convenient to lift such a lobe with an Ellis or Babcock clamp, and to continue the incision of the mucosa under the intravesical lobe. The index finger of the dominant hand is then inserted into the internal urethral meatus of the bladder neck, and with a forceful motion upwards, the anterior commissure is split down to the capsule in the mid-prostate (31.3d). This fissure is then continued cranially until it extends into the bladder and connects there with the incision of the mucosa carried out previously. At this time, the self-holding retractor should be removed to facilitate the enucleation under digital control. By using the index finger of the dominant hand, the plane between the adenoma (i.e. transition zone) and the surgical capsule (i.e. compressed peripheral zone) must be clearly identified. It is imperative to perform the enucleation at this level, as otherwise either adenomatous tissue is left behind or, by perforating through the surgical capsule or the peripheral zone, it is possible to remove the posterior structures, including the seminal vesicles, together with the adenoma. The feeling should be that of having the smooth surgical capsule always lateral or outward and peeling the meat, i.e. the adenomatous tissue, of the surgical capsule as the finger glides around the 12 o'clock position on the right and left side towards the 6 o'clock position (31.3e). The urethra can be divided at the apex by pinching it between two fingers. If this is not possible, a sharp transection of the urethra is better than a forceful ripping of the urethra: this can be accomplished with sharply bent Torek scissors (31.3f). At this time, the adenomatous tissue can be lifted out of the prostatic fossa and held up with a Babcock clamp or ring forceps (31.3f). Often, at this stage, the adenomatous tissue is still connected at the bladder neck and blunt or sharp dissection is needed to complete the enucleation of the gland. A large intravesical lobe often requires sharp dissection at the level of the bladder neck;

great care is necessary in order that neither the ureteral orifices nor the ureters are injured.

Following the removal of the adenomatous tissue, the fossa is carefully palpated to ensure that all adenomatous tissue has been removed. Once this has been accomplished, two figure-of-eight sutures are placed at the 5 and 7 o'clock positions, the ureteral orifices being carefully avoided in order to control the bleeding that is usually heaviest at these positions. It is often advantageous to suture the mucosa just cranial from the bladder neck into the prostatic fossa, in order to establish a straight plane through which the catheter is inserted into the bladder. This can be done by using 2/0 chromic sutures and sewing the mucosa into the floor of the prostatic fossa, thus avoiding the 'step up' effect (31.3g). All bleeders within the prostatic fossa can usually be coagulated with electrocautery, but occasionally individual suture ligatures are needed. The anterior portion of the bladder neck can be sutured down with 2/0 chromic interrupted stitches to narrow and reconstruct the bladder neck (31.3h). At this time, a 26 or 28 Fr suprapubic tube is pulled through a separate stab wound into the bladder and secured with a pearl string suture. Following this, the bladder is closed in two layers in the standard fashion and both catheters are irrigated to assure patency. A single Jackson–Pratt drain is placed in the retropubic space and brought out through a separate stab wound. Wound closure is completed in the usual fashion. The Foley catheter may be removed as soon as the urine begins to clear, while the suprapubic tube should be clamped after approximately 5–7 days. Once the patient is able to void, the suprapubic tube may be removed.

Retropubic prostatectomy (Fig. 31.4)

The principle of retropubic prostatectomy is that the adenomatous tissue is removed through an incision in the surgical capsule of the prostate, rather than through an opening in the bladder. Therefore, no incision is made in the bladder, thus obviating the need for suprapubic catheter drainage in most cases. The incision in the capsule allows for improved exposure and inspection of the prostatic fossa to control bleeding. This is offset by an increased risk of intraoperative problems due to injury and bleeding from the dorsal vein complex of Santorini.

(a)

(b)

(c)

(d)

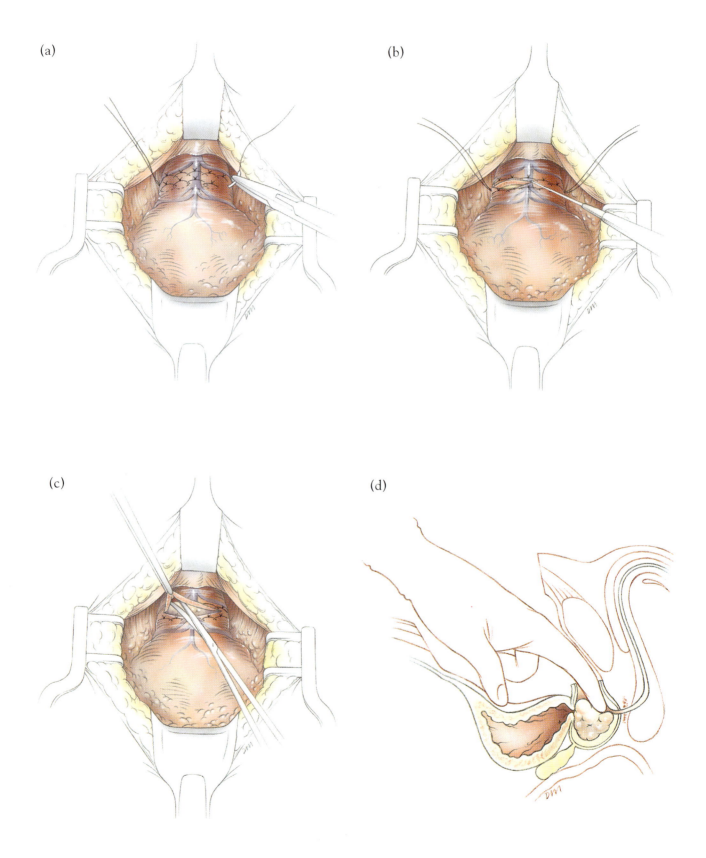

Figure 31.4. *Retropubic prostatectomy.*

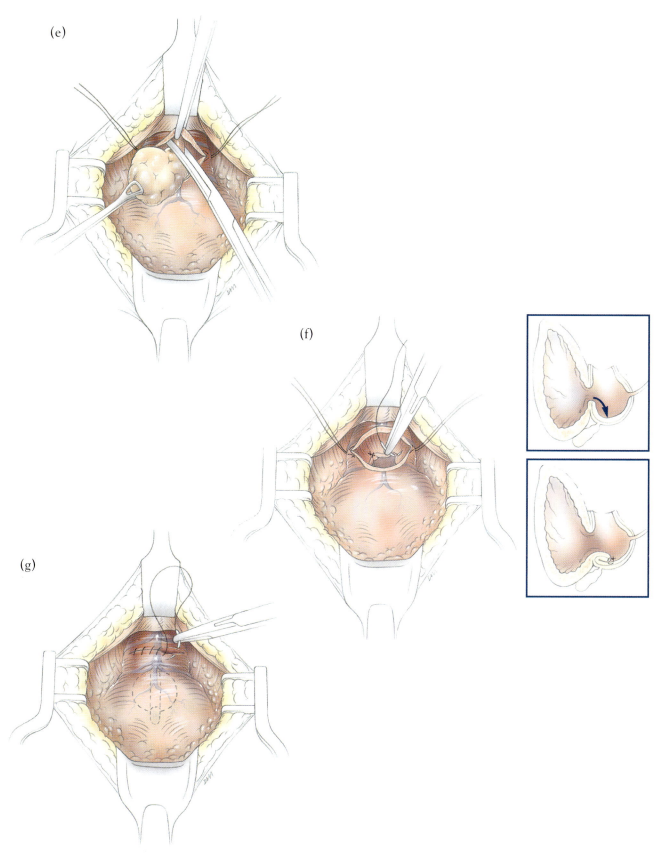

Figure 31.4. *Retropubic prostatectomy.*

Both a vertical midline incision and a Pfannenstiel incision are acceptable. A self-retaining retractor (Balfour or Bookwalter with bodywall blades) is useful to allow exposure of the anterior surface of the prostate. Ventral veins of the dorsal vein complex are divided between suture ligatures. The fatty tissue overlying the anterior prostate and the puboprostatic ligaments can be bluntly pushed down and laterally using either a sponge stick or a scraping action with a moist sponge. To reduce bleeding, it is advantageous to place two rows of sutures (2/0 chromic) approximately 5 mm apart in a transverse orientation (31.4a). These rows of sutures should be overlapping, to encompass all veins running on top of the prostate in a craniocaudal orientation. The lateral sutures can be used for traction purposes. Thereafter, the capsule is incised in a transverse orientation with electrocautery (31.4b). It is of the greatest importance to carry the incision deep enough to extend through the surgical capsule into the adenoma. It is imperative that, at this point, the plane between the surgical capsule (i.e. peripheral zone) and the adenomatous tissue (i.e. transition zone) is identified correctly to facilitate enucleation of the adenoma. If needed, curved scissors are used to develop the plane between the capsule and the adenomatous tissue (31.4c). However, in general the index finger of the dominant hand is used to enucleate the adenoma and shell it out of the capsule (31.4d). As is the case in a suprapubic prostatectomy, sharply bent Torek scissors can be useful to transect the urethra (31.4e). Furthermore, once the distal aspect of the adenoma is developed, it is possible to lift the adenoma out of the wound with the help of ringed forceps or Babcock clamps, facilitating either blunt or sharp dissection and transection of the adenoma at the bladder neck.

Two figure-of-eight 2/0 chromic sutures are placed at the 5 o'clock position through the bladder neck to control bleeding. Care should be taken to avoid getting too close to the ureteral orifices or the ureters. The mucosa cranial to the bladder neck can be sutured to the floor of the prostatic capsule with advantage, thus avoiding the 'step up' effect (31.4f). This leads effectively to the re-trigonization of the raw area of the bladder neck, making the passage of the catheter and the postoperative course more comfortable, while at the same time being helpful in controlling bleeding. All

remaining bleeders in the prostatic fossa can be controlled either by electrocautery or by figure-of-eight suture ligatures. At this time, a 22 or 24 Fr Foley catheter is inserted through the urethra into the bladder and the balloon is inflated. The transverse incision of the capsule is then closed with appropriate suture material (chromic or vicryl); this may be done in one or two layers (31.4g). Care should be taken not to puncture the balloon at this stage, which may be left only partially inflated during this part of the operation. If excessive bleeding is noted, it may be advantageous to place a suprapubic tube through a separate stab wound. Lastly, a Jackson–Pratt drain is placed in the retropubic space and brought out through a separate stab wound. Usually, it is not necessary to perform either intermittent or continuous bladder irrigation.

The Foley catheter may be removed between postoperative days 3 and 5, when the urine has become clear.

Treatment outcomes

When evaluating surgical treatment modalities for BPH, it is important to assess the impact each treatment has on both the indirect (peak urinary flow rate and residual urine) and direct outcomes, the latter being those outcomes that are of greater relevance to the patient as they more or less directly affect either the extent or quality of his life.[32] The following discussion of the outcomes is expanded from the analyses carried out for the AHCPR Guidelines.[13] Outcome estimates are derived from a combination of outcomes reported in the peer-reviewed literature following OPSU,[33–61] TURP[8,15,47,53,55,56,58,60–81] and TUIP.[8,9,71–74,76,80,82–87] Additional reports published since these analyses were performed are discussed in the individual sections if they contain data pertinent to the outcomes considered.

Urinary flow rate

Among the parameters obtained from flow rate recordings, the peak urinary flow rate (Q_{max}) is most widely utilized as an outcome parameter of BPH treatment. There are considerable problems associated with the interpretation of the peak urinary flow rate, such as a significant intra-individual variability from recording to recording,[88,89] a dependency of Q_{max} on the voided volume,[13] electronic reading artefacts of most commercial flow rate meters,[90] and, lastly, the fact that peak urinary flow rates do not correlate with the symptoms and bother of lower urinary tract symptoms.[91] Considering the large number of prostatectomies performed, the documentation of flow rate changes following the traditional treatments of OPSU and TURP is disappointingly low. Figure 31.5 depicts the combined analysis of mean pre- and postoperative peak urinary flow rates, as well as the percentage change from baseline for the three surgical treatment modalities.

Recently, Wasson et al.[92] published a 3-year follow-up of a prospective, randomized, trial comparing watchful waiting with TURP in men with moderate symptoms of BPH. In the group of 280 men who underwent TURP, the peak flow rate improved from 11.6±6.4 to 17.8±9.1 ml/s (+54%), of note being the somewhat higher baseline mean peak flow rate resulting from the inclusion criteria of the trial and causing a rather lower percentage improvement than reported in retrospective TURP series. Riehman et al.[93] prospectively randomized 120 patients with prostates of more than 20 g resectable weight to TURP (n=56) and TUIP (n=61). Comparable improvements in peak flow rates were seen for both treatment modalities for up to 72 months of follow-up.

Post-void residual urine

The post-void residual urine volume has severe limitations as an outcome parameter in the evaluation of BPH treatments. It shows significant intra-individual variability,[94,95] and only very limited predictive value with regard to treatment outcomes.[92] Furthermore, the correlation between residual urine volume and symptoms is practically non-existent.[91] Although all treatment modalities are capable of reducing the residual urine volume by more than 50%, comparison of the various therapies is difficult because of the vastly different baseline mean residual urine volume (Fig. 31.6). In the TURP arm of the prospective study by Wasson et al.,[92] mean residual urine volume decreased from 109±74 to 51±54 ml (–55%).

Symptom improvement

When patients are asked which outcome from treatment for BPH is of greatest significance to them, the overwhelming majority will rank symptom relief as the most important factor in choosing a treatment.[13] Symptom relief can be measured by counting the number of patients who have either an improvement, no change, or worsening of their symptoms by global subjective assessment following the treatment, or by assessing the magnitude of the change in symptoms

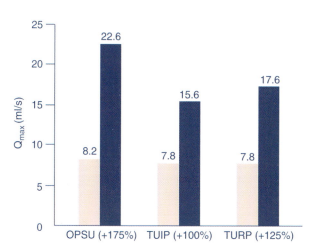

Figure 31.5. *Combined analysis of preoperative ( ) and postoperative (■) peak urinary flow rate (Q_{max}) and percentage change from baseline for open surgery (OPSU), transurethral incision (TUIP) and transurethral resection (TURP) of the prostate.*

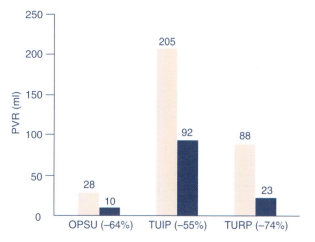

Figure 31.6. *Combined analysis of preoperative ( ) and postoperative (■) post-void residual urine volume (PVR) and percentage change from baseline for open surgery (OPSU), transurethral incision (TUIP) and transurethral resection (TURP) of the prostate.*

using pre- and post-treatment symptom scores (see Chapter 12).

All three surgical interventions give the patient a mean probability of symptomatic improvement of over 80% (Fig. 31.7), with OPSU being slightly superior to the endoscopic interventions. However, as no direct comparisons between OPSU and TUIP/TURP are available, this could reflect a patient selection bias, favouring those patients who are more symptomatic at baseline to be treated by OPSU, who then have a greater probability of perceiving improvement.

When expressing the magnitude of the improvement as the drop in symptom severity score normalized to 100%, the interventions achieve between a 73 and 85% drop from baseline, and all lower the symptom score to about 10% of the total achievable score (this would be about 3.5 points on the seven-item 35-point American Urological Association Symptom Index) (Fig. 31.8). The TURP-treated patients in Wasson's study[92] experienced a drop in symptom score from 14.6±3.0 to 4.9±4.0 points with a drop of –9.6 points, or from 54 to 18% of the 27-point scale (64% drop). In a direct comparison, no differences were noted between pre- and post-treatment mean symptom scores in up to 72 months of follow-up between TURP- and TUIP-treated patients, while in both groups the symptoms scores were significantly better at all follow-up visits.[93]

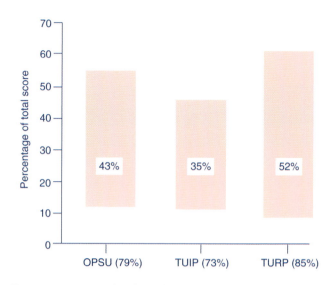

Figure 31.8. *Combined analysis of magnitude of symptom improvement expressed as drop in symptom score following OPSU, TUIP and TURP. The upper extent of each box indicates the mean pretreatment score expressed as a percentage of the total possible score, and the lower extent of the box indicates the mean post-treatment score. The number in each box indicates the difference between the pre- and post-treatment scores, and the numbers in parentheses on the x-axis the percentage drop in symptom score from baseline.*

Perioperative morbidity

The superior symptom improvement effected by surgical treatment of BPH must be balanced with the associated morbidity and mortality. An abundance of data are available regarding perioperative complications, secondary interventions for bleeding problems (such as clot evacuation and re-exploration), the need for blood transfusions, and two specific infectious complications, namely postoperative urinary tract infections and epididymitis.

General perioperative complications are those complications listed by the respective authors and are not grouped by presumed severity. They include wound infection and other wound-related problems, catheter problems, temporary retention, transitory incontinence, pneumonia, urine leakage and fistulae, osteitis pubis, deep venous thrombosis and pulmonary emboli, cardiovascular complications, and other less commonly reported events. Combined analyses are shown in Table 31.3. The mean probability varies from 12% for TUIP to 25% for suprapubic transvesical prostatectomy (OPSS). The mean probability for complications, of 15% following TURP, may be contrasted with the

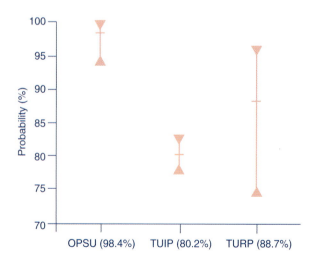

Figure 31.7. *Combined analysis of probability of experiencing symptomatic improvement following OPSU, TUIP and TURP [90% CI (▼ and ▲) and mean probability indicated by the horizontal lines and noted in parentheses on the x-axis].*

Table 31.3. *Combined* analyses for the probability of selected perioperative complications following open enucleation by suprapubic (OPSS) or retropubic (OPSR) prostatectomy, TUIP and TURP. OPSU represents the combined probabilities for OPSS and OPSR*

Modality	n	Bleeding intervention (%)[†]	Surgical complications (%)[‡]	Epididymitis (%)[‡]	Urinary tract infection (%)[‡]	Perioperative mortality (%)[‡]
OPSR	6249	1.7	18.7 (5.7–39.8)	2.5 (0.8–5.5)	2.6 (0.1–12.9)	1.8 (0.7–3.8)
OPSS	3588	1.2	25.2 (9.5–47.5)	3.6 (0.4–12.6)	12.5 (5.0–24.3)	3.8 (3.2–4.4)
OPSU	9538	1.5	21.0 (7.0–42.7)	2.6 (0.4–8.2)	13.4 (2.1–31.6)	2.3 (1.0–4.6)
TUIP	1243	0.5	12.1 (2.2–33.3)	3.0 (0.1–16.3)	12.5 (1.6–38.3)	0.5 (0.2–1.5)
TURP	11693	2.2	15.0 (5.2–30.7)	1.1 (0.1–4.5)	15.5 (3.4–38.3)	1.5 (0.5–3.3)

*The combination was done using the Confidence Profile Method and the software program FAST*PRO (ref. 163). †Weighted average. ‡Mean (and 90% CI).

contemporary series reported by Wasson et al.,[92] who reported that 9% of patients suffered from a perioperative complication in the first 30 days postoperatively. In a contemporary series of 240 suprapubic prostatectomies, Meier et al.[96] reported an overall early complication rate of 19.6%. Postoperative complications following TURP are more common in patients with renal insufficiency (25 vs 17%, respectively) and in patients presenting in retention (24 vs 15.7%, respectively).[15]

The need for blood transfusion is probably vastly overestimated in the older literature. The estimates range from 1.1% (TUIP) to 49% (retropubic prostatectomy; OPSR). The reasons for these high transfusion rates are the fact that many series were reported prior to the concern about hepatitis and AIDS (acquired immune deficiency syndrome) virus transmission by blood products. In a contemporary series of 280 patients undergoing TURP at Veterans Administration (VA) Medical Centers, the transfusion rate was only 3/280 or 1%,[92] a probability more likely to reflect current trends, although patients not specifically selected for a randomized trial comparing watchful waiting with TURP are probably more likely to have co-morbidities leading to a slightly higher need for transfusion. Similarly, the transfusion rate for a contemporary series of 240 open prostatectomies was 4.6%, of which 2.1% were believed to be medically justified.[96]

Secondary interventions for bleeding have a mean probability ranging from 0.5% (TUIP) to 2.2% (TURP) (Table 31.3) in the literature, and it is not likely that these are significant overestimates. In fact, Meier et al.[96] reported a 2.9% rate for reoperation for clot retention following contemporary open prostatectomy.

Two specific infectious postoperative complications are epididymitis and urinary tract infections (Table 31.3). The mean probabilities range from 1.1% (TURP) to 3.6% (OPSS) for the former, and from 2.6% (OPSR) to 15.5% (TURP) for the latter. These data are probably biased — by the time of sampling the urine for a culture and by whether (and for how long) patients received perioperative antibiotics.

Perioperative mortality

According to the US Life Tables, the probability of a 67-year-old man — which is the average age of men undergoing treatment for BPH in the USA — dying within the next year is 3.2%, or 0.8% in the next 3 months. Perioperative mortality, defined as death due to any cause within 90 days (or 3 months) of the surgical procedure, ranges from 0.5% (TUIP) to 3.8% (OPSS) (Table 31.3). There is no correlation between the number of patients in each series and the mortality rates for TURP and OPSU, thus making surgical expertise not a very likely explanatory variable.[13] For open surgical procedures there is no correlation between the mortality rates and the date at which the studies were published. A recent report of a contemporary series of 240 consecutive patients treated by OPSS in Nigeria, however, reported no mortality.[96] For TURP, on the other hand, there is a trend towards reduced mortality in more recent reports (Fig. 31.9). In large retrospective studies, mortality rates have fallen from 2.5%[97] to 1.3%[64] and finally to 0.2%.[15] Roos et al.[78] reported 1989

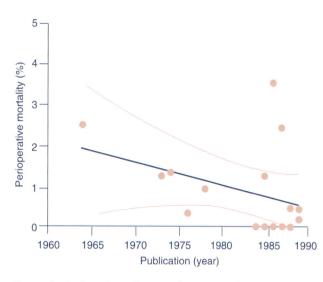

Figure 31.9. *Correlation between the year of publication of results and the incidence of perioperative mortality following TURP, indicating a trend towards lower mortality in more recent reports (r= –0.35).*

perioperative mortality rates following OPSU and TURP in three geographic regions, namely in Denmark, Manitoba (Canada) and the Oxford region in England, based on hospital claims data. Mortality rates in Denmark were 2.66 and 2.47%, in Manitoba 1.58 and 1.73%, and in the Oxford region 3.21 and 4.38% for OPSU and TURP, respectively. The same group of investigators reported earlier an insurance claims data-based analysis in which the adjusted odds ratio for 90 days mortality of open prostatectomy over TURP was 1.27 [95% confidence interval (CI) 0.89–1.80].[98] The difference in perioperative mortality cannot be explained by differences in patients' age or the fraction of patients in urinary retention or with renal failure, although it has been suggested that mortality rates following TURP are higher for azotaemic patients (0.7 versus 4.1%, respectively).[66]

Lu-Yao et al.[99] used claims data to examine 30-day mortality rates among Medicare patients undergoing TURP from 1984 to 1990. Within this time period, mortality rates decreased in all age groups, and overall from 1.2 to 0.77% (linear trend, $p=0.0001$). The average 30-day mortality following TURP was 0.39% for men 65–69 years old, 0.67% for those 70–74 years old, 1.10% for those 75–79 years old, 1.92% for those 80–84 years old, and 3.54% for those over 85 years of age.

Incontinence

Urinary incontinence is defined as the involuntary loss of urine. With regard to surgical treatment for BPH, two types of incontinence are of relevance — namely total urinary incontinence, which indicates the inability of a person to control his urination at all under any conditions, and stress urinary incontinence, which refers to the loss of urine under stress conditions, such as coughing, sneezing, lifting or changing position. Urge incontinence refers to the involuntary loss of urine associated with the uncontrollable urge to void. Urgency and even urge incontinence is not uncommon in patients with BPH. It represents the clinical symptom of the urodynamic finding of detrusor instability (DI), which is found in about two-thirds of patients prior to surgery for BPH.[13] Postsurgical urgency or urge incontinence is rarely reported in the literature. It may be due to the irritation from the surgery itself or the indwelling catheter associated with the surgery, or it may be a symptom indicating persistent DI.

In reviewing the literature for data on incontinence following surgical treatment for BPH, the authors' information regarding incontinence was taken at face value. Several potential sources of error may exist. Authors may report incontinence rates at different time points following surgery, and thus some of the reported incontinence may be only temporary. On the other hand, it was assumed that if an author reported a certain rate of stress incontinence but gave no information on total incontinence, the incidence of total incontinence, in fact, was zero. This assumption is based on the theory that an author who reported on incontinence issues at all would certainly report if total incontinence occurred in his patient population. Thus, several partially offsetting biases may affect the analysis of the literature.

Overall, data are available from 18 series of OPSU, nine series of TUIP and 13 TURP series (Table 31.4). The median probability for stress incontinence ranges from 1.75% for TUIP to 2.59% for OPSS, while for total incontinence it ranges from 0.09% for TUIP to 0.98% for TURP. No correlations were noted in the OPSU and TURP studies between the weight of the resected specimen and incontinence rates, the number of patients in each of the studies who were in urinary retention with indwelling catheters prior to treatment, the age of the patients, or any other analysed variable.

Given the nature of the surgical intervention, it should not come as a surprise that the differences in the rates of stress incontinence following the various procedures are not significant, whereas the rate of total incontinence is clearly lower for TUIP than for any of the other modalities, and it is significantly higher for TURP than for any of the other modalities. Stress incontinence is not uncommon in elderly men with or without prostatic disease, and it is particularly prevalent in nursing home residents. Tinetti et al.[100] found in a 1-year study of 927 men aged 72 and older, an incontinence rate (defined as at least one episode of incontinence per week) of 16%. In the presented literature review, it is impossible to determine the exact percentage of patients who had a similar degree of incontinence prior to the surgical procedure. Wasson et al.[92] reported in the VA cooperative trial, that four of 280 men after TURP and four of 276 after watchful waiting had 'persistent' incontinence, with a relative risk of 0.99 (0.25–3.90) after 3 years of follow-up. Nevertheless, there is little doubt that surgical procedures, and in particular uncontrolled resection of the apical tissue of the prostate, can result in incontinence of varying severity. Total incontinence, indeed, is a very debilitating complication of surgery. In the absence of any definite contemporary studies of this problem, rates of total incontinence of 0.1% for TUIP, 0.5% for OPSU and 1.0% for TURP, as shown in Table 31.4, represent best estimates and should be discussed with the patient.

Bladder neck contracture and urethral stricture

Two complications resulting from surgical treatment of BPH are clearly defined and reported separately in many of the studies in the literature. These are the development of a urethral stricture or a bladder neck contracture (BNC) following either open or transurethral prostate surgery. Although in some cases no treatment may be necessary, other patients have to undergo either dilatation of the stricture or BNC, or a surgical revision in the form of a visual internal urethrotomy or a BNC resection, requiring anaesthesia and at least a day-surgery procedure.

There are 18 studies reporting the incidence of urethral stricture and/or BNC following open surgical enucleation of the prostate. These studies comprise a

Table 31.4. *Combined* analyses for the probability of stress and total urinary incontinence following open enucleation by OPSS or OPSR, TUIP and TURP. OPSU represents the combined probabilities for OPSS and OPSR*

Modality	n	Percentage probability (mean and 90% CI)	
		Stress urinary incontinence	Total urinary incontinence
OPSR	5384	1.6 (0.3–4.7)	0.5 (0.3–0.8)
OPSS	2329	2.6 (0.5–7.2)	0.3 (0.1–0.8)
OPSU	7962	1.9 (0.4–5.2)	0.5 (0.4–0.8)
TUIP	1200	1.8 (1.4–2.2)	0.1 (0.02–0.5)
TURP	7055	2.2 (1.8–2.5)	1.0 (0.7–1.4)

*As in Table 31.3.

total of 8634 patients, 5271 of whom were treated by OPSR while 3080 were treated by OPSS. The mean age of the population in these groups was 67.8 years, and was 67.7 and 67.6 years for the subgroups of OPSR and OPSS, respectively. In three series, the mean weight of the prostate was reported, the average mean weight being 46.7 g. No meaningful conclusion can be drawn from the correlation between the weight of the prostate and the incidence of the complications, since only three of the total of 18 studies reported the mean weight, which ranged from 42 to 51 g in those studies in which it was reported.

The mean probability of developing urethral stricture disease following OPSR is 1.0% (Table 31.5), wheras for OPSS it is 5.1%. This higher probability results from one study involving 32 patients, 25% of whom developed urethral stricture disease, and another study involving 179 patients, of which 10.06% of whom developed urethral stricture disease.[42,55] There is one other study reporting on 309 patients with an incidence of 9.06% patients who developed urethral stricture disease.[48] Although two of the studies are rather old and were published in 1970[42] and 1976,[48] the smallest series[55] stems from 1984 and is carefully reported and documented. Overall, open surgical enucleation of the prostate resulted in urethral stricture disease in 181 of 8634 patients, for a mean probability of 2.6 with (2.8–9.4)% (Table 31.5).

Table 31.5. *Combined* analyses for the probabilities of urethral stricture, bladder neck contracture (BNC), or either one of the two complications, following open enucleation by OPSS or OPSR, TUIP and TURP. OPSU represents the combined probabilities for OPSS and OPSR*

| Modality | n | Percentage probability (mean and 90% CI) | | |
		Urethral stricture	BNC	Combined
OPSR	5271	1.0 (0.2–2.7)	1.0 (0.2–3.5)	1.9 (0.3–5.7)
OPSS	3080	5.1 (0.5–18.4)	2.9 (0.3–10.5)	7.7 (1.0–24.9)
OPSU	8634	2.6 (2.8–9.4)	1.8 (0.2–6.1)	4.3 (0.6–14.1)
TUIP	1218	1.7 (1.2–2.5)	0.4 (0.1–1.0)	1.9 (1.3–2.7)
TURP	12003	3.1 (0.5–9.7)	1.7 (1.3–2.1)	3.7 (0.7–10.1)

*As in Table 31.3.

In nine TUIP studies, 21 of 1218 patients developed a urethral stricture with a mean probability of 1.7 (1.2–2.5)%. Seventeen studies reported the incidence of urethral stricture disease following TURP. These studies total 12 003 patients with an average age of 67.6 years. A total of 269 patients developed urethral stricture disease with a mean probability of 3.1 (0.5–9.7)%. Three studies reported relatively high incidences of 16%,[76] 16.3%[55] and 13%;[60] however, they are carefully documented and contemporary. In six studies the average weight of tissue removed was reported (mean 21.1 g; range 7–57 g). There is no correlation between the weight of tissue resected and the incidence of stricture formation. The problem associated with urethral stricture formation following TURP has been recognized at an early stage during the use of this procedure. Warres[101] reported on the use of hydrocortisone ointment topically applied to the urethral mucosa in 75 of 173 patients undergoing TURP; in the remaining patients, no ointment was used: the incidence of stricture postoperatively was 6.0% in the non-hydrocortisone ointment group versus 6.2% in the hydrocortisone ointment group. The author concluded, therefore, that the topical application of hydrocortisone does not prevent or decrease the incidence of stricture formation. He did, however, state that prophylactic meatotomy will reduce the incidence of postoperative urethral stricture formation although no data are reported. Aimed[102] reported on a total of 1036 patients undergoing TURP between 1952 and 1961 at the Mayo Clinic. All these men underwent

preliminary internal urethrotomy or meatotomy or both, if calibration up to 30 Fr was found to be difficult. This manoeuvre was necessary in 24.8% of 2550 consecutive TURPs during this time period. Follow-up data are available on 494 of 648 (76%) patients. Postoperatively, the authors found evidence of urethral stricture in seven of 632 cases (1.2%). The authors conclude that, in order to eliminate the incidence of postoperative stricture, the anterior portion of the urethra must be enlarged by internal urethrotomy or bypassed by performing the TURP through a perineal urethrostomy. Lentz et al.[67] found an incidence of urethral stricture postoperatively of 6.3% (97/1539). These strictures were detected at an average of 4.2 months after the TURP. The distribution of the strictures was as follows: meatal strictures 17.5%, post-navicular 23.7%, penile scrotal 11.3%, deep bulbous urethral 32.9%, and multiple 14.4%. The authors found that during the procedure, residents had a higher incidence of (in particular) meatal strictures than teaching staff. The length of the surgical procedure and the amount of tissue removed played no apparent part. It appeared that larger catheters (26 Fr) were associated with a higher incidence of stricture, although this was not significant. The length of catheterization following the procedure did not have any influence on the incidence of stricture, neither did preoperative urinary tract infection predict those patients who would develop a stricture. The authors conclude from their analysis, that the important factors were (1) initial calibration of the urethra to determine the anatomical adequacy prior to instrumentation, (2) gentle dilatation of the urethra,

(3) the use of perineal urethrostomy in patients with a stricture noted at the time of initial endoscopy (n=142), and (4) the size of the urethral catheter used postoperatively (not significant). Lundhus et al.[103] investigated whether the extent of transurethral prostatic section had an impact on the incidence of stricture formation: in a group of men with a median weight of resected prostatic tissue of 7 g (range 1–40 g) four of 72 (5.5%) developed a urethral stricture, while of 68 men with a median resected prostatic weight of 18 g (range 4–118 g), eight developed a urethral stricture (12%) (not significant).

Two studies address the issue of urethral stricture formation after TURP in a controlled randomized fashion.[104,105] Schultz et al.[104] studied stricture formation after TURP in a randomized clinical trial including 185 patients. The patients were allocated to either a 2-day urethral catheter dilatation or internal urethrotomy by the Otis method, and at the same time the operation was performed with either an uninsulated metal resectoscope sheath or a polytetrafluoroethylene (PTFE)-coated resectoscope sheath. Urethral stricture was defined as an obstruction resulting in a Q_{max} of less than 15 ml/s and not permitting the passage of a 21 Fr cystoscope sheath. The authors found that the frequency of stricture formation was significantly lower after internal urethrotomy (0.4%) than after a 2-day urethral catheter dilatation (16%). Coating the resectoscope sheath with PTFE did not significantly alter the incidence of stricture formation (0.8 vs 12%). The incidence of stricture formation was not related to age, duration of pre- or postoperative catheterization, operating time, and/or the presence of urinary tract infection. Hammarsten et al.[105] examined the role of the catheter in a randomized controlled trial. Two hundred and five patients following TURP were randomly assigned to drainage with a suprapubic latex catheter versus a transurethrally placed siliconized latex catheter. At follow-up, 6–12 months after the procedure, 17% of patients in the transurethral group had developed a urethral stricture, versus only 0.4% in the group of patients treated by a suprapubic drainage catheter. This difference was significant at $p<0.01$. The location of the stricture was equally divided in the TURP group between the external meatus, the foci navicularis, the penile scrotal urethra and the bladder neck, while in the suprapubic group the majority of strictures were located at the bladder neck.

Wasson et al.[92] reported that, at 3-years follow-up in a contemporary series of 280 patients following TURP, nine (3.2%) had developed a urethral stricture requiring dilatation, a probability almost identical to the calculated mean probability of 3.1% in the older literature. Riehman et al.[93] reported that eight of 56 patients (14.3%) initially treated by TURP in their randomized trial had to undergo a transurethral incision or resection of a BNC, a considerably higher probability than that estimated from the literature review. Contemporary data for open prostatectomy are, unfortunately, not available.

BNC following open prostatectomy occurs with a mean probability of 1.0% (OPSR), 2.9% (OPSS) and 1.8 (0.2–6.1)% (OPSU) for both procedures combined (Table 31.5). The previously mentioned report by Beck,[42] with a 12.8% incidence of BNC, is mainly responsible for the higher rate following OPSS.

Of all the reports describing long-term complications following TUIP, only one study[83] reported that two of 646 patients developed a BNC, with a mean probability of 0.4% only.

Only nine of the studies reporting urethral stricture development following TURP presented data on BNC following the same intervention. The incidence ranges from 0 to 7.1%, with a raw average of 1.4%. Overall, 61 of 4152 patients had this complication, with a mean probability of 1.7 (1.3–2.1)%. There was no correlation between the amount of tissue resected and the incidence of BNC, although it had been postulated that BNC is more likely to occur after resection of less than 10 g tissue. In one report of 388 patients, the average weight was 57 g and the incidence of BNC was 0.77,[8] while in another report of 84 patients the average weight was 23.5 g and the incidence 7.14%.[70] In three studies totalling 52 patients with average resected weights of less than 20 g, no patient developed BNC.[71–73] These data do not justify the conclusion that there might not be a correlation between the amount of tissue resected and the incidence of BNC.

It has been stated that BNC occurs after resection of BPH tissue of less than 20 g. The bladder neck was incised at the conclusion of the TURP by using a cold knife incision of the vesicle neck at the 6 o'clock position extending from the mid-trigone verumontanum. The complication is believed to be secondary to excessive resection of an undilated bladder neck. Kulb et al.[30] performed prophylactic bladder neck incisions very similar to TUIP in conjunction with TURP on 114 patients with BPH tissue weighing less than 20 g (Table 31.6). BNC occurred in only one patient (0.87%), compared with 12 BNCs found in 161 patients (7.5%) who underwent TURP alone; this difference was significant (p<0.05). It should be noted that TURP alone resulted in an incidence of BNC of 4.7% (12/253 patients), when all patients were considered, whereas the incidence was (as previously stated) 7.5% in those men with prostates weighing less than 20 g. The additional incision of the bladder neck did not have an impact on the incidence of BNC in those men that had prostates larger than 20 g (Table 31.6).

In the VA cooperative trial, nine of the 280 men (3.2%) undergoing TURP, with a mean resection weight of 14 g, had to undergo an endoscopic procedure for a BNC at 3 years of follow-up.

If one assumes that, for the patient, the actual type of complication he develops is less important than the fact that some complications require active surgical intervention, it is reasonable to combine the numbers for urethral stricture and BNC into a total representing the total number of patients suffering one of these complications requiring surgical intervention. For OPSR, a total of 125 of 5271 patients required such an intervention, with a mean probability of 1.9%.

Following OPSS, 160 of 3080 patients developed such complications, with a mean probability of 7.7%. For the entire group of patients undergoing open prostatectomy, 301 of 8634 men developed these complications, with a mean probability of 4.3 (0.6–14.1)%. Following TUIP, 23 of 1218 men developed one of these complications, with a mean probability of 1.9 (1.3–2.7)% and, following TURP, 330 of 12 003 men developed them, with a mean probability of 3.7 (0.7–10.1)%.

Given the fact that contemporary surgical series have similar or even higher incidence rates for these long-term complications, it appears unlikely that the mean probabilities listed in Table 31.5 will be significantly improved by minor modifications in the surgical technique.

Sexual function

Impotence

Although BPH is a disease of ageing men, maintaining or restoring sexual function is of increasing importance to patients suffering from BPH. A variety of studies can be utilized to assess the prevalence of impotence in the normal ageing man, based on a total of 7316 men.[106–110] Pearlman and Kobashi reported not only on the frequency of intercourse in men but also on the prevalence of impotence seen in patients with BPH (n = 1095).[110] Figure 31.10 shows the range of

Table 31.6. *Incidence of BNC following TURP depending on whether simultaneous incision of the bladder neck was performed.*

| | | | BNC | |
Procedure	Patients	n	No.	%
TURP with incision	All	137	1	0.72
	Resected weight < 20 g only	114	1	0.9*
TURP without incision	All	253	12	4.7
	Resected weight < 20 g only	161	12	7.5

Asterisk denotes statistically significant difference from non-incised subgroup of patients with resected weight < 20 g (*p<0.05). (From ref. 30 with permission.)

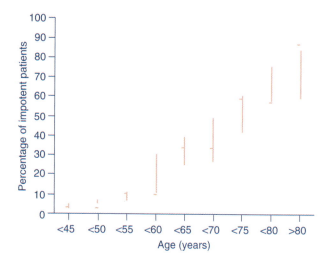

Figure 31.10. *Range (vertical lines) of reported prevalence of erectile dysfunction in the general male population stratified by age. The horizontal dashes indicate the prevalence of erectile dysfunction noted by Pearlman and Kobashi[110] in 1095 men with BPH.*

impotence reported in the general population within the five studies, as well as the reported prevalence of impotence in the BPH population.[110] Men with BPH apparently do not differ from the general population of ageing men with regard to the prevalence of impotence. Similarly, among patients presenting for surgical treatment for BPH, the prevalence of erectile dysfunction ranges from 20.8 to 42.1%.

Before discussing the probability of suffering from erectile dysfunction as a result of surgery for BPH, one must acknowledge that in most of the available literature the assessment of erectile function was crude at best, usually based only on a loosely structured and poorly defined physician assessment or interview, while sophisticated means of determining potency status, such as standardized questionnaires and nocturnal penile tumescence measurement, were rarely used

A total of 24 studies[107,109–129] were identified in the literature that reported in some detail on potency before and after surgical treatment for BPH. Some of the studies include several arms. For example, several authors compared the rate of impotence following TURP or open prostatectomy, while others compared the rate of impotence following general surgical procedures (cholecystectomy or hernia repair) with that after surgery for BPH.[116,118,126] Following general surgical procedures, 1.0% of men claimed to have changed from being potent to impotent (Table 31.7), whereas following TUIP the rate was 4.6%. Following TURP, a rate of 13.6% was noted, whereas following

open surgical procedures including perineal prostatectomy, the rate ranged from 15.6 to 31.5%.

Concerning the rate of impotence following TUIP, four of the five studies available (n = 49) report no new onset of impotence after the procedure, while in one study,[84] three of 13 preoperatively potent patients complained of 'deteriorated sexual performance'. The author of this study used a technique of two deep incisions. The most recent report from Riehman et al.[93] compared TUIP and TURP in a randomized fashion: all 22 patients who were potent prior to TURP remained potent after surgery, and all 23 patients potent prior to TUIP remained potent as well. Wasson et al.[92] found that 19% in the TURP group and 21% in the watchful waiting group reported, at 3 years follow-up, worsening of their sexual performance. However, the difference between the two groups was not significant ($p=0.92$).

A study of great significance in the overall context of this particular problem has been conducted by Libman et al.,[130] who examined 72 married men after a transurethral prostatectomy. Socioeconomic status, personal and demographic variables, symptom check-list, psychological status [Brief Symptom Inventory (BSI)] and marital function [Locke Wallace Marital Adjustment Scale (MAS)] were assessed and a variety of tests to evaluate sexual functions were performed. These tests included the sexual history form (SHF), Goal for Sex Therapy Scale (GSTS), Sexual Self-efficacy Scale — erectile functioning (SSES), Sexual Interaction

Table 31.7. *Potency and ejaculatory status before and after general surgical procedures and various surgical procedures for BPH*

Treatment	n	Mean age (years)	Follow-up (months)	Before surgery Potent n	%	Impotent n	%	After surgery Potent n	%*	Impotent n	%*	Retrograde ejaculation (%)*
GENSU	186	66.0	30	174	93.7	12	6.3	168	97.0	6	3.0	1.0
TUIP	144	63.7	14	62	57.9	828	42.1	59	95.4	3	4.6	38.8
TURP	1543	65.1	24	989	77.5	603	21.5	736	86.4	224	13.6	70.4
OPSR	784	67.4	14	542	76.2	269	23.8	441	84.4	101	15.6	65.0
OPSS	647	65.5	22	558	79.2	109	20.8	444	83.6	114	16.4	80.8
PERP	98	n.a.	n.a.	53	61.0	37	39.0	36	68.5	17	31.5	n.a.

GENSU, general surgical procedures; PERP, perineal prostatectomy; n.a., not assessed. *Expressed as a percentage of those previously potent.

Inventory (SII), and additional sexual measures (SHF-A). The authors found that pre- and postsurgery scores correlated highly for all parameters measured, apart from satisfaction with the current sexual relationship. Men with good presurgical sexual adjustment had a better outcome after surgery than those with poor adjustment. Younger men were more prone to retain good sexual capability and confidence than older men. However, older men with good couple scores were more likely to remain in the well-functioning range regarding couple behaviour and adjustment after surgery. There was an overall decrease in the frequency of intercourse, reduced variability, decrease in sexual desire, erectile capability, and self-confidence, while an increase was noted in the prevalence of retrograde ejaculation. However, of greatest importance is the fact that the ratings of general couple satisfaction and harmony were not adversely affected by the surgery. This study emphasizes the fact that the effects of prostate surgery may differ greatly, depending on whether the focus is on individual sexual functioning or the sexual relationship within a well-functioning adjusted couple. This indicates that these two aspects of sexuality are independent and must be evaluated separately.

It probably is safe to say that for very few of the BPH treatment data was such careful and detailed analysis performed. It must be assumed that in the majority of these studies the men were asked only about their individual sexual functioning, without taking into consideration the couple's sexual relationship.

It is of interest in this regard that a recent study[129] also demonstrated the impact of a permanent partner in sexual function. Of 58 men reporting presurgical impotence, 20 (34.4%) had no permanent partner whereas only six of 152, or 3.9%, of those patients who were potent prior to surgical treatment had no permanent partner. The difference between these percentages was highly significant ($p<0.001$). Following surgery, the ratio was unchanged (29.3 vs 2.7%). These authors conclude that the risk of postoperative impotence is dependent on the patient's age, as well as the presence of a partner.

Retrograde ejaculation

Another area of concern is the incidence of retrograde ejaculation resulting from the destruction of the bladder neck mechanism. The pathophysiology of retrograde ejaculation is believed to be a failure of the bladder neck to close during ejaculation, allowing the semen to flow back into the bladder which, in this case, is the line of least resistance. Under normal circumstances, the bladder neck closes during ejaculation under sympathomimetic influence as a result of the alpha-adrenergic innervation. It is a well-known and accepted risk of any surgical procedure performed for BPH that the patient may develop retrograde ejaculation. Although some patients are not, apparently, particularly worried about the possibility of this occurring, it is of concern that some patients do not understand the difference between impotence and retrograde ejaculation. These patients tend to claim that the surgery left them impotent because they do not have emission during intercourse, although they may be able to have an orgasm. It is the duty of the physician to counsel the patient, prior to treatment, about the difference between impotence and retrograde ejaculation, as well as to inform him about the probability of either of these outcomes.

The risk of retrograde ejaculation developing after general surgical procedures is 1%, whereas for any surgical procedure that involves the bladder neck the risk is significant, ranging from 38.8% for TUIP to 80.8% for OPSS (Table 31.7). In a contemporary randomized study retrograde ejaculation was found in 15 of 22 patients (68%) after TURP and in eight of 23 patients (35%) after TUIP ($p=0.02$).[93] These numbers are very comparable to those found in the older literature (Table 31.7).

Treatment failure and re-treatment

Treatment failure and the need for re-treatment represent some of the most important outcomes from both a patient's point of view and from that of health-care economics. Patients who have undergone a certain treatment strategy for BPH have, in essence, invested in this therapy, either by buying medication or by paying their surgeon, the anaesthetist and the hospital. If the therapy fails to provide long-lasting relief of symptoms and additional treatment becomes necessary, additional cost are invariably incurred.

When attempting to calculate treatment failure and re-treatment rates, one is faced with several potential sources of bias. First, few studies in the literature report on these outcomes. When comparing the re-treatment rates of different treatment strategies, one has to ask whether the patient populations at baseline were, indeed, comparable. For example, it may be assumed that patients selected for a medical therapy are less symptomatic — and thus less likely to fail therapy — than those selected for surgical treatment. Moreover, even if re-treatment rates are reported, it is not always clear which proportion of the original study population was followed, and whether those patients lost to follow-up behaved in a way similar to those patients for whom follow-up data were available. Lastly, failure to relieve symptoms is not identical to re-treatment, nor are failure rates identical to re-treatment rates. For example, in trials of medical therapy, failure is usually defined by the investigators by arbitrarily setting a certain threshold for improvement in symptom score or peak urinary flow rate. However, patients who fail to achieve that level of improvement do not necessarily agree with this assessment, and many of them will, in fact, not undergo re-treatment.

Although some of these considerations are not relevant in surgical treatment modalities, where a re-treatment rate can be clearly defined as the fraction of patients who undergo a second surgical procedure, other interpretational problems remain. A certain fraction of patients reported in claims data-based analyses to have undergone a second TURP will, in fact, have undergone this procedure in an attempt to stage an incidentally found prostatic carcinoma. About 10% of TURP specimens contains prostate carcinoma, and in an unknown percentage of these the treating physician may elect to undertake a second TURP to document the presence or absence of more carcinomatous tissue in the prostate. Furthermore, some procedures with the aim of correcting problems such as BNC may be coded in such a way that a claims data review will not be able to separate them from true re-treatments for recurrent or persistent BPH.

These latter considerations are less relevant for the patient than they are from a health-care economics point of view. To the patient, the precise indication for the anaesthesia and surgery does not matter as much as the fact that he has to submit to another surgical procedure.

TUIP

Eight reports are available for assessment of the treatment failure rate and the need for re-treatment following TUIP. Hellström et al.[71] compared 13 men with BPH treated with TURP with 11 men with BPH treated by TUIP. Patients were estimated to have a prostate gland weighing less than 30 g. Over a follow-up period of 6 months, none of the men treated by TUIP required re-treatment for failure of symptomatic relief. Dorflinger et al.[73] compared 21 men with BPH and prostate glands estimated to weigh less than 20 g, treated by TURP, with 17 similar patients treated by TUIP. During the follow-up period of 3 months, three patients in the TUIP group required a TURP and were deemed treatment failures. Larsen et al.[72] compared 18 men with BPH and prostates estimated to weigh less than 20 g, treated by TURP, with 19 men treated with TUIP in a randomized trial. Follow-up was available over 12 months. None of the men treated with TUIP required re-treatment during this period of follow-up. Only one patient in the TUIP group had no improvement in symptoms, but cystoscopy showed that he had a wide open bladder neck; he did not undergo re-treatment. Nielsen[76] documented a failure rate of three of 24 men treated with transurethral prostatotomy in a randomized trial compared with 25 men treated by TURP; the follow-up was 12 months. Delaere et al.[82] utilized TUIP in 32 men with either mechanical or functional bladder outlet obstruction. These men were followed over a mean of 18 months, during which period three required re-treatment. This report poses a problem in that it mixes men with mechanical and functional outlet obstruction. However, the mean age was 60 years and therefore close to the average age of men treated for symptomatic BPH. The exact definition of functional obstruction is difficult to ascertain and the data from this study are included in the re-treatment calculation. Katz et al.[87] treated 66 men with BPH, with prostates estimated to weigh less than 15 g, with TUIP; these men were followed up for 24 months, during which five of the 64 men available for follow-up required re-treatment. Mobb and Moisey[85] treated 94 men with BPH with TUIP and had follow-up data available on 75 men at 60 months; during this time, six patients had required re-treatment. Edwards et al.[8] treated 700 patients with BPH and have follow-up data from 3 months to 7 years. Of these patients, 388 were treated by TURP and the remaining 312 patients, with prostates estimated to weigh less than 35 g, were treated by TUIP. Over the extended follow-up, five of these 312 men required re-treatment because of failure of TUIP to relieve symptoms. On several occasions, Orandi has published details of his personal experience with patients undergoing TUIP.[11,83,84,131–133] Recently, he reviewed his experience with TUIP for the treatment of BPH and presented re-treatment data in tabulated form over a maximum follow-up period of 18 years (total number of procedures 753).[133] The data presented allow accurate calculation of the total number of patients at risk for any given period, the incidence density or failure rate for the period extending from 3 months to 60 months and the cumulative failure rate at any given interval. The cumulative failure rate up to 5 years is plotted in Fig. 31.11. Up to 5 years no clear decrease in the failure rate is noticeable; however, the highest failure rate occurred within the first year following treatment, according to the raw data. The failure rate then remains steady, with a minor decrease only through years 2–5 (failure rates 0.00288, 0.00264, 0.00219, 0.00215, respectively). Although the data are not shown for the following years, it appears that this failure rate holds steady over the next 5 years up to 10 years of

follow-up. The reported failure rates in this series by Orandi and for the other series discussed above are plotted in Fig. 31.11. On the basis of the information available from Orandi's series, projected re-treatment or cumulative failure rates for 60 months were calculated for all studies for which they were not already available. Using the actual as well as the projected data, the mean probability for the need for re-treatment and the 90% CI were calculated. The mean probability for the need for re-treatment was 12.9% (90% CI 4.7–26.5) and is indicated as a vertical line in Fig. 31.11. If only those studies that actually report 5-year follow-up data[8,85,133] are used, the mean re-treatment probability is 8.9% (CI 1.2–28.1%). Whereas the point estimate is lower than if all actual and projected data are utilized, the CI remains virtually unchanged.

TURP and OPSU

Excellent data concerning failure and re-treatment rates are available for OPSU and TURP. Treatment data have been reported for 44 832 patients treated by TURP and 17 065 patients treated with OPSU (either OPSS or OPSR). The individual data points are plotted in Fig. 31.12. Roos and Ramsey[61] reported re-treatment data on 1855 patients following TURP, 621 patients following OPSS, and 223 patients following OPSR. The data are derived from the Universal Health Insurance System in Manitoba, Canada, and follow-up was available for up to 8 years after the initial procedure. By the end of the follow-up period, 16.8% of TURP patients had undergone a second prostatectomy, compared with 7% or less of those who initially underwent an open procedure. The TURP patient group required an additional prostatic operation at a constant rate of approximately 2% per year. Roos et al.[78] reported on re-treatment rates following TURP and open prostatectomy in Denmark (n = 36 703), in Oxfordshire, England (n = 5284) and in Manitoba (n = 12 090). Patients were identified retrospectively through administrative data and followed for up to 8 years. The cumulative probabilities of undergoing a second prostatectomy, according to the type of initial prostatectomy, were reported for 1, 5 and 8 years: the 8-year probabilities for TURP ranged from 5.0 (Denmark and Oxford region) to 15.5% (Manitoba), whereas for open prostatectomy the 8-year re-treatment probability

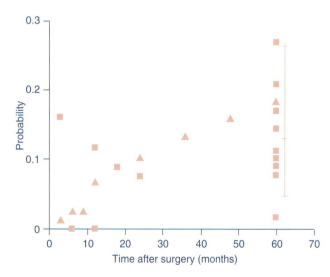

Figure 31.11. *Actual (solid symbols) and projected (open symbols) re-treatment rates following TUIP. Cumulative failure rates up to 5 years, for Orandi's series (▲) and all series (■). Mean probability and 90% CI are shown as a vertical bar and are based on all data.*

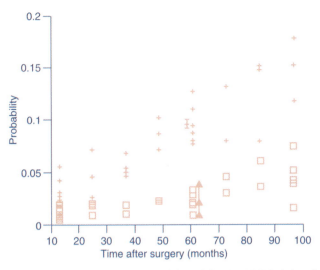

Figure 31.12. *Re-treatment probabilities following TURP (+) and OPSU (□). Mean probabilities and 90% CI indicated at 60 months by vertical bars (— TURP; ▲, OPSU).*

ranged from 1.8% (Oxford region) to 4.5% (Denmark). Taylor and Krakauer[134] presented data from a random sample of 3641 Medicare-enrolled patients who underwent prostatectomy in 1985. Of these, a subsample of 2617 patients had a diagnosis of BPH; 2449 of whom were treated by TURP (93.6%) while 168 underwent open prostatectomy. The probability of having a repeat prostatectomy after 2 years of follow-up was 4.7% following a TURP and 1.84% following an open prostatectomy (difference not statistically significant). Singh et al.[63] reported re-treatment rates on 935 patients following TURP and 217 patients following open prostatectomy (198 OPSR and 19 OPSS). Within 1 year of the initial operation, 2.8% in the TURP group required re-treatment versus 0.5% in the open prostatectomy group. Several smaller series are also available for assessment of re-treatment data. Ball and Smith[53] followed for 5 years 38 patients who underwent TURP, and reported that two required re-treatment within 5 years of follow-up. Aalkjer[62] reported re-treatment rates in 110 patients following TURP, and compared them with a similar group of patients who underwent dilatation of the prostatic urethra with the Deisting dilator. The cumulative probability for re-treatment at 5 years was 8.2% in this series, which represents the oldest evidence available. Stephenson et al.[135] studied the outcome of surgery for BPH in

Rochester, Minnesota between 1980 and 1987. During this time, 330 men underwent prostatectomy for BPH. The likelihood of re-operation within 6 years of the initial surgery was 15.1% (95% CI 9.7–20.6). The probability of re-operation at 5 years was 12.9%, which therefore represents the highest reported rate of any of the listed studies. Lastly, Meyhoff and Nordling[60] reported on 38 men who underwent TURP for BPH and found a re-treatment rate of 7.9% at the 5-year follow-up. It is specifically noted that an important piece of evidence presented by Wennberg et al.[98] is not used in the calculation of the re-treatment probability. This publication from 1987 reports re-treatment rates up to 8 years for patients having undergone TURP and open prostatectomy for BPH and is based on data from the Manitoba Health Services Commission Claims Data System. These data relating to the Manitoba population are contained in a later publication by the same group[78] and are therefore not listed separately in the analysis.

Several other reports cite a certain rate of re-treatment at a certain follow-up time. However, the quality of the data and the accuracy of follow-up information are inferior to those in the studies utilized and these studies were therefore not included. In this context, however, it is interesting to observe that, in a national survey of all American urologists (n = 2716 urologists) the mean percentage of patients who underwent TURP and who had previously undergone a TURP was 8.1%.[12] This figure is remarkably similar to that reported by Mebust et al.[15] who found in a cooperative study of 13 participating institutions evaluating 3885 patients that 8% of all patients undergoing TURP had already done so. This is, again, remarkably similar to the mean probability of 9.7% estimated for the likelihood of undergoing a second prostatectomy within 5 years of follow-up. There is one important caveat, however: claims data and other administrative data do not necessarily separate those patients who undergo re-operation because of recurrent or persistent disease from those who undergo surgery to correct BNC or a urethral stricture (see earlier). Nevertheless, the main interest for the patient is whether he has to undergo repeat surgery, rather than what is the precise underlying problem. The same is true of those patients who may have undergone repeat TURP for accurate staging because an incidental prostatic carcinoma was found in the first TURP. The majority of the large claims data-based series exclude this patient population, however, and focus the analysis on those patients with histological BPH.

Most recently, Lu-Yao et al.[99] used a 20% sample of Medicare beneficiaries to update re-operation rates in the Medicare population between 1984 and 1990. The overall risk for a second TURP was 7.2% over the study period, whereas it was 5.5% when the indication for a second TURP was restricted to BPH only. Age was not a major factor in the re-operation rates, as the risk was 5.7% for those over 75 years and 5.4% for those under 75 years of age. Limitations of this dataset are the absence of men under 65 years of age, and the reliance on claims data.

The cumulative re-treatment probabilities obtained from the literature at 60 months were converted into numbers of patients of the original population that had failed at this time point, and were used to calculate the mean probability and confidence limits for the need of re-treatment. Because of the large number of patients involved in these studies, the confidence limits are rather narrow and the data appear to be stable (TURP: 9.75%; 90% CI 9.36–10.6; OPSU: 2.25%; 90% CI 1.06–4.11) (shown as vertical bars in Fig. 31.12). The mean probability estimates and confidence intervals are plotted as vertical lines (mean probability indicated by a horizontal bar) for the three surgical treatment modalities assessed in Fig. 31.13. OPSU clearly has the lowest probability of treatment failure and/or need for re-treatment within 5 years. The probability distributions for the need for re-treatment following OPSU versus TURP do not overlap and there is, therefore, a significant difference between these two treatment modalities in this respect.

The individual data points for TURP and OPSU can be analysed further. For the TURP re-treatment data, the best fit is represented by the formula y = a + b·x [slope (b) = 0.138; intercept (a) = 1.295] with the correlation coefficient r = 0.89. Figure 31.14 demonstrates the linear relation between duration of follow-up and probability of re-treatment, and the 95% CI over the entire duration of follow-up: the probability of re-treatment remains constant throughout at least 8 years of follow-up. This is in some contrast to the data available for balloon dilatation, watchful waiting and

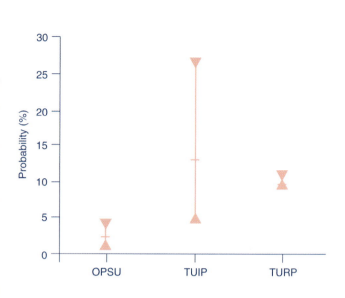

Figure 31.13 *Re-treatment probabilities (mean and 90% CI) following TUIP, TURP and OPSU.*

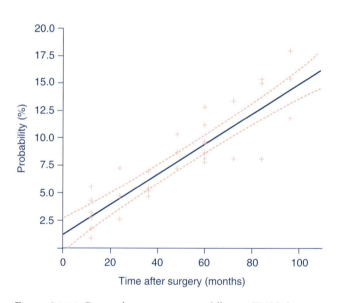

Figure 31.14. *Reported re-treatment rates following TURP for up to 8 years of follow-up. Correlation coefficient (r)=0.89 (y=a+bx); CD=0.79; R²=0.95. Dotted lines indicate 95% CI.*

TUIP, which demonstrate a very high failure rate in the first year and a subsequent decrease in failure rate throughout the remainder of the follow-up to 5 years. A similar analysis of the re-treatment data for OPSU reveals a somewhat different situation. The correlation coefficient for the linear curve fitting (y = a + b·x) [slope (b) = 0.046; intercept (a) = 0.26) is r = 0.798. A better fit is obtained using the formula $y = a \cdot e^{bx}$ (slope = 0.019; intercept = 0.779; e = base of the natural logarithm). The correlation coefficient $r = 0.827$. The data with the best fit curve are shown in Fig. 31.15. It appears that the re-treatment probability following OPSU remains very low for the initial 5 years, but that the failure rate increases somewhat faster thereafter. Theoretically, it seems possible that the re-treatment rate for recurrent BPH following open enucleation of the entire adenoma remains very low after the surgery and that it will take several years for recurrent disease to cause obstructive symptoms and necessitate re-treatment. At the same time, it is quite likely that TURP tends not to remove tissue as completely and that, therefore, the re-treatment rate during the first 5 years is, in fact, significantly higher than after OPSU.

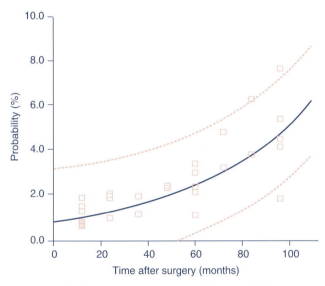

Figure 31.15. *Reported re-treatment rates following OPSU for up to 8 years of follow-up. Correlation coefficient (r)=0.827 ($y=a.e^{ex}$); CD=0.68; R²=0.84. Dotted lines indicate 95% CI.*

Delayed mortality following TURP and OPSU

Perioperative mortality is an important outcome to be considered in the discussion of any major surgical procedure. However, in recent years it has been suggested that there are differences in delayed mortality following TURP and OPSU (for the purpose of this discussion, OPSS and OPSR are considered jointly). The urological community responded to the challenge by attempting to explain the observed differences in terms of patient selection biases. Patients selected for TURP, so the argument goes, differ from those selected for open prostatectomy with regard to their general health status, associated diseases, and anaesthetic and surgical risks. In short, patients selected for TURP are less fit than those selected for OPSU and have a higher co-morbidity index; they thus have a shorter life expectancy, independent of the actual surgical procedure. Although data regarding co-morbidity are virtually absent from the older literature, most studies addressing the problem of delayed mortality attempt to correct for co-morbidities, using a variety of techniques.

As described in the previous section, Roos et al.[78] reported mortality up to 8 years following TURP or OPSU in three geographical areas (Denmark, Oxfordshire, England and Manitoba, Canada). The analysis is based on existing computerized databases: these are the Oxford Record Linkage Study in England, the National Hospital Patient Registry in Denmark and provincial claims data in Manitoba. The Manitoba data were adjusted for claims-based co-morbidity data such as concomitant diagnoses and previous hospitalizations. The age-adjusted cumulative risk of death per 100 patients after TURP or OPSU according to geographic location is presented in Table 31.8. A separate analysis of patients from the University of Manitoba teaching hospital revealed that the relative risk (RR) of dying within 5 years following TURP versus OPSU was 1.45 (95% CI 1.15–1.84) before and after age and co-morbidity adjustment. This finding, of a higher RR of dying following TURP, remained unchanged when the data were adjusted using a wide variety of risk strata (general health status, age, prior diagnosis of cancer, nursing home resident, on digitalis, high risk diagnosis, etc.), both from claims data and a separate, concurrent prospective study of anaesthetic risk. The size of the prostate gland enucleated during OPSU was not a statistically significant predictor of subsequent survival. An analysis of the causes of death showed that the excess mortality following TURP was mainly due to cardiovascular causes, especially acute myocardial infarction (Table 31.9).

Malenka et al.[136] re-evaluated a subset of the patient population that had previously been reported by Roos et al.[61,78] The purpose was to identify whether differences in

Table 31.8. *Age-adjusted cumulative risk of death (per 100) after TURP or OPSU according to geographic region*

Time	Denmark			Manitoba			Oxford		
	TURP (27 911)*	OPSU (8782)	RR	TURP (8995)	OPSU (3095)	RR	TURP (2171)	OPSU (3113)	RR
90 days	2.47	2.67	0.93	1.73	1.57	1.10	4.39	3.21	1.37
1 year	7.55	5.76	1.31	5.97	4.18	1.43	10.32	7.64	1.35
5 years	31.05	25.49	1.22	25.37	21.14	1.20	35.42	26.45	1.34
8 years	46.5	39.78	1.17	39.25	33.53	1.17	49.49	38.42	1.29

*Numbers in parentheses indicate number of patients in arm. RR, relative risk. (From ref. 78 with permission.)

case-mix unidentified by data previously available explained the increased mortality following TURP. To this end, a chart review was performed by six trained abstracters (registered nurses), blinded to the purpose of the study, at the Manitoba Health Science Centre, Winnipeg, Canada. The chart review included 485 patients who underwent prostatectomy between 1974 and 1980 (236 OPSU and 249 TURP). The crude RR of dying in the 5 years following TURP/OPSU in this subset was 1.58 (95% CI 1.07–2.33). This RR decreased slightly after controlling for patient age to a RR of 1.48 (95% CI 1.09–2.01). Further adjustment using co-morbidity data from the chart review, including the Charlson weighted co-morbidity index[137] and the Karnovsky score, did not change the results significantly.

Table 31.9. *Multivariate relative risk of death according to cause after TURP or OPSU (Manitoba dataset only)*

Patients	Cause of death	RR	95% CI
All (n=2965)	All causes	1.42	1.22–1.65
	Cardiovascular	1.51	1.20–1.90
	All other	1.51	1.20–1.91
	Acute MI	2.50	1.59–3.93
	Cerebrovascular accident	1.25	0.73–1.78
Low-risk patients (n = 586)	All causes	1.63	0.98–2.73
	Cardiovascular	2.92	1.20–7.06
	All other	1.06	0.46–2.42
	Acute MI	5.50	1.26–24.41
	Cerebrovascular accident	0.69	0.12–4.20

MI, myocardial infarction. (From ref. 78 with permission.)

Concato et al.[138] conducted a retrospective cohort study at Yale-New Haven Hospital involving 252 men undergoing TURP (n = 126) or open prostatectomy (n = 126) for BPH from 1979 through 1981 and assessed 5-year mortality adjusted for age and severity of co-morbidity at the time of surgery. Co-morbidity was measured by the methods of Kaplan and Feinstein[139] and Charlson et al.[137] Data were extracted from charts using explicit abstraction instructions. At least one abstracter was blinded with regard to the procedure. In a sample of 30 records abstracted by two abstracters, an almost perfect concordance was found with respect to co-morbidity scores. At 5 years after surgery, 17.5% (22/126) patients after TURP had died versus 13.5% (17/126) after OPSU. The RR of 1.29 (TURP/OPSU) (95% CI 0.72–2.31) is not statistically significant, but is similar to the unadjusted RR in the originally reported Manitoba dataset (n = 1284) (RR 1.27, 95% CI 1.03–1.57).[140] The 5-year mortality rates increased with increasing Kaplan–Feinstein co-morbidity grade, from 7% (7/101) for grade 'none', and 18% (24/134) for 'intermediate' grade, to 47% (8/17) for 'severe' grade [total 16% (39/252)]. A comparison of the Kaplan–Feinstein co-morbidity grade revealed a higher proportion of TURP patients with more severe co-morbidity grades (Table 31.10). The point estimate for the RR of dying (TURP/OPSU) at 5 years decreases and becomes essentially 1.0 after adjustment for co-morbidity using the two methods mentioned (Table 31.11). A proportional hazard analysis revealed that increasing age was associated with a RR of 1.71 (95% CI 1.08–2.69) and the Kaplan–Feinstein co-morbidity grade with a RR of 2.47 (95% CI 1.40–4.34). After

Table 31.10. *Comparison of treatment groups in relation to Kaplan–Feinstein co-morbidity grade*

Kaplan–Fernstein grade	TURP (n=126) n*	OPSU (n=126) n*	Percentage of TURP in Kaplan–Fernstein grade
None	37(29)	64(51)	37
Intermediate	75(70)	59(47)	56
Severe	14(11)	3(2)	82

*Percentages in parentheses. (From ref. 138 with permission.)

taking both these factors into account, the type of surgery did not significantly affect 5-year survival (RR TURP/OPSU 0.91, 95% CI 0.47 –1.75, $p = 0.77$).

A group of Danish investigators[141] studied survival through linkage of hospital discharge data with mortality data for the entire male population of Denmark (1977–1985). For a maximum of 10.5 years (minimum 2 years), 38 067 patients were followed, of which 28 991 had a TURP while 9076 had OPSU surgery. After adjustment for age only, the RR for dying (TURP/OPSU) within 10.5 years was 1.24 (95% CI 1.20–1.29). After adjustment for age *and* co-morbidity, the RR (TURP/OPSU) was 1.19 (95% CI 1.15–1.24) for all patients, while it was 1.11 (95% CI 1.03–1.19) for the subgroup of healthiest men. Thus, the additional adjustment for co-morbidity did not significantly change the increased risk of dying following TURP versus OPSU, although the indicators of co-morbidity employed contributed in a multivariate (Cox regression) analysis significantly as predictors of death. During the time frame of the study, the fraction of patients treated by TURP changed from 40% (1977–1979) to 81% (1983–1985). However, this gradual change was not associated with a change in the *relative* health status of the TURP and OPSU patients. Overall, however, the health status of TURP patients improved over the period of time when diffusion of the new technology of TURP was being completed. The causes of death underlying the higher probability of dying following TURP versus OPSU differed from those in the previously mentioned studies (Table 31.12). The RR of dying from an acute mycardial infarction after TURP/OPSU was estimated at 1.08 (95% CI 0.99–1.18, $p = 0.07$). The excess risk of death was therefore due mainly to death resulting from respiratory complications, namely chronic obstructive pulmonary disease (COPD) and other respiratory causes. This is interpreted by the authors as a clue in favour of a selection bias hypothesis, in that vulnerable patients with chronic conditions such as COPD were considered for TURP rather than for OPSU.

Table 31.11. *Effects of data source and co-morbidity classification on relative risk TURP versus OPSU*

Method of grading co-morbidity	Mortality rate for entire group (n)*	RR (TURP/OPSU)[†]
Discharge diagnoses Charlson sum		
0	30/219 (14)	1.20
≥ 1	9/33 (27)	(0.63–2.26)
Medical record review Charlson sum		
0–1	27/217 (12)	1.12
≥ 1	12/35 (34)	(0.57–2.10)
Charlson sum		
0	17/154 (11)	
1	10/63 (16)	1.03
2	7/24 (29)	(0.51–2.07)
≥ 3	5/11 (45)	
Kaplan–Feinstein grade		
None	7/101 (7)	
Intermediate	24/134 (18)	0.97
Severe	8/17 (47)	(0.51–1.86)

*Percentage rate in parentheses. [†]Range in parentheses. (From ref. 138 with permission.)

Table 31.12. *Cause of death among 13 700 prostatectomy patients who died between 1977 and 1987 according to age and surgical approach (RR TURP/OPSU)*

Cause of death	Age of patient (years)		
	55–64	65–74	75–99
Malignancies	0.98	0.97	0.99
Total cardiovascular	0.89	0.96	0.98
Acute MI	0.88	0.96	0.89
Heart disease	0.87	0.97	0.99
Cerebrovascular accident	1.05	1.09	1.13
Other vascular	0.82	0.91	1.05
Total respiratory	1.44	1.24	1.11
Pneumonia	0.91	0.81	1.03
COPD	1.70	1.59	1.19
Other respiratory	1.29	1.18	1.11
Urological	0.79	0.81	0.80
Other causes	1.23	1.14	1.12

COPD, chronic obstructive pulmonary disease; MI, myocardial infarction. (From ref. 141 with permission.)

Taylor and Krakauer[134] analysed data from a pilot project undertaken by the Health Care Finance Administration and seven peer review organizations, and found a co-morbidity-adjusted RR of mortality at 2 years following TURP/OPSU of 1.68 (95% CI 0.89–3.17). However, this increased risk associated with undergoing TURP was not statistically significant in the analysis controlling for other variables associated with mortality. The most important predictors of mortality following prostatectomy were a history of metastasis from cancer (RR 5.74), congestive heart failure (RR 3.56), cancer (RR 3.15), renal insufficiency indicated by elevated blood urea nitrogen (RR 2.75), serum albumin of less than 3 mg% (RR 2.69), atrial fibrillation (RR 2.33), lung infiltrates (RR 2.22), COPD (RR 2.17) and a history of diabetes (RR 2.04). In the subsample of 2449 TURP patients and 168 OPSU patients with a histological diagnosis of BPH, the cumulative probability of mortality at 2 years was 14.31% (TURP) and 7.09% (OPSU).

Hooten et al.[142] drew from a large database of 2005 men who entered a urological health screening programme a sample of 25 men who underwent TURP and a group of 50 age-matched control men with symptoms of prostatism. Patients were followed for 6 years. There were four deaths (16%) in the 25 TURP patients, while there were five deaths (10%) in the 50 control men. Although TURP did account for a significant amount of the variability of survival after 5 years of follow-up, a far greater proportion of the variance in survival was explained by other variables such as age, preoperative risk factors, co-morbidity factors and postoperative urinary disease. The authors conclude that the negative effect of TURP on survival, noticeable after 5 years of follow-up, makes a cause–effect relationship appear to be only speculative.

Sidney et al.[143] assessed the incidence of re-operation and mortality after TURP and open prostatectomy in 8219 men in the Kaiser Permanente Medical Care Program, Northern California Region. The vast majority (7771, or 94.5%) received TURP. Of the open prostatectomies, 211 (49%) were done suprapubically and 138 (31%) retropubically. In 89 (20%) the technique was not known. The age-adjusted RR of dying (TURP/OPSU) was most pronounced during the first 5 years after surgery (RR 1.8, 95% CI 1.3–2.5), and declined to 1.1 (95% CI 0.8–1.6) for deaths occurring after the first 5 years. The authors did not attempt a formal adjustment for co-morbidity in this population.

The RR ratios for 5-year mortality following TURP/OPSU, from those four studies that include some attempt to adjust for co-morbidity, were combined using the hierarchical Bayes formula (FAST*PRO). Table 31.13 reflects the RR and 95% CI for the individual studies and the combined RR. The study by Sidney et al.[143] did not attempt co-morbidity adjustment. On including the results of this study, the combined RR of dying (TURP/OPSU) increases to 1.34 (95% CI 0.98–1.83). On including the study by Meyhoff,[144] without age or co-morbidity adjustment, the RR of dying (TURP/OPSU) increases to 1.4 (95% CI 0.85–2.33).

On the basis of the data available, it appears that, despite an attempt to correct for age and co-morbidities, there remains a concern that the RR of dying following TURP is greater than that following open surgery for BPH. Only one study found no increased risk for TURP over OPSU after adjusting by means of several co-morbidity indices. The impact of adjusting for age appeared clear in all studies; however, the impact of a co-morbidity adjustment was not noticed by all

Table 31.13. *Relative risk and 95% CI of 5-year mortality following TURP and OPSU for four individual studies and combined analysis*

Reference no.	Source, adjustments	RR and 95% CI
138	Yale-New Haven Hospital Co-morbidity (Kaplan–Feinstein), age Chart review data	0.91 (0.47–1.76)
141	Male Danish population Co-morbidity, age Database data	1.19 (1.15–1.24)
78	Subset from University Hospital Co-morbidity Database data	1.45 (1.15–1.83)
136	Subset from Health Science Center, Winnipeg Co-morbidity (Charlson), age Chart review data	1.48 (1.09–2.01)
Combined	Hierarchical Bayes	1.26 (0.99–1.59)

investigators. All studies presented are based on a retrospective review of either administrative databases or medical records, or on data collected prospectively to answer other research questions. Administrative databases are created and maintained with purposes in mind that differ greatly from the retrospective assessment of the risk of dying following certain interventions. Furthermore, entries in medical records are not meant to be used for such data analysis. Rather, entries into medical records by surgeons and anaesthetists reflect the thoughts of the attending physician at the time of entry as to whether the patient in question can withstand a certain procedure with its associated risk. The assessment of the magnitude of the risk varies from physician to physician. Consequently, the entries may be more (or less) complete, depending on the perceived seriousness of the intervention (bias in favour of reporting co-morbidity in OPSU patients) and opinion among specialists as to the risk involved with the procedure (bias in favour of reporting co-morbidity in OPSU patients). The studies using a detailed review of medical records, rather than databases, do not come to the same conclusions, but differ in their assessment of the adjusted RR of dying. Whether this is due to differences in the patient population at the various

hospitals, the methods and thoroughness of abstracting, or other unidentified factors, is unknown. It is interesting, however, that the type of hospital may have an impact on the risk of dying. Wennberg et al.[98] found no difference in mortality rates between TURP and OPSU in teaching hospitals, and concerns have been raised that possibly the surgeons in some of the geographic regions from which patients were analysed were more familiar with one type of surgery than another. Another factor that may have to be taken into account was pointed out by Adell and Grabe.[145] In a 7-year follow-up study of 189 men after TURP, they found that preoperative treatment with an indwelling catheter (for urinary retention) was associated with a RR of 2.0 ($p=0.06$) of dying in the follow-up period, while age (more than, or less than, 70 years) was associated with an even greater RR of 3.3 ($p<0.001$) (Cox proportional hazard multivariate analysis of survival). It appears that most retrospective studies utilizing databases did not include the use of information on retention and indwelling catheters. The cumulative probability of dying within 8 years after TURP was clearly higher in the Oxford region (49.49%) than in Manitoba (39.25%).[78] On the basis of the differences in the health-care systems in both countries during the observation period, it is quite likely that more patients were treated while in retention and wearing an indwelling catheter in England than in Manitoba. As it is not known to what degree the presence or absence of an indwelling catheter influences survival after OPSU, no firm conclusion can be drawn regarding this variable. Another important observation is that although the magnitude of the effect was similar in the various studies, the main cause leading to the increased mortality was vastly different: in the Roos study the excess mortality was due to cardiovascular causes, mainly acute myocardial infarction, whereas in the Andersen study it was due to respiratory problems.

The lack of a consistent difference in specific causes of death among men exposed to TURP and open prostatectomy raises serious questions about the biological plausibility of the finding. It is clear that no retrospective study can match the thoroughness of data collection in a prospective study;[134] accordingly, several investigators have taken the position that the evidence demands the initiation of such a prospective study.[134,136]

Faced with the immediate dilemma of explaining the seemingly implausible fact that patients treated with TURP run a greater long-term risk of dying than those treated with open surgery for BPH, investigators have developed an interest in some of the basic pathophysiological reactions to TURP. The following discussion focuses on those aspects of TURP that are unique to the procedure itself and that might conceivably explain the observed long-term mortality difference. These aspects are (1) hypothermia occurring during TURP, (2) a combination of blood loss and/or circulatory overload due to absorption of irrigation fluid and the effect on cardiovascular performance, (3) haemolysis induced by certain irrigants, (4) other systemic effects induced by the absorption of certain irrigants, (5) metabolic effects exerted by absorbed irrigant, and (6) effects attributable to the lithotomy position.

Hypothermia during TURP has received little attention in the literature. Allen altered the temperature of the irrigation fluid from 68 to 100°F in 60 patients and documented a progressively lower body temperature in all patients except those in whom the fluid was kept close to body temperature.[146] Carpenter monitored rectal temperatures in 16 men before and at least 6 h after TURP and showed a decrease to a mean nadir of 96°F (35.6°C) at 3 h after surgery. The cardiovascular system is particularly sensitive to hypothermia, and certain electrocardiograph (ECG) changes pathognomonic for hypothermia may occur at 35.6°C that are known to precede ventricular fibrillation. If shivering occurred to compensate for heat loss, it would increase oxygen consumption significantly, again putting the cardiovascular system at additional risk; however, in most cases the use either of muscle relaxants or of a spinal block will abolish the ability to shiver and therefore will aggravate the hypothermia.

It is beyond the scope of this discussion to explore the vast body of literature dealing with the issue of fluid absorption during TURP and its impact on haemolysis, cardiovascular changes, TURP syndrome and mortality. The use of sterilized water has, in most countries, been replaced by the use of isotonic irrigation fluids, thus reducing the risk of haemolysis due to the absorption of hypotonic solutions. The irrigation fluids currently used contain sugars such as glycine, sorbitol or mannitol in varying concentrations. The amount of fluid absorbed depends on the experience of the resectionist, the duration of time of the resection, the hydrostatic pressure of the irrigation fluid and the presence or absence of any surgically induced capsular perforation or opened venous sinuses. A modern technique to measure absorption of fluid is to tag it with 1% ethanol and measure the ethanol concentration in the expired breath. Using this method, two investigators found vastly different amounts of fluid absorbed in similar patient populations. Hahn[147] studied 70 patients, in whom a mean of 29 g tissue was resected in an average of 51 min (range 20–135 min); blood loss averaged 490 ml; fluid absorption averaged 1300 ml (range 200–4300 ml). On the other hand, Hultén[148] described 20 men (duration of surgery 42±15 min, prostate weight 31±21 g, blood loss 555±483 ml) with an average absorption of only 552±460 ml. The impact of the choice of the irrigation fluid on short-term outcome is evident from an old study by Emmett et al.[149] After these investigators had switched from the use of water to that of a non-haemolytic isotonic irrigation fluid, the rate of mortality following TURP at the Mayo Clinic dropped from about 1.0% to less than 0.5%. Although in most countries isotonic non-haemolytic solutions (mannitol, sorbitol, glycine) are used during TURP, in some institutions sterile water may still be in use. Whether choice of irrigation fluid has a role in the long-term mortality of TURP versus OPSU is unknown, as the studies available did not report on this factor.

In an early study Mebust et al.[150] reported that 90% of patients (n = 30) experienced a decrease in cardiac output by a mean of 17.5% during TURP. De Angelis et al.[151] observed haemodynamic changes occurring in an unpredictable fashion in nine men during TURP. Pulmonary capillary wedge pressure increased in four of the nine patients, and was not always indicated by an increase in central venous pressure. Systemic vascular resistance decreased significantly in six cases. Evans et al.[152] studied haemodynamic changes during routine TURP. They noted that heart rate and stroke volume fell progressively over the first 30 min of surgery, resulting in a steady-state reduction in cardiac output over time. At the same time, a significant increase in left ventricular afterload was noted. The authors interpreted these findings as demonstrating the occurrence during TURP of haemodynamic responses not detectable by conventional monitoring methodology. In particular, the increased left ventricular afterload indicates increased myocardial workload and oxygen demand, possibly resulting in myocardial ischaemia. Overall, these effects may be part of a link with the increased cardiovascular morbidity and mortality observed following TURP. In this study, the cardiac risk index was assessed using the Goldman Classification and a standardized anaesthetic technique, including intubation and intermittent positive pressure ventilation, was used. For the actual procedure, intermittent irrigation using a 1.5% glycine solution at room temperature, delivered through a fast-flow glass set from a reservoir at 60 cm above the pubic symphysis, was utilized. Beyond the usual monitoring, total fluid balance was determined by a system of transducers placed under the operating table to give a continuous read-out of the weight of the patient and the operating table (accuracy ± 50 g at a load of 275 kg). Haemodynamic data were obtained with an oesophageal Doppler ultrasound transducer. Mannitol blood pressure and Doppler wave parameters were recorded throughout the procedure at 10 min intervals. The average age of the ten patients in the study was 68 ± 3.5 years, and the average cardiac risk index was 4.6 ± 1.7. The resected prostate weight averaged 22 ± 2.5 kg, the duration of the procedure was 40 ± 2.7 min, average blood loss was 203 ± 39 ml, and fluid load averaged 856 ± 492 ml. During the procedure, the heart rate decreased by an average of 8.5 ± 4.5%. The minute distance (the product of the stroke distance and the heart rate, representing a linear index of cardiac output) decreased by 29 ± 2.6%, and systemic vascular resistance increased by 47 ± 6.4%. No relationship was detected between the magnitude of the haemodynamic changes and either the surgeon, the age of the patients, the resected prostate weight, the length of the operation, the estimated blood loss or the load of irrigation fluid. The authors speculate that among the factors contributing to the unexpected haemodynamic responses during TURP were the irrigation fluid absorption, haemorrhage, the use of anaesthetic agents, the absorption of glycine, hyperammonaemia, sympathetic responses to the surgery, or the response to heat loss. In a follow-up controlled study, the same group of authors compared haemodynamic parameters in 20 men undergoing TURP with those in eight men undergoing hernia repair and five men who underwent testicular exploration.[153] Mean arterial pressure fell in the 13 control patients by 11% (95% CI 5–17), whereas in the TURP patients it increased by 16% (95% CI 5–27). In the TURP patients, cardiac output fell by 21% (95% CI 10–32), and the index of systemic vascular resistance increased by 46.8% (95% CI 28–66) at the end of the TURP. All parameters observed differed statistically between the controls and the TURP patients (arterial pressure: $p<0.5$; cardiac output: $p<0.005$; systemic vascular resistance: $p<0.0005$). The authors speculate that these responses may be due to the rapid central cooling observed during TURP (core temperature fell by a mean of 0.8 (0.6–1.0)°C.

Bearing in mind these considerable haemodynamic effects occurring during TURP, it is of interest to review a study by Ashton et al.[154] These authors obtained ECGs preoperatively and on the first three postoperative days in 206 men undergoing TURP. The occurrence of cardiac events was monitored and assessed by measurement of creatinine kinase isoenzymes during the first three postoperative days, and by review of the entire clinical course. Although 21% of patients developed postoperative ECG changes, mostly involving the T-wave, none had cardiac symptoms or sustained creatinine kinase isoenzyme elevation. The changes were not significantly more common in men known to have coronary disease. In the one patient who suffered a perioperative myocardial infarction, no ECG changes were noted. Only one of the 21% of patients who had postoperative ECG changes had a cardiac event in the year after surgery. This low likelihood of a cardiac event, in only one of 44 patients followed throughout the 12 months after TURP, provided empirical evidence of the limited clinical significance of the ECG changes commonly seen in patients undergoing this procedure. In view of the finding of increased delayed mortality following TURP, this report is of interest in that it documents a high frequency of ECG changes (21%) that not do seem to have any consequences in the year following surgery.

Several reports that might possibly shed some light on the puzzling delayed mortality effect examine the effects of glycine, a commonly used irrigant. Glycine acts as an inhibitory neurotransmitter in the spinal cord, brain stem and central nervous system.[155] Investigators have documented visual aberrations during or following TURP as a result of the absorption of glycine resulting from its specific role as an inhibitory neurotransmitter in the retina.[156–158] The same group of investigators also demonstrated significant haemodynamic responses to glycine infusion in dogs.[158] Although immediate cardiac output increased and systemic vascular resistance and mean arterial pressure decreased, later both cardiac output and mean arterial pressure decreased significantly, while systemic vascular resistance returned to normal. In a study in human subjects, seven healthy volunteers received an intravenous infusion of 1 l of 2.2% (isosmotic) glycine over 20 min.[159] This infusion elicited a significant increase in the plasma vasopressin level, by 60% (±13%) above the baseline level. Only in the patient who developed signs of glycine toxicity, however, did the serum cortisol level increase. The results of the study may be interpreted as showing that a glycine solution has water-retaining properties by stimulation of vasopressin secretion, but usually not by increasing the cortisol secretion. The same authors had previously reported that during transurethral prostatic surgery, the secretion of vasopressin and cortisol increased once the irrigant solution containing glycine had been taken up into the circulation through severed prostatic veins.[160,161] However, in the clinical study of TURP in which an increase in the serum cortisol level was reported, glycine absorption was, on average, 30% greater than the amount of glycine given by intravenous infusion in the experimental study. It is possible, therefore, that either the litre of isomorphic glycine solution infused was insufficient to elicit the effect in these healthy volunteers, or that effects occurring during TURP other than the infusion of glycine cause the stimulation of cortisol secretion. What remains, however, is the fact that a stress-related hormone —namely, cortisol — increases during TURP, whether because of the absorption of irrigant fluid containing glycine or through some other mechanism. It is evident that a significant increase in the plasma level of this hormone might affect the cardiovascular system, thus being partially responsible for the haemodynamic changes observed .

Although, overall, none of the studies discussed convincingly explain the increased risk of mortality following TURP over OPSU they do underline some of the unique features associated with transurethral resection versus open surgical enucleation of the prostate. It is apparent that the awareness level has increased and much more attention is paid to these aspects of prostate surgery. There will probably be a number of investigations attempting to address these issues in a scientific and systematic fashion, which may help to explain the retrospective findings. Meanwhile, it is evident that there is a possibility that features unique to TURP that are not captured in either administrative databases or during chart reviews may have an important role, if there is really an increased risk of long-term mortality following this procedure. Unmeasured co-morbidity among TURP patients, however, still seems the most likely explanation for these findings. Prospective studies may, indeed, be the only way to settle this question.

References

1. Bellfield W T. Operations on the enlarged prostate with a tabulated summary of cases. Am J Med Sci 1890; 100: 439
2. Fuller E. Six successful and successive cases of prostatectomy. J Cutan Genitourin Dis 1895; 13: 229
3. Freyer P. A new method of performing prostatectomy. Lancet 1900; 1: 774
4. Millin T. Retropubic prostatectomy: new extravesical technique. Report on 20 cases. Lancet 1945; 2: 693
5. Millin T. Retropubic prostatectomy. J Urol 1948; 59: 267–274
6. Nesbit R M. A history of transurethral prostatectomy. Rev Mex Urol 1975; 35: 349–62
7. Iglesias J J, Sporer A, Gellman A C. New Iglesias resectoscope with continuous irrigation, simultaneous suction and low intravesical pressure. J Urol 1975; 114: 929–933
8. Edwards L E, Bucknall T E, Pittam M R et al. Transurethral resection of the prostate and bladder neck incision: a review of 700 cases. Br J Urol 1985; 57: 168–171
9. Hedlund H, Ek A. Ejaculation and sexual function after endoscopic bladder neck incision. Br J Urol 1985; 57: 164–167
10. Keitzer W A, Chervantes L, Demaculang A. Transurethral incision of bladder neck for contracture. J Urol 1961; 86: 242
11. Orandi A. Transurethral incision of the prostate. J Urol 1973; 110: 229–231
12. Holtgrewe H L, Mebust W K, Dowd J B et al. Transurethral prostatectomy: practice aspects of the dominant operation in American urology. J Urol 1989; 141: 248–253
13. McConnell J D, Barry M J, Bruskewitz R C et al. Benign prostatic hyperplasia: diagnosis and treatment. Clinical Practice Guideline, Number 8. Rockville, Md: Agency for Health Care Policy and Research, Public Health Service, US Department of Health and Human Services, 1994
14. Cockett A T K, Aso Y, Denis L et al. Recommendations of the International Consensus Committee. In: Cockett A T K, Khoury S, Aso Y et al. (eds) The 2nd International Consultation on Benign Prostatic Hyperplasia (BPH). Jersey, Channel Islands: SCI, 1993: 553–564

15. Mebust W K, Holtgrewe H L, Cockett A T K, Peters P C. Transurethral prostatectomy: immediate and postoperative complications. A cooperative study of 13 participating institutions evaluating 3885 patients. J Urol 1989; 141: 243–247

16. Cockett A T K, Khoury S, Aso Y et al. The 2nd International Consultation on Benign Prostatic Hyperplasia (BPH). Jersey, Channel Islands: SCI, 1993.

17. McGowan S, Smith G. Anaesthesia for transurethral prostatectomy: a comparison of spinal introduced anaesthesia with two methods of general anaesthesia. Anesth Analg 1980; 35: 847

18. Nielson K, Anderson K, Asbjorn J. Blood loss in transurethral prostatectomy: epidural versus general anaesthesia. Int Urol Nephrol 1987; 19: 287

19. Moffat N A. Transurethral prostatic resections under local anaesthesia. J Urol 1977; 118: 607–608

20. Sinha B, Haikel G, Lange P H et al. Transurethral resection of the prostate with local anaesthesia in 100 patients. J Urol 1986; 135: 719–721

21. Birch B R, Gelister J S, Parker C J et al. Transurethral resection of prostate under sedation and local anaesthesia (Sedoanalgesia). Urology 1991; 38: 113–118

22. Graversen P H, Gasser T C, Larsen E H et al. Transurethral incisions of the prostate under local anaesthesia in high-risk patients: a pilot study. Scand J Urol Nephrol Suppl 1987; 104: 87–90

23. Loughlin K R, Yalla S V, Belldegrun A. Transurethral incisions and resections under local anaesthesia. Br J Urol 1987; 60: 185

24. Orandi A. Urological endoscopic surgery under local anaesthesia: a cost reducing idea. J Urol 1984: 132: 1146–1147

25. Hugosson J, Bergdahl S, Norlen L, Ortengren T. Outpatient transurethral incision of the prostate under local anaesthesia: operative results, patient security and cost effectiveness. Scand J Urol Nephrol 1993; 27: 381–385

26. Riehman M, Bruskewitz R C. Transurethral incision of the prostate and the bladder neck. J Androl 1991; 12: 415

27. Nesbit R M. Transurethral prostatic resection. In: Campbell L, Harrison J (eds) Urology. Philadelphia: Saunders, 1970: 2479

28. Mebust W K. Transurethral resection of the prostate and transurethral incision of the prostate. In: Lepor H, Lawson R K (eds) Prostate diseases. Philadelphia: Saunders, 1993: 150–163

29. Nesbit R M. Transurethral prostatectomy. Springfield: C. C. Thomas, 1943

30. Kulb T B, Kamer N, Lingeman J E, Foster R S. Prevention of postprostatectomy vesical neck contracture by prophylactic vesical neck incision. J Urol 1987; 137: 230–231

31. Mebust W K, Foret J D, Valk W L. Transurethral surgery. In: Harrison JH, Walsh PC, Perlmutter AD et al. (eds) Campbell's urology. Philadelphia: Saunders, 1979: 2361–2381

32. Eddy D M. Clinical decision making: from theory to practice. Comparing benefits and harms: the balance sheet. JAMA 1990; 263: 2493–2505

33. Lich R. Retropubic prostatectomy: a review of 678 patients. J Urol 1954; 72: 434–438

34. Taylor W N, Kaylor W M, Taylor J N. Retropubic and suprapubic prostatectomy: comparative clinical study. J Urol 1955; 74: 129–131

35. Blue G D, Campbell J M. A clinical review of one thousand consecutive cases of retropubic prostatectomy. J Urol 1958; 80: 257–259

36. Salvaris M. Retropubic prostatectomy: an evaluation of 1200 operations. Med J Aust 1960; 370–376

37. Macky W. Hryntschak prostatectomy: experiences with 300 consecutive cases. Br J Urol 1961; 33: 19–23

38. Stearns D B. Retropubic prostatectomy, 1947–1960: a critical evaluation. J Urol 1961; 85: 322–328

39. Lenko J, Cieslinski S. Millin's retropubic prostatectomy: report of 233 cases. Br J Urol 1965; 37: 450–454

40. Beck A D. Benign prostatic hypertrophy and uraemia. A review of 315 cases. Br J Surg 1970; 57: 561–565

41. Beck A D, Gaudin H J. The Hryntschak prostatectomy. 3. A modified technique of closing the vesical neck and prostatic cavity. J Urol 1970; 104: 739–744

42. Beck A D The Hryntschak procedure: II. A late review of 179 cases. J Urol 1970; 103: 778–782

43. Beck A D, Gaudin H J. The Hryntschak prostatectomy. I. A review of 1326 cases. J Urol 1970; 103: 637–640

44. Arvola I, Lilius H G. Transvesical prostatectomy a.m. Hryntschak. Ann Chir Gynaecol Fenn 1972; 61: 74–78

45. Singh B, Singh B, Singh J. Modified suprapubic prostatectomy (a report of 30 cases). J Indian Med Assoc 1974; 63: 392–395

46. Bollmann J, Zingg E. Retropubic prostatectomy. Prog Clin Biol Res 1976; 6: 59–65

47. Lund B L, Dingsor E. Benign obstructive prostatic enlargement. A comparison between the results of treatment by transurethral electro-resection and the results of open surgery. Scand J Urol Nephrol 1976; 10: 33–38

48. Hohenfellner R. Suprapubic prostatectomy. Prog Clin Biol Res 1976; 6: 49–57

49. Lenko J. Millin's retropubic prostatectomy. A clinical study. Int Urol Nephrol 1977; 9: 25–32

50. Nicoll G A, Riffle G N, Anderson F O. Suprapubic prostatectomy. The removable purse string: a continuing comparative analysis of 300 consecutive cases. J Urol 1978; 120: 702–704

51. Davillas N E, Miliaresis A, Katsoulis A, Katatigiotis S. Observations on 1,000 Millin prostatectomies. Eur Urol 1978; 4: 100–102

52. Gregoir W. Haemostatic prostatic adenomectomy. Eur Urol 1978; 4: 1–8

53. Ball A J, Smith P J. The long-term effects of prostatectomy: a uroflowmetric analysis. J Urol 1982; 128: 538–540

54. Ball A J, Powell H. Prostatectomy trends in the Bristol area. Br J Urol 1982; 54: 539–541

55. Meyhoff H H, Nordling J, Hald T. Urodynamic evaluation of transurethral versus transvesical prostatectomy. A randomized study. Scand J Urol Nephrol 1984; 18: 27–35

56. Meyhoff H H, Nordling J, Hald T. Clinical evaluation of transurethral versus transvesical prostatectomy. A randomized study. Scand J Urol Nephrol 1984; 18: 201–209

57. Magasi P, Vegh A. One thousand cases of prostatectomy. Acta Chir Hung 1984; 25: 63–74

58. Meyhoff H H, Nordling J, Hald T. Transurethral versus transvesical prostatectomy. Physiological strain. Scand J Urol Nephrol 1985; 19: 85–91

59. Lesiewicz H, Cieslinski S. Millin's retropubic prostatectomy: a clinical study. Int Urol Nephrol 1985: 17: 341–348

60. Meyhoff H H, Nordling J. Long term results of transurethral and transvesical prostatectomy. A randomized study. Scand J Urol Nephrol 1986; 20: 27–33

61. Roos N P, Ramsey E W. A population based study of prostatectomy: outcomes associated with differing surgical approaches. J Urol 1987; 137: 1184–1188

62. Aalkjer V. Transurethral resection/prostatectomy versus dilatation treatment in hypertrophy of the prostate II. Urol Int 1965; 20: 17–22

63. Singh M, Tresidder G C, Blandy J P. The evaluation of transurethral resection for benign enlargement of the prostate. Br J Urol 1973; 45: 93–102

64. Melchior J, Valk W L, Foret J D, Mebust W K. Transurethral prostatectomy: computerized analysis of 2,223 consecutive cases. J Urol 1974; 112: 634

65. Melchior J, Valk W L, Foret J D, Mebust W K. Transurethral prostatectomy and epididymitis. J Urol 1974; 112: 647–650

66. Melchior J, Valk W L, Foret J D, Mebust W K. Transurethral prostatectomy in the azotemic patient. J Urol 1974; 112: 643–647

67. Lentz H C, Mebust W K, Foret J D, Melchior J. Urethral strictures following transurethral prostatectomy: review of 2223 resections. J Urol 1977; 117: 194–196

68. Abrams P H, Farrar D J, Turner-Warwick R T et al. The results of prostatectomy: a symptomatic and urodynamic analysis of 152 patients. J Urol 1979; 121: 640–642

69. Chilton C P, Morgan R J, England H R et al. A critical evaluation of the results of transurethral resection of the prostate. Br J Urol 1978; 50: 542–546

70. Bruskewitz R C, Larsen E H, Madsen P O, Dorflinger T. 3-year followup of urinary symptoms after transurethral resection of the prostate. J Urol 1986; 136: 613–615

71. Hellström P, Lukkarinen O, Kontturi M. Bladder neck incision or transurethral electroresection for the treatment of urinary obstruction caused by a small benign prostate? A randomized urodynamic study. Scand J Urol Nephrol 1986; 20: 187–192

72. Larsen E H, Dorflinger T, Gasser TC et al. Transurethral incision versus transurethral resection of the prostate for the treatment of benign prostatic hypertrophy. A preliminary report. Scand J Urol Nephrol Suppl 1987; 104: 83–86

73. Dorflinger R, Oster M, Larsen J F et al. Transurethral prostatectomy or incision of the prostate in the treatment of prostatism caused by small benign prostates. Scand J Urol Nephrol Suppl 1987; 104: 77–81

74. Li M K, Ng A S. Bladder neck resection and transurethral resection of the prostate: a randomized prospective trial. J Urol 1987; 138: 807–809

75. Kadow C, Feneley R C, Abrams PH. Prostatectomy or conservative management in the treatment of benign prostatic hypertrophy? Br J Urol 1988; 61: 432–434

76. Nielsen H O. Transurethral prostatotomy versus transurethral prostatectomy in benign prostatic hypertrophy. A prospective randomised study. Br J Urol 1988; 61: 435–438

77. Malone P R, Cook A, Edmonson R et al. Prostatectomy: patients perception of long-term follow up. Br J Urol 1988; 61: 234–238

78. Roos N P, Wennberg J E, Malenka D J et al. Mortality and reoperation after open and transurethral resection of the prostate for benign prostatic hyperplasia. N Engl J Med 1989; 320: 1120–1124

79. Bandhauer K. Transurethral prostatectomy — complications. New Dev Biosci 1989; 5: 81–87

80. D'Ancona C A L, Netto N R Jr, Cara A M, Ikari O. Internal urethrotomy of the prostatic urethra or transurethral resection in benign prostatic hyperplasia. J Urol 1990; 144: 918–920

81. Lepor H, Rigaud G. The efficacy of transurethral resection of the prostate in men with moderate symptoms of prostatism. J Urol 1990; 143: 533–537

82. Delaere K P J, Debruyne F M J, Moonen W A. Extended bladder neck incision for outflow obstruction in male patients. Br J Urol 1983; 55: 225–228

83. Orandi A. Transurethral incision of prostate (TUIP): 646 cases in 15 years — a chronological appraisal. Br J Urol 1985; 57: 703–707

84. Orandi A. Transurethral incision of prostate compared with transurethral resection of prostate in 132 matching cases. J Urol 1987; 138: 810–815

85. Mobb G E, Moisey C U. Longterm follow-up of unilateral bladder neck incision. Br J Urol 1988; 62: 160–162

86. Kelly M J, Roskamp D, Leach G E. Transurethral incision of the prostate: a preoperative and postoperative analysis of symptoms and urodynamic findings. J Urol 1989; 142: 1507–1509

87. Katz P G, Greenstein A, Ratliff J E et al. Transurethral incision of the bladder neck and prostate. J Urol 1990; 144: 694–696

88. Golomb J, Lindner A, Siegel Y, Korczak D. Variability and circadian changes in home uroflowmetry in patients with benign prostatic hyperplasia compared to normal controls. J Urol 1992; 147: 1044–1047

89. Barry M J, Girman C J, O'Leary M P et al. Using repeated measures of symptom score, uroflowmetry and prostate specific antigen in the clinical management of prostate disease. J Urol 1995; 153: 99–103

90. Grino P B, Bruskewitz R, Blaivas J G et al. Maximum urinary flow rate by uroflowmetry: automatic or visual interpretation. J Urol 1992; 149: 339–341

91. Barry M J, Cockett A T, Holtgrewe H L et al. Relationship of symptoms of prostatism to commonly used physiological and anatomical measures of the severity of benign prostatic hyperplasia. J Urol 1993; 150: 351–358

92. Wasson J H, Reda D J, Bruskewitz R C et al. A comparison of transurethral surgery with watchful waiting for moderate symptoms of benign prostatic hyperplasia. The Veterans Affairs Cooperative Study Group on Transurethral Resection of the Prostate. N Engl J Med 1995; 332: 75–79

93. Riehman M, Knes J M, Heisey D et al. Transurethral resection versus incision of the prostate: a randomized, prospective study. Urology 1995; 45: 768–775

94. Birch N C, Hurst G, Doyle P T. Serial residual urine volumes in men with prostatic hypertrophy. Br J Urol 1988; 62: 571–575

95. Bruskewitz R C, Iversen P, Madsen P O. Value of postvoid residual urine determination in evaluation of prostatism. Urology 1982; 20: 602–604

96. Meier D E, Tarpley J L, Imediegwu O O et al. The outcome of suprapubic prostatectomy: a contemporary series in the developing world. Urology 1995; 46: 40–44

97. Holtgrewe H L, Valk W L. Factors influencing the mortality and morbidity of transurethral prostatectomy: a study of 2015 cases. J Urol 1962; 87: 450–459

98. Wennberg J E, Roos N, Sola L et al. Use of claims data systems to evaluate health care outcomes. JAMA 1987; 257: 933–936

99. Lu-Yao G L, Barry M J, Chang C H et al. Transurethral resection of the prostate among Medicare beneficiaries in the United States: time trends and outcomes. Prostate Patient Outcomes Research Team (PORT) (Review). Urology 1994; 44: 692–698

100. Tinetti M E, Inouye S K, Gill T M, Doucette J T. Shared risk factors for falls, incontinence, and functional dependence. JAMA 1995; 723: 1348–1353

101. Warres H L. Urethral stricture following transurethral resection of the prostate. J Urol 1958; 79: 989–993

102. Emmet J L, Rous S N, Greene L F et al. Preliminary internal urethrotomy in 1036 cases to prevent urethral stricture following transurethral resection; caliber of normal adult male urethra. J Urol 1963; 89: 829–835

103. Lundhus E, Dorflinger T, Moller-Madsen B et al. Significance of the extent of transurethral prostatic resection for postoperative complications. Scand J Urol Nephrol 1987; 21: 9–12

104. Schultz A, Bay-Nielsen H, Bilde T et al. Prevention of urethral stricture formation after TURP: a controlled randomized study of Otis urethrostomy versus urethral dilation and the use of polytetrafluoroethylene coated versus the uninsulated metal sheath. J Urol 1989; 141: 73–75

105. Hammarsten J, Lindqvist K, Sunzel H. Urethral stricture following transurethral resection of the prostate. The role of the catheter. Br J Urol 1989; 63: 397–400

106. Kinsey A C. Sexual behavior in the human male. Philadelphia: Saunders, 1948

107. Finkle A L, Moyers T G, Tobenkin M I. Sexual potency in aging males. I. Frequency of coitus among clinic patients. JAMA 1959; 170: 1391–1393

108. Newman G, Nichols C R. Sexual activities and attitudes in older persons. JAMA 1960; 173: 33–35

109. Bowers L M, Cross R R, Lloyd F A. Sexual function and urologic disease in the elderly male. J Am Geriatr Soc 1963; 11: 647–652

110. Pearlman C K, Kobashi L I. Frequency of intercourse in men. J Urol 1972; 107: 298–301

111. Dahlen C P, Goodwin W E. Sexual potency after perineal biopsy. J Urol 1957; 77: 660–669

112. Finkle A I, Moyers T G. Sexual potency in aging males: IV. Status of private patients before and after prostatectomy. J Urol 1960; 84: 152–157

113. Finkle A L, Prian D V. Sexual potency in elderly men before and after prostatectomy. JAMA 1966; 196: 125–129

114. Finkle A L, Moyers T G. Sexual potency in aging males: V. Coital ability following open perineal prostatic biopsy. J Urol 1960; 84: 649–653

115. Freeman J T. Sexual capacities in the aging male. Geriatrics 1961; 16: 37–43

116. Gold F G, Hotchkiss R S. Sexual potency following simple prostatectomy. N Y State J Med 1969; 69: 2987–2989

117. De Nicola P, Peruzza M. Sex in the aged. J Am Geriatr Soc 1974; 22: 380–382

118. Windle R, Roberts J B M. Ejaculatory function after prostatectomy. Proc R Soc Med 1974; 67: 1160–1162

119. Finkle J E, Finkle P S, Finkle A L. Encouraging preservation of sexual function postprostatectomy. Urology 1975; 6: 697–702

120. Madorsky M L, Ashamalla M G, Schussler I et al. Post-prostatectomy impotence. J Urol 1976; 115: 401–403

121. Zohar, Meiraz D, Maoz B, Durst N. Factors influencing sexual activity after prostatectomy: a prospective study. J Urol 1976; 116: 332–334

122. DeBacker E, Lauwerijns A, Willem C. Sexual behavior after prostatectomy. Eur Urol 1977; 3: 295–298

123. Hargreave T B, Stephenson T P. Potency and prostatectomy. Br J Urol 1977; 49: 683–688

124. Hauri D. Life after prostatectomy. Urol Int 1982; 37: 271–276

125. Moller Nielsen C, Lundhus E, Moller-Madsen B et al. Sexual life following 'minimal' and 'total' transurethral prostatic resection. Urol Int 1985; 40: 3–4

126. Bolt J W, Evans C, Marshall V R. Sexual dysfunction after prostatectomy. Br J Urol 1986; 58: 319–322

127. Libman E, Fichten C S, Prostatectomy and sexual function (Review). Urology 1987; 29: 467–478

128. Vereecken R L. Sexual activity of men presenting with prostatism: effect of prostatectomy. Eur Urol 1989; 16: 328–332

129. Lindner A, Golomb J, Korzcak D et al. Effects of prostatectomy on sexual function. Urology 1991; ???

130. Libman E, Fichten C S, Creti L et al. Transurethral prostatectomy: differential effects of age category and presurgery sexual functioning on postprostatectomy sexual adjustment. J Behav Med 1989; 12: 469–485

131. Orandi A. A new method for treating prostatic hypertrophy. Geriatrics 1978; 33: 58–60, 64–65

132. Orandi A. Transurethral incision of prostate. Seven year follow-up. Urology 1978; 12: 187–189

133. Orandi A. Transurethral resection versus transurethral incision of the prostate. Urol Clin North Am 1990; 17: 601–612

134. Taylor Z, Krakauer H. Mortality and reoperation following prostatectomy: outcomes in a Medicare population. Urology 1991; 38: 27–31

135. Stephenson W P, Chute C G, Guess H A et al. Incidence and outcome of surgery for benign prostatic hyperplasia among residents of Rochester, Minnesota: 1980–87. Urology 1991; 38: 32–42

136. Malenka D J, Roos N, Fisher ES et al. Further study of the increased mortality following transurethral prostatectomy: a chart-based analysis. J Urol 1990; 144: 224–228

137. Charlson M E, Pompei P, Ales K L, MacKenzie C R. A new method of classifying prognostic co-morbidity in longitudinal studies: development and validation. J Chronic Dis 1987; 40: 373–383

138. Concato J, Horwitz R I, Feinstein A R et al. Problems of comorbidity in mortality after prostatectomy. JAMA 1992; 267: 1077–1082

139. Kaplan M H, Feinstein A R. The importance of classifying initial co-morbidity in evaluating the outcome of diabetes mellitus. J Chronic Dis 1974; 27: 387–404

140. Le Duc A, Cariou G, Baron C et al. A multicenter, double-blind, placebo-controlled trial of the efficacy of prazosin in the treatment of dysuria associated with benign prostatic hypertrophy. Urol Int 1990; 45 (suppl 1): 56–62

141. Folmer Andersen T, Bronnum-Hansen H, Sejr T, Roepstorff C. Elevated mortality following transurethral resection of the prostate for benign hypertrophy! But why? Med Care 1990; 28: 870–879

142. Hooten M E, Finnstuen K, Thompson I M. Multivariate case–control study of survival following transurethral resection of the prostate. Urology 1992; 39: 111–116

143. Sidney S, Quesenberry C P, Sadler M C et al. Reoperation and mortality after surgical treatment of benign prostatic hypertrophy in a large prepaid medical care program. Med Care 1992; 30: 117–125

144. Meyhoff H H. Transurethral versus transvesical prostatectomy. Clinical, urodynamic, renographic and economic aspects. A randomized study. Scand J Urol Nephrol Suppl 1987; 102: 1–26

145. Adell L, Grabe M. Long term survival after transurethral resection of the prostate — influence of preoperative bacteriuria and indwelling catheter treatment on late mortality. Scand J Urol Nephrol 1991; 25: 9–13

146. Allen T D. Body temperature changes during prostatic resection as related to the temperature of the irrigating solution. J Urol 1973; 110: 433–435

147. Hahn R G. Blood ammonia concentrations resulting from absorption of irrigating fluid containing glycine and ethanol during transurethral resection of the prostate. Scand J Urol Nephrol 1991; 25: 115–119

148. Hultén J, Sarma V J, Hjertberg H, Palmquist B. Monitoring of irrigating fluid absorption during transurethral prostatectomy. Anaesthesia 1991; 46: 349–353

149. Emmett J L, Gilbaugh J H, McLean P. Fluid absorption during transurethral resection: comparison of mortality and morbidity after irrigation with water and non-hemolytic solutions. J Urol 1969; 101: 884–889

150. Mebust W K, Brady T W, Valk W L. Observations of cardiac output, blood volume, central venous pressure, fluid and electrolyte changes in patients undergoing transurethral prostatectomy. J Urol 1970; 103: 632–636

151. De Angelis J, Chang P, Kaplan J H et al. Hemodynamic changes during prostatectomy in cardiac patients. Crit Care Med 1982; 10: 38–40

152. Evans J W H, Singer M, Chapple C R et al. Haemodynamic evidence for per-operative cardiac stress during transurethral prostatectomy. Br J Urol 1991; 67: 376–380

153. Evans J W H, Singer M, Chapple C R et al. Haemodynamic evidence for cardiac stress during transurethral prostatectomy. Br Med J 1992; 304: 666–671

154. Ashton C M, Thomas J, Wray N P et al. The frequency and significance of ECG changes after transurethral prostate resection. J Am Geriatr Soc 1991; 39: 575–580

155. Pycock C J, Kerwin R W. Minireview. The status of glycine as a supraspinal neurotransmitter. Life Sci 1981; 28: 2679–2686

156. Mantha S, Rao S M, Singh A K et al. Visual evoked potentials and visual acuity after transurethral resection of the prostate. Anaesthesia 1991; 46: 491–493

157. Wang J M, Creel D J, Wong K C. Transurethral resection of the prostate, serum glycine levels, and ocular evoked potentials. Anesthesiology 1989; 70: 36–41

158. Wang J M, Wong K C, Creel D J et al. Effects of glycine on hemodynamic responses and visual evoked potentials in the dog. Anesth Analg 1985; 64: 1071–1077

159. Hahn R G, Stalberg H P, Gustafsson S A. Vasopressin and cortisol levels in response to glycine infusion. Scand J Urol Nephrol 1991; 25: 121–123

160. Hahn R G. Influence of the fluid balance on the cortisol and glucose responses to transurethral prostatic surgery. Acta Anaesthesiol Scand 1989; 33: 638–641

161. Hahn R G, Rundgren M. Vasopressin responses during transurethral resection of the prostate. Br J Anaesth 1989: 330–336

162. Holtgrewe L. The economics of BPH. In: Cockett A T K, Khoury S, Aso Y et al. (eds) The 2nd International Consultation on Benign Prostatic Hyperplasia (BPH). Jersey, Channel Islands: SCI, 1993: 35–45

163. Eddy D M, Hasselblad V. FAST*PRO. Software for meta-analysis by the confidence profile method. San Diego: Academic Press/ Harcourt Brace Jovanovich, 1992

32

Laser prostatectomy
B. S. Stein

Introduction

It has been many years since Malcolm McPhee referred to surgical lasers as 'machines in search of a disease', yet in urology this remained true until the recent upsurge in interest generated by the promise of laser treatment of benign prostatic hyperplasia (BPH).[1] The development of right-angle-delivery fibres enabled the physician to deliver energy that could be aimed directly at the lateral lobes of the prostate. The new fibres promised something for everybody. For the patient, the word 'laser' promised rapid and effective treatment, with no healing time needed and no complications. For the physician, the laser promised a treatment that could be very easily learned, took only about 10 min, and produced a satisfied patient. For third-party payers there was the promise of less expensive therapy for the number two surgical procedure under Medicare reimbursement, namely transurethral resection of the prostate (TURP). Enough experience has now been gained with the laser to separate reality from 'hype' and to decide, like McPhee, whether the laser is still searching for its niche.

Types of lasers

Many types of lasers are currently available (Table 32.1). The laser most widely used to treat BPH (albeit not the ideal laser) is the neodymium:yttrium aluminium garnet (Nd:YAG) laser. The ideal properties of a laser used to treat BPH should include the ability to bring about a high degree of vaporization, so that tissue is removed cleanly at the time of treatment. It should also have the ability to coagulate blood vessels as large as those found in the prostatic fossa. The laser should be able to be passed through thin fibres and should not be significantly absorbed by fluids. The laser wavelength should not be associated with post-treatment oedema and should allow for the bending of the laser energy by 90 degrees.

Table 32.1. *Commercially available lasers*

Carbon dioxide
Argon
KTP
Diode
Holmium
Nd:YAG
Excimer
Pulsed Dye

Types of fibres

Four types of fibre systems have been used to treat the prostate, namely bare fibres, right-angled fibres, contact tips and interstitial fibres. Kandel and associates reported on using the bare fibres to treat the prostate in the canine model.[2] They used 100 W and attempted to vaporize the gland by dragging the fibre through the prostate. This proved to be slow and ineffective and was abandoned. Shanberg reported on a similar technique, used to perform laser transurethral incision of the prostate.[3] He, too, found this to be a slow procedure, and used several fibres per treatment. At about the same time, contact tips were used in an attempt to vaporize prostatic lobes. These initial efforts used sapphire tips to change a coagulating laser into a cutting laser. However, the small size of the tips and the low power that they could tolerate translated into slow treatments of small glands.

The ability to deliver higher-power energy at right angles to tissue increased the interest in using Nd:YAG lasers to treat BPH. The initial fibres that were available included the TULIP and the Bard Urolase. The TULIP is composed of a right-angled fibre within a dilating balloon (and guided by transurethral ultrasound). The Urolase fibre is composed of a bare fibre that ends in an open metal cavity with a prism. This system is used under cystoscopic guidance, leading to the term visual laser-assisted prostatectomy (VLAP). Later VLAP fibres included a bare fibre ending in a plastic-enclosed cavity in which the laser energy is bent by air refraction. Both these latter types of VLAP fibres are currently commercially available. Contact tips have also been improved over the years. Each year there are reports from investigators using larger and higher power tips, capable of delivering greater energy, to allow for vaporization of larger glands. Lastly, of recent interest are interstitial fibres, which are placed transurethrally directly into the prostatic lobes, sparing the urethra from injury. The remainder of this chapter focuses on the VLAP fibres, as these are the most widely used and concerning which there is the greatest experience to draw upon.

Right-angle fibre physics

The VLAP fibres, although all similar in the principle of deflecting the laser beam, have decidedly different properties, making it imperative to understand the physics of the fibres. The two unique properties of these fibres include the angle of deflection and the angle of divergence.

Angle of deflection

The angle of deflection is the angle at which the beam is bent with respect to the forward direction. The laser energy in all VLAP fibres is delivered through a bare fibre, and is bent at the terminal end to a (more or less) right angle. In order to treat the lateral lobes, the ideal bend of the laser to give the smallest spot size and thus the greatest energy density would be a true 90 degree bend (Fig. 32.1a). However, this is seldom the actual case, as the fibre beam is commonly deflected to more or less than 90 degrees. A bend of less than 90 degrees (Fig. 32.1b) means that greater care should be taken in the bladder neck/orifice area, since the laser is directed slightly forwards. A bend of more than 90 degrees (Fig 32.1c) means that greater care should be taken near the sphincter area since the laser is directed slightly backwards. Understanding the angle of deflection can help prevent inadvertent injury.

Angle of divergence

The angle of divergence relates to the spread of the laser beam as it leaves the fibre. If a bare fibre is used, the laser beam spread will be approximately 8 degrees. The

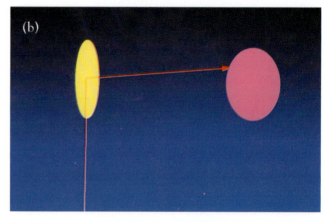

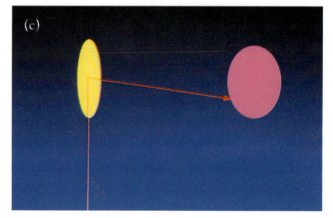

Figure 32.1. *Right-angled fibres: (a) true 90 degree bend; (b) bend of less than 90 degrees showing forward projection; (c) bend of more than 90 degrees showing retrograde projection.*

various VLAP fibres produce a wide variety of angles of divergence. The greater the angle of divergence, the wider the area of tissue affected by the laser, but the less the power density will be (Fig. 32.2). Von Swol et al. studied the effect of the angle of divergence on the tissue effect.[4] They also studied the effect of technique

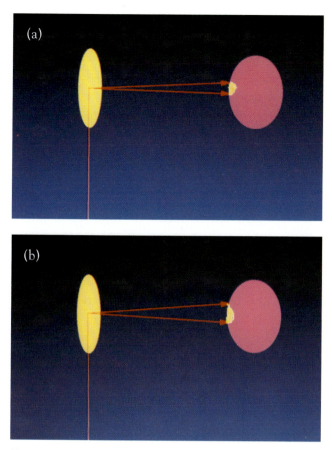

Figure 32.2. *Angles of divergence: (a) narrow; (b) wide.*

(such as static treatment versus painting) on ultimate tissue effect. In general, the metal cavity (reflective) fibres are of lower power density owing to the wider angle of divergence, while the air-refractive fibres are of higher power density. The differences in power density may be as much as tenfold at the same power. Since the refractive fibres can tolerate higher power settings than can the reflective fibres, this difference is potentially even greater. In addition, those authors concluded that the difference in tissue necrosis was up to five times higher with the painting technique than with the static treatment technique. It becomes apparent that using refractive fibres can allow for high power density treatment, especially with the painting technique, whereas the reflective fibres allow for lower power density treatment with static techniques. Thus, understanding fibre physics will allow one to choose the ideal fibre for the type of treatment that is desired.

Types of treatment

The two methods of treating BPH using VLAP fibres are coagulation and vaporization. Coagulative necrosis can be achieved by using low power and long pulse durations; vaporization requires high power settings, and shorter pulse durations. Thus, although 100 W for 1 s, 50 W for 2 s and 25 W for 4 s all produce 100 J, that produced by 25 W for 4 s will give rise to the greatest depth of penetration since all of the laser energy will be converted into coagulative necrosis. The choice of 100 W for 1 s will produce the least penetration, since the higher power and shorter pulse duration will result in surface vaporization, with a concomitant decrease in coagulative necrosis. Thus, two treatment potentials are apparent — high power density (using refractive fibres for vaporization) and low power density (using reflective fibres for coagulation) — although both treatments produce some degree of both effects. With coagulative necrosis, temperature changes ranging from 60 to 70°C are expected, producing coagulative necrosis with little surface vaporization.[5] There will be grey-white discoloration of the tissue, with the maximum possible depth of penetration. Tissue ablation requires secondary sloughing of tissue, taking weeks to occur, with early tissue oedema. By contrast, with vaporization temperature changes on the surface well in excess of 100°C can be expected, with immediate tissue ablation. There will be far less depth of penetration, since most of the laser energy is directed to the surface. As a result, there will be less oedema postoperatively and less slough, since there is insignificant coagulative necrosis. The actual depth of prostate treated will, however, ultimately be less with this technique.

Surgical technique

Coagulation treatment

As previously described, this treatment is based upon low power and long pulse duration. Thus, the metal reflective fibres would be ideal for this type of treatment. The majority of studies have used between 40 and 60 W, although some laboratory studies have suggested that even lower power settings should be used.[6] The majority of the investigators have actually increased power settings from 40 to 60 W. Pulse durations may vary from 30 to 120 s. Currently, the most common combination is 60 W for 60 s to each of four treatment areas starting just outside the bladder neck. The four areas are at 2, 4, 8 and 10 o'clock and a second treatment at similar locations is undertaken for larger glands. It is advisable to re-check the fibres after the first four-quadrant treatment, since the power delivery may have decreased significantly. As this method produces the equivalent of a thermal burn, and produces much tissue oedema, prolonged catheter drainage is required, usually for a week or more.[7] This treatment can be performed under local anaesthesia with pudendal block.[8]

Two interesting papers afford insight into the healing process after VLAP by the coagulation technique. Marks presented seven patients who underwent VLAP and subsequently were studied by serial video-endoscopy.[9] He found that in the early weeks after treatment there were typical findings of coagulative necrosis, i.e. the prostate appeared shaggy, white and irregular. No patient demonstrated healing in less than 6 weeks. By 3–4 months, some patients had undergone considerable healing, while others still appeared to be actively sloughing tissue. By 3 months, some degree of post-prostatectomy defect was noted in all patients; some had a completely clean fossa, while others had residual tissue. Costello and colleagues studied the histological changes in the prostate after VLAP in six patients who underwent TURP and one patient who underwent radical prostatectomy, from 24 h to 10 months after VLAP.[10] Costello et al. found that in the first days after VLAP the findings were similar to those of a thermal burn. As days turn to weeks after treatment, the effect of the VLAP became more pronounced and extensive coagulative necrosis took place. This slough continued until, after 1 month or more, regenerating glandular cells appeared and squamous metaplasia became evident. Ten months after VLAP some denatured tissue remained in a central location.

Vaporization treatment

This treatment requires higher power density and shorter pulse duration, and is best undertaken with refractive fibres. Power settings of 80–100 W are most commonly employed, as is the painting technique. In the painting technique, the median lobe is first treated, using tangential laser energy delivery. After vaporization of the median lobe, the fibre is placed just outside the bladder neck (to preserve antegrade ejaculation) and slowly dragged through the lateral lobe to the verumontanum, care being taken to avoid treating beyond this area. The drag rate should be slow enough to ensure adequate vaporization (as determined visually). After four troughs have been created at the 2, 4, 8 and 10 o'clock areas, any remaining untreated tissue is then lasered in the same fashion until the entire prostate has been treated. Owing to the charring and tissue colour change, attempts to re-treat areas already vaporized do not result in deeper penetration. Approximately 1000 J of laser energy per gram of tissue are delivered in this technique. A catheter will be required, although usually for a shorter period than after coagulation. To the author's knowledge, this has not been performed under pudendal block, but no doubt could be.

Results

Coagulation technique

The first paper to appear on the use of VLAP fibres in humans was published in 1992 by Costello et al.[11] They described the use of the Lateralase fibre (Trimedyne) in treating four men with outlet obstruction due to BPH, employing 60 W for 60 s at four quadrants. The initial results were promising, with all four patients showing improvement in flow rates. In addition, one patient underwent VLAP treatment prior to radical prostatectomy for cancer. Histological examination of the radical prostatectomy specimen revealed a zone of necrosis extending 2.5 cm deep, with an intact capsule. Using an improved fibre, Costello reported on his results with 33 men undergoing VLAP for BPH.[12] This study included two patients treated while receiving anticoagulant therapy. The protocol was identical to that in Costello's first study, except that a second round of treatments was added for men with prostatic lengths greater than 3.0 cm. Treatment was continued until all obvious adenoma had been lased. The results of this study are summarized in Table 32.2. The catheter was routinely removed by 48 h, and all but seven patients required recatheterization owing to burn oedema at the bladder neck. Three patients (9%) failed to void and

Table 32.2. *Results of coagulation using VLAP fibres in 33 men with BPH*

Parameter	Before treatment	After treatment
Peak flow rate (ml/s)	8.5	15.2
AUA-SS*	21.5	9.5

*AUA-7 symptom score. Values are means. (From ref. 12 with permission.)

Table 32.3. *Results of a prospective randomized trial of TURP vs VLAP in 115 patients with BPH*

Group	Peak flow rate (ms/s) Before	After[†]	AUA-SS* Before	After[†]
Laser (n=56)	8.9	14.2	18.7	9.7
TURP (n=59)	9.5	16.5	20.8	7.5

*AUA-6 symptom score. [†]12 months after procedure. Values are means. (From ref. 13 with permission.)

Table 32.4. *Adverse effects after VLAP or TURP in 115 patients with BPH*

Complication	VLAP (n=56)	TURP (n=59)
Impotence	3(5.4)	2(3.4)
Urinary tract infection	3(5.4)	1(1.7)
Stenosis/stricture	1(1.8)	12(20.4)
Clot retention	0	3(5.1)
Transfusion	0	2(3.4)
Post-TURP syndrome	0	2(3.4)
Incontinence	0	2(3.4)
Urinary retention	17(30.4)	5(8.5)
Haematuria	9(16.1)	9(15.3)
Dysuria/pain	10(17.9)	13(22.1)
Urgency	0	3(5.1)
Dribbling	1(1.8)	0

Values are numbers of patients, with percentages in parentheses. (From ref. 13 with permission.)

cystoscopic examination showed no laser effect; these patients underwent TURP. The laser was found to be faulty and was blamed for this failure.

The first US trial of VLAP was sponsored by C.R. Bard.[13] The study was a prospective, randomized trial of TURP versus VLAP. A total of 115 patients were randomized, with 59 in the TURP arm and 56 in the laser arm. There were no differences between the two arms in terms of age, prostate size, post-void residual or preoperative peak flow rates. American Urological Association (AUA)-6 symptom scores differed statistically, the TURP group having patients with higher preoperative scores (20.8 vs 18.7 for VLAP). Eight of the patients were in urinary retention. This protocol used 40 W in four quadrants (3, 6, 9 and 12 o'clock). The pulse durations were 30 s at the 6 and 12 o'clock positions and 60 s at the 3 and 9 o'clock positions. A second set of pulses was used for prostate glands over 4 cm in length. Increases in peak flow rates and decreases in post-void residual and AUA symptom scores were noted in both groups, but were more pronounced in the TURP group (Table 32.3). Six of the 56 patients in the VLAP arm (11%) had a second operation within 6 months. Two had a repeat laser treatment because of laser malfunction, and four underwent TURP owing to unsatisfactory results. Adverse effects were minimal in the laser group (Table 32.4). The largest problem in this group of patients was delayed time to void, but this was not considered to constitute an adverse effect. About one-third or 30% of the men had bouts of urinary retention, requiring repeat catheterization, and 15% experienced irritative symptoms and/or a poor initial flow. Retrograde ejaculation did not occur in the laser group, but was universal in the TURP group. The 1 year data were

examined in a subgroup of this study, of which nine patients underwent laser treatment as described above, and ten underwent TURP.[14] Five of these patients were in retention at the start of this study, of whom two were in the TURP arm and three in the VLAP arm. Both patients in the TURP arm did well, and voided with low post-void residuals. Of the three patients with retention in the VLAP arm, two failed and required TURP, after which both voided well. As in the entire trial, the patients in the subgroup showed improvements in the AUA symptom scores and peak flow rates after treatment, but such improvements were greater in the TURP arm than in the VLAP arm (Fig. 32.3). Three of the nine laser patients underwent TURP by 1 year.

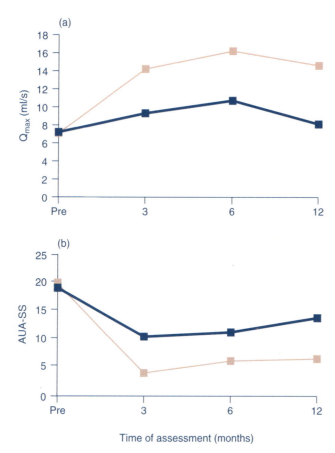

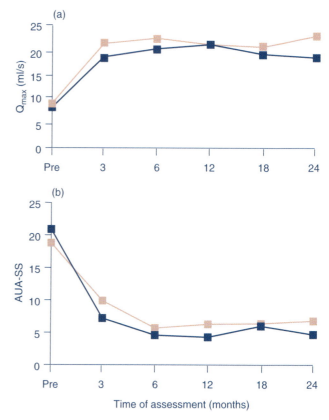

Figure 32.3. *Results from a subgroup of a randomized trial of TURP (■; n=10) versus VLAP (■; n=9) using the Urolase laser: (a) peak flow rates (Q$_{max}$); (b) AUA-6 symptom scores (AUA-SS). (From ref. 14.)*

Figure 32.4. *Results from another subgroup of a randomized trial of TURP (■; n=12) versus VLAP (■; n=13) using the Urolase laser: (a) peak flow rates (Q$_{max}$); (b) AUA-6 symptom scores (AUA-SS). (From ref. 16 with permission.)*

Results from another subset of this multicentre study, with 13 patients in the VLAP group and 12 in the TURP arm, have been published by Kabalin and colleagues.[15,16] By 6 months the peak flow in the laser group had increased from 8.5 to 20.5 ml/s while the AUA symptom score decreased from 20.9 to 4.6. By contrast, in the TURP arm the peak flow rate increased from 9.0 to 22.9 ml/s and the AUA symptom score decreased from 18.8 to 5.7 (Fig. 32.4). Kabalin also reported on cystoscopic findings on the VLAP patients at 3 months, even though this was not part of the overall protocol: the TURP patients were all found to have open prostatic fossas; the VLAP patients uniformly had residual tissue, with two appearing to have obstructed lobes, despite good uroflow rates and low symptom scores. The only complications in the VLAP arm were in two

patients, in whom repeat retention necessitated re-catheterization.

Norris et al. reported on a total of 108 patients treated with the Urolase fibre:[17] 60 W was delivered for 60 s to each lateral lobe, as well as to the roof and floor. Further applications were given as needed to blanch the lateral lobes completely. Entry criteria were AUA symptom scores of 15 or more, and peak flow rates of 10 ml/s or less. The uroflow rates improved from 7.5 to 12 ml/s and AUA symptom scores fell from 22.3 to 9.23. The major complication was the need for repeat catheterization, in from 17 to 38% of patients, depending upon which day the catheter was removed, despite the use of 1 mg terazosin postoperatively for 2 weeks in 70 patients. Four of the six patients who presented in retention required a second operation (three TURPs and one repeat laser).

Leach and associates reported on a subset of patients treated with a similar 60 W protocol, but under local anaesthesia as outpatients.[8] A total of 46 men underwent VLAP in this fashion, five of whom were treated while on Coumadin. A periprostatic block with a 50/50 mixture of 1% xylocaine and 0.5% bupivacaine was used, as well as Versed i.v. sedation. By 6 months the peak flow rates had improved from 8.1 to 13.0 ml/s and the AUA-6 symptom score had decreased from 21 to 9.4. Only one patient required a second surgical procedure — a bladder neck incision for contracture.

Shanberg et al. reported on two sequential series of patients: the first 25 were treated with the above protocol, and the second 25 were treated by multiple pulses over the entire prostate until all pink tissue was ablated.[18] The first group was treated with the Urolase or Prolase fibre, while the second group was treated with the Laserscope ADD fibre. All patients were discharged on Toradol and Hytrin for 10 days. Table 32.5. summarizes these results. No differences between the groups were noted in improvements in AUA symptom scores or uroflow rate improvements. However, there were six failures in the first group and only one failure in the second group; ultimately, three of the 50 patients underwent TURP.

Lastly, Malek and associates from the Mayo Clinic have reported on their experience with 47 men treated with VLAP for BPH.[19] Like Shanberg, they used the Urolase fibre in 25 patients, and the Laserscope ADD fibre in 22 patients. They used a protocol identical to that of Norris et al.[17] but reduced the power to 40 W for smaller glands.

Preoperative values are not given for flow rates or AUA symptom scores, but percentage improvements are given: the AUA symptom score improved by 54 and 78%, and the peak flow improved by 65 and 97% in groups I and II, respectively. Urinary retention developed in 26% of patients, taking up to 60 days to resolve. Ten patients were no better after treatment than before, and three of these underwent TURP 6 months after VLAP, with removal of 35–55 g tissue.

In summary, the coagulation technique is simple and rapid; it has several disadvantages, however. The patients have a prolonged time to void and their initial voiding is often associated with a poor stream and severe irritative complaints that may take months to resolve.

Table 32.5. *Results of coagulative VLAP treatment with the Urolase or Prolase fibre (group I) or with the Laserscope ADD fibre (group II) in men with BPH*

Group	Peak flow rate (ml/s)		AUA-SS*	
	Before	After	Before	After
I (n=25)	5.7	13.5	26.5	7.8
II (n=25)	6.5	14.5	25.6	5.2

*AUA-7 symptom score. Values are means. (From ref. 18 with permission.)

The improvements in symptom scores and flow rates are, in most comparative studies, poorer than those seen in the TURP arm. In addition, reoperation rates in the first year approximate 5–10%. For patients presenting in retention, the need for a second operation (usually TURP) is even greater, making this VLAP technique a poor choice for these patients. This technique may still have a place for patients on anticoagulant therapy and from whom this medication cannot safely be withdrawn, even for short periods.

Vaporization techniques

To date, the only published experience with the vaporization technique is that of Narayan and associates,[20] who treated 61 men with BPH. Entrance criteria included an AUA symptom score of more than 8 and a peak flow rate of less than 15 ml/s or patients in retention. The size of the glands ranged from 20 to 97 g. A refractive fibre and power settings of 60–80 W were used, the technique employed being as described earlier. A total of 32 000–225 000 J was delivered. The catheter was removed on day 2 in 43 and on days 3–7 in 18 patients; only five patients required recatheterization. Two of the 61 patients required a TURP for residual adenoma. All 12 patients in retention voided well. Urinary tract infection was the only significant complication, seen in 4.9% of patients. Results are summarized in Table 32.6. The experience of the present author and colleagues with this technique has been identical; they have also used Hytrin lead-in (1–5 mg/day) for 3 weeks before and 3 weeks after laser treatment. This may help the patient over the initial period of oedema and, in the author's experience, has reduced the need for recatheterization. Long-term

Table 32.6. *Results of the vaporization procedure in 61 men with BPH*

Parameter	Pre-treatment	3 months	6 months	12 months
		Assessment		
Peak flow rate (ml/s)	9.3	15.5	13.2	24.6
AUA-SS*	27.5	8.0	6.6	8.0

*AUA-7 symptom score. Values are means. (From ref. 20 with permission.)

follow-up is needed to ascertain whether reoperation rates are lower with this technique.

Several presentations on this technique have been accepted for the 1995 AUA meeting, and have been published as abstracts. Krautschick et al. studied 112 patients treated with an identical technique to that described above.[21] Twenty-three of the patients were in retention preoperatively. Peak flow rates improved from a mean of 6.9 to 19.3 at 3 months, and the AUA symptom scores dropped from 32 to 5. Significant delayed time to catheter-free status was noted. Gottfried and associates reported the results of a European multicentre study using the same techniques at 60 W.[22] AUA symptom scores declined from 26 to 6 at 1 year, and peak flow rates improved from a mean of 7.5 to 19.8 ml/s. Most patients noted irritative voiding symptoms for 2–4 weeks after treatment. Narayan and associates expanded their series to 100 patients and evaluated outcomes based on initial prostate size.[23] No difference was noted in results for patients grouped on this basis. These authors also compared 20 patients treated with this technique with 20 treated with the coagulation technique: the vaporization group was noted to have superior improvements in peak flow and a lesser incidence of prolonged retention.

Conclusions

TURP took approximately 40 years to become the gold standard, from its initial development in 1926. The initial report on TURP included a 25% mortality rate. A report from 1933 was entitled 'TURP without the moonlight and roses', and was a compendium of TURP problems of the day. VLAP is only 3 years old and is still under development. The initial studies should be considered as just that, and within that context the laser actually appears to have potential. Much needs to be done in order to develop this promising technology, with new lasers, new fibres and new methods of treatment on the horizon.

References

1. McPhee M S, Mador D, Tulip J, Lakey W H. Surgical lasers: machines in search of a disease? Mod Med Can 1982; 37: 1445–1449
2. Kandel L B, Harrison L H, McCullough D L et al. Transurethral laser prostatectomy in the canine model. Lasers Surg Med 1992; 12: 33–42
3. Shanberg A M, Tansey L A, Baghdassarian R. The use of Nd:YAG in prostatectomy. Poster 331, American Urological Association, Atlanta, May 1985
4. Von Swol C F P, Verdassdork R M, Van Vliet R J et al. Side-firing devices for laser prostatectomy. World J Urol 1995; 13: 88
5. Stein B S, Kendall A R. Lasers in urology. I. Laser physics and safety. Urology 1984; 23: 405–410
6. Orihuela E, Motamedi M, Pow-Sang M et al. Low-power laser radiation for the treatment of benign prostatic hyperplasia: initial clinical experience. J Endourol 1994; 8: 301–304
7. Stein B S (personal experience)
8. Leach G E, Sirls L, Ganabathi K et al. Outpatient visual laser-assisted prostatectomy under local anesthesia. Urology 1994; 43: 149
9. Marks L S. Serial endoscopy following visual laser ablation of prostate (VLAP). Urology 1993; 42: 66–71
10. Costello A J, Bolton D M, Ellis D, Crowe H. Histopathological changes in human prostatic adenoma following neodymium:YAG laser ablation therapy. J Urol 1994; 152: 1526–1529
11. Costello A J, Johnson D E, Bolton D M. Nd:YAG laser ablation of the prostate as a treatment for benign prostatic hypertrophy. Lasers Surg Med 1992; 12: 121–124
12. Costello A J, Shaffer B S, Crowe H R. Second-generation delivery systems for laser prostatic ablation. Urology 1994; 43: 262–266
13. Cowles R S, Kabalin J N, Childs S et al. A prospective randomized comparison of transurethral resection to visual laser ablation of the prostate for the treatment of benign prostatic hyperplasia. Urology 1995; 46: 155–160
14. Stein B S, Zabbo A (personal experience)
15. Kabalin J N. Laser prostatectomy performed with a right angle firing neodymium:YAG laser fibre at 40 watts power setting. J Urol 1993; 150: 95–99
16. Kabalin J N, Gill H S, Bite G, Wolfe V. Comparative study of laser versus electrocautery prostatic resection: 18-month followup with complex urodynamic assessment. J Urol 1995; 153: 94–98
17. Norris J P, Norris D M, Lee R D, Rubenstein M A. Visual laser ablation of the prostate: clinical experience in 108 patients. J Urol 1993; 150: 1612–1614
18. Shanberg A M, Lee I S, Tansey L A, Sawyer D E. Extensive neodymium-YAG photoirradiation of the prostate in men with obstructive prostatism. Urology 1994; 43: 467–471
19. Malek R S, Barrett D M, Dilworth J P. Visual laser ablation of the prostate: a preliminary report. Mayo Foundation for Medical Education and Research 1995; 70: 28
20. Narayan P, Leidich R, Fournier G et al. Transurethral evaporation of prostate (TUEP) with Nd:YAG laser using a contact free beam

technique: results in 61 patients with benign prostatic hyperplasia. Urology 1994; 43 813–820

21. Krautschick A W, Weber H M, Benken N et al. VLAP — single centre experience with more than 110 patients. J Urol 1995; 153: 416A

22. Gottfried H W, Frohneberg D, de la Rosette J J M C H et al. Transurethral laser ablation of prostate (TULAP) — experience of a European multicenter study using Ultraline fibre. J Urol 1995; 153: 230A

23. Narayan P, Ashutosh T, George F et al. Impact of prostate size and techniques of laser prostatectomy (evaporation vs coagulation) on the outcome of therapy for benign prostatic hyperplasia. J Urol 1995; 153: 231A

33

Interstitial laser coagulation
T. A. McNicholas M. Al-Sudani

Introduction

The user of laser energy to treat benign prostatic hyperplasia (BPH) has emerged as the main challenge to the 'gold standard' of transurethral resection of the prostate (TURP). This chapter reviews the interstitial method of applying laser energy for BPH treatment. This refers to the use of laser light as a means of transferring energy into the prostate where it will have either a thermal or a photochemical effect.

Reports of the therapeutic use of heat date back to ancient Egypt (circa 1700 BC).[1] When tissue is heated to a temperature range of 41–45°C there is some degree of selectivity of the effect on normal and malignant tissues, with the latter being somewhat more sensitive. Above 50°C (and probably above 45°C) this selectivity is lost, with an equal thermal effect and irreversible cellular damage occurring in normal and malignant tissue. At temperatures at or above 60°C coagulative necrosis occurs with sloughing or reabsorbtion of necrotic tissue later. At 100°C vaporization occurs with acute disruption of tissue due to steam formation. Higher temperatures are associated with tissue burning and carbonization and immediate tissue removal may be seen endoscopically on the treated surface.

Currently, research effort is being devoted to the destruction of BPH by three laser techniques. Two are predominantly thermal and the third invokes a photochemical process. All are delivered to the target tissues by the same fibreoptic mechanisms, namely:

1. Photodynamic therapy (PDT) by endoscopic and interstitial methods.
2. Endoscopic laser coagulation (ELC).
3. Interstitial laser coagulation (ILC).

Photodynamic therapy

PDT involves the use of lasers to produce light of pure wavelengths chosen to activate previously administered photosensitizing agents to cause cell injury by a non-thermal mechanism. Ideally, the photosensitizing drug is taken up or retained to a greater degree by the target tissue than by other tissues. The precise mechanism by which cells are killed is unclear but probably involves the liberation of oxygen radicals and toxic effects on small blood vessels.[2]

PDT research has largely been directed at malignant disease but attention has recently turned to BPH.[3] It is too early to predict whether there will be any role for PDT in BPH, although experiments are approaching clinical application.

Endoscopic laser coagulation

The neodynium:yttrium aluminium garnet (Nd:YAG) laser beam can be directed at high intensity at the prostatic adenoma under direct vision to perform visual laser ablation of the prostate (VLAP) by three methods: (a) the bare fibre method; (b) use of a transurethral endoscopic fibre with a specialized tip; and (c) use of a transurethral endoscopic fibre with various beam-deflecting devices alone or contained within a transurethral balloon.

The development of right-angle beam delivery devices[4] and laser balloon devices[5] both increase the efficiency of laser transmission into the prostate and improve transurethral access to all areas of the prostate and have greatly extended the role of endoscopic laser coagulation for BPH. High total energies can be more readily and easily applied by these devices than by bare fibre methods. The laser energy is applied to the walls of the prostatic cavity either by a continuous passage of the beam over the surface or by intermittent firing of the laser at multiple spots.

Laser prostatectomy by these methods appears to be safe and rapid, and is an acceptable treatment option for men with bladder outlet obstruction due to BPH. However, problems remain, as follows. First, apical tissue is relatively spared in order to avoid sphincteric injury, and it may cause a degree of residual obstruction. It may take up to 3 months or more for the full benefit to occur. VLAP appeals to the urologist, as the application of laser effect appears to be under endoscopic control, however, once within the prostate the process is largely invisible. These laser processes are not predictable in terms of tissue effect compared with TURP. Once laser light strikes the prostatic urethral lining it will undergo variable degrees of reflection, absorbtion, scattering and transmission, resulting in a relatively uncontrolled process. Symptoms of bladder irritability are often severe and may relate to the prolonged presence of necrotic prostatic tissue within the prostatic urethra in contact with the urinary stream. Finally, large adenomas are more difficult to treat by VLAP than smaller ones and the response is slower and less complete.

Interstitial therapy, i.e. the insertion of the chosen laser energy delivery source directly into the tissue to be treated, offers the possibility of controlled deep tissue heating. Temperatures well above 45°C are achievable, allowing short treatment durations and localized tissue destruction while preserving the prostatic urethral lumen. Intraprostatic necrotic tissue is separated from the urinary stream and is resorbed by the normal processes of tissue repair. For these reasons the use of interstitially delivered laser energy via a small-calibre fibre placed into the target tissue has attracted attention recently.

Interstitial laser coagulation of the prostate

ILC is the endoscopic or percutaneous interstitial application of laser energy using a bare or modified fibre to achieve tissue coagulation by a thermal process.

The advantage of the interstitial laser technique is that only relatively low power Nd:YAG or diode laser light (2–10 W) is needed to cause localized coagulative necrosis of prostate tissue since all the laser energy is available for scattering and absorbtion and little is lost by reflection or transmission. This energy is easily directed into the tissue, either transurethrally, transrectally or percutaneously, through a thin fibre. Several groups have subsequently investigated whether sources of laser light can be placed within the prostate gland to cause precise, controlled necrosis of a size that might be useful for the treatment of BPH. Initial work involved the transrectal or transperineal approach but most interest now focuses on the transurethral approach

to ILC, with the fibre being delivered to the prostatic urethra through a cystoscope and then inserted through the mucosa into the adenoma (Fig. 33.1).

The laser energy can be introduced into prostatic tissue by the following methods:

1. *A simple bare fibre*. This is cheap and easily repairable but the fibre cladding may not resist the very high intraprostatic temperatures that may develop, leading to the cladding burning and damaging the fibre and leading to breakage of the silica glass fibre itself within the prostate. The fibre and tissue heating effects are readily visible by transrectal ultrasonography (TRUS).
2. *A more complex fibre with a distal 'diffusor tip' attached*. This acts to diffuse the emitted laser light over a relatively large surface area and so should prevent excessive heat build-up on the tip surface. There is a mechanical 'weak point' at the junction of the fibre and diffusor tip that may be prone to failure. The fibre may be inserted into the prostate within a protective outer plastic sheath and is visible by TRUS; however, as yet no real-time TRUS-visible tissue heating changes have been described.
3. A recent compromise between these two basic fibre types is a *bare fibre within a cannula* through which saline flows to protect the cannula, the cladding and the fibre, similar in size to the diffusor tip fibre. Current experiments show characteristic TRUS-visible changes during prostatic heating, although these differ from those that develop during bare fibre ILC.

Experimental background

Nd:YAG laser light was suggested for the purpose of creating focal areas of tissue coagulation within a solid organ.[6] Nd:YAG laser light distributed in the tissue causes a predominantly thermal effect. When delivered by a fine transmitting fibre inserted within the tissue, the Nd:YAG laser energy results in a well-demarcated cytotoxic effect, as shown in previous experimental studies performed on animal liver and gut.[7,8] Matthewson et al.[7] placed single bare fibres in the rat liver and described areas of coagulation, approximately 15 mm in diameter, surrounding the fibre. Subsequent

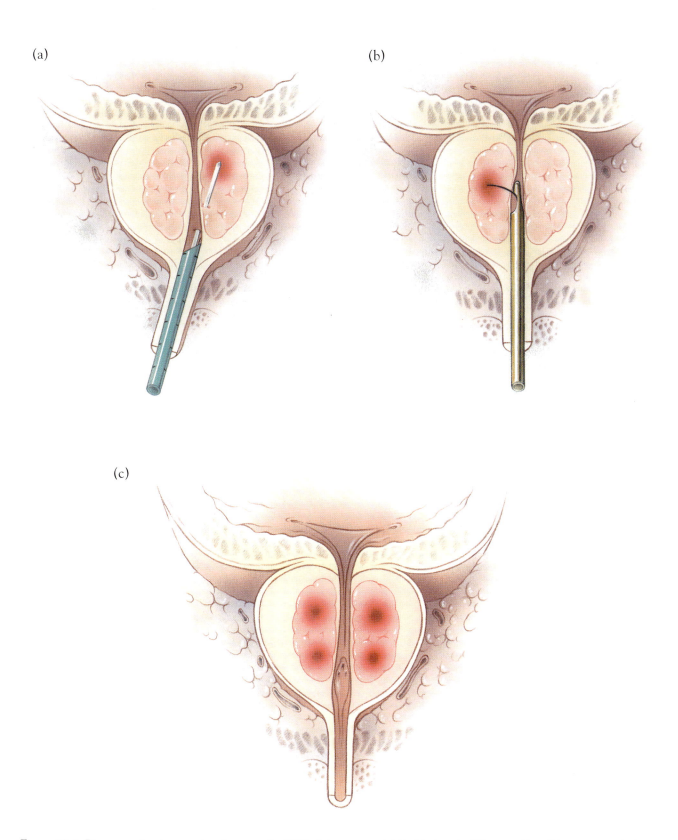

Figure 33.1. *Diagrammatic representation of transurethral ILC of the prostate. (a) Positioning of a diffusor tip fibre, (b) positioning of a bare, saline cooled fibre: the urethra is preserved; the fibre is TRUS visible in each case; in (b) the heating effect is also TRUS visible; positioning can be adjusted according to the size of the adenoma. (c) Effect of treatment: the adenoma is partially replaced by cystic echogenic zones.*

studies in larger animals, particularly the dog, have confirmed that single bare fibres can cause homogeneous areas of necrosis in the canine pancreas and liver varying from 8 to 12 mm in maximum diameter and larger lesions could be created using multiple fibres.[9] The same group[10] have implanted fibres in rats bearing a transplantable fibrosarcoma, and have treated cohorts of rats with varying combinations of power and exposure times and a similar amount of energy, 675–1500 J. This makes the concept of the delivery of a 'dose' of laser energy causing a predictable amount of thermal necrosis an attractive proposition. Why similar results should be obtained in different organs in different animals is not entirely clear. The thermal and optical properties of the prostate, pancreas and liver differ with regard to optical density (colour) and therefore light penetration. They also have different thermal diffusion and blood flow characteristics, all of which in theory should alter the tissue response to low-power laser irradiation and alter energy absorbed per unit volume of tissue. If charring occurs at the fibre tip, this area always acts as a point heat source, rather than a light source, with thermal diffusion away from that point into the surrounding tissue in all tissues at a similar rate.

Hashimoto et al.[11] described what appears to have been the first clinical application of Bown's[6] suggested technique. They inserted a quartz glass fibre, the end of which was altered to give a hemispherical shape to produce diffuse emission of light. Under ultrasonic imaging, tumours of the liver were identified and their volume calculated, and the fibre was inserted into the centre of the identified tumour. Using a continuous-wave YAG laser at a power of 15 W, they administered energy according to a protocol of 1000 J/cm^3 of tumour. A pronounced fall in tumour markers followed treatment. On ultrasonographic (US) scanning the characteristic low-echo areas of tumour were gradually replaced by high echoes, presumably related to local gas formation.

Similar hyperechoic changes were seen in other tissues[12] and in the canine and human prostate by McNicholas et al.[13] using a simple bare fibre, and were thought to aid in the control of the heating process. Muschter et al.[14] used a complex fibre with a larger-calibre 'diffusor tip', which achieves different tissue temperatures, and did not produce hyperechoic changes on US.

ILC of the prostate: canine studies

Initial experimental studies[15–17] showed that large or small lesions could be produced in the canine prostate, which healed with fibrocystic degeneration.

McNicholas et al.[16,18] implanted 150–400 mm fibres within the substance of elderly male beagle prostates. Nd:YAG laser energy was transmitted through the fibre(s) using longer exposures (200–1500 s) and lower powers (1–5 W) than used in routine endoscopic laser therapy. Well-defined areas of coagulative necrosis were created without extensive tissue charring or damage to the fibre. For any energy dose of 1000 J, a lesion ± 1 cm in diameter resulted at 4 days. There appeared to be a threshold of approximately 650–700 J below which tissue necrosis was negligible. Treatments were well tolerated. At 6 weeks following treatment, healing was by fibrosis surrounding an area of cystic degeneration.

A multifibre system was developed, allowing the simultaneous treatment of a much larger volume of tissue within an acceptable treatment time. In practice, however, clinical studies have shown that single-fibre systems can readily create large-volume necrosis within the human prostate by making a number of punctures sequentially within a reasonable time span.[19]

Littrup et al.[15] have described the ablation of canine prostate in a manner similar to that described above but using higher powers (15–60 W) for 5 s, giving total energy doses of 75–300 J. They also compared the effects of percutaneous injection of absolute ethanol or Nd:YAG laster 'hyperthermia' via a fibre, with both being inserted under TRUS guidance. This procedure was feasible under TRUS control in dogs and their results are very similar to those described by McNicholas et al.[16,18] The tissue effects were much better controlled when produced by the laser than by ethanol.

Hoopes et al.[20] used a prototype saline-cooled fibre in the canine prostate and showed fibre preservation, US-visible changes during treatment that correlated with acute and chronic pathological changes, and high tissue temperatures localized to the zones of US-visible change.

These studies suggested that, with low-power or medium-range Nd:YAG laser energy, it was possible to cause reproducible areas of thermal necrosis in the normal canine prostate that healed over time with little harm to the animal. Various stages of the process and the lesions themselves could be seen with ultrasound.

Feasibility studies to assess the application of canine results to man

There are significant differences between the soft, glandular canine prostate and the complex, vascular human gland, which is more resistant to heating. Further experiments and the application to the more challenging human prostate have been described.[13,21]

McNicholas et al.[13] concluded that, in man, bare fibres (0.15–0.4 mm diameter) and carrying needles inserted transurethrally or transrectally into the prostate were seen on TRUS and could be placed accurately. The heating process itself had characteristic TRUS appearances, thereby allowing the operator to titrate the treatment according to the tumour (or adenoma) volume, adding to the margin of safety. Therapeutically useful temperatures were generated within the prostate and could be expected to lead to significant tissue death. Coagulative necrosis could be produced immediately and was more extensive at 1 week. On follow-up of patients there were distinct changes visible within the target area on TRUS at 6 weeks to 3 months. The mixed pattern of hyperechogenic changes and hypoechogenic small cystic spaces has not been reported for any other heating modality and did suggest a distinct physical effect of the laser energy on a significant volume of human prostatic tissue. Similarly encouraging preliminary results were reported by Muschter et al.[14] using higher powers transmitted via larger (1.6–1.7 mm diameter) specialized interstitial fibres that were inserted through a percutaneous transperineal approach.

Current clinical experience

More recently, Muschter[22] has described results of the use of several diffusor tip fibres in 172 men treated by the transperineal or the transurethral interstitial approach. American Urological Association symptom scores (AUA-SS) fell from a mean of 25.1 to 5.7 and peak flow rates rose from a mean of 5.8 to 16.2 ml/s at 6 months.[22] Orovan et al.[23] reported 16 men treated transurethrally with a power of 7 W for 10 min for each lateral lobe and for 5 min for the median lobe, and

found that the AUA-SS fell from 16.3 to 5.8 and flow rates increased from 8.8 to 11.9 ml/s at 3 months, with minimal side effects. Irritative symptoms were less common than with other laser procedures. Ultrasound changes were not described.

The present authors' recent experience is with a transurethrally delivered saline-cooled interstitial laser fibre in 25 patients with symptomatic BPH. The mean age was 69 (61–77) years; the mean prostatic volume was 40 (24–72) cm^3. The mean total energy given was 11 400 J (5560–17 600) J at powers of 5–10 W over a mean laser exposure time of 22 (6.5–45) min. Postoperative bladder drainage in the first ten men was by an 8 Fr suprapubic catheter; subsequently, catheters were dispensed with and the patients were taught intermittent clean self-catheterization (ICSC). Patients were discharged home on the first postoperative day to be reviewed 1 week after treatment, to allow removal of the suprapubic catheter or for general review. Patients were then reviewed at 4 weeks and at 3, 6 and 12 months, with measurement of symptom score, flow rate and residual volume. Intraprostatic changes were monitored by TRUS.

Eight patients managed to void satisfactorily a few days after the treatment, and the suprapubic catheter was removed on postoperative day 7. Five patients showed slower improvement and the suprapubic or urethral catheter needed to remain in situ for 3 weeks. Twelve patients had their bladder drained with a urethral catheter, which was removed on postoperative day 1. The patients started to use self-catheterization, if necessary, with an average of 3 days of ICSC being required. Preoperative mean AUA-SS of 22 (18–29) fell to 5.4 and peak flow rates increased from a mean of 9.5 to 13.8 ml/s at 3 months (Table 33.1).

Table 33.1. *Pre- and postoperative (3 month) outcome parameters of 25 men undergoing transurethral ILC with a saline-cooled fibre*

Parameter	Preoperative	3 months
AUA-SS	22 (18–29)	5.4 (3–9)
Peak flow rate (ml/s)	9.5 (6.7–14.7)	13.8 (8.3–18.5)
Post-void residual (ml)	116 (35–500)	88 (0–281)

Values are means, with ranges in parentheses.

Most of the patients tolerated the treatment very well and the majority required only mild oral analgesia in the immediate postoperative days. One patient developed severe dysuria in the immediate postoperative period and required transurethral resection. The pre-resection TRUS indicated a large volume of necrosis at the site of coagulation, which was confirmed endoscopically and by histological examination of the prostatic tissue removed. However, no other patient had these symptoms, despite US evidence of similar or greater tissue destruction. Most of the patients noticed improvement in their symptoms as well as their flow rate at week 4 post-treatment. Complications were otherwise minor. As with most other laser applications, there were no effects on ejaculation.

TRUS during treatment showed the cannula in situ and the thermal changes within the adenoma as heating progressed (Figs 33.2, 33.3). TRUS at 4 weeks after treatment showed a zone of mixed hyper- and hypo-echoic areas corresponding to the site of coagulation. By week 6, cystic changes had appeared in the centre of the treatment zone, surrounded by a rim of hyperechoic tissue. By month 3 after treatment these characteristic changes had become very distinct, with the cystic changes becoming larger and extending along the entire length of the adenoma (Figs 33.4, 33.5).

Further work should focus on the development of devices to allow safe and even more accurate fibre insertion and treatment control. Although the studies described above were largely directed at the treatment

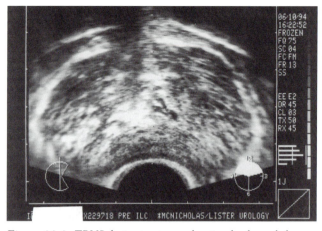

Figure 33.3. *TRUS during treatment showing the thermal changes (white areas) within the adenoma as heating develops.*

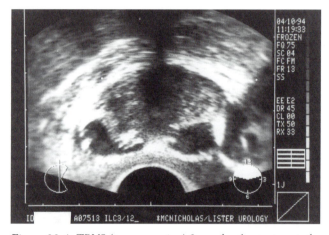

Figure 33.4. *TRUS (transverse view) 3 months after treatment: the characteristic changes become very distinct, with the cystic changes becoming larger within the adenoma.*

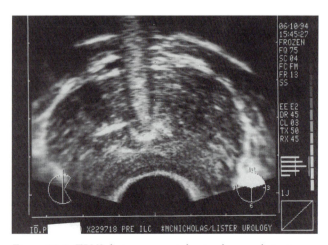

Figure 33.2. *TRUS during treatment showing the cannula in situ.*

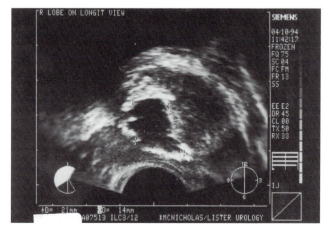

Figure 33.5. *TRUS (longitudinal view) 3 months after treatment: cystic changes extending along the entire length of the adenoma.*

of BPH, Amin et al.[24] have recently treated an area of recurrent or residual prostatic adenocarcinoma in this manner after failure of initial radiotherapy.

Discussion

Higher-power methods of destruction of focal liver lesions have been described that involve a much shorter exposure period. Godlewski et al.[25] described an interstitial laser method using a 5 mm diameter probe to carry a fibre to the target tissue (liver) but using a much higher power (80 W) for a shorter period (10 s). They produced lesions 12–18 mm in diameter in pig liver, with marked central cavitation and charring.

Although a treatment time of 5 s seems attractive compared with the 600–1500 s exposures of the lower-power method, a slower treatment will allow adjustment of the position(s) of the fibre(s), particularly if the laser effect is seen to extend into an undesirable area. Multiple-fibre systems available now and in the foreseeable future cannot cope with the high powers quoted[15,25] and, indeed, clinical Nd:Yag lasers are not available that will produce enough laser power to supply a four-fibre system with 60 W each.

The 'slow cooking' method may allow observation of the evolution of the lesion, with readjustment of the position of the fibre(s) if necessary. It is not yet clear whether either method differs in terms of patient perception of pain. Prostatic needle insertion (and biopsy) is performed as part of urological practice with minimal or no sedation. It appears that transurethral prostatic heating by VLAP can be tolerated under local prostatic block[26] and the same may be true for ILC.

There are two ways by which laser light of a coagulating wavelength may have a thermal effect. The first is optical penetrance of the tissue, with the light being absorbed by the cells with concomitant thermal damage. Alternatively, light is absorbed around the fibre by blood, which coagulates and forms a char that then absorbs the laser light, from which point there is thermal diffusion through the tissue with the laser fibre acting as a point heat source. Which method of heating occurs depends on the trauma of insertion of the fibre and the colour of tissue under treatment. In dark tissue containing a great deal of pigment and blood, such as the liver, the latter method most probably applies, whereas in a paler structure such as the pancreas (and, possibly the prostate), optical penetrance may play a greater part, as the prostate — in vitro at least —has been shown to be relatively 'transparent' to laser wavelengths.[27]

There is much debate as to whether charring is essential to the process of ILC. This is important because if affects the design and complexity of the fibre systems required. If charring is to be avoided, then a fibre with a large emitting surface is needed to reduce the power density, in order to diffuse the Nd:YAG laser light into the tissues.[14,21,28] This should avoid raising the temperature of the body fluids adjacent to the fibre surface to the level that would cause carbonization (whereupon laser light distribution falls sharply, since the light is now intensely absorbed by the adjacent charred tissue acting as a 'black body' rather than being highly scattered into the surrounding tissues).

Sapphire tips are more complicated to use and are more traumatic to insert, owing to their larger size. Van Eeden et al.[29] showed that the diameter of necrosis that can be produced in liver around a sapphire-tipped probe is less than that around a bare fibre for the equivalent laser powers and exposure times. Karanov et al.[30] using transplanted tumour in mice, have found that the extent of coagulation necrosis created by 1200 J delivered by a sapphire tip 'contact' system was significantly less than that resulting from the same energy delivered by external beam irradiation or a bare fibre interstitial method. Nolsoe et al.[28] measured the size of lesions created by Nd:YAG light passed through either a simple bare fibre system or by a larger-calibre fibre with a 'diffusor tip', but were unable to show any statistically significant advantage for the larger fibre. Until convincing evidence is forthcoming it would seem appropriate to use simpler fibre systems, which have the advantage of being cheaper as well as less disruptive to the tissues through which they must pass.

It may even be the case that charring or carbonization is essential to achieving a larger volume effect. Some charring was seen in all animal and human studies performed at the authors' institution, even at very low powers. This is probably inevitable and may be beneficial in achieving larger volume lesions. The charred zone (however small), having absorbed light energy, acts as a heat emitter. If this is a substantial contribution to the total thermal effect, then it raises the possibility that the laser light itself (and certainly the wavelength) is not crucial to the process, and would suggest that the same thermal process could be produced by other non-laser heating methods. Even if this does prove to be the case, the use of laser light through fine-calibre fibres will remain a very elegant and minimally invasive method of applying the original energy.

For this method to be successful it is necessary to have a laser capable of producing low powers reliably in a stable manner. The Nd:YAG laser technology used in this study is widely available and is becoming cheaper. With the availability of multiple-fibres couplers, the standard Nd:YAG laser can be used both for 'traditional' high-power applications and for multiple-fibre low-power interstitial uses by a range of different specialities, as long as that particular laser will produce a stable power output at the lower end of its power range. Alternatively, smaller and cheaper Nd:YAG lasers are becoming available. At the low powers used in this study there is little need for complex electrical or cooling arrangements and the lasers are more likely to be truly portable.

Relatively tiny tough and viable 'diode' lasers producing coagulative wavelength light are already available. The authors have found the effect of the Diomed 805 nm wavelength diode laser in the human prostate in vivo to be identical to that of the Nd:YAG laser. Their experiments with the Cytocare Diolase 950 nm diode laser for VLAP showed very similar effects and long-term results when compared with those with the Nd:YAG laser[31] and they expect the interstitial effects also to be similar.

The ILC method produces much higher temperatures than are usually seen in conventional hyperthermia, but this does not seem to be a problem either in the authors' animal or clinical BPH studies, or in the clinical studies reported in gastroenterology,[32] as long as the energy is appropriately and precisely directed to where the necrotic effect is intended. In liver and pancreatic studies, even when there was evidence of microvaporization and therefore high temperatures on ultrasound, this was not associated with patient discomfort. If the operator can see (ultrasonically) the end of the fibre he can assess where the region of high temperature will be. This does not diminish the need to develop sensitive thermometry methods to accompany the safe use of interstitial laser hyperthermia, and a

combination of TRUS and thermometry would appear to be safest.

Conclusions

Controlled tissue coagulation can be produced by low-power laser light transmitted by fine fibres inserted interstitially by percutaneous transperineal, transrectal and endoscopic routes to destroy prostatic tissue. Clinical studies have shown the following:

1. ILC can be applied accurately and safely under TRUS or endoscopic control.
2. Therapeutically useful temperatures in a significant volume can be achieved in the human prostate.
3. Significant tissue changes can be created and these are visible on TRUS.
4. Symptomatic and flow rate changes are similar to those after other methods of laser prostatectomy.
5. There is only a suggestion that the early postoperative problems of dysuria and obstruction are less problematic.
6. The possibility exists of making laser prostatectomy a more controlled and therefore a more predictable process by exploiting the TRUS visibility of ILC.
7. The longer 'slow cooking' method is advantageous, rather than using a much higher powered and shorter exposure, because the slower technique allows repositioning of the fibre during treatment as and when necessary to achieve total coagulation of the target zone, without the extensive tissue disruption resulting from the explosive production of superheated steam that occurs with higher powers.
8. The ideal fibre for ILC is as yet undetermined. The diffusor tip fibres do not appear to give rise to TRUS-visible thermal changes during therapy which might indicate that this is an important means of controlling energy deposition and heating.

References

1. Breasted J H. The Edwin Smith Surgical Papyrus, Vol 1. Chicago: University of Chicago, 1930
2. Selman S H. Transurethral photodynamic ablation of benign canine prostate. J Urol 1994; 151: 335 (abstr 429)
3. Star W M, Marijnissen H P A, van der Berg-Blok A E et al. Destruction of rat mammary tumour and normal tissue

microcirculation by haematoporphyrin derivative photoradiation observed in vivo in sandwich observation chambers. Cancer Res 1986; 46: 2532–2540

4. Costello A J, Johnson D E, Bolton D M. Nd-YAG laser ablation of the prostate as a treatment for benign prostatic hypertrophy. Lasers Surg Med 1992; 12: 121–124

5. Assimos D G, McCullough D L, Woodruff R D et al. Canine transurethral laser induced prostatectomy. J Endourol 1991; 5: 145–149

6. Bown S G. Pathotherapy of tumours. World J Surg 1983; 7: 700–709

7. Matthewson K, Coleridge-Smith P, O'Sullivan J P et al. Gastroenterology 1987; 93: 550–557

8. Barr H, Tralau C J, MacRobert A J et al. PDT in the normal rat colon with phthalocyanines sensitization. Br J Cancer 1987; 56: 111–118

9. Steger A C, Bown S G, Clark C G. Interstitial laser hyperthermia — studies in the normal liver. Br J Surg 1988; 75: 598

10. Matthewson K, Barr H, Tralau C, Bown S G. Low power interstitial Nd YAG laser photocoagulation: studies in a transplantable fibrosarcoma. Br J Surg 1989; 76: 378–381

11. Hashimoto D, Yabe K, Uedera Y. Ultrasonic guided lasers and spheric lasers. In: Riemann J F, Ell C (eds) Lasers in gastroenterology (international experiences and trends). Stuttgart; Georg Thieme Verlag, 1989: 134–138

12. Steger A C, Shorvon P, Walmsley K et al. Ultrasound features of low power interstitial laser hyperthermia. Clin Radiol 1992; 46: 88–93

13. McNicholas T A, Pope A J, Timoney A et al. Hyperthermia of the prostate by interstitial laser coagulation. J Urol 1992; 147: 345A

14. Muschter R, Hofstetter A, Hessel S et al. Hi-tech of the prostate: interstitial laser coagulation of benign prostatic hypertrophy. SPIE 1992; 1643 (laser surgery): 25–34

15. Littrup P J, Lee F, Borlaza G S, Sacknoff E J. Percutaneous ablation of canine prostate using transrectal ultrasound guidance. Absolute ethanol and Nd:YAG laser. Invest Radiol 1988; 23: 734–739

16. McNicholas T A, Steger A C, Charig C, Bown S G. Interstitial Yag laser coagulation of the prostate. Lasers Med Sci 1988; (abstracts issue): abstr 446

17. McNicholas T A, Steger A C, Bown S G. Interstitial laser coagulation of the prostate: an experimental study. Br J Urol 1993; 71: 439–444

18. McNicholas T A, Steger A C, Pope A et al. Interstitial laser coagulation of the prostate: experimental studies. In: Proc Int Soc Optical Engineering. SPIE's Biomedical optics, Vol 1421: Lasers in urology, laparoscopy and general surgery. Bellingham, WA: SPIE Optical Engineering Press, 1991; 30–35

19. McNicholas T A, Hoopes J P, Williams J et al. Interstitial laser coagulation (ILC) of the canine prostate with ultrasound and thermal monitoring. SIU meeting, Sydney, Sept 1994: abstr 319

20. Hoopes J P, Williams J, Harris R et al. Interstitial laser coagulation (ILC) of the canine prostate with ultrasound and thermal monitoring. J Urol 1994; 151: 334A (abstr 425)

21. Muschter R, Hofstetter A, Hessel S et al. Interstitial laser prostatectomy — experimental and first clinical results. J Urol 1992; 147: 346A

22. Muschter R, Zellner M, Hessel S, Hofstetter A. Lasers and benign prostatic hyperplasia — experimental and clinical results to compare different application systems. J Urol 1994; 151: 230A (abstr 11).

23. Orovan W L, Whelan J P. Neodynium YAG laser treatment of BPH using interstitial thermometry: a transurethral approach. J Urol 1994; 151: 230A (abstr 12)

24. Amin Z, Lees W R, Bown S G. Technical note: interstitial laser photocoagulation for the treatment of prostatic cancer. Br J Radiol 1993; 66: 1044–1047

25. Godlewski G, Sambuc P, Eledjam J J et al. A new device for inducing deep localised vaporisation in liver with the Nd-YAG laser. Lasers Med Sci 1988; 3: 111–117

26. Leach G E, Sirls L, Ganabathik K et al. Outpatient visual laser-assisted prostatectomy under local anaesthesia. Urology 1994; 43: 149–153

27. Pantelides M, Whitehurst C, Moore J V et al. Photodynamic therapy for localised prostate cancer: light penetration in the human prostate gland. J Urol 1994; 143: 398–401

28. Nolsoe C P, Torp-Pedersen S, Holm H H et al. Ultrasonically guided interstitial Nd:YAG laser diffuser tip hyperthermia: an in vitro study. Scand J Urol Nephrol 1991; 137(suppl): 119–124

29. Van Eeden P J, Steger A C, Bown S G. Fibre tip considerations for low power laser interstitial hyperthermia. Lasers Med Sci 1988; 3: A336

30. Karanov S, Karaivanova M, Getov H, Karanova S. External beam, sapphire tip contact and interstitial Nd-YAG laser therapy at 1.064 μm on a transplanted adenocarcinoma in mice: a comparative study. Lasers Med Sci 1992; 7: 483–486

31. Alsudani M L, Aslam M, Akbar M et al. A comparison of diode and Nd YAG laser therapy for symptomatic benign prostatic hyperplasia (BPH). J Urol 1995; 153(4): 416A

32. Steger A C, Lees W R, Walmesley K, Bown S G. Interstitial laser hyperthermia: a new approach to local destruction of tumours. Br Med J 1989; 299: 362–365

Introduction

Transurethral resection of the prostate (TURP) is the conventional therapy for the relief of bladder outflow obstruction due to benign prostatic hyperplasia (BPH). In 75% of patients, the indication for performance of this procedure in the United States is relief of the symptoms of prostatism.[1] TURP has resulted in symptomatic improvement in 85% of patients in whom it is performed.[2] Complications and side effects, although seldom severe, include incontinence, the need for blood transfusion, urinary tract infection, urethral stricture, bladder neck contracture, retrograde ejaculation and impotence in some cases. In addition, age and co-morbidities of patients undergoing the procedure increase anaesthetic and surgical risk. These concerns, the increasing number of ageing men and the economics of BPH have led to a virtual explosion of investigation into medical and minimally invasive device therapies during the last decade.

Several devices have been introduced to heat the prostate using either a transurethral or transrectal probe. The treatments are performed on an outpatient basis without general or regional anaesthesia. Hyperthermia is a term that has become associated with heat treatment of the prostate, but it was first used in the treatment of malignancies. Hyperthermia is defined as raising tissue temperature to 42–44°C. At these temperatures, malignant tissue is supposedly more susceptible to heat damage than is benign tissue.[3] There are no current data to suggest that stromal or glandular tissues in BPH are more sensitive to such temperatures than normal tissue. At least one hyperthermia device seeks to raise tissue temperatures above 45°C.[4]

Since 1982, local microwave hyperthermia has been proposed as a treatment for patients with prostatic diseases.[5] Early treatments using hyperthermia, including its use in prostatic diseases, were directed at malignancies.[5–9] At temperatures below 40°C, neither malignant nor normal cells are affected to an appreciable extent. At temperatures above 45°C, both malignant and normal cells are affected by heat, and cell death can occur. The differential effect of heat on tumour versus normal cells is estimated to temperatures between 40 and 43°C. Part of the increased susceptibility to heat in malignant cells is due to the type of vascularity found in such tissue. There is a high resistance to blood flow in the neovascularity associated with malignant tumours, and these vessels do not respond to heat with vasodilatation, as is the case in normal tissue. In general, blood supply to the tumour cells is much poorer than that to normal cells. Heat applied to malignant tissue cannot be dissipated by use of the mechanisms found in the normal vasculature. Another advantage of heat treatment for tumour cells is that cells in the S-phase of the cell cycle are very sensitive to heat, whereas they are fairly resistant to X-rays. Hypoxic cells, often found in tumour cells, are sensitive to heat destruction. It is also theorized that the use of local hyperthermia may enhance the immunological response to tumour.[5]

It appears that the transmission of microwaves or radiofrequency waves is the most practical way to produce local deep hyperthermia.[3,6] A microwave antenna or antennae in a probe produce an electromagnetic field interaction, which causes oscillation of ions in the tissue or a change in magnetic orientation of molecules, which is converted to heat. The penetration of electromagnetic waves depends on the frequency of the waves and the tissue composition. The higher the frequency of the wave source, the less deep is the penetration. Satisfactory heating is limited to depths of 2–3 cm.[3]

Permanent or irreversible tissue damage is time and temperature dependent. As mentioned above, both malignant and normal cells can be destroyed at temperatures above 45°C, and the important differential response to heat between significant cell death in malignant tissue compared with normal tissue appears to occur at about 43°C over 1 h.

Figure 34.1a represents tissue heating as a function of distance from the treatment applicator.[3] The tissues closest to the applicator achieve the highest temperature and the drop in radial temperature away from the applicator is rather precipitous. If the surface is cooled, the tissue closest to the applicator is maintained at normal or below-normal temperatures. This allows the 'hot point' to shift deeper into the tissue, and the integrity of the tissue closest to the applicator can be maintained (Fig. 34.1b). This principle is used in some transrectal devices to protect the rectal wall, and in one transurethral device to protect the urethra and to achieve higher temperatures deeper within the lateral lobes of the prostate.

Animal studies

The first article describing the use of microwave hyperthermia to treat prostate tissue in an animal study was that by Magin et al in 1980 using eight dogs with urinary diversion.[10] The experiments aimed at total thermodestruction of the canine prostate with temperatures of 60°C for 15 min. To protect the structures and tissues adjacent to the prostate, a complicated shielding device was used. Four animals were killed at 1 week and four at 6 months after treatment, which was found to have produced almost complete destruction of the prostate. In 1985, a preliminary study was presented by Harada et al. describing the use of a transurethral microwave applicator for prostate thermodestruction in 20 dogs.[11]

A study to determine tolerable temperatures for hyperthermic treatment of the prostate in 20 dogs by a water-cooled transrectal probe was reported in 1986 by Lieb et al.[6] Each of the animals had six sequential treatments, with time between treatments varying from 48 to 72 h. The conclusion of this study was that heating to temperatures up to 42.5°C (± 0.5°C) for 90 min was safe. Astrahan et al. described an applicator to heat the prostate gland, using a transurethral approach in a 38 kg German shepherd dog.[12] This was a study of longitudinal temperature distributions measured in situ at the applicator–urethral interface and the longitudinal radial temperature distribution measured in a normal canine prostate. These authors described a technique capable of elevating temperatures to above 42°C in a cylindrically symmetrical volume up to 5 cm in length and 0.5 cm radial penetration surrounding the applicator. Roehrborn et al. noted that in dogs treated with a transurethral microwave antenna, temperatures

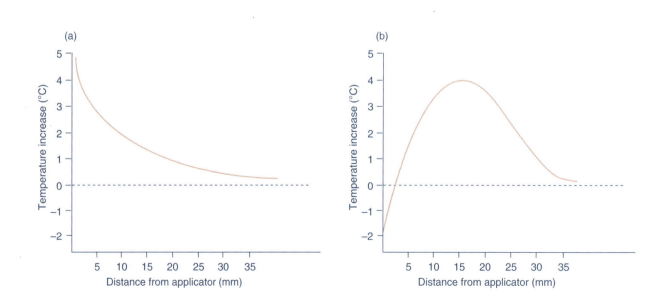

Figure 34.1. *Presentation of heating patterns in tissue as a function of distance from the treatment applicator: (a) without cooling of tissue surface; (b) with cooling of tissue surface. (From ref. 3 with permission.)*

of 42°C were noted in periurethral tissue. However, there was a 1°C decrease in temperature per 3 mm distance from the treatment applicator.[13]

Biophysics of human prostate microwave hyperthermia

The location of the prostate deep within the pelvis makes it easily accessible by applicators of energy sources via the transrectal or transurethral route. Radiative heating of the prostate is thus possible with a number of high-frequency (434, 915 and 2450 MHz) microwave applicators. With increasing distance from the applicator, however, radiative heating dissipates in proportion to the frequency of the wavelength being used: the higher the wavelength, the less penetration can be achieved. In addition, individual variations in anatomy such as urethral blood supply of the urethra and the rectum, prostate size, vascularity and variations in prostate histomorphology all affect radiative heating.

Energy is delivered to the tissue by conductive, convective and absorptive mechanisms. The microwaves interact with cellular molecules to transfer kinetic energy. Specific interstitial data on microwave hyperthermia by either the transrectal or transurethral route to the prostate have not been reported, and most of the current information is extrapolated from published oncology data.[14] Because of fear of injury to non-target tissue, temperatures achieved within the prostate are generally kept at 43–45°C.

A major advantage of the transrectal route is the comfortable positioning and patient acceptance of a transrectal probe. However, exact positioning to ensure contact against the rectal wall is often difficult owing to patient movement during the course of the procedure. In addition, variations in rectal vault size and in thickness of the rectal wall will produce uncertainty as to the correct positioning of the probe. Using standard applicators, maximal penetration of the microwave is probably limited to less than 2 cm.[13] A criticism of transrectal hyperthermia therefore is that maximum deposition of energy is to the peripheral zone of the prostate gland and not to the transition zone — the main location of BPH. For this reason, cooling of the anterior rectal wall was introduced to promote the penetration of energy into the prostate and to protect

the rectal wall.[14] Multiple treatment sessions (five to ten) for at least 1 h have been performed in the hope of overcoming these logistical problems.

The transurethral route appears to be a better approach in terms of proximity to transition zone tissue. Placement of the urethral catheter causes more patient discomfort, which may be offset by the improvement in symmetrical heating of the prostate gland, as a Foley balloon placed on the trigone ensures proper placement and accurate positioning during the treatment session. Thermosensors on the treatment applicators have measured temperatures of up to 45°C within the urethra, which are well tolerated by the patient.[4] Transurethral hyperthermia systems are designed to operate without urethral cooling: the urethral tissue in closest proximity to the applicator receives the highest output of energy, and there is a steep gradient of temperature decrease away from the applicator. Thus, multiple transurethral treatment sessions are required for these devices to produce the desired clinical results.

Clinical reports of use of microwave hyperthermia in BPH

Table 34.1 lists commercially available transrectal and transurethral hyperthermia devices, individual features and published series by authors using the device.

Transrectal devices

Yerushalmi et al.[15] in 1985 reported on 29 patients between the ages of 50 and 81 years at poor operative risk, who underwent localized deep microwave hyperthermia for the treatment of BPH via a water-cooled transrectal probe (2450 MHz). Treatment was given twice weekly for 1 h and the number of treatments per patient varied from four to 18. Of the 29 patients, 27 were able to complete the treatment. One patient died during the treatment cycle, but not because of the treatment, and one discontinued the treatment because of discomfort and inability to tolerate it. Eight of the 11 patients with indwelling catheters for 1–10 months before treatment were catheter free after hyperthermia. Yerushalmi recently updated this series (in 1992) to include 89 patients over an 8-year period.[16] A total of 13% have undergone transurethral resection and 12 patients have undergone a second series of

Table 34.1. *Transrectal (TR) and transurethral (TU) hyperthermia devices*

| Device | Frequency used (MHz) | Sessions | | Route | Published series |
		Length (h)	No.		
Prostathermer® (Biodan Medical Systems Ltd, Israel)	915	1	6–10	TR	Yerushalmi[5,15,16] Servadio[7,17,19] Saranga[20] Strohmaier[24] Montorsi[27] Watson[23]
Primus® (Technomatix Medical, Antwerp, Belgium)	915	1	6–10	TR	Kaplan[28] vanErps[21] Fabricius[26] Watson[23]
BSD® (BSD Medical, Salt Lake City, Utah)	915	1	3–10	TU	Baert[36,–39] Sapozink[35] Astrahan[12,32]
LEO Microthermer® (Laser Optics, London)	915	1	1	TU	Bdesha[41]
Thermex II® (Direx, Israel)	915	1	5–10	TU	Vanden Bossche[49,50] Watson[23] Meier[57] Corica[51] Nissenkorn[53]

treatments; 65% of men in this series have not required subsequent therapy.[16]

In 1987, Lindner et al.[3] reported on six patients between the ages of 60 and 78 years who were in urinary retention (indwelling catheter in place for 1–6 months) and who underwent microwave treatment to the prostate via a water-cooled rectal probe. The patients received five to ten outpatient treatments of 60 min each, once or twice weekly. At 6 months follow-up, five of the six patients were catheter free. One patient, however, required phenoxybenzamine after his catheter removal, in order to empty his bladder completely. One patient developed a stricture of the mid-urethra and another, a meatal stenosis. Pretreatment mean peak flow rate for the entire group was 6.7 ml/s, increasing to 18 ml/s after treatment. When the one treatment failure was eliminated from the evaluation, the improvement in each peak flow rate was from 7.5 to 22.4 ml/s.

Servadio et al.[17] reported in 1987 on 37 patients with BPH who were at poor surgical risk: 29 were

treated with microwave hyperthermia via a water-cooled rectal probe (915 MHz) and compared with eight controls. Treatment was for 1 h once or twice weekly for six to ten sessions per patient. Eight of 13 patients with indwelling catheters were rendered catheter free after microwave hyperthermia, after a follow-up of 24 months.

In 1990, Lindner et al.[18] presented a long-term follow-up of 72 patients between the ages of 58 and 92 (mean 76.7) years, all presenting in urinary retention. Patients had a 1 h treatment via a water-cooled transrectal probe (915 MHz) that raised the temperature of the prostate to 42 ± 1.5°C. They were divided into four groups: group 1 received five sessions of microwave hyperthermia; group 2 had three to five sessions plus 50 mg tid cyproterone acetate; group 3 had six to ten sessions of microwave therapy; and group 4 had six to ten sessions of microwave therapy plus the same dose of cyproterone acetate. The patients were evaluated at 1 month and 1 year. Thirty-six patients were catheter free at 1 month for a 50% response rate; 29 were without a catheter at 1 year for a 40% response rate.

The patients with more treatment sessions appeared to have better outcomes. Of the short-term treatment patients in groups 1 and 2, 33% were rendered catheter free versus 60% of the long-term patients in groups 3 and 4. Patients who received both long-term treatment and cyproterone acetate had a higher catheter-free rate (74%) than any of the other groups, compared with long-term treatment without cyproterone acetate (50%). There was no significant difference between the catheter-free rate of group 1 compared with group 2. Complications consisted of fever to at least 38°C in ten patients, rectal pain in 12, diarrhoea in three and haematuria in 11. Although the patients were treated as outpatients, four were hospitalized — two with severe haematuria, one for pain and one with bacteraemia.

Servadio et al.[19] reported in 1990 a 1-year follow-up of 124 patients who were treated with the same transrectal water-cooled probe used by those authors in their earlier studies. Random assignment to different protocols included variables of high (41–43°C) or low (39–41°C) temperatures; treatment courses of 3 or 5 weeks; treatment sessions lasting 30 or 60 min; individual treatments given once or twice a week; and administration to some of patients of cyproterone acetate, 50 mg tid, during the course of hyperthermia treatment. Patients were evaluated at 3, 6, 9 and 12 months. In assessing the variables, higher temperature treatment for 3 weeks with individual sessions of 60 min twice weekly appeared to produce the best results. The addition of cyproterone acetate did not seem to affect results. An objective improvement was observed in 63 of 124 patients (51%), mostly in those presenting with severe symptoms. An analysis of objective parameters (a combination product score of peak flow rate and residual urine volume) showed that, when improvement occurred, it was primarily as a decrease in the residual urine component.

Another report on the effect of local microwave hyperthermia via a water-cooled transrectal probe (915 MHz) in the treatment of BPH was published by Saranga et al.[20] in 1990. One group of 83 patients between the ages of 67 and 91 (average age 81 years) had obstructive symptoms only. The second group of 31 patients, between the ages of 70 and 87 (average age 77 years), had catheters indwelling for 1–13 months. There had been an attempt to remove the catheter in each patient, which had failed. Those patients who had obstructive symptoms only had a weekly 16 min treatment session on four to seven occasions. Those in the catheter group had twice-weekly treatment for a total of eight to ten sessions each 60 min in length. The temperature of the prostate was raised in both groups to 42.5 ± 1°C. Of the 83 patients with obstruction, only 71 completed treatment: six withdrew for personal reasons, one withdrew because of high fever and urinary tract infection, one developed gross haematuria necessitating an immediate prostatectomy, and four had a myocardial infarction during treatment. Of these 71 patients, 20 (28%) were considered successful for subjective criteria improvement, such as symptom score and for objective changes such as measurement of prostate size and flow rate; in 38 of these patients (54%) treatment was considered to have failed; 13 patients (18%), benefited in only subjective or objective categories but not both. Of the 31 patients in urinary retention, one patient abandoned treatment for unknown reasons and one died during the treatment protocol from causes unrelated to the microwave hyperthermia; of the 29 patients remaining, 19 were able to remove their catheters, for a catheter-free rate of 65%. Follow-up was incomplete and only eight patients were seen at 6 and 12 months.

Using a Primus transrectal applicator, which uses 915 MHz microwaves at 40 W without a transurethral temperature probe, vanErps et al. treated 60 patients with treatments twice a week for 5 weeks (ten total).[21] Objective improvement was noted in 21 (35%) and subjective improvement in 41 (68%). Therapy was delivered without complications. These authors noted no objective decrease in size of the prostate or elevation in serum prostate-specific antigen (PSA) values.[21] This study confirmed the finding of Lindner et al.,[22] that transrectal hyperthermia does not cause prostatic destruction to the point of elevating serum PSA. Watson[23] used the Primus device to treat 17 patients at a target temperature of 42–44°C for six 1 h treatments. He reported symptom score reduction of 38% and improved peak flow rate from 7.8 to 10.4 ml/s at 6 months.

Strohmaier et al.[24] in 1990 reported a phase II study using a transrectal water-cooled probe (915 MHz) in 30 patients (25 with symptoms of prostatism only and five in urinary retention). A total of eight sessions of 60 min each was administered twice weekly. Only 28 of the 30 patients were evaluable at 4 weeks after treatment. Objective improvement in voiding parameters occurred only in two of the 28 patients (7.1%), and only one of five patients in retention became catheter free.

Zerbib et al.[25] conducted a prospective randomized trial comparing transrectal hyperthermia (n=38) with sham treatment (n=30). The protocol used was weekly treatments for 5 weeks at 43°C. They reported subjective and some objective improvement only in the active therapy group versus subjective improvement in the sham treatment group. This report has been criticized for differences in pretreatment parameters in both groups (the peak flow rate in the active treatment group was 7.6 ml/s compared with 10.6 ml/s in the sham group). Thus, the active treatment group had a wider margin to demonstrate improvement.

Fabricius et al.[26] reported a placebo-controlled study using transrectal hyperthermia and demonstrated minimal differences between the two groups. Montorsi, et al.[27] had reported long-term results in 191 patients followed for up to 2 years and reported sustained improvement in subjective scores, but no objective improvement. According to peak flow rate nomograms, all patients were still obstructed after the procedure, but post-void residual urine was reduced significantly. Light and electron microscopy showed no irreversible damage to glandular epithelium in patients in whom treatment failed and who subsequently underwent surgery. However, chronic inflammatory infiltrates were noted when compared with non-heated controls.[27]

Kaplan et al.[28] studied 30 patients who underwent transrectal hyperthermia with a Primus device in ten weekly 1 h sessions. A total of 29 patients completed the 6 month follow-up. Improvement in mean peak flow rate was from 5.0 ml/s at baseline to 15.2 ml/s. Correspondingly, more than 50% of the patients had a more than 50% reduction in symptom score. The authors pointed out that the thermal distribution was clearly related to the distance from the applicator dipole, i.e. a temperature of over 43°C was achieved only at distances of less than 2.5 cm.[28]

Conclusions regarding transrectal hyperthermia

The varied results reported with transrectal hyperthermia (Table 34.2) can be related to a number of

issues including improperly designed and uncontrolled studies, variations in wavelength, differences in device design, treatment protocol and the confounding natural history of BPH. Proper multi-institutional studies to include randomization versus sham and other alternative therapies such as drug therapy or TURP have not been performed. Transrectal hyperthermia is a relatively safe procedure, as demonstrated by many authors. Lindner reported a complication rate of 6.6% in 435 patients treated with the Prostathermer.[29] In addition, these complications were apparently minor: urinary tract infection, minor haematuria and epididymitis accounted for 51% of the complications.[29] Watson[23] reported reduced complications using the Primus machine without transurethral manipulation. At temperatures of 42–44°C, no rectourethral fistulae or anorectal abnormalities occurred in the absence of a transurethral temperature probe. There have been no reports of sexual dysfunction related to therapy, and Rigatti et al.[30] demonstrated no change in semen analysis or in measurable biochemical constituents after transrectal hyperthermia. It is encouraging that the devices are safe and produce some subjective improvement, but long-term follow-up studies to define the optimal protocol, proper patient selection, efficacy and re-treatment rates for transrectal hyperthermia would be necessary to enable these devices to find their proper place in the treatment armamentarium.

Transurethral devices

In 1985, the use of transurethral microwave radiation treatment (2450 MHz) was reported by Harada et al.[11] in six patients with prostate obstruction. It was not clear from this early report how many of these patients were obstructed by BPH and how many had prostate cancer. Patients were treated with 100 W for 60 s, which was repeated two or three times for several minutes in each patient. A catheter was left in place for 7–14 days after treatment. Five of these six patients voided after removing the catheter, having been in urinary retention before that time.

In 1987, Harada et al.[31] described microwave surgery via a transurethral probe as a tool for improving prostate electroresection. A comparative study was made of 16 patients with bladder neck obstruction treated with microwave coagulation, compared with 19 patients who

Table 34.2. *Efficacy of transrectal hyperthermia in non-randomized studies*

Series	Instrument	Sessions Length (h)	Sessions No.	Target temperature (°C)	No. of patients	Subjective improvement (%)	Objective improvement (%)	Longest follow-up (months)
Yerushalmi 1985[15]	Prototype	1	1–18	43	18	57	–	23
Servadio 1987[17]	Prostathermer	1	5–10	43	16	48	48	24
Saranga 1990[20]	Prostathermer	1	4–7	42.5	11	19	28	12
Servadio 1990[19]	Prostathermer	1	8	42	140	–	47	12
Watson 1992[23]	Prostathermer	1	6	44.5	19	50	55	12
Watson 1991[23]	Primus	1	6	44	17	38	32	6
Stawarz 1991[54]	Prototype	0.5	6	43	16	51	189	3
Strohmaier 1990[24]	Prostathermer	1	8	42.5	23	24	10	4
Yerushalmi 1992[16]	Prostathermer	1	8–20	43	89	80	27	96
Montorsi 1992[27]	Prostathermer	1	5–10	43	118	n/a	n/a	24
Kaplan 1993[28]	Primus	1	10	43.5	30	65	33	6

had a conventional transurethral resection. Both groups were analysed for the amount of blood loss, irrigant absorption and frequency of complications. The hyperthermic group had a significant reduction of blood loss and no complications. The authors concluded that the combination procedure of microwave coagulation can minimize the disadvantage of a formal TURP or may be of value in the treatment of a patient with both prostatic obstruction and haemorrhagic diathesis, as well as high-risk patients.

Astrahan et al.[12] have studied two prototype transurethral antennae and tested them on tissue equivalent. In the first design, a three-dipole applicator was incorporated into a modified Foley catheter, while a later design consisted of a flexible helical antenna around a modified Foley catheter. Both applicators appeared to be similar in terms of the heating characteristics. However, the helical design produced a more cylindrical heating pattern with a broader and more consistent hot spot compared with the early design (Fig. 34.2). These authors showed that this applicator was well suited for heating a cylindrical volume of approximately 4 cm in length and 0.5 cm in radial depth around the applicator.[12] The same group carried out interstitial thermometry in canine prostates during transurethral microwave hyperthermia (915 MHz). The selective cylindrical heating produced by phantom studies was confirmed in the dog model.[32] The radial heat penetration showed a hot spot near the longitudinal set of the applicator at about 0.5 cm from the applicator with a dissipation gradient of approximately –7°C/cm. Histological examination of the canine prostates revealed dilated glands surrounded by interstitial oedema. The lumen of the glands was filled with sludged, epithelial material and necrosis of glandular elements was evident.[32] Tissues obtained by transurethral resection in patients who failed transurethral microwave hyperthermia have shown

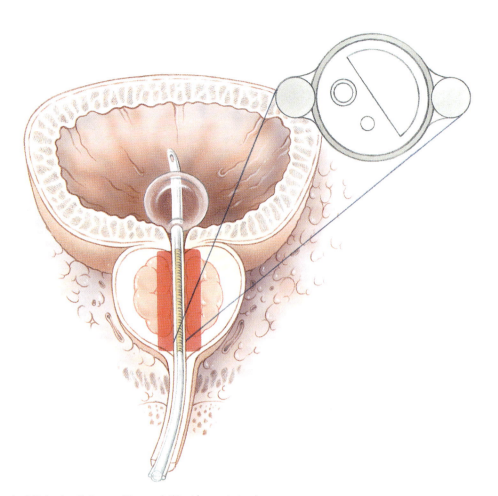

Figure 34.2. *Transurethral (helical coil) device. (From ref. 58 with permission.)*

interstitial haemorrhages, blood vessel thrombosis and coagulative and haemorrhagic necrosis in the periurethral prostate.[33] The depth of penetration of these lesions correlates well with the heating profile of the helical applicator.[33] It is believed that selective shrinking or retraction of the prostate tissue dilates the urethra and reduces or eliminates outflow obstruction.[34]

Sapozink et al.[35] published in 1990 a report on 21 patients with biopsy-proven BPH who underwent treatment with a pilot protocol involving intracavitary transurethral radiation microwave hyperthermia without extrinsic cooling (630 MHz in 12 patients, 915 MHz in nine patients). Interstitial thermometry demonstrated a mean temperature of 44.1°C, mean maximal temperature of 47.7°C and a maximal temperature of 49°C. There were highly significant increases in mean peak flow rate (44%) and a decrease in post-void residual urine (49%). A decrease in urinary

frequency (30%) and nocturia (44%) was also observed. Median follow-up in these patients was 12.5 months, and only three required subsequent prostatic resection. Complications included bladder spasms in 26% of patients, haematuria in 23% and dysuria in 9%.[35]

Recently, Baert et al.[36] demonstrated a doubling of peak flow rates in patients treated with five to ten sessions of transurethral microwave hyperthermia without cooling (915 MHz). This same group, in a more recent publication, reported on the results of 31 patients who had at least 12 months of follow-up and an additional seven patients who failed hyperthermia and underwent surgical therapy.[37] The reported group were taken from a total of 79 patients (seven of these had discontinued their treatment) who were scheduled to receive five 60 min sessions with temperature controlled on the urethral surface at 45.5°C (915 MHz). The Boyarsky symptom score in the 61 patients decreased from 15.1 to 7.7, mostly in the obstructive categories. Mean peak flow rate increased from 8.8 to 11.5 ml/s. Of those seven patients in whom hyperthermia failed, five had a median lobe and one a median bar. Significant improvement occurred in 73% of those with lateral lobe hyperplasia and in only 30% with median lobe hyperplasia.[37]

In a study of over 74 patients, Baert et al.[38] showed an overall objective response rate of 70%. The importance of anatomy was again pointed out as patients with bilobar versus trilobar hyperplasia showed an improvement from 9.8 to 13.6 ml/s ($p<0.0056$) and from 7.1 to 11.1 ml/s ($p<0.09$) respectively. A greater than 50% subjective response rate in terms of symptom score was obtained in 75% of patients. Patients with primarily obstructive symptoms achieved the best response. Of 32 patients in urinary retention, 25 patients had bilobar symmetrical hyperplasia, and seven had asymmetrical median lobe enlargement. None of the seven median lobe patients resumed spontaneous voiding. However, 72% of the bilobar hyperplasia patients were urinating at 12 months after transurethral microwave hyperthermia.[38] Histological examination of specimens from patients who underwent TURP revealed coagulative necrosis of urethral and periurethral tissue at depths of 6 mm radially. The same group has recently reported a prospective randomized trial comparing three and six sessions.[39] Of a total of 28 BPH patients, 80% of the patients who underwent three sessions (group 1) experienced subjective improvement, compared with 86% of those in group 2 who underwent six sessions. Total symptom score improved by 21.4% in the first group and by 51.1% in the second group ($p<0.006$). There was a statistically significant difference between the two groups in the mean peak flow rate: the first group improved by 8.4% whereas the second group increased the rate by 51.1% ($p<0.001$). These investigators concluded that six sessions of transurethral microwave hyperthermia using this device were more effective than three sessions.[39] Bladder atony, prostate asymmetry and median lobe hyperplasia are most detrimental to the efficacy of transurethral hyperthermia.

Petrovich et al.[40] studied the relationship of response to transurethral hyperthermia to prostate volume in BPH patients. They studied 63 patients and compared those with small (<50 g) and large (>50 g) glands. Of 40 patients with small prostates, 10% experienced failure, versus 9% of the 23 patients with large prostates. The authors concluded that the prostate gland size was not an important predictor of response to transurethral microwave hyperthermia.[40]

Sham studies are important in device studies and are analogous to placebo-controlled drug studies. Scientifically, however, they are different in that there cannot be a placebo lead-in period with device trials. Bdesha et al.[41] recently reported a sham-controlled but unblinded trial of transurethral microwave hyperthermia involving 40 patients. After active therapy, an American Urological Association (AUA) symptom score improvement of 63% (from 19.2 to 7.1) versus only marginal improvement (from 18.8 to 16.7) following sham treatment ($p<0.001$) was noted. Mean peak flow rates improved by 2.3 ml/s and post-void residual decreased by 50% after active therapy, but no improvement was noted after sham therapy. Sham-treated patients were then offered active therapy, and the results mirrored the original active treatment arm. The side effects were minimal with no sexual dysfunction reported. The authors concluded that the instrumentation effect of the therapy was minimal.[41] Although blinded, sham-controlled, randomized device studies are rare, a statistically significant and therapeutic response has been noted in approximately one-quarter to one-third of patients.[42–45] These results underline the importance of carrying out double-blind studies for device trials to account for instrumentation or sham effects.

Billebaud et al.[46] in 1994 presented data from a multi-centre sham study using a transurethral microwave hyperthermia device at 44°C (Medi-Therm Ltd, France). Twenty-four patients were randomized to receive transurethral microwave hyperthermia and 31 received sham treatments at 37°C (placebo) at five different general hospitals in the Ile de France region. Treatment consisted of three 1 h outpatient sessions every 48 h. The study demonstrated that the act of treatment leads to an objective improvement in the peak flow rate at 3 months and improvement in daytime frequency at 6 months. Apparently, the objective response was not durable at 6 months, although subjective improvement was maintained. Table 34.3

Table 34.3. *Efficacy of transurethral hyperthermia in reported studies*

Series	Instrument	Sessions Length (h)	Sessions No.	No. of patients	Subjective improvement (%)	Objective improvement (%)	Longest follow-up (months)
Sapozink 1990[35]	BSD	1	10	21	43	45	12
Baert 1990[36]	BSD	1	5–10	12	65	98	12
Stawarz 1991[54]	BSD	0.5	3–6	14	77	79	12
Baert 1992[37]	BSD	1	5	79	49	30	12
Watson 1992[23]	Thermex II	3	1	68	40	n.s.	1
Vanden Bossche 1993[49]	Thermex II	1	1	191	65	45	–
Viguier 1993[52]	Thermex II	1	1	50	68	n.s.	12
Bdesha 1994[41]	LFO Micro-thermer*	1	1	40	63	n.s.	3

*Laser Optics, London, UK. n.s., not significant.

summarizes the results of reported series of transurethral hyperthermia for BPH.

It is apparent that transurethral microwave hyperthermia is a safe procedure. The treatment toxicity is mild with bladder spasms (14.5%), local pain (16%) and mild haematuria (7.4%) being the most common side effects.[33,47] Transient urinary retention is usually seen in less than 5% of patients, and the use of routine antibacterial therapy appears to prevent urinary tract infection.[47] The reported late complications include urethral stricture formation in 4.8% of patients.[47] However, no sphincter dysfunction, sexual dysfunction or incontinence have been reported.[33,47]

Transurethral hyperthermia of the prostate has recently also been accomplished by using radiofrequency (0.5–10 MHz) rather than microwave energy (300–3000 MHz). Penetration of electromagnetic waves depends on its frequency. Thus, investigators consider that the use of low radiofrequency waves gives a deeper and more uniform penetration than microwaves (Fig. 34.3). Two-to three-fold increases in PSA 1 day after treatment and histological examination indicate periurethral prostatic destruction.[48] Evidence of prostatic destruction by increases in serum PSA indicates therapeutic temperatures above 45°C and thus this therapy is defined by the International Consensus Conference (ICC) organized by the World Health Organization (WHO) on BPH held in Paris, 1991, as *thermotherapy* (>45 °C target tissue temperature) as opposed to *hyperthermia* (<45°C target tissue temperature).[48]

The Thermex II is a transurethral prostate device that uses a capacitative diathermy to heat the prostate.[23,49–53] The electrode is placed on a modified Foley catheter and positioned in the prostatic urethra. Two grounding plates are placed on the upper inner thighs. Target temperatures of 44.5–47°C for one 3 h session produces necrosis of periurethral tissue. Watson treated 100 patients with the device and reported 9-month follow-up data for 68 of the total group.[23] An increase in peak flow rate by 2 ml/s, a decrease in post-void residual volume from 100 to 67 ml and a drop in symptom score by approximately 40% was noted. Side effects were minimal but 19 (19%) patients subsequently underwent TURP.

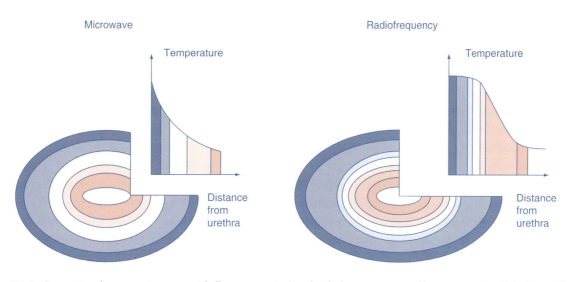

Figure 34.3. *Comparison between microwaves (shallow penetration) and radiofrequency waves (deep penetration, high thermal dose). From ref. 59 with permission.)*

Vanden Bossche et al.[49] also used the Thermex II device in 191 patients at various temperatures (44.5 and 47–48°C) in one session. At 44.5°C, 60% of patients were subjectively better and 71% at 47–48°C. Of the patients in retention, 58% were rendered catheter free. No statistically significant improvement in peak flow rate was noted at either temperature. In an earlier study, these authors noted no change in prostate volume by ultrasound or magnetic resonance imaging.[50] However, serum PSA increased two- to three-fold on the day following therapy and returned to pretherapy levels at 1 month. Histopathological examination revealed a periurethral necrotic area measuring 15×10×10 mm.[50]

Viguier et al.[52] reported on 50 patients treated with a Thermex II. They also noted no change in prostate volume but modest improvements in peak flow rates (not statistically significant). Symptom score improved in 68% of the patients, with a more pronounced effect on irritative as opposed to obstructive symptoms. The authors recommend therapy for prostates of 40 g or less.[52] Other authors have demonstrated subjective improvement of 70% with increases of peak flow rate of up to 4 ml/s.[51–53] This has also been shown to be an effective treatment option for patients in urinary retention, as up to 58% are rendered catheter free after a single office-based session.[52,53] Complications are rare, and urinary retention is seen in approximately 10% after treatment.[53]

Comparative studies

A non-parallel, non-randomized comparison of transrectal hyperthermia and transurethral hyperthermia was reported recently.[54] Twenty-two patients had transrectal hyperthermia treatment with a water-cooled probe (2450 or 434 MHz) in six 30 min sessions twice weekly, and 14 patients had transurethral hyperthermia without urethral cooling (2450 MHz) in from three to six 30 min sessions twice weekly (ten patients had all six scheduled treatments). Follow-up ranged from 10 to 28 months (mean 19 months) for the transrectally treated group, and from 7 to 16 months (mean 10 months) for the transurethral group. Toxicity was higher in the transurethrally treated groups (27 vs 8%). Three of the transurethrally treated patients underwent surgery during the treatment period, all in chronic urinary retention. At 3 months there was a greater symptom score improvement in the transurethral group than in the transrectal group (79 vs 41%). Prostate volume decreased in 45% of the transrectal group and 79 in the transurethral group. There was significant improvement in mean peak urinary flow rate in both groups, and post-void residual urine volume decreased, with no significant difference between the two groups. These authors also reported a high failure rate in patients with median lobe hyperplasia.[54]

Abbou et al.[55] devised a double-blind, randomized multicentre study to compare transrectal and transurethral hyperthermia and sham in the treatment of patients presenting with obstructive BPH. From ten centres, 216 patients were randomized. Five different transurethral devices and five transrectal microwave hyperthermia machines were used. Selection criteria were as follows: age above 50 years; symptom duration more than 3 months; no suspicion of cancer; peak flow rate of 15 ml/s or less; prostate weight of 30–80 g. Although a detailed analysis was not presented in this abstract, the conclusions of the authors were that transurethral and transrectal microwave hyperthermia provided no improvement in objective criteria and that only the transurethral approach improved the subjective symptoms. The authors questioned the efficacy of hyperthermia in general as a treatment alternative to surgical therapy.[55]

Perlmutter et al.[56] recently published a non-randomized pilot study of 134 patients with symptomatic BPH, comparing transrectal and transurethral hyperthermia. Nineteen patients underwent transrectal hyperthermia with the Prostathermer and 15 with the Primus machine. One hundred patients underwent therapy with the transurethral device, Thermex II. All patients were candidates for TURP, but were encouraged to undergo no further therapy for 1 year. Although 16 of 19 (84%) Prostathermer and 14 of 15 (93%) Primus-treated patients experienced initial improvement in symptoms at 6 weeks, only seven of 19 (37%) and six of 15 (40%), respectively, had not sought additional therapy at the 30 month follow-up. Improvement was mostly related to symptom reduction, and was seldom due to significant increases in peak flow rate (Table 34.4). Of the 100 patients treated by the Thermex II device, 93% had initial satisfactory results at 6 weeks, but only 55% at 1 year. At 1 year, 40% of Thermex II patients had not undergone TURP. Sustained improvement was achievable in symptom scoring, with minimal sustained improvement in peak flow rate. All devices were well tolerated and periprocedural complications were few: four Prostathermer (21%) and four Thermex II patients (4%) experienced urinary tract infection; two Prostathermer (10%) and two Thermex II (2%) patients experienced urinary retention; two Prostathermer and two Thermex II patients experienced syncope. Bladder spasm was most severe with the Thermex II and persistent rectal burning was seen with the Prostathermer and Primus devices in two patients each.[56]

Conclusions regarding transurethral hyperthermia

Many of the criticisms of transrectal microwave hyperthermia can be applied to transurethral microwave hyperthermia as well. Sham-controlled, blinded,

Table 34.4. *Pretreatment parameters amd comparison of initial parameters in successful* and unsuccessful treatments*

Instrument	Patient outcome	No. of patients	Patient age (years)	Prostate volume (cm³)	Symptoms Irritative	Symptoms Obstructive	Symptoms Total	Peak flow (ml/s)	Post-void residual (ml)
Biodan	All	19	68	40	5.3	6.5	11.8	7.3	136
	Successes	7	71	35	5.2	6.8	12.0	7.8	140
	Failures	12	66	43	5.5	6.2	11.7	7.0	134
Primus	All	15	67	43	5.5	5.3	10.8	8.3	118
	Successes	6	69	49	5.4	4.4	9.8	10.0	130
	Failures	9	66	39	5.8	5.7	11.5	7.0	110
Thermex II	All	10	66	34	4.5	5.3	9.8	8.8	110
	Successes	55	67	35	4.5	6.5	11.0	9.4	80
	Failures	40	65	33	4.3	4.0	8.3	8.0	165

*Success is defined as a patient who remains in the study with sufficient improvement to avoid further intervention. Failure is defined as a patient who requires additional treatment. (From ref. 56 with permission.)

randomized multi-institutional studies that account for the sham effect, and that compare conventional treatments, with long-term follow-up, have not been conducted. It is apparent that many patients will either fail the therapy or require re-treatment. It is difficult to compare series as patient populations are different, and the clinical results are expressed in different ways in terms of peak flow rate, average flow rate and various symptom scores. Lack of uniformity in response criteria makes it difficult to compare results with different devices and various protocols.[57] Not withstanding these differences, the results of most studies show similar results in terms of improvement in subjective symptoms, with modest improvement in objective parameters such as peak flow rate and residual urine volume. It appears that these devices are safe, but because of the lack of rigorous studies under multi-institutional protocols, it is difficult to compare the results of transurethral microwave hyperthermia with those of transrectal hyperthermia or other modalities. Use of these devices for symptoms of BPH should be considered investigational until longer follow-up and results of comparative trials are available.

References

1. Mebust W K, Holtgrewe H L, Cockett A T K et al. Transurethral prostatectomy immediate and postoperative complications: a cooperative stuudy of thirteen participating institutions evaluating 3,885 patients. J Urol 1989; 141: 243–247

2. Mebust W K. Transurethral prostastectomy. Urol Clin North Am 1990; 17: 575–585

3. Lindner A, Golomb J, Siegel Y et al. Local hyperthermia of the prostate gland for the treatment of benign prostatic hypertrophy and urinary retention. Br J Urol 1987; 60: 567–571

4. Devonec M, Berger M D, Perrin P. Transurethral microwave heating of the prostate — or from hyperthermia to thermotherapy. J Endourol 1991; 5: 129

5. Yerushalmi A, Servadio C, Leib Z et al. Local hyperthermia for treatment of carcinoma of the prostate: a preliminary report. Prostate 1982; 3: 623–630

6. Lieb Z, Rothern A, Lev A et al. Histopathological observations in the canine prostate treated by local hyperthermia. Prostate 1986; 8: 93–102

7. Servadio C, Leib Z. Hyperthermia in the treatment of prostate cancer. Prostate 1984; 5: 205–211

8. Servadio C, Leib Z, Lev A. Further observations on the use of local hyperthermia for the treatment of diseases of the prostate in man. Eur Urol 1986; 12: 38–40

9. Szmigielski S, Zielinski H, Stawarz B et al. Local microwave hyperthermia in treatment of advanced prostatic adenocarcinoma. Urol Res 1988; 16: 1–7

10. Magin R L, Fridd C W, Bonfiglio T A et al. Thermal destruction of the canine prostate by high intensity microwaves. J Surg Res 1980; 29: 265–275

11. Harada T, Etori K, Kumazaki T et al. Microwave surgical treatment of diseases of prostate. Urology 1985; 26: 572–576

12. Astrahan M A, Sapozink M D, Cohen D et al. Microwave applicator for transurethral hyperthermia of benign prostatic hyperplasia. Int J Hyperthermia 1989; 5: 283–296

13. Roehrborn C G, Krongrad A, McConnell J D. Temperature mapping in the canine prostate during transurethrally applied local microwave hyperthermia. Prostate 1992; 20: 97

14. Ameye F, Baert L. Critical evaluation of treatment modalities and localized hyperthermia of the prostate. In: Petrovich Z, Baert L (eds) Innovations in the management of benign prostatic hyperplasia. Berlin: Springer-Verlag, 1994: 329–359

15. Yerushalmi A, Fishelovitz Y, Singer D et al. Localized deep microwave hyperthermia in the treatment of poor operative risk patients with benign prostatic hyperplasia. J Urol 1985; 133: 873–876

16. Yerushalmi A, Singer D, Katsnelson R et al. Localised deep microwave hyperthermia in the treatment of benign prostatic hyperplasia: long-term assessment. Br J Urol 1992; 70: 178–182

17. Servadio C, Leib Z, Lev A. Diseases of prostate treated by local microwave hyperthermia. Urology 1987; 30: 97–99

18. Lindner A, Braf Z, Golomb J et al. Local hyperthermia of the prostate gland for the treatment of benign prostatic hypertrophy and urinary retention. Br J Urol 1990; 65: 201–203

19. Servadio C, Braf Z, Siegel Y et al. Local thermotherapy of the benign prostate: a 1-year follow-up. Eur Urol 1990; 18: 169–173

20. Saranga R, Matzkin H, Braf Z. Local microwave hyperthermia in the treatment of benign prostatic hypertrophy. Br J Urol 1990; 65: 349–353

21. vanErps PM, Dourcy B, Denis LJ. Transrectal hyperthermia in benign prostatic hyperplasia (BPH). J Urol 1991; 145: 263A (abstr 203)

22. Lindner A, Siegel Y I, Korczak, D. Serum prostate-specific antigen levels during hyperthermia treatment of benign prostatic hyperplasia. J Urol 1990; 144: 1388–1389

23. Watson G. Minimally invasive therapies of the prostate. J Min Invas Ther 1992; 1: 231–240

24. Strohmaier W L, Bichler K-H, Flüchter S H et al. Local microwave hyperthermia of benign prostatic hyperplasia. J Urol 1990; 144: 913–917

25. Zerbib M, Steg A, Conquy S et al. Localized hyperthermia versus sham procedure in obstructive benign prostatic hyperplasia of the prostate: a prospective randomized study. J Urol 1992; 147: 1048

26. Fabricius P G, Schäfer J, Schmeller N et al. Efficacy of transrectal hyperthermia for benign prostatic hyperplasia: a placebo-controlled study. J Urol 1991; 145: 363A (abstr 602)

27. Montorsi F, Galli L, Gauazzoni G et al. Transrectal microwave hyperthermia for benign prostatic hyperplasia: long-term clinical, pathological and ultrastructural patterns. J Urol 1992; 148: 321–325

28. Kaplan S A, Shabsigh R, Soldo K A et al. Transrectal hyperthermia in the management of men with prostatism: an algorithm for therapy. Br J Urol 1993; 72: 195–200

29. Lindner A, Siegel Y I, Saranga R et al. Complications in hyperthermia treatment of benign prostatic hyperplasia. J Urol 1990; 144: 1390–1392

30. Rigatti P, Buonaguidi A, Grasso M et al. Morphodynamic and biochemical assessment of seminal plasma in patients who underwent local prostatic hyperthermia. Prostate 1990; 16: 325–330

31. Harada T, Tsuchida S, Nishizawa O et al. Microwave surgical treatment of the prostate: clinical application of microwave surgery as a tool for improved prostastic electroresection. Urol Int 1987; 42: 127–131

32 Astrahan M A, Sapozink M D, Cohen D et al. Microwave applicator for transurethral hyperthermia of benign prostatic hyperplasia. Int J Hyperthermia 1989; 5: 283–296

33. Ameye F, Baert L. Urological effects of local microwave hyperthermia of prostate tissues. In: Petrovich Z, Beart L (eds) Innovations in the management of benign prostatic hyperplasia. Berlin: Springer-Verlag 1994: 239–274

34. Lauweryns J, Baert L, Vandenhove J et al. Histopathology of prostatic tissue after transurethral hyperthermia. Int J Hyperthermia 1991; 7: 221–230

35. Sapozink M D, Boyd S D, Astrahan M A, et al. Transurethral hyperthermia for benign prostatic hyperplasia: preliminary clinical results. J Urol 1990; 143: 944–950

36. Baert L, Ameye F, Willemen P et al. Transurethral microwave hyperthermia for benign prostatic hyperplasia: preliminary clinical and pathological results. J Urol 1990; 144: 1383

37. Baert L, Willemen P, Ameye F et al. Treatment response with transurethral microwave hyperthermia in different forms of benign prostatic hyperplasia: a preliminary report. Prostate 1992; 18: 315–320

38. Baert L, Ameye F, Astrahan M. Transurethral microwave hyperthermia for benign prostatic hyperplasia: the Leuven clinical experience. J Endourol 1993; 7: 61–69

39. Baert L, Ameye F, Pike M, Petrovich Z. Optimization of transurethral hyperthermia. Number of treatments. Urology 1994; 43: 567–571

40. Petrovich Z, Ameye F, Pike M et al. Relationship of response to transurethral hyperthermia and prostate volume in BPH patients. Urology 1992; 40: 317–321

41. Bdesha A S, Bunce C J, Snell M E, Witherow R O. A sham controlled trial of transurethral microwave therapy with subsequent treatment of the control group. J Urol 1994; 152: 453–458

42. Lepor H, Sypherd D, Machi G et al. Randomized double-blind study comparing the effectiveness of balloon dilatation of the prostate and cystoscopy for the treatment of symptomatic benign prostatic hyperplasia. J Urol 1992; 147: 639–644

43. Debruyne F M J, Bloem F A G, de la Rosette J O M C H et al. Transurethral thermotherapy (TUMT) in benign prostatic hyperplasia: placebo versus TUMT. J Urol 1993; 149: 146A (AUA syllabus)

44. Ogden C W, Reddy P, Johnson H et al. Sham versus transurethral microwave thermotherapy in patients with symptoms of benign prostatic outflow obstruction. Lancet 1993; 341: 14

45. Blute M L, Patterson D E, Segura J W et al. Transurethral microwave thermotherapy versus sham: a prospective double blind randomized study. J Urol 1994; 151 :752A

46. Billebaud T, Mechali P, Astier L et al. Transurethral microwave hyperthermia for benign prostatic hyperplasia: is it effective? Results of a multicentric randomized prospective study versus placebo with six month followup. J Urol 1994; 151: 760A

47. Baert L, Ameye F, Astrahan M, Petrovich Z. Transurethral microwave hyperthermia for benign prostatic hyperplasia: the Leuven clinical experience. J Endourol 1993; 7: 61–69

48. Smith P, Shase C, Conart P et al. Report of the committee on other nonmedical treatment. In: Cockett A T K, Aso Y, Chatelain C et al (eds) International Consultation on Benign Prostatic Hyperplasia. Jersey: SCI Ltd, 1992: 223–257.

49. Vanden Bossche M, Peltry A, Schulman C C. (TURF) Transurethral radiofrequency heating for benign prostatic hyperplasia at various temperatures with Thermex II: clinical experience. Eur Urol 1993; 23: 302–306

50. Vanden Bossche M, Noël J C, Schulman C C. Transurethral hyperthermia for benign prostatic hypertrophy. World J Urol 1991; 9: 2–6

51. Corica A, Marianetti A, Anchelerguez R et al. Transurethral radio frequency thermotherapy for symptomatic benign prostatic hyperplasia. Eur Urol 1993; 23: 312–317

52. Viguier J L, Dessouhi T, Corlebo A et al. Benign prostatic hypertrophy treatment by transurethral radiofrequency hyperthermia with Thermex II. Eur Urol 1993; 23: 318–321

53. Nissenkorn I, Rotbard M, Slutzker D, Bernheim J. The connection between the length of the heating antenna and volume of the prostate in transurethral thermotherapy for benign prostatic hyperplasia. Eur Urol 1993; 23: 307–311

54. Stawarz B, Szmigielski S, Ogrodnik J et al. A comparison of transurethral and transrectal microwave hyperthermia in poor surgical risk benign prostatic hyperplasia patients. J Urol 1991; 146: 353–357

55. Abbou C C, Colombel M, Payan C e tal. Transrectal and transurethral hyperthermia versus sham to treat benign prostatic hyperplasia: a double blind, randomized, multicenter study. J Urol 1994; 151: 761A

56. Perlmutter A P, Verdi J, Watson G M. Prostatic heat treatments for urinary outflow obstruction. J Urol 1993; 150: 1603–1606

57. Meier A H P, Weil E H J, van Waalwijk van Doorn E S C et al. Transurethral radio frequency heating or thermotherapy for benign prostatic hypertrophy: a prospective trial on 65 consecutive cases. Eur Urol 1992; 22: 39–43

58. Astrahan M A, Ameye F, Oyenh R et al. Interstitial temperature measurements during transurethral microwave hyperthermia. J Urol 1991; 145: 305

59. Schulman C C, Vanden Bossche M. Hyperthermia and thermotherapy of benign prostatic hyperplasia: a critical review. Eur Urol 1993; 23(suppl 1): 54`

Transurethral thermotherapy

M. A. Devonec

Introduction

The aim of heat therapy is to destroy benign prostatic hyperplasia (BPH) tissue without damaging the structures surrounding the treated organ, namely the sphincter, bladder wall, rectum and urethra. Tissue destruction results from coagulative necrosis caused by heating the target area to over 44°C. These two features characterize transurethral microwave thermotherapy (TUMT)[1–4] and distinguish it from hyperthermia using microwaves[5,6] or transurethral radiofrequency (TURF).[7]

Interstitial thermometry

Interstitial thermometry data[3,4,8] are essential in understanding the mechanism of heat therapy for BPH. Temperature mapping in the transition zone differentiates hyperthermia from microwave thermotherapy: during hyperthermia treatment, intraprostatic temperatures remain below 44°C, whereas TUMT elevates the temperature of the transition zone well above 44°C.

An analysis performed by Carter and Ogden[8] of the temperature distribution in the horizontal plane calculated as a function of the distance from the urethra showed a maximum temperature of 65.2°C measured at a distance of about 6 mm. Temperatures exceeding 44°C are achieved at distances ranging from 5 to 18 mm lateral to the urethra. These distances correspond to the configuration of the transition zone. The variability of temperature increase among different prostates is presumed to be related to individual prostates anatomy (tissue composition and vascularization). When the urethra is properly cooled, the intraprostatic temperature reaches a maximum inside the prostatic tissue. The location of this maximum value is estimated to be at 6 mm from the urethra. Hence, owing to the effect of the cooling, the temperature curve has a steep ascending slope (2–3°C/mm) and a smooth descending slope (0.4°C/mm), characteristic of the thermotherapy

principle (Fig. 35.1). These interstitial thermometry data corroborate earlier pathological data reported by Devonec et al.:[9] the hottest areas, in which coagulation necrosis develops, are symmetrically located at a distance of 6 mm from the prostatic urethra on either side (Fig. 35.2).

The temperature distribution in a vertical plane encompassing the prostatic urethra shows that temperatures above 44°C are generated 4–20 mm distal to the bladder neck.

Peak rectal and urethral temperatures are continuously monitored throughout the TUMT procedure and these values are compared with preset safety thresholds of 42.5 and 44.5°C, respectively. If these thresholds are reached, microwave power output is downregulated. Monitoring of rectal and urethral

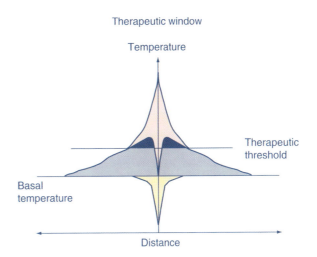

Figure 35.1. *Transurethral microwave thermotherapy concept: the x-axis represents the distance from the antenna in the urethra; the y-axis represents the temperature. The combination of deep radiative heating and superficial conductive cooling leads to an asymmetrical temperature profile, with steep ascending slope and progressive descending slope. Because of the cell toxicity threshold, periurethral tissue is preserved as long as the temperature stays below the therapeutic threshold. Tissue coagulation (dark area) is obtained as soon as the ascending slope crosses therapeutic threshold and is maintained until the descending slope crosses it.*

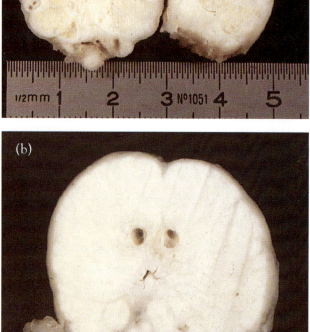

Figure 35.2. *The hottest areas on a transverse section of the prostate are symmetrically situated at a distance of 6 mm from the urethra. (a) Human prostate: the hottest areas are lateral to the urethra; (b) dog prostate: the hottest areas are anterior to the urethra.*

temperatures allows the delivery of large amounts of energy to the prostate while preventing any damage to these structures. When no microwaves are emitted, the periurethral tissue is cooled to 0–5.5°C below the patient baseline temperature at 5–15 mm from the urethra. The estimated 'characteristic cooling depth' is of the order of 5 mm. Hence, urethral cooling is an efficient protective mechanism in the periurethral zone.

Higher intraprostatic temperatures correlate only moderately with a greater decrease in symptom score (Table 35.1). However, higher intraprostatic temperatures are associated with greater improvement in peak flow rate (PFR) (Table 35.1). The positive regression coefficient (slope) provides an estimate for the rate of change of PFR per unit change of time-averaged temperatures of approximately 0.5 ml/s/°C.

Pathological results (e.g. the sharp delineation between the treated and non-treated areas and the bell-shaped temperature curve) support the existence of a therapeutic temperature threshold. The mean change in prostatic temperature (6.8 ± 2.4°C) of patients with improved symptom score differs significantly ($p < 0.02$) from that of the unimproved group (4.7 ± 1.5°C). The mean change in time-averaged temperature (7.3 ± 2.5°C) in patients with improved PFR also differs significantly ($p < 0.02$) from that of the unimproved group (5.4 ± 2.1°C). This indicates that higher average temperatures are associated with a clinically significant improvement in PFR.

Both basic and clinical research have shown that TUMT is a safe treatment and that the clinical outcome is related to the thermal dose. Depending on the vascularization, the shape and tissue composition of the

Table 35.1. *Intraprostatic temperature versus clinical outcome*

Intraprostatic temperature (°C)	No. of patients	Peak flow rate		Symptom score*	
		Percentage increase	Pre- vs post-treatment mean (ml/s)	Percentage decrease	Pre- vs post-treatment mean (ml/s)
Low: 43.8	13	34	7.4–9.9	73	14.7–4.0
Medium: 47.5	16	43	7.4–10.6	76	15.0–3.6
High: 53.2	10	79	7.5–13.4	90	13.5–1.3

*See ref. 33. (From ref. 21 with permission.)

prostate, and also on clinical expectations, higher-energy protocols may be developed in order to tailor the treatment to the needs of each patient.

Thermotherapy pathology

Coagulative necrosis of the transition zone is achieved by TUMT at 915 or 1296 MHz as soon as the therapeutic temperature threshold over 44°C is reached.[3,4,9] Examination of the prostate at 1 week reveals a brownish symmetrical area extending 15–20 mm from the urethra (Fig. 35.3). Microscopic examination shows coagulative necrosis of the treated area within the transition zone. Acinar and smooth muscle cells are totally destroyed. Although small blood vessels are thrombosed, large blood vessels and the urethra are preserved. The lesion is sharply defined and its margins clearly show the boundary between normal and necrotic tissue. Close examination of this border area suggests that smooth muscle cells are slightly more sensitive to heat than are glandular cells.

After 2–3 weeks, the oedematous reaction diminishes and collagen deposition is observed. At the periphery of the lesion, neo-angiogenesis with mild lymphohistiocytic infiltrate is seen.

Long-term pathological studies have not shown regeneration of acini or smooth muscle in the treated area, where collagen bands and fibroblasts are abundant. Coagulation necrosis of the transition zone with a butterfly shape parallel to that of the isotherm curve

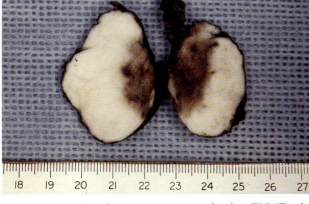

Figure 35.3. *Coagulative necrosis 1 week after TUMT: the transverse section of a large adenoma shows the sharp delineation of the thermal lesion.*

distribution is the feature that differentiates TUMT from hyperthermia using microwave or radiofrequency. At most, a superficial necrosis of the urethra or randomly distributed small coagulation areas (corresponding to hot spots) are observed with the two latter techniques.[10]

Clinical results

Hyperthermia has been tested in randomized, sham-controlled multicentre, double-blind studies.[11] No difference was found between results obtained with active versus sham treatment. Following the recommendations of the 2nd International Consultation on BPH, hyperthermia should no longer be used for the treatment of BPH.[12]

Clinical results of TUMT in BPH are reported using the Prostatron device operating at 1296 MHz. The early use of 915 MHz for TUMT, a frequency allegedly less adapted to prostate anatomy, has resulted in a limited number of papers.[3,4]

TUMT (1296 MHz) versus sham (European studies)

Four prospective randomized and controlled clinical trials have been conducted to compare TUMT with sham (simulated treatment without heat application (Table 35.2).[13–16] The objectives of these studies were (a) to demonstrate that post-TUMT results differ significantly from those after sham treatment and (b) to evaluate the safety of TUMT by determining the extent of adverse events attributable to TUMT and to catheterization alone.

The difference in symptom score improvement between TUMT and sham treatment varied from 29 to 60% and the improvement in PFR compared with the sham treatment varied from 33 to 45% (Table 35.2). A significant difference was noted ($p < 0.001$) between the TUMT and sham treatment results and between baseline values and TUMT treatment results.

TUMT (1296 MHz) versus sham (US study)

The TUMT/sham treatment conducted at the Mayo Clinics (Rochester and Jacksonville) is the only study using a double-blind protocol with a 2:1 (TUMT:sham) randomization.[17]

Table 35.2. *Results of European sham-controlled TUMT studies: percentage changes relative to baseline in symptom score and PFR*

Study	No. of patients (TUMT/sham)	Percentage change in symptom score		Percentage change in PFR	
		TUMT	Sham	TUMT	Sham
Perrin et al.[13]	12/11	48	19	23	–18
Ogden et al.[14]	21/19	70	10	52	7
de la Rosette et al.[15]	25/25	74	24	49	16
Devonec et al.[16]	184/61	52	22	29	–6

After 3 months, a significant difference ($p \leq 0.0001$) in the Madsen symptom score was noted between TUMT and sham treatment. Significant differences were observed in the obstructive and irritative components of the score between the two groups, and the improvement in the TUMT group was nearly twice that of the sham group (Table 35.3). A significant difference ($p < 0.01$) in PFR change between TUMT and sham treatments (58 and 27%, respectively) was also observed.

The various sham studies are consistent and demonstrate a significant placebo and/or instrumentation effect. Significant changes from baseline were observed in the sham group in both Madsen symptom score and, to a lesser extent, in PFR. A significant effect on the serum prostate-specific antigen (PSA) level was noted after 1 week in the TUMT group (+ 470% from baseline), whereas only a slight variation was noted in the sham group. This clinically significant difference confirms the histological effect in patients receiving therapeutic heating.

There was no statistically significant difference ($p > 0.5$) between the two groups in the incidence of treatment-related side effects. However, the incidence of acute urinary retention requiring catheterization differed significantly between the two groups ($p < 0.001$). If success is defined as a Madsen symptom score of 3 or less, or a decrease of more than 8 points from baseline, and/or a PFR increase of at least 4 ml/s or at least 50% from baseline, 72% of the TUMT patients are categorized as having had a successful treatment, compared with 40% of the sham group. As this difference is significant, the TUMT effect differs from that of instrumentation alone.

Table 35.3. *Results of US sham-controlled TUMT study: percentage changes relative to baseline in symptom score, PFR and serum PSA*

Parameter	TUMT (n=75)			Sham (n=35)			p-value
	Baseline	Follow-up*	Percentage change	Baseline	Follow-up*	Percentage change	
Madsen symptom score (total)	13.9	6.3	–55	14.9	10.8	–28	<0.0001
Irritative	4.2	2.5	–41	4.7	3.7	–21	<0.01
Obstructive	9.7	3.8	–61	10.2	7.1	–30	<0.0001
PFR (ml/s)	7.2	11.5	+58	7.4	9.4	+27	<0.01
PSA (ng/ml)	3.3	18.8	+470	2.9	3.7	+28	<0.0001

*Follow-up assessment at 3 months for all parameters except serum PSA (1 week). (From ref. 17 with permission.)

TUMT (1296 MHz) versus TURP (Swedish study)

The TUMT/transurethral resection of the prostate (TURP) study was conducted to compare the efficacy and morbidity of TUMT with TURP. Randomization was achieved using a 1:1 ratio at one site, the Sahlgrenska Hospital in Göteborg, Sweden.[18]

Statistically significant improvements in the Madsen symptom score were observed at 24 months in both the TUMT and the TURP groups. The difference in the changes from baseline between treatment groups, and the difference in the obstructive component did not achieve statistical significance (Table 35.4).

Improvements in PFR differed significantly between TUMT (46%) and TURP (106%) at 24 months. There was also a statistically significant improvement in PFR from baseline in both groups, whereas the difference in post-void residual volume reduction between the two groups was not significant.

In conclusion, although the change in Madsen symptom score is almost equivalent in two groups, the improvement in PFR is less pronounced in the TUMT group. The main difference between the two treatments is the morbidity: TUMT produces fewer serious and minor complications, and can be performed on an ambulatory basis, whereas TURP entails all the risks associated with spinal or general anaesthesia and prostatic resection (see Chapter 31).

TUMT (1296 MHz): responders versus non-responders

In order to identify the ideal candidate and treatment parameters, a retrospective analysis was conducted in patients treated at eight centres.[19] Before treatment, no significant differences in patient profile were found between the two groups. However, significant differences in the treatment parameters were found. The total energy delivered to the prostate was 121 kJ in the responder group compared with 102 kJ in the non-responders. The total time with a urethral temperature greater than rectal temperature was 31 min in responders compared with 24 min in non-responders; the serum PSA increase 1 week after treatment was 1300% in responders compared with 150% in non-responders. The analysis shows that, as yet, there is no ideal patient profile, because no significant differences between the groups were found before treatment. However, treatment outcome is heat-dose dependent and probably is linked to the individual's prostate histomorphology and blood supply.[20] The significant difference in serum PSA levels after 1 week suggests that the responders achieve greater tissue damage than the non-responders.

Urodynamic studies and patient selection

The degree and type of obstruction as shown by pressure–flow studies is an important factor in determining the outcome of TUMT. Tubaro et al.[21] recently demonstrated a significantly better outcome for patients with predominantly constrictive obstruction, defined by the slope of the linear PURR (passive urethral resistance relation)[22] and minimal voiding pressure, as opposed to compressive obstruction. Between the two groups, patients with constrictive obstruction had an equivalent improvement in symptoms but a significantly better increase in mean PFR to 14.7 ml/s (compared with

Table 35.4. Results of randomized study comparing TUMT and TURP: percentage changes relative to baseline in system score, PFR and post-void residual (PVR)

Parameter	TUMT			TURP		
	Baseline	24 months	Percentage change	Baseline	24 months	Percentage change
Madsen symptom score	12.7	2.3	+82	13.6	1.2	+91
PFR (ml/s)	8.4	12.3	+46	8.3	17.1	+106
PVR (ml)	97	47	−51	104	27	−74

(From ref. 18 with permission.)

10.4 ml/s in the compressive obstructive patients) at 6 months. A similarly significant larger decrease in post-void residual urine was seen in constrictive patients. The fact that there appears to be a differential response to TUMT in the two types of obstruction suggests a multifactorial aetiology of the symptoms of prostatism.

Moderate versus high-energy TUMT (1296 Mhz)

The dose-dependence of the clinical response to microwave energy has led to an increase in the thermal dose delivered to improve the efficacy of TUMT[23] in obstructed patients.

The results of two therapeutic regimens have been compared,[24] namely, the results of a higher-energy TUMT protocol 2.5 (maximum dose of energy 219 kJ) versus results of the standard TUMT protocol 2.0 (maximum dose of energy 194 kJ). A comparison of the two protocols demonstrates that the increase in the thermal dose delivered by protocol 2.5 results in a superior clinical outcome (Table 35.5, Fig. 35.4).

Following protocol 2.5, PFR is greater than that of age-matched controls without symptoms of BPH (13 ml/s at the age of 70 years).[25] This clinical study confirms the hypothesis that 'the higher the energy, the

better the results'. No serious complications were observed at the level of the upper urinary tract, rectum or striated sphincter. However, side effects are significantly more pronounced than after protocol 2.0: urinary retention is more frequent and the inflammatory reaction lasts longer.

The choice between treatment protocol 2.0 or 2.5 should therefore be made according to the patient profile: significant BPH obstruction should preferably be treated using the higher-energy TUMT protocol 2.5, whereas a patient who has mild obstruction or is predominantly symptomatic should preferably be treated using the 'conservative' standard protocol 2.0.

Response rate

Clinical studies reporting mean values of parameters at follow-up, often do not fully disclose the clinical benefit in terms of the number of patients within the group who were treated effectively. Perhaps one of the most useful aspects of the guidelines for assessment of new treatments for BPH[26] is the suggestion that outcomes should be reported for both individual parameters of symptom score and PFR, as well as a combination of both, categorically stratified as improvements of at least 75, 50 or 25%. This classification of 'responders' may enable comparisons among different clinical studies.

Table 35.5. *Results of TUMT at 3 months: percentage changes relative to baseline in mean Madsen and AUA symptom scores and in mean PFR for protocol 2.0 versus higher-energy protocol 2.5*

Parameter	Assessment	Treatment protocol 2.0 (n=163)	2.5 (n=72)	p-value
Madsen symptom score	Before	14.1	17.5	<0.001
	3 months	6.8	6.5	ns
	Percentage change	−52	−63	<0.001
AUA symptom score	Before	17.6	22.6	<0.001
	3 months	9.0	8.3	ns
	Percentage change	−49	−63	<0.001
PFR (ml/s)	Before	10.5	9.2	<0.001
	3 months	12.7	15.2	<0.001
	Percentage change	+21	+65	<0.001

(From ref. 24 with permission.) ns, not significant.

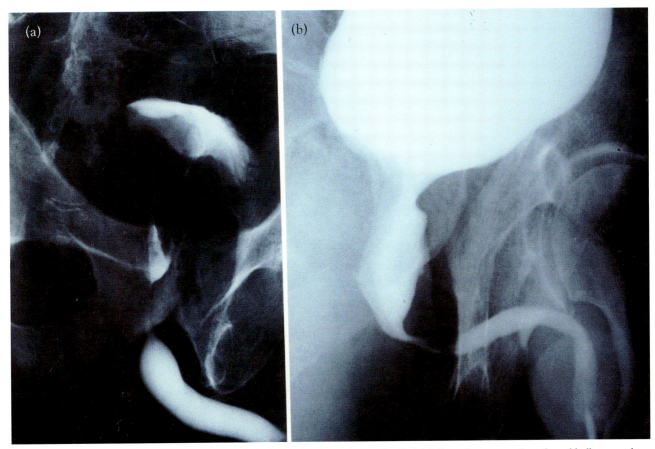

Figure 35.4. *TUMT cavity: retrograde urethrocystogram 3 months after protocol 2.5. (a) Filling phase: normal penile and bulbous urethra; (b) voiding phase: wide-open bladder neck and prostatic cavity.*

Table 35.6 enumerates the response rates for different TUMT studies and shows the advantage of case selection by urodynamic criteria and the benefit of higher temperatures achieved in the prostate.

Place of TUMT among other treatment modalities

The question is no longer whether TUMT has a therapeutic effect, but whether its effect is of clinical

Table 35.6. *Percentage of the study population with at least a 75% improvement in symptom score (SS) and PFR in studies using TUMT protocol 2.0*

	Percentage with a 75% improvement			
Study	SS	PFR	SS or PFR	SS and PFR
Compressive obstruction[21]	44	11	n.a.	16
Constrictive obstruction[21]	59	55	n.a.	41
Low temperature 2.0[8]	75	8	54	8
High temperature 2.0[8]	90	50	100	40

n.a., not assessed.
(From ref. 21 with permission)

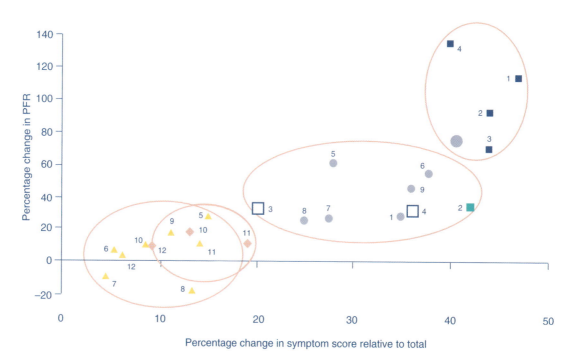

Figure 35.5. *Place of TUMT among other treatment modalities: efficacy is defined by the percentage change in symptom score, normalized to total scale of the score (x-axis) and by the percentage change in peak flow rate relative to baseline (y-axis). Each of the 12 randomized studies mentioned in the text is represented by two points, one for each arm of the study (for further explanation see text):* ■, *TURP;* ●, *TUMT 2.0* (●, *TUMT 2.5 is an (unnumbered) non-randomized study);* □, *VLAP;* ■, *TUIP;* ◆, *drugs;* ▲, *sham or placebo.*

value when compared with the two other standard treatments — drugs and TURP.

Although there are no prospective studies comparing the results of drug therapy with TUMT, several randomized studies have compared drugs with placebo,[27–29] TUMT with sham,[13–17] TUMT with TURP,[18] transurethral incision of the prostate (TUIP) with TURP[30] and visual laser ablation of the prostate (VLAP) with TURP,[31] using both symptom score and PFR as outcome parameters. The results of peer-reviewed studies and the results of TUMT are shown in Figure 35.5.[32] In order to eliminate the bias due to the use of different symptom score scales, the change in symptom score is expressed as a percentage of the total scale of the score. Four (encircled) regions with increasing degree of efficacy are clearly identified:

1. Lower left: the placebo arms of drug studies and sham arms of thermotherapy studies.
2. Central left position: effective treatment with drugs.

3. Central right: effective treatment with TUMT protocol 2.0, VLAP and TUIP.
4. Upper right: TURP.

The non-randomized TUMT protocol 2.5 (large unnumbered dot) is located in the fourth region and is approaching the efficacy of TURP.

Conclusions

Treatment of BPH is a trade-off between patient expectations concerning improvement in the quality of life, and the perception of risks. TUMT is a compromise between the limited efficacy of drug treatment and the invasiveness of surgery. The concept of clinical utility, which takes into account all parameters of a treatment, has never been applied to the treatment of BPH. Long-term, controlled, prospective studies comparing various treatment alternatives for BPH including thermotherapy, are needed to determine the clinical utility of these therapies.[34]

References

1. Devonec M, Berger N, Perrin P. Transurethral microwave heating of the prostate from hyperthermia to thermotherapy. J Endourol 1991; 5: 129–135

2. Carter S, Patel A, Reddy P et al. Single-session transurethral microwave thermotherapy for the treatment of benign prostatic obstruction. J Endourol 1991; 5: 137–144

3. Trachtenberg J. High temperature thermotherapy of the prostate creates TUR defect without anaesthesia. J Urol 1994; 151: 416A

4. Larson T R, Coricka A, Bostwick D. Extent of thermal cell death correlated to accurate interstitial temperatures of ten pathologic prostate specimens using urologix T3 microwave transurethral thermal therapy unit. In: Proc XIth Congr Eur Assoc Urol, Berlin 1994: 335

5. Strohmaïer W L, Bichler K H, Flüchter S H, Wilbert D M. Local microwave hyperthermia of benign prostatic hyperplasia. J Urol 1990; 144: 913–917

6. Sapozink M D, Boyd S D, Astrahan M A et al. Transurethral hyperthermia for benign prostatic hyperplasia: preliminary clinical results. J Urol 1990; 143: 944–950

7. Vanden Bossche M, Noel J C, Schulman C C. Transurethral hyperthermia for benign prostatic hypertrophy. World J Urol 1991; 9: 2–6

8. Carter S St C, Ogden C. Intraprostatic temperature versus clinical outcome in TUMT. Is the response heat-dose dependent? J Urol 1994; 151: 416A

9. Devonec M, Cathaud M, Dutrieux-Berger N et al. Histology of thermal injury induced by transurethral microwave thermotherapy of benign prostatic hyperplasia. In: Bichler K H, Strohmaïer W L, Wilbert D M (eds) Hyperthermia of the prostate. State of the art. Frankfurt: Verlagsgruppe, 1992: 98–103

10. Lauweryns J, Baert L, Vandenhove J, Petrovich Z. Histopathology of prostatic tissue after transurethral hyperthermia. Int J Hyperthermia 1991; 7: 221–230

11. Abbou C C, Colombel M, Payan C et al. Transrectal and transurethral hyperthermia versus sham to treat benign prostatic hyperplasia: a double blind, randomized, multicentric study. J Urol 1994; 151: 418A

12. Smith P, Marberger M, Conort P et al. Other non-medical therapies (excluding lasers) in the treatment of BPH. In: Cockett A T K, Khoury S, Aso Y et al. (eds) 2nd International Consultation on Benign Prostatic Hypertrophy. Jersey: SCI, 1993: 453–491

13. Perrin P, Devonec M, Fendler J P et al. Thermotherapy versus SHAM treatment in benign prostatic hypertrophy. Prog Urol 1992; 2(suppl): A50

14. Ogden C, Reddy P, Johnson H et al. Sham versus transurethral microwave thermotherapy in patients with symptoms of benign prostatic outflow obstruction. Lancet 1993; 341: 14–17

15. de la Rosette J, de Wildt M, Alivazatos G et al. Transurethral microwave thermotherapy (TUMT) in benign prostate hyperplasia: placebo versus TUMT. Urology 1994; 44: 58–63

16. Devonec M, Houdelette P, Colombeau P et al. A multicenter study of sham versus thermotherapy in benign prostatic hypertrophy. J Urol 1994; 151: 415A

17. Blute M L, Tomera K M, Hellerstein D K et al. Transurethral microwave thermotherapy for the management of benign prostatic hyperplasia: results of the United States Prostatron Cooperative study. J Urol 1993; 10: 1591–1596

18. Dahlstrand C, Geirsson G, Walden M, Pettersson S. Transurethral microwave thermotherapy versus transurethral resection for benign prostatic hyperplasia: a prospective randomized study with a two-year follow-up. Urology 1995; Br J Urol 1995; 76: 614–618

19. Berg C, Choi N, Colombeau P et al. Responders versus non-responders to thermotherapy in BPH: a multicenter retrospective analysis of patient and treatment profiles. J Urol 1993; 149: 251A

20. Devonec M, Berger N, Fendler J P et al. Thermoregulation during transurethral microwave thermotherapy: experimental and clinical fundamentals. Eur Urol 1993; 23: 63–67

21. Tubaro A, Ogden C, de la Rosette J et al. The prediction of clinical outcome from thermotherapy by pressure–flow study. Results of a European multicenter study. World J Urol 1994; 12: 352–356

22. Schäfer W. Urethral resistance? Urodynamic concepts of physiological and pathological bladder outlet function during voiding. Neurourol Urodyn 1985; 4: 161–201

23. Devonec M, Ogden C, Perrin P, Carter S S. The clinical response to transurethral microwave thermotherapy is thermal-dose dependent. Eur Urol 1993; 23: 267–274

24. Perrin P, Devonec M, Houdelette P et al. Single-session transurethral microwave thermotherapy: comparison of two therapeutic modes in a multicenter study. In: Marberger M (ed) Application of newer forms of therapeutic energy in urology. Oxford: Isis Medical Media, 1995: 35–39

25. Girman G J, Panser L A, Chute C G et al. Natural history of prostatism: urinary flow rates in a community-based study. J Urol 1993; 150: 887–892

26. American Urological Association New Technology Assessment Committee. Guidance for clinical investigations of devices used for treatment of benign prostatic hyperplasia. J Urol 1993; 150: 1588–1590

27. Lepor H, Auerbach S, Puras-Baez A et al. A randomized, placebo-controlled multicenter study of the efficacy and safety of terazosin in the treatment of benign prostatic hyperplasia. J Urol 1992; 148: 1467–1474

28. The Finasteride Study Group. Finasteride (MK-906) in the treatment of benign prostatic hyperplasia. Prostate 1993; 22: 291–299

29. Jardin A, Bensadoun H, Delauche-Cavallier M C, Attali P. Alfuzosin for treatment of benign prostatic hypertrophy. Lancet 1991; 337: 1457–1461

30. Christensen M M, Aagaard J, Madsen P O. Transurethral resection versus transurethral incision of the prostate. A prospective randomized study. Urol Clin North Am 1990; 17: 621–630

31. Dixon C M, Lepor H. Lasers add a glow to the search for BPH therapies. Contemp Urol 1993; 5: 44–62

32. Devonec M, Carter S S, Tubaro A et al. Microwave thermotherapy. Current opinion in Urology 1995; 5: 3–9

33. Madsen P, Iversen P. A point system for selecting operative candidates. In: Hinman F (ed) Benign prostatic hypertrophy. New York: Springer-Verlag, 1983: 763–765

34. Kaplan S A, Olsson C A. State of the art: microwave therapy in the management of men with benign prostatic hyperplasia: current status. J Urol 1993; 150: 1597–1602

Transurethral needle ablation of the prostate

C. C. Schulman A. R. Zlotta

Introduction

Benign prostatic hyperplasia (BPH) is a particularly common feature of male ageing and is considered to be responsible for urinary symptoms in a large group of men over the age of 50 years.[1]

It is commonly estimated that nearly one in every five males will sooner or later require an operation to relieve symptoms due to BPH.[2] A considerable percentage of individuals are bothered by their symptoms but are unwilling to encounter the risks of surgery. Recent reports have claimed that at least 15–20% of patients undergoing a transurethral resection of the prostate (TURP) will develop a significant complication such as incontinence, impotence, urethral stricture or bleeding necessitating transfusion.[3] The reintervention rate after TURP is estimated as 10–15% of cases within 10 years.[4]

For this reason, in the last decade, a multitude of alternative treatments for BPH have emerged, such as medical therapy (5 alpha-reductase inhibitors or alpha-adrenergic agents), or non-medical alternatives such as urethral stents, balloon dilatation, laser therapy, thermal treatments and cryosurgery. The majority of the new technologies have focused on delivering thermal energy to the prostate. As an objective improvement in flow rates had not been observed after hyperthermia (45°C),[5] raising the temperature delivered to the prostate without increasing the side effects has been the goal of different new thermal devices.

Transurethral needle ablation (TUNA™) is a new anaesthesia-free, outpatient method for treatment of BPH. It uses low-level radiofrequency (RF) energy that is delivered directly into selected prostatic areas, producing large necrotic lesions inside the prostatic parenchyma while sparing the urethral mucosa. In the authors' department, 130 patients have been treated since March 1993 with this technique. Histopathological and clinical studies have been conducted in order to assess the efficacy of this new procedure for treatment of BPH.

Animal and ex vivo human prostate studies

Prior to human treatments, Goldwasser et al.[6] created 1 cm necrotic lesions in the prostate dog using the TUNA system with no resultant damage to the rectum, bladder base or distal prostatic urethra. Similar lesions were observed in an ex vivo human prostate study by the same authors.[7] As this had been shown to be a safe elective treatment in animal studies, it was subsequently investigated in humans.

TUNA technique in patients with BPH

TUNA was explored as a fast minimally invasive procedure that could be performed on an outpatient basis.[8] Low-level RF power is delivered directly into the prostate, through a special catheter fitted with adjustable needles placed in selected tissue areas.

TUNA achieves temperatures above 100°C in selected prostatic areas, as measured by infrared and interstitial measurements, and produces major necrotic lesions in 3–5 min. The TUNA system consists of a special 22 Fr urethral catheter connected to a RF generator. The catheter tip contains two needles that deploy at an acute angle to each other and to the catheter (Fig. 36.1). The needles and covering shields (used to protect the urethra if desired) advance and retract by controls on the catheter handle. Thermosensors at the end of the shields, at the tip of the catheter and eventually in the rectum, measure prostatic and periprostatic temperatures during ablation. The catheter is advanced and positioned in the prostate using direct fibreoptic vision or (if desirable) ultrasound control. By rotating the shaft with the deploying needles towards the selected prostatic area, both lateral lobes can be treated in two or three planes, starting 1 cm from the bladder neck to 1 cm proximal to the verumontanum (Fig. 36.1). The length of needles and

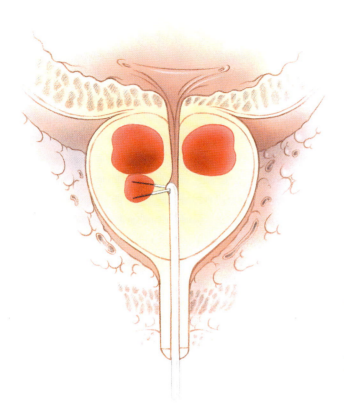

Figure 36.1. *TUNA™ procedure: the catheter is advanced and the needles are deployed inside the prostatic parenchyma.*

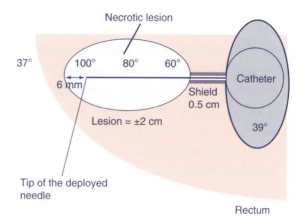

Figure 36.2. *Scheme of temperature distribution and lesion size with TUNA.*

the deployment of the shields is determined by measuring the transverse section of the prostate using transrectal ultrasonography (TRUS).

Patients are treated under topical lidocaine hydrochloride anaesthesia with intravenous sedation if required, in most cases. On average, the TUNA procedure takes 30–40 min, with 4–15 W applied for 5 min. Proximal lesion temperatures measured at the shield range from 45 to 72°C and urethral temperatures average 41°C, while central lesion temperatures are estimated to be around 110°C (Fig. 36.2), as confirmed by infrared and interstitial measurements.[9] The temperature at the shield by the end of the procedure should be 50°C at least, in order to achieve maximal lesions. All patients have tolerated the procedure very well, reporting total absence of pain to mild discomfort. No treatment has ever been stopped because of intolerable pain. At the completion of the procedure, no catheter is left in situ and patients are discharged home. Patients in chronic retention prior to the treatment are usually hospitalized for 1 or 2 days after the procedure before being discharged, as the average delay to recovery of voiding is about 7 days.

Human pathological studies

An initial study on 25 patients was conducted to assess the safety, tolerance and lesions produced by TUNA. Patients were treated with TUNA prior to scheduled retropubic prostatectomy. Prostate weight varied from 14 to 88 g.

Macroscopic examination of the surgical prostatic specimen (Fig. 36.3) recovered from 1 day to 3 months after TUNA demonstrated localized necrotic lesions with a sharp demarcation between treated and untreated areas.[8] These lesions averaged 12 × 7 mm and 18 × 12 mm after 3 and 5 min treatment, respectively. Microscopic examination revealed necrotic lesions with extensive coagulation up to 30 × 15 mm. Specific immunohistochemical staining showed destruction of all tissue components, glandular cells being slightly more thermoresistant than stromal tissue.

Magnetic resonance imaging showed necrotic lesions corresponding to those seen in the recovered surgical specimens.[10] Gadolinium contrast agent was reinforced at the periphery of the lesion and absent in the central zone of the necrotic lesion.

Surgery in three of the authors' patients that did not improve after the TUNA procedure (6–10 months after TUNA) with subsequent histological examination revealed a fibrotic process with the absence of necrotic lesions.

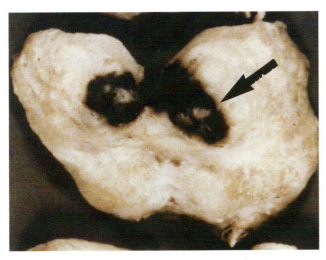

Figure 36.3. *Macroscopic appearance of necrotic lesions in a step-sectioned prostate specimen 15 days after the TUNA™ procedure.*

Clinical studies

Over 700 patients have been treated in different centres and a multicentre European and an American study are in progress. In the authors' department, 130 patients have been treated with different protocols from March 1993 to December 1995 (pathological study, patients in chronic retention, clinical study). In the clinical study, 46 patients have been treated and evaluated, with a follow-up of up to 2 years.

Inclusion criteria were as follows: International Prostate Symptom Score (I-PSS) and quality-of-life (scores) greater than 15 and 3, respectively; peak flow rate less than 15 ml/s (voided volume over 125 ml); post-void residual volume less than 200 ml; prostate size less than 90 cm³. Table 36.1 summarizes the data of the patients treated by TUNA and with a follow–ip to two years.

Effectiveness

Symptom score and quality of life were assessed at 1, 3 and 6, 12 and 24 months after treatment (Fig. 36.4). A significant improvement was noted in I-PSS, from 20.7 before treatment to 8 at the 3 month follow-up and to 7.8 at the 6 month follow-up and 9.7 at the 12 month follow-up. A total of 88% of the patients showed an increase greater than 75% in their symptom score.[7]

Uroflowmetry

The mean peak flow rate increased significantly from 9.9 ml/s before treatment to 15.3 ml/s at 6 months follow-up and 16.2 at the 12 month follow-up. Patients that did have an improvement in flow at 3 months maintained this improvement at 12 and 24 months. In terms of percentage of increase in flow rate, 60% of patients at the 6 months follow-up had an increase of over 50% in their flow rate (Fig. 36.5).

Ultrasonography

Mean prostatic volume decreased from 37.5 to 31.0 cm³ but this difference was not statistically significant. Examination of the prostate revealed in some patients a modification of the echogenicity (hypoechoic areas or creation of a cystic cavity) in the transitional zone but this finding was not constant and not correlated with clinical outcome. In some patients, a TURP-like defect was seen in the areas surrounding the urethra, but this was not a constant finding.

Adverse reactions/complications

The most frequent complication was haematuria, which occurred in all patients. Mild dysuria was noted in all treated patients, lasting 24–96 h; this was treated successfully with anti-inflammatory agents. A total of 35% of the patients experienced urinary retention

Table 36.1. *Summary of the clinical evolution (uroflow, symptom score and quality of life) after TUNA (Brussels) with up to two year follow–up.*

Follow–up period	No. of patients	Uroflow (ml/s)	Symptom score	Quality of life
Pre-treatment	46	10.0	21.0	4.5
3 months	36	15.8	9.1	2.2
6 months	25	15.3	8.1	1.8
12 months	19	16.2	9.7	1.9
24 months	6	16.2	8.0	2.0

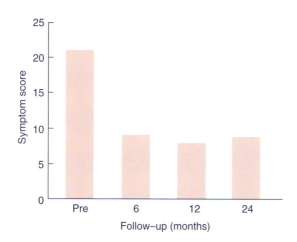

Figure 36.4. *Evolution in symptom score (maximum defavorable = 35) after TUNA in Brussels with up to 2 year follow–up.*

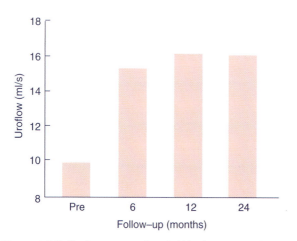

Figure 36.5. *Evolution in uroflow (ml/s) after TUNA (Brussels). with up to two year follow–up.*

(28%) lasting from 2 to 21 days (median 4 days), but resolving spontaneously. Two patients in the clinical study and one in the retention study developed prostatitis, which was treated with antibiotics. In no case was urethral stricture, urinary incontinence, retrograde ejaculation or impotence observed in this clinical series. All complaints appeared to be transient and limited: no complaints or adverse reactions were reported at 30 days.

TUNA treatment for patients in chronic retention

Chronic retention was defined as retention due to BPH that was present for more than 2 weeks. All patients had a suprapubic catheter, and attempts at catheter removal had failed. Patients in acute retention were excluded from this study. Patients with a past history of prostate surgery, proven prostate cancer or neurological disease were excluded from this group. Patients in this group were generally disabled and six were classified as ASA IV anaesthesia risk. To date, 26 of the 34 patients in chronic retention prior to TUNA treatment voided after the procedure and clinical evaluation showed sustained improvement in flow rate at 6 months follow-up. Mean peak flow at 6 months follow-up was 10.6 ml/s in this group of patients successfully treated with TUNA.

Discussion and conclusions

The TUNA procedure uses a thermoablation device that achieves temperatures above 100°C inside the prostatic parenchyma, producing major necrotic lesions in 3–5 min. A major feature of this method is that it is a true outpatient procedure performed with urethral anaesthesia and, in some patients, intravenous sedation. The low-level radiofrequency energy used with the TUNA device produces very localized, selective and controlled coagulative lesions. The lesions seen after TUNA are much larger than all others reported in published thermotherapy studies.

The clinical experience acquired with the TUNA procedure is recent, as the first patients were treated less than 2 years ago. The results, as well as the techniques and technology, are rapidly evolving as lessons are learned from this clinical experience. Given the fact that there is no control group or any extensive long-term data, the clinical results should be analysed with caution. Current experience has demonstrated the ease of the procedure, which has been proven safe for treatment of BPH.

The clinical outcome after TUNA is very encouraging, as demonstrated by the significant increase in peak flow rate and improvement in symptom score.

When comparing the current data with the authors' initially published clinical experience,[11] clinical failures were observed mainly in patients treated with insufficient length of needle deployment within the prostate. This seems logical, as the size of the lesions created correlates with the length of needle deployment.

The authors' current opinion is that the minimal length of needle deployment within the prostate should be 10 mm. The data reviewed here concern patients with this length of needle deployment during TUNA treatment.

TUNA appears to be highly effective and is of particular interest in the treatment of poor-risk patients in chronic retention due to BPH. Apart from the high-risk group of patients that certainly can benefit from this new outpatient anaesthesia-free procedure, an increasing number of patients without absolute indications for surgery seek relief of their prostatic symptoms with minimal discomfort and complications. The acceptable retention rate, the short duration and few side effects of treatment, together with a significant improvement in both objective and subjective parameters of micturition, make TUNA an attractive alternative for treatment of BPH.

As with all thermal ablation devices, necrosis of prostatic hyperplastic tissue is the primary objective of the treatment. It remains unclear which part of the prostate is best ablated for the best therapeutic effect. The authors have attempted to produce necrotic lesions very close to the urethra but with preservation of the prostatic mucosa. Pathological studies have shown that the necrotic lesions are only 2–3 mm away from the urethra, the shielding simply preventing the sloughing of the urethral mucosa. The coagulative necrosis gradually changes to a retractile fibrous scar. This could result in a decrease in the volume of the treated area, although the entire prostatic volume would not change, and/or a decrease in the tonus of the periurethral tissues, thus affecting both dynamic and static components of obstruction by destruction of nerve receptors.

Temperatures as high as 100°C have been obtained without any discomfort for the patient and no general anaesthesia. This absence of pain is probably explicable in terms of (a) the relative poverty in nerve sensory endings in the prostatic parenchyma, and (b) the rapidity with which the temperatures are attained, which brings about rapid destruction of those nerve endings.

Early experience with TUNA has demonstrated that this technique is a promising, easy and safe, low-morbidity, anaesthesia-free outpatient treatment for symptomatic BPH. It produces improvements in both objective and subjective parameters. Enthusiasm is no substitute for objective data, however, and longer follow-up is required to ascertain the durability of the initial response. Further randomized studies comparing TUNA and TURP are planned to establish the place of TUNA for the non-surgical management of BPH in the urologist's armamentarium.

References

1. Walsh P C. Benign prostatic hyperplasia. In: Walsh P, Retick A, Stamey T, Vaughn E Jr (eds) Campbell's Urology, 6th ed. Philadelphia: Saunders, 1992: 1007–1027
2. Arrighi H M, Guess H A, Metter E J et al. Symptoms and signs of prostatism as risk factors for prostatectomy. Prostate 1990; 16: 253–261
3. Mebust W K, Holtgrave H L, Cockett A T K. Transurethral prostatectomy: immediate and postoperative complications. A cooperative study of 13 participating institutions evaluating 3855 patients. J Urol 1989; 141: 243–247
4. Roos N P, Wennberg I C, Malenka D J et al. Mortality and reoperation after transurethral resection of the prostate for benign prostatic hyperplasia. N Engl J Med 1989; 320: 1120–1124
5. Schulman C C, Vanden Bossche M. Hyperthermia and thermotherapy of benign prostatic hyperplasia: a critical review. Eur Urol 1993; 23(suppl 1): 53–59
6. Goldwasser B, Ramon J, Engelberg S et al. Transurethral needle ablation of the prostate using low-level radiofrequency energy: an animal experimental study. Eur Urol 1993; 24: 400–405
7. Ramon J, Goldwasser B, Shenfeld O et al. Needle ablation using radio-frequency current as a treatment for benign prostatic hyperplasia: experimental results in ex vivo human prostate. Eur Urol 1993; 24: 406–410
8. Schulman C C, Zlotta A R, Rasor S R et al. Transurethral needle ablation (TUNA): safety, feasibility and tolerance of a new office procedure for treatment of benign prostatic hyperplasia. Eur Urol 1993; 24: 415–423
9. Rasor J S, Zlotta A R, Edwards S D, Schulman C C. Transurethral needle ablation: gradient mapping and comparison of lesion size in a tissue model and in patients with benign prostatic hyperplasia. Eur Urol 1993; 24: 411–414
10. Schulman C C, Zlotta A R. Transurethral needle ablation of the prostate: pathological, radiological and clinical study of a new office procedure for treatment of benign prostatic hyperplasia using low-level radiofrequency energy. Semin Urol 1994; 3: 205–210
11. Schulman C C, Zlotta A R. Early clinical experience with a new procedure for treatment of BPH (TUNA). Urology 1995; 45: 28–33

High-intensity focused ultrasound
S. Madersbacher M. Marberger

Introduction

The majority of recently developed minimally invasive treatment alternatives for benign prostatic hyperplasia (BPH) make use of the therapeutic effect of heat.[1] There is a close correlation between the temperature achieved and the historical effect observed.[1] In BPH, moderate heating below 45°C does not cause irreversible histological or ultrastructural cell damage.[2] In the borderline temperature range of 47–50°C, the degree of cellular necrosis depends mainly on the time frame of temperature exposure.[1] Therapeutic temperatures exceeding 50°C lead to irreversible cell destruction and above 80–90°C ('thermoablation') cystic cavities comparable to those after transurethral resection of the prostate (TURP) can be induced.[1,3,4] High-intensity focused ultrasound (HIFU) is the only currently available means permitting contact- and irradiation-free in-depth thermoablation.[4–6] HIFU therefore enables intraprostatic tissue ablation to be achieved without urethral or intraprostatic manipulation.

Physics of HIFU

A beam of ultrasound waves can be brought to a tight focus at a selected depth within the body, thus producing a region of high-energy density (Fig. 37.1). Biological tissues, like all common media, transform the mechanical energy of the ultrasound beam in part into heat.[4–6] With HIFU, therapeutic temperatures in the range of 80–200°C are induced. This sharp heat impulse leads to the immediate death of all cellular elements within the beam focus.[4–6] As the HIFU beam is focused, thermal damage to intervening tissue can be avoided. The source of HIFU is a piezoceramic transducer, which has the property of changing its thickness in response to an applied voltage, generating an ultrasound wave with a frequency equal to that of the voltage applied.[4–6] Frequencies used for HIFU therapy range between 0.5 and 10 MHz. Focusing of the HIFU beam is achieved either by placing a lens in front of the transducer, or by

using a transducer that itself has the shape of a part of a spherical bowl.[4–6] The site intensity has to be above the temperature threshold, yet below the cavitation threshold, as tissue cavitation is known to result in uncontrollable tissue destruction.[4–6] In most experimental designs and clinical trials to date, the respective site intensities are between 1000 and 3000 W/cm[2]. All HIFU devices currently being used for clinical trials damage an ellipsoidal tissue volume of several cubic millimetres.[4–6] In order to obtain a clinically useful treatment volume, a series of laterally or axially displaced lesions can be generated by physical movement of the sound head or by electronically sweeping the focused beam.[4–6]

HIFU instrumentation

To ablate prostatic tissue by HIFU, an extracorporeal or a transrectal approach are theoretically possible. For anatomical reasons, the transabdominal approach is poorly suited, as the prostate is shielded by the bony pelvis making it almost inaccessible to the HIFU beam.[4] In contrast, the vicinity of transducer and target tissue using the transrectal approach facilitates the procedure

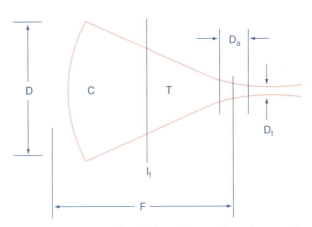

Figure 37.1. *Geometry of HIFU beam. D, transducer diameter; C, coupling; T, tissue; D_a, beam focal length; D_t, beam focal diameter; I_f, interface; F, focal length. (Adapted from ref. 5.)*

from the technical standpoint. Owing to this close proximity, shorter HIFU focal lengths can be used that minimize thermal damage to intervening structures. Currently, two transrectal HIFU devices are available both of which incorporate an imaging and therapy transducer in a single transrectal probe. In one device the same 4.0 MHz transducer is used for imaging and therapy (Fig. 37.2).[4,7–9] The focal lengths depend on the transducer used and at present are available at 2.5, 3.0, 3.5 and 4.0 cm. The site intensity can be varied from 1260 to 2200 W/cm^2. The second transrectal device uses two separate transducers, one for imaging operating at 7.5 MHz and one for HIFU therapy operating at 2.25 MHz (focal length 3.5 cm).[4,10,11] Site intensities in this system have been reported to range between 700 and 2200 W/cm^2. For this device, clinical data for BPH have not been reported. In both systems, the probe is covered by a condom, which is filled with degassed water after insertion into the rectum to provide air-free coupling of the HIFU beam to tissue.

Experimental data

For human BPH, the best animal model currently available is the canine prostate. Consequently, the histological impact of HIFU on this organ has been studied intensively. Foster et al.[7] determined the histological effect of transrectal HIFU on 26 prostates from dogs that were killed between 2 and 12 weeks following HIFU. Within the first 72 h after HIFU, the

treated areas appeared microscopically as dark brownish lesions. Histologically, they consisted of a typical coagulative necrosis. After 14 days, early formation of cystic cavities was identified and after 3 months, these cavities were consistently present, lined with urothelium and connected with the urethra. In all animals, surrounding structures such as rectal wall and prostate capsule were invariably intact. A similar study was conducted by Gelet et al.[11] As in the study by Foster et al., intraprostatic coagulative necrosis was consistently present, which subsequently formed a cystic cavity within 4 weeks.[11] These canine studies proved the feasibility, safety and efficacy of transrectal HIFU in inducing contact-free intraprostatic coagulative necrosis via the transrectal approach.

Transrectal HIFU procedure

To date, the clinical efficacy of transrectal HIFU for human BPH has been reported only with the device using the same crystal for imaging and therapy (Fig. 37.2).[8,9,12] The procedure is usually carried out under general or spinal anaesthesia. A subgroup of patients have also been successfully treated under intravenous sedation.[9] Therapy is performed in the lithotomy position. After diagnostic cystoscopy, a suprapubic 10 Fr cystostomy tube is inserted. Subsequently, a 16 Fr transurethral balloon catheter is introduced to allow exact identification of urethra, bladder neck and verumontanum during the imaging phase of the procedure. The HIFU transducer is covered by a condom, lubricated with gel and inserted into the rectum. The condom is inflated with about 30 ml degassed water for precise air-free coupling of HIFU to tissue. The HIFU transducer is positioned under direct ultrasound guidance using the imaging mode so that the prostatic urethra and bladder neck are located with the target zone. Longitudinally, the treatment zone comprises an area from the bladder neck to the verumontanum. Once the optimal position is obtained, the transducer is immobilized with a locking arm device. HIFU treatment is started after removal of the transurethral catheter. After the initial zone is treated in the 12 o'clock position, the transducer rotates laterally and creates another zone in the far lateral aspect of the transverse plane (Fig. 37.3). Ultimately seven to nine

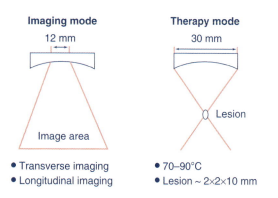

Figure 37.2. Imaging and HIFU modes of a transrectal HIFU transducer. By electronic modification of the piezoceramic crystal, the same transducer operating at 4.0 MHz can be used for imaging and therapy.[8,9]

(a)

(b)

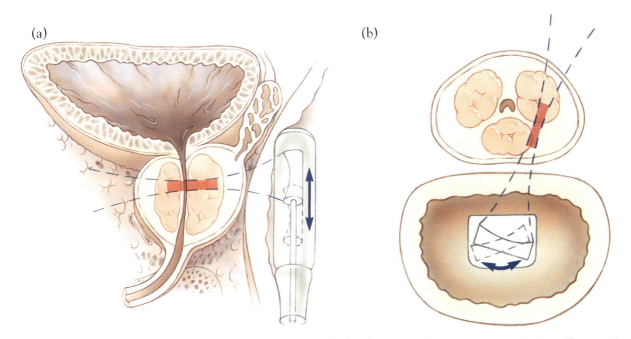

Figure 37.3. *Volume lesion generation by transrectal HIFU. The single focal lesion is very distinct comprising only a few millimetres. By moving the focal zone under computer control in a longitudinal (a) and transverse (b) mode, a lesion of clinically significant size is generated.*[8,9]

sectors are subjected to therapy, in the transverse plane (Fig. 37.3). Once HIFU therapy is completed, the condom is deflated and the transducer is removed.

Histological impact of transrectal HIFU on the human prostate

Despite the encouraging animal data, it should be stressed that the histological impact of heat on the canine and human prostate are not comparable.[3] In addition, there are significant anatomical differences, particularly regarding the relation of the adenomatous tissue to the urethra. It is mandatory, therefore, to determine the histological impact on the human prostate. A total of 54 human prostates were treated at the authors' institution in vivo with transrectal HIFU prior to surgical removal.[8,13,14] After surgery, detailed histological analyses including whole-mount prostatic sections and electron microscopy were performed. Thermolesions in good correlation with the computer-defined segment were identified in all specimens (Fig. 37.4).[8,13,14] Fresh lesions (at a maximum of 3 h after HIFU) could be identified only microscopically. Epithelial cells showed small, pyknotic and heavily discoloured nuclei. The surrounding cytoplasm was small and irregularly vacuolated. Cells were detached from the basal membrane, cell-to-cell contacts were disrupted, and the interstitial connective tissue revealed massive oedematous alterations. Within 5–7 days after HIFU, the treated tissue segments presented as typical

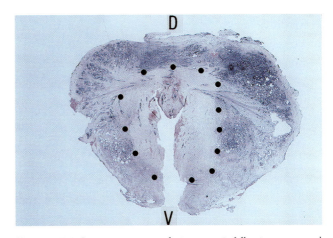

Figure 37.4. *Intraprostatic coagulative necrosis following transrectal HIFU. The tissue segment circumscribed by the black circles indicates the coagulative necrosis induced by transrectal HIFU. The prostate was surgically removed 3 h after HIFU by radical prostatectomy. D, dorsal; V, ventral.*

coagulative necrosis. The border between viable and necrotic tissue was very sharp, comprising only five to seven cell layers.[8,13]

Electron microscopy revealed massive alterations at the cellular level, including destruction of the cell organelles and ruptured membranes. These changes are considered as signs of definitive cell death ('point of no return').[13]

The extent of histologically evident coagulative necrosis correlated well with the computer-defined tissue segment to be treated.[8,13,14] There was a close correlation between power input, focal length and lesion volume. The enlargement of the HIFU zone with higher site intensities and longer focal length is not symmetrical around the midpoint of the lesion, but mainly extends towards the HIFU transducer in the direction of the ultrasound beam, Hence the lesion 'drifts' towards the transducer under these conditions.[8,14] These data demonstrate that transrectal HIFU permits safe, predictable and effective intraprostatic tissue ablation.

Clinical efficacy of transrectal HIFU for BPH

To date, worldwide approximately 250 BPH patients have been treated with transrectal HIFU in an international phase II clinical trial.[4,8,9,12] Inclusion/ exclusion criteria were uniform [peak flow rate $\leq$ 15 ml/s: American Urological Association (AUA) symptom score $\geq$ 18: prostate volume $\leq$ 75 ml; serum prostate-specific antigen (PSA) $\leq$ 10 ng/ml]. After HIFU, patients were followed at regular time intervals on an outpatient basis. Outcome parameters included symptom score, flow rate recording, residual volume, transrectal ultrasonography and serum PSA.

At the Department of Urology, University of Vienna, 86 patients underwent this procedure and the clinical results of the first 50 patients were presented in detail.[4,8] The total treatment time was a mean of 40.2 $\pm$ 14.1 min, including both diagnosis and therapy. Serum PSA rose from a mean of 2.05 $\pm$ 2.7 ng/ml to 11.2 $\pm$ 8.5 ng/ml within 24 h after HIFU and returned to baseline within 4–6 weeks. All other laboratory parameters remained without statistically significant changes throughout the observation period. Significant clinical

improvements were observed in both the subjective (AUA score, quality of life; Fig 37.5) and objective (uroflow, residual volume; Fig 37.6) BPH parameters. After 12 months (n=20), the peak flow rate improved by 47% and the subjective symptoms were reduced by a mean of 55%. More than a 50% reduction of the AUA symptom score was noticed in 77% of all patients.

Bihrle et al.[9] recently reported the initial US experience of 15 patients and noticed after 3 months an increase of the mean peak flow rate from 9.3 to 14.0 ml/s; within the same period, the AUA symptom score decreased from 31.2 to 15. Ebert et al.[12] treated a total of 22 patients, eight of whom were in urinary retention, and reported similar results, i.e. an improvement in mean peak flow rate from 6.1 to 14.1 ml/s, a decrease in the International Prostate Symptom Score (I-PSS) from 16 to 8.5 and of the post-void residual volume from 165 ml (preoperative) to 46 ml at 3 months.

Intraprostatic cystic cavities, comparable to those resulting from a TURP, were demonstrable by transrectal ultrasonography (7.5 MHz) in approximately 25% of patients.[8,9] These cavities appear as early as 6 weeks after HIFU and are still present 1 year after HIFU.

The urodynamic impact of transrectal HIFU has been assessed recently in a group of patients (n=28), who underwent multichannel pressure–flow studies before and 3–6 months (mean 4.2 months) after HIFU.[15] The detrusor opening pressure (cmH$_2$0) decreased from 70 $\pm$ 20 to 57 $\pm$ 20 ($p<0.005$), the maximum detrusor pressure (cmH$_2$0) from 76 $\pm$ 20 to 63 $\pm$ 20 ($p>0.005$) and linear passive urethral resistance relation (linear PURR/Schäfer obstruction score) from 3.5 $\pm$ 0.9 to 2.3 $\pm$ 0.8 ($p<0.005$). Overall, a decrease of the linear PURR of at least one degree was seen in 68% of all patients. Analysis according to the Abrams–Griffiths nomogram revealed similar data: whereas 86% of patients were obstructed preoperatively, this percentage dropped to 24% after HIFU. However, only 16% were clearly unobstructed after HIFU according to the Abrams–Griffiths nomogram. These data indicate that transrectal HIFU is capable of relieving the infravesical obstruction in a significant percentage of patients.

Overall, HIFU treatment is well tolerated, with a short postoperative hospitalization period.[8,9] The

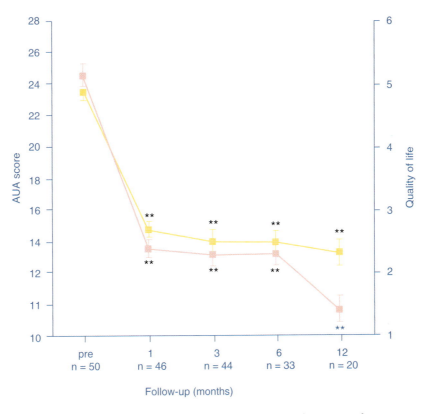

Figure 37.5. *AUA symptom score (■) and quality of life (■) before and after transrectal HIFU. Both parameters improved significantly (**p<0.001) after the procedure.*

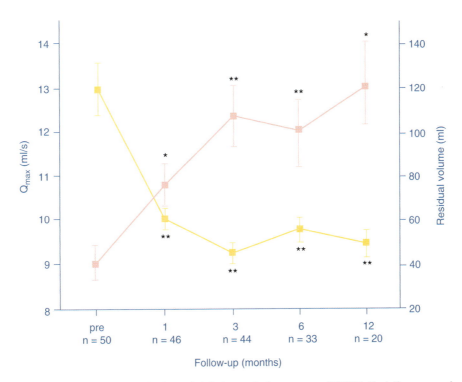

Figure 37.6. *Peak flow rate (■) and post-void residual volume (■) before and after transrectal HIFU. Peak flow rate and post-void residual volume improved significantly (*p < 0.01; **p < 0.001); follow-up data indicate a therapeutic effect up to 12 months.*

majority of patients underwent a rectoscopy immediately after the procedure, which yielded normal results in all patients. None of the patients had postoperative complaints in the anal region. The predominant side effect, observed in almost all patients, was urinary retention.[8,9] At the authors' institution, a 10 Fr cystostomy catheter is routinely inserted intraoperatively, which is usually removed on an outpatient basis after a mean of 6 days.[8] The majority of sexually active patients reported haematospermia, which always disappeared spontaneously after 4–6 weeks.[8,9]

Focused extracorporeal pyrotherapy

If shock waves are generated at high frequency (more than 10 shots/s), tissue cavitation within the focal zone can be induced with sufficient power for immediate cell death.[4,16–18] Vallancien et al. recently reported on an extracorporeal device for in-depth tissue ablation based on this principle, which is basically a modification of a piezoelectric lithotriptor.[16–18] Site intensities within the focal zone have been quoted as exceeding 10 000 W/cm^2, but precise data are not available. During therapy, tissue cavitation within the focal zone increases progressively and leads to mechanical disruption of cells within the target zone. Although both technologies [HIFU and focused extracorporeal pyrotherapy (FEP)] permit contact-free in-depth tissue ablation, the physical principles are somewhat similar but not identical:[4] whereas HIFU employs thermal effects of ultrasound if operated below the cavitation threshold, the therapeutic effect of FEP seems to be predominantly mechanical by tissue cavitation. This device has been tested under experimental conditions and, in preliminary human trials involving kidney, prostate and bladder, in-depth tissue ablation was successfully induced.[16–18]

FEP has also been used to ablate prostatic tissue.[16–17] Although intraprostatic coagulative necrosis was demonstrable, the transabdominal approach proved to be poorly suited. The lesion size was poorly reproducible and it was difficult to define the right dosage. As a consequence of these drawbacks, damage to non-target tissues such as skin and rectal wall were present. Vallancien et al. could target the prostate adequately for

FEP therapy in only 50% of cases.[16,17] Clinical data for BPH using this approach have not been reported.

Conclusions

Several experimental and clinical studies have demonstrated the feasibility, safety and efficacy of thermoablation of the prostate by transrectal HIFU. The histological data confirm that this technique is capable of destroying prostatic tissue while preserving non-target structures such as the rectal wall and posterior prostate capsule.[7,8,11,13,14] The advantage of transrectal HIFU over other currently tested minimally invasive treatment options for BPH (transurethral microwave thermotherapy: side firing, contact or interstitial laser techniques) is that the treatment is contact free.[19–21] It is, therefore, feasible to coagulate periurethral tissue selectively via the transrectal route, avoiding the side effects and risks associated with urethral or intraprostatic manipulation. As the clinical experience with this novel technique is still limited, it is currently premature to predict the future role of transrectal HIFU as a minimally invasive treatment option for BPH. However, clinical data of phase II trials and the long-term follow-up exceeding 12 months allow some conclusions to be drawn.[8,9,12] HIFU treatment for BPH is associated with very little postoperative morbidity. The therapeutic effect of this minimally invasive treatment modality is comparable to that of other treatment alternatives such as transurethral microwave thermotherapy at high therapeutic temperatures (Prostasoft 2.5 software) and laser devices.[19–21] Clinical data indicate a therapeutic effect up to 12 months. Nevertheless, the definitive future role of transrectal HIFU can be assessed only in a prospective, randomized phase III trial against TURP.

There is also considerable room for further improvement. The optimal anaesthetic protocol still needs to be defined. The majority of patients have been treated either under general or spinal anaesthesia. At the University of Indiana, four of five patients were successfully treated under i.v. sedation.[9] Patients were operated on as outpatients with no anaesthetic recovery-room time. The possibility of prostatic block as an anaesthetic regimen is currently being evaluated. In addition, the impact of intraprostatic lesion volume and location on the clinical outcome is currently being determined. The most important technical improvement would be the availability of a phase-array HIFU transducer with variable focal length. Zanelli et al.[22] recently presented a 10 cm annular array HIFU transducer, operating at 1.25 MHz, designed for extracorporeal application. This extracorporeal transducer prototype is capable of focusing the HIFU beam between 8 and 12 cm by phasing the array. Once these transducers are to hand it should be possible to simply mark the target zone identified in two planes on the computer screen and the respective area will be precisely ablated. The availability of varying focal sizes and shorter duty cycles would help to shorten treatment time.

HIFU represents an exciting new method of minimally invasive surgery without affecting intervening tissue. Although many reports demonstrate its efficacy in the treatment of BPH in phase II trials, it is obvious that HIFU will have a major impact in the field of minimally invasive surgery (e.g. extracorporeal, transrectal, transvaginal) for the treatment of malignant tumours.[23–26] Theoretically, all organs accessible for ultrasound are potentially suitable for this kind of therapy.[4,6]

References

1. Smith P H, Marberger M, Conort P et al. Other non-medical therapies (excluding lasers) in the treatment of BPH. In: Cockett A T K, Khoury S, Aso Y et al. (eds) 2nd International Consultation on Benign Prostatic Hyperplasia (BPH). Jersey, Channel Islands: Scientific Communications International, 1993: 453–491

2. Montorsi F, Gallin L, Guazzoni G et al. Transrectal microwave hyperthermia for benign prostatic hyperplasia: long-term clinical, pathological and ultrasound patterns. J Urol 1992; 148: 321–325

3. Devonec M, Berger N, Fendler J P et al. Thermoregulation during transurethral microwave thermotherapy: experimental and clinical fundamentals. Eur Urol 1993; 23(suppl 1): 63–67

4. Madersbacher S, Marberger M. Therapeutic applications of ultrasound in urology. In: Marberger M (ed) Application of newer forms of therapeutic energy in urology. Oxford: ISIS Medical Media, 1995: 115–136

5. Fry F J. Intense focused ultrasound in medicine. Eur Urol 1993; 23(suppl 1): 2–7

6. Ter Haar G. Focused ultrasound therapy. Curr Opin Urol 1994; 4: 89–92

7. Foster R S, Bihrle R, Sanghvi N et al. Production of prostatic lesions in canines using transrectally administered high-intensity focused ultrasound. Eur Urol 1993; 23: 330–336

8. Madersbacher S, Kratzik C, Susani M, Marberger M. Tissue ablation in benign prostatic hyperplasia with high intensity focused ultrasound. J Urol 1994; 152: 1956–1961

9. Bihrle R, Foster R S, Sanghvi N T et al. High intensity focused ultrasound for the treatment of benign prostatic hyperplasia: early United States clinical experience. J Urol 1994; 151: 1271–1275

10. Gelet A, Chapelon J Y, Margonari J et al. High-intensity focused ultrasound experimentation on human benign prostatic hyperthrophy. Eur Urol 1993; 23: 44–47

11. Gelet A, Chapelon J Y. Margonari J et al. Prostatic tissue destruction by high intensity focused ultrasound: experimentation on canine prostate. J Endourol 1993; 7: 249–253

12. Ebert T, Miller S, Schmitz-Draeger B, Ackermann R. High intensity focused ultrasound (HIFU) in patients with benign prostatic hyperplasia. J Urol 1994; 151(suppl): 399A

13. Susani M, Madersbacher S, Kratzik C et al. Morphology of tissue destruction induced by focused ultrasound. Eur Urol 1993; 23(suppl 1): 34–38

14. Marberger M, Susani M, Madersbacher S et al. Effect of high intensity focused ultrasound on human prostate cancer. J Urol 1994: 151(suppl): 436A

15. Madersbacher S, Klingler C H, Schmidbauer C P, Marberger M. Fokussierter Ultraschall zur Behandlung der benignen Prostatahyperplasie: Einjahresergebnisse und urodynamische Untersuchungen. Urologe (A) 1994; (suppl 1): S94

16. Vallancien G, Chartier-Kastler E, Chopin D et al. Focused extracorporeal pyrotherapy: experimental results. Eur Urol 1991; 20: 211–219

17. Vallancien G, Harouni M, Veillon B et al. Focused extracorporeal pyrotherapy: feasibility study in man. J Endourol 1992; 6: 173–181

18. Vallancien G, Chartier-Kastler E, Bataille N et al. Focused extracorporeal pyrotherapy. Eur Urol 1993; 23(suppl 1): 48–52

19. Ogden C W, Reddy P, Johnson H et al. Sham versus transurethral microwave thermotherapy in patients with symptoms of benign prostatic bladder outflow obstruction. Lancet 1993; 341: 14–17

20. Devonec M, Carter S S C, Tubaro A et al. Microwave therapy. Curr Opin Urol 1995; 5: 3–9

21. Boon T A, Lepor H, Muschter R, McCullough D L. Laser treatment of benign prostatic hyperplasia (BPH) workshop. In: Kurth K, Newling D W W (eds) Benign prostatic hyperplasia: recent progress in clinical research and practice. New York: Wiley-Liss, 1994: 534–544

22. Zanelli C I, Hennige C W, Sanghvi N T. Design and characterisation of a 10 cm annular array transducer for high intensity focused ultrasound (HIFU) applications. IEEE Symposium 1994; 3: 1887–1990

23. Yang R, Reilly C R, Rescorla F J et al. Effects of high-intensity focused ultrasound in the treatment of experimental neuroblastoma. J Pediatr Surg 1992; 27: 246–251

24. Chapelon J Y, Margonari J, Vernier F et al. In vivo effects of high-intensity focused ultrasound on prostatic adenocarcinoma Dunning R3327. Cancer Res 1992; 52: 6353–6357

25. Moore W E, Lopez R, Matthews D E et al. Evaluation of high-intensity therapeutic ultrasound irradiation in the treatment of experimental hepatoma. J Pediatr Surg 1989; 24: 30–33

26. Ter Haar G R, Rivens I, Chen L, Riddler S. High-intensity focused ultrasound for the treatment of rat tumours. Phys Med Biol 1991; 36: 1495–1501

J. A. Vale T. J. Christmas

Introduction

Benign prostatic hyperplasia (BPH) is a major cause of morbidity in elderly men, and is reported to have an incidence of 88% among men in their nineties.[1] With advances in other fields of medicine and increasing longevity, the number of patients requiring treatment for this complaint will inevitably increase. Already it is estimated that a 50-year-old man has a 20–25% chance of requiring a prostatectomy during his lifetime,[2] and more than 300 000 prostatectomies are performed in the United States annually.[3] This represents an enormous financial burden to health services and private insurance companies. Moreover, there have been recent concerns about the safety of transurethral resection of the prostate (TURP),[4] with long-term morbidity including retrograde ejaculation in a majority of patients,[5] and impotence variably reported in the range of 4–40%.[6–8] There is, therefore, a need to develop and evaluate alternatives to prostatectomy. The aim of this chapter is to review the current status of balloon dilatation of the prostate.

History of prostatic dilatation

Techniques for the transurethral dilatation of the prostate (TUDP) have been in existence for centuries. However, the first instrument developed specifically for this purpose was that described by Guthrie in 1836,[9] and others followed shortly thereafter. The degree of dilatation attainable with these early dilators was limited by urethral access. In 1956, Deisting[10] introduced a special metal dilator for the prostate that overcame this problem by opening within the prostate (Fig 38.1). He reported excellent results in a series of 324 patients: 95% of patients were cured initially and 83, 74 and 48% were asymptomatic at 3, 5 and 8 years, respectively. However, this study did not compare transurethral dilatation with prostatectomy on a prospective randomized basis and when such a study was performed within the same centre,[11] open prostatectomy

and TURP yielded significantly better long-term results and were associated with fewer complications.

TUDP using a balloon was first reported in 1984 when Burhenne et al.[12] demonstrated that the diameter of the cadaveric male prostatic urethra could be increased by inflating a 24 Fr angioplasty balloon within

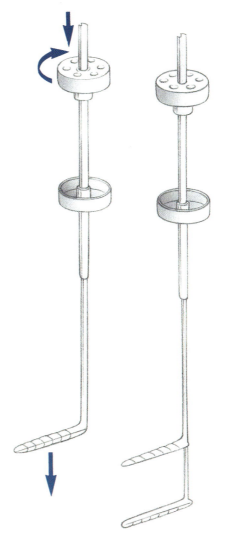

Figure 38.1. *Deisting dilator. The instrument was introduced into the prostate per urethram, and then the blades were separated by twisting the hand wheel. A characteristic 'give' was felt as anterior commissurotomy occurred.*

the prostate for 30 s. To illustrate the potential value of this finding, Burhenne performed balloon dilatation on his own prostate, and recorded an increase in his urinary stream which persisted at 4 weeks. Subsequent studies in dogs[13] demonstrated that a balloon diameter of at least 20 mm and an inflation period of 10 mm were required to produce an increase in urethral diameter that was still present at 14 months. Since then, a number of studies of balloon dilatation in patients with BPH have been published.

Mechanism of balloon dilatation of the prostate

Any successful treatment for BPH must act by reducing the bladder outflow resistance caused by the prostate. There are three main theories as to how TUDP might achieve this. The first is the ischaemic atrophy theory, which proposes that the inflated balloon causes a reduction in blood flow of sufficient duration and magnitude to cause tissue necrosis and subsequent prostatic shrinkage. This mechanism is supported by findings on magnetic resonance imaging (MRI) of an increase in periurethral T2 signal intensity after TUDP, followed by an early return to normal signal intensity and a reduction in prostatic volume in some cases.[14] The prostatic capsule and surrounding tissues appeared normal on all images. However, these MRI findings have not been corroborated by other studies, and histological sections of dog prostate immediately after TUDP showed minimal changes, apart from some inevitable urothelial denudation.[13]

The second proposed mechanism of action of TUDP is that it stretches the prostatic capsule, and that there is some loss of elastic recoil during the procedure. There can be little doubt that capsular stretching does occur on inflation of the balloon; it probably accounts for the pain felt by patients when the procedure is performed under local anaesthesia, and an increase in capsular circumference has been confirmed by performing TUDP on fresh surgical specimens.[15] A loss of elastic recoil is more difficult to prove, but would be consistent with the finding that there is often a gradual loss of balloon pressure during dilatation.[15]

The final theory is that a successful TUDP produces a disruption of the anterior and/or posterior commissures

of the prostate. This was the mechanism of action of the Deisting dilator, and using this instrument there was a characteristic 'give' when disruption occurred. That this may occur during TUDP is beyond doubt: it can be observed cystoscopically,[16] and has been suggested as a hallmark of satisfactory dilatation.[17] However, other studies have demonstrated no association between commissurotomy and clinical outcome of TUDP.[18,19]

Thus, the mechanism of TUDP remains controversial. However, the apparent short-term success of the Deisting dilator would be more consistent with the theories of capsular stretching and/or commissurotomy than with the concept of ischaemic atrophy.

Technique of transurethral balloon dilatation of the prostate

TUDP can be performed under fluoroscopic or cystoscopic control. The fluoroscopic technique has the advantage that the instrumentation is flexible and therefore lends itself to local anaesthesia. The endoscopic approach has the advantage that the length of balloon can be measured precisely and the verumontanum can be visualized, thus minimizing the risk of sphincter damage.

The authors have had most experience with the ASI Uroplasty balloon (90 Fr), the procedure being performed under regional or general anaesthesia. In order to select the correct balloon length, the distance between the bladder neck and external urethral sphincter is measured cystoscopically using the calibration catheter supplied. The 26 Fr ASI disposable sheath is then passed and the balloon catheter is advanced through the sheath until the first mark on its shaft is visible; this places the distal tip of the catheter in the bladder, and the distal balloon is inflated and snugged down against the bladder neck (Fig. 38.2). A 0 or 30 degree telescope is passed through the sheath alongside the catheter, and the sheath is withdrawn until the second mark on the catheter is seen. This indicates the distal limit of the balloon, and should be sited just superior to the sphincter. The balloon is inflated to its full diameter of 30 mm (90 Fr) at 4 atm (404 kPa; Fig. 38.2) using the positive displacement pump provided. There is a tendency for the balloon to

(a)

(b)

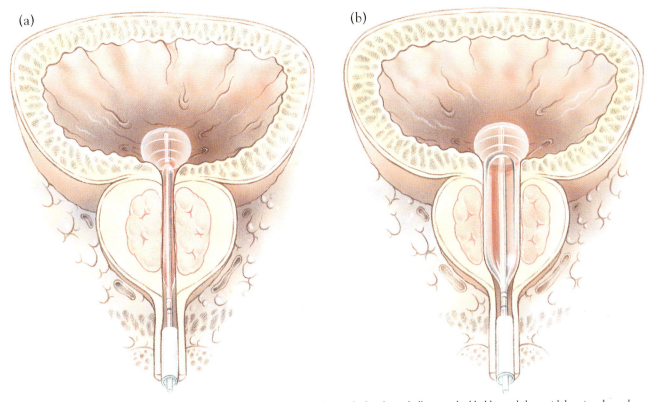

Figure 38.2. *(a) The balloon dilator has been localized correctly by inflating the localizing balloon in the bladder and then withdrawing the catheter until it catches on the bladder neck. (b) The dilatation balloon has been inflated to 4 atm (404 kPa; 90 Fr).*

ride up into the bladder during inflation, and this can be prevented by gentle traction. Its position can be checked by rectal examination. The balloon is left inflated for 10 min, and then deflated and withdrawn into the sheath for removal. A 22 Fr Foley catheter is inserted and left in situ for 72 h.

Other balloons differ in their instrumentation. The American Medical Systems (AMS) Optilume balloon (90 Fr), which has also been used by the authors, is inserted over a guidewire and does not require calibration of the prostatic urethra. Correct positioning of this catheter relies upon a 1 ml capacity balloon below the dilating balloon. This small localizing balloon is inflated within the bladder and then the catheter is withdrawn until this balloon is palpable per rectum at the apex of the prostate. It is then withdrawn a further 1.5–2 cm so that the localizing balloon lies below the external sphincter and the lower limit of the dilatation balloon is palpable at the apex of the prostate as it is inflated to its full 30 mm diameter (90 Fr).

Balloon dilatation under fluoroscopic control can be performed on patients in the supine position. It is essentially similar to the technique described above, except that the sphincter and bladder neck are localized on a urethrogram, thus permitting urethrographic calibration of the prostatic urethra, and the position of the dilatation balloon is demonstrated by inflation with contrast.

Results of balloon dilatation of the prostate

Multiple case series of TUDP with very conflicting results have been published. One of the main factors contributing to this conflict is the difficulty of standardizing the diagnosis of bladder outflow obstruction, and assessing the outcome of intervention objectively. Results of some early series have been encouraging, with overall response rates of about 70% for symptomatic and flow rate improvement.[15,20–23]

However, other studies, particularly those with urodynamic assessment, have been less favourable. Gill et al.[18] reported the results of TUDP using 20 and 25 mm diameter balloons in 48 patients with urodynamically proven obstruction. Less than half reported symptomatic improvement in terms of stream and nocturia, and 89% remained obstructed by urodynamic criteria on repeat cystometrograms 3–11 months after dilatation. A possible explanation for these disappointing results was the use of relatively small 20 mm balloons in half of the patients; there is good evidence that smaller balloons may be ineffective.[13,24] However, a further series has been published recently from the same centre using a balloon of 35 mm diameter (105 Fr).[19] Three months following TUDP, 19/27 patients (70%) with bladder outflow obstruction were improved symptomatically and 13/27 patients (48%) were unobstructed, as judged by urodynamic criteria. However, this objective benefit from dilatation was short-lived: by 6 months after dilatation only three of the 13 patients who had been rendered unobstructed remained so. This latter study is important; the symptomatic response rate of 70% is similar to that of the most promising studies of TUDP, but not all of the symptomatically improved patients were unobstructed. This illustrates the difficulty of assessing outcome following treatments for BPH and the possible contribution of a placebo response. Lepor et al.[25] have compared TUDP with cystoscopy, and found the latter to be equally effective in terms of symptomatic response.

Another possible explanation for the relatively poor results in some series might be poor patient selection, and some authors have suggested that certain criteria are associated with a poor outcome. These include prostates over 40 g, prominent median lobe hypertrophy, chronic retention and detrusor instability.[26] Patients in acute retention also fare poorly.[20–23] The authors have performed TUDP on 28 patients (mean age 57.6 years) with symptomatic BPH, an obstructed flow rate (peak urinary flow rate less than 15 ml/s on a voided volume greater than 150 ml), prostate size less than 50 g and no evidence of median lobe hypertrophy on cystoscopy.[27] Dilatation was performed using the ASI Uroplasty balloon (90 Fr) in 23 patients and the AMS Optilume dilator (90 Fr) in the remaining five. Follow-up of at least 1 year is available on 20 patients: the mean maximum flow rate of these patients was 10.5 ml/s (SD 4.0), with a mean ultrasound residual volume of 106 ml (SD 57).

With respect to their symptom scores,[28] nine patients were improved and were very satisfied with the outcome of treatment. Their mean symptom score before treatment was 12.8 (SD 3.1) which reduced to 3.8 (SD 3.0) 1 year after TUDP. However, only four of these patients showed any objective improvement in their urinary flow rate, and the mean rise in maximum flow rate for the group was 2.2 ml/s. Ultrasound residual volumes showed a more consistent change, with eight of the nine patients showing a reduction in residual volume; the mean preoperative residual volume was 107 ml (SD 62), compared with 37 ml (SD 41) 1 year after dilatation. This was significant at a p-value of 0.0136 (Mann–Whitney U-test).

Of the remaining 11 patients, two showed an initial improvement at the 6 week follow-up; one showed a reduction in his symptom score from 14 to 8, and the other from 13 to 6 points. There was a concomitant improvement in urinary flow rate in both patients. However, this benefit was short-lived: one patient required a TURP at 6 months and the other was awaiting TURP 1 year after dilatation. The other nine patients showed no improvement at all.

There were no differences in preoperative characteristics, including prostatic size, between the patients who were improved by TUDP and those who were not. There were no serious complications: one patient had a brief period of urinary incontinence following the procedure, which resolved over 1 month. He was one of the first patients treated, and the incontinence probably resulted from a rather distal balloon placement causing transient dilatation of the external sphincter. No patient developed retrograde ejaculation as a consequence of the procedure.

These results are rather disappointing, despite the fact that the patients were selected on the basis of criteria suggested previously as correlating with a more favourable outcome.[26] Less than half of the patients demonstrated sustained improvement following TUDP, and by 1 year after dilatation 11 out of 20 patients had undergone or were awaiting TURP. In the authors' opinion, the failure of TUDP can be explained by its probable mechanisms of action — either capsular stretching or rupture of the anterior commissure — with a gradual return to the pretreatment situation postoperatively.

Conclusions

Balloon dilatation appears to be of limited value in the treatment of BPH; response is unpredictable, only half of the patients treated can expect symptomatic improvement, and most objective evidence suggests that TUDP is not a very effective means of relieving obstruction. However, it is amenable to day surgery, provided that the patient is willing to go home with a catheter in situ for 72 h, and it is safe: there have been no serious complications in any of the series reported to date. TUDP may have a role in providing symptomatic relief in the younger patient who wishes to avoid or delay TURP, as it does not cause retrograde ejaculation, but here it may be replaced by microwave thermotherapy or endoscopic laser ablation of the prostate. TURP remains the most effective treatment for BPH.

A final note of caution is necessary. As with many new treatments for BPH, no tissue is taken during TUDP. It is therefore essential before treatment to exclude carcinoma of the prostate by digital rectal examination, serum prostate-specific antigen and/or transrectal ultrasound with ultrasound-guided biopsy. The patient must be informed also that he may require a prostatectomy in the future if balloon dilatation is unsuccessful in the longer term.

References

1. Berry S J, Coffey D S, Walsh P C et al. The development of human benign prostatic hyperplasia with age. J Urol 1984; 132: 474–479
2. Birkhoff J J. Natural history of benign prostatic hypertrophy. In: Hinman F (ed) Benign prostatic hypertrophy. New York: Springer-Verlag, 1983
3. Utilization of short stay in hospitals. Vital Health Stat 1980; 80: 1797
4. Roos N P, Wennberg J E. Malenka D J et al. Mortality and reoperation after open and transurethral resection of the prostate for benign prostatic hyperplasia. N Engl J Med 1989; 320: 1120–1124
5. Libman E, Fichten C B. Prostatectomy and sexual function. Urology 1987; 29: 467
6. Hargreave T B, Stephenson T P. Potency and prostatectomy. Br J Urol 1977; 49: 683
7. Bruskewitz R C, Larsen E H, Madsen P et al. 3-year follow-up of urinary symptoms after transurethral resection of the prostate. J Urol 1986; 136: 613–615
8. Holtgrewe H L, Valk W L. Late results of transurethral prostatectomy. J Urol 1964; 92: 51
9. Guthrie G J. On the anatomy and diseases of the urinary organs. London, 1836 (cited in: Hinman F (ed) Benign prostatic hypertrophy. New York: Springer-Verlag, 1983)
10. Deisting W. Transurethral dilatation of the prostate: a new method in the treatment of prostatic hypertrophy. Urol Int 1956; 2: 158–171
11. Aalkjaer V. Transurethral resection/prostatectomy versus dilatation treatment in hypertrophy of the prostate II: a comparison of the late results. Urol Int 1965; 20: 17–22
12. Burhenne H J, Chisholm R J, Quenville N F. Prostatic hyperplasia: radiological intervention. Radiology 1984; 152: 655–657
13. Castaneda F, Lund G, Larson B W et al. Prostatic urethra: experimental dilation in dogs. Radiology 1987; 163: 645–648
14. Johnson S D, Kuni C C, Castaneda F et al. MR imaging of patients undergoing prostatic balloon dilatation. Radiology 1987; 165: 332
15. Wasserman N F, Reddy P K, Zhang G et al. Experimental treatment of benign prostatic hyperplasia with transurethral balloon dilatation of the prostate: preliminary study in 73 humans. Radiology 1990; 177: 485–494
16. Isorna S, Maynar M, Belon J L et al. Prostatic urethroplasty: endoscopic findings. Semin Intervent Radiol 1989; 6: 46–56
17. Klein L A. Balloon dilatation of the prostate as compared with transurethral resection of the prostate for treatment of benign prostatic hypertrophy. World J Urol 1991; 9: 29–31
18. Gill K P, Machan L S, Allison D J, Williams G. Bladder outflow tract obstruction from benign prostatic hypertrophy treated by balloon dilatation. Br J Urol 1989; 64: 618–622
19. McLoughlin J, Keane P F, Jager R et al. Dilatation of the prostatic urethra with a 35 mm balloon. Br J Urol 1991; 67: 177–181
20. Daughtry J D, Rodan B A, Bean W J. Balloon dilatation of prostatic urethra. Urology 1990; 36: 203–209
21. Baert L, Werbrouck P, Bamelis B et al. Balloon dilatation of the prostate. Urol Int 1991; 47: 74–76
22. Dowd J B, Smith J J. Balloon dilatation of the prostate. Urol Clin North Am 1990; 17: 671–677
23. Goldenberg S L, Perez-Marrero R A, Lee L M, Emerson L. Endoscopic balloon dilatation of the prostate: early experience. J Urol 1990; 144: 83–87
24. Klein L A, Lemming B. Balloon dilatation for prostatic obstruction. Urology 1989; 33: 198–201
25. Lepor H, Sypherd D, Machi G, Derus J. Randomized double-blind study comparing the effectiveness of balloon dilation of the prostate and cystoscopy in the treatment of symptomatic benign prostatic hyperplasia. J Urol 1992; 147: 639–644
26. Klein L A, Perez-Marrero R A, Bowers G W et al. Transurethral cystoscopic balloon dilatation of the prostate. J Endourol 1990; 4: 183–191
27. Vale J A, Miller P D, Kirby R S. Balloon dilatation of the prostate — should it have a place in the urologist's armamentarium? J R Soc Med 1993; 86: 83–86
28. Boyarsky S, Jones G, Paulson D F, Prout G R. A new look at bladder neck obstruction by the Food and Drug Regulators: guidelines for the investigation of benign prostatic hypertrophy. Trans Am Assoc Genitourin Surg 1977; 68: 29–32

Temporary stents

J. Nordling

39

Introduction

The insertion of a stent to relive infravesical obstruction due to benign prostatic hyperplasia (BPH) was first described in 1980 by Fabian (Prostacoil or Urocoil).[1,2] Almost 10 years later, Nissenkorn[3] reported on a silicone stent (intraurethral catheter, IUC), Nordling et al.[4] on a gold-plated coil (Prostakath) and Williams et al.[5] on a stent of woven stainless steel (Urolume). Subsequent development in this area has increased rapidly. Stents have been described as temporary (removable) or permanent (incorporated into the tissue) but the distinction between the two groups is becoming less clear, as the temporary stents might be left in situ for several years, and often patients die with the stent in situ. The internal diameters of the stents differ, however, and permanent stents have the advantage that cystoscopy can be carried out through the stent, although this may also be possible through the second generation of temporary stents. This chapter deals with the temporary stents, which have been divided into first- and second-generation stents (Table 39.1).

First-generation temporary stents

Urospiral

The initial stent was introduced by Fabian[1] (Fig 39.1). This device is a coil of stainless steel. It consists of three parts. The body lies in the prostatic urethra and protrudes 10–15 mm into the bladder. The length of the body ranges from 45 to 75 mm to fit the length of the

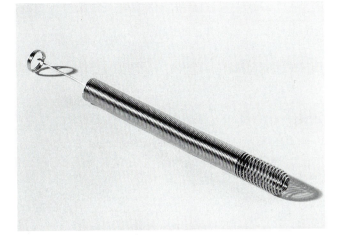

Figure 39.1. *Urospiral.*

sphincteric urethra. The neck is 20 mm long and should be positioned in the sphincteric urethra; the head is 2 mm long, and lies in the bulbous urethra distal to the sphincter. Before insertion of the stent, prostatic urethral length is measured either endoscopically or by either abdominal or rectal ultrasound. It is the author's experience, that these methods give quite different results. Endoscopic length is often quite short, partly because measurement is normally to the verumontanum and not to the apex, which may be 1–2 cm further distal in the urethra. Using the rigid endoscope, the straight distance from the bladder neck is also measured, whereas the prostatic urethra is normally curved, at least posteriorly where the stent preferably should be positioned.

The urospiral is inserted under endoscopic guidance using a special grasping forceps. A 7 Fr ureteral catheter used as a guidewire considerably facilitates insertion. Insertion is performed under sedo-analgesia or using urethral gel containing local analgesic. Insertion through a cystoscope sheath,[6] guided by fluoroscopy[7] or by rectal ultrasound,[8] have been described. Occasionally, insertion is not possible because of a urethral stricture.

Table 39.1. *Temporary stents*

First generation	Second generation
Urospiral	Memokath
Prostakath	Prostacoil
Intraurethral catheter	

Symptomatic outcome

A 'success' rate of about 70% is reported within the first year after insertion (Table 39.2), but only sparse information exists on symptom scores. Guazzoni et al.[17] reported a postinsertion mean Boyarsky symptom score of 11.1 (3 months), 13.2 (6 months) and 13.5 (12 months) in 20 patients, all of whom were in urinary retention before stent insertion.

Effect on obstruction

An increase in peak urinary flow rate is reported, although actual figures are scarce, especially before stent insertion, as a majority of patients were in retention. A peak flow rate of about 10–15 ml/s up to 1 year after insertion has been reported.[6,7,18] No data exist on pressure–flow evaluation.

Complications

The most common complications are bacteriuria (Table 39.2), migration, encrustation, incontinence and urethral stricture. Bacteriuria is normally not a serious problem and many patients become clear of infection with time.[2] The longest reported follow-up with the Urospiral is in most reports 24 months. Possible complications after this time are unknown.

Prostakath

This device is shaped like the Urospiral but is covered with gold to prevent encrustations.[19] A special detachable catheter makes insertion much easier and not too different from inserting an indwelling catheter (Fig. 39.2). A 7 Fr ureteral catheter is recommended as a guidewire during insertion and is also provided with the stent. The stent is most easily inserted under ultrasonic guidance (Fig. 39.3).[4] The Prostakath comes in lengths from 35 to 95 mm and also has an outer diameter of 21 Fr (Fig 39.4). Insertion is performed as an outpatient procedure using a urethral gel with local analgesic.

Symptomatic outcome

The 'success rate' of about 70% is very much like that of the Urospiral (Table 39.3) but the reported follow-up time is much longer (up to 5 years). Thomas et al.[23] demonstrated a much better outcome in patients with acute retention (success rate 89%) then in patients in chronic retention (success rate 30%) in a study with up to 4 years' follow-up. In a small controlled study[24] a modified Madsen–Iversen score decreased from 8 to 5, 4 months after insertion of the Prostakath; in the control group, the symptom score decreased from 8.5 to 7. After transurethral prostatectomy, symptom scores decreased

Table 39.2. *Results of studies using the Urospiral*

Reference	No. of patients	Age (years) [median (range)]	Follow-up (months)	Success rate (%)	Complications (number)
Fabian[1]	2	(75–79)	5–12	100	
Fabian[2]	48	80 (53–92)	≤ 30	88	
Langkopf et al.[9]	15		< 3	45	
Fabricius et al.[10]	15		≤ 12	30	Migration (6) Encrustation (4)
Rohl et al.[11]	11	75.4 (63–93)	≤ 12	45	Incontinence (6)
Flier and Seppelt[12]	49	(62–93)	≤ 24	70	Dislocation (5) Too short (6) Encrustation (1)
Schops and Kierfeld[13]	7		?	100	
Langemeyer and Ferwerda[14]	11	77 (62–91)	≤ 7	90	Encrustation (1)
Roth and Rathert[15]	8	?	≤ 12	25	
Garbit et al.[16]	26	(61–94)	≤ 24	80	
Guazzoni et al.[7]	20	85 (78–92)	6	95	Incontinence (1)
Parker et al.[6]	36	75 (50–98)	1–18	67	Pain/dysuria (2) Migration (2) Encrustation (2)

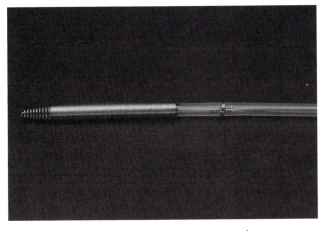

Figure 39.2. *Prostakath mounted on an insertion catheter.*

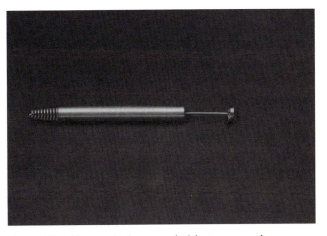

Figure 39.4. *Prostakath after removal of the insertion catheter.*

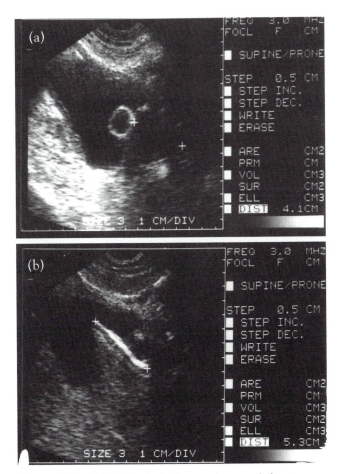

Figure 39.3. *(a) Abdominal ultrasound scan of the prostate. Prostatic urethral length 4.1 cm; (b) Prostakath: 55 mm long body is seen in place.*

outlined in Table 39.4. As can be seen, most of these quite elderly patients have no, or only minor, voiding symptoms with the stent in situ. The most bothersome symptoms are persistent frequency and urgency in 15–30% of all patients. Within this long observation period, the stent was removed in 150 patients, while 48 patients died with a functioning stent. Reasons for stent removal are outlined in Table 39.5.

Effect on obstruction

Only two papers report on pressure–flow studies with the Prostakath.[24,25] They only include a small number of patients, but the first is randomized and controlled and patients in both groups ultimately had a transurethral prostatectomy (TURP). In the latter,[25] eight patients were evaluated at a median of 61 days after stent insertion and detrusor pressure at this time was 46 cmH$_2$O (median) or in the middle of the equivocal area. In the first study,[24] detrusor pressure at peak flow rate decreased from 74 cmH$_2$O before stent insertion to 60 cmH$_2$0 4 months after stent insertion, which is in the obstructed area. In the observation group, detrusor pressure increased slightly during 4 months' observation. After TURP, all patients became unobstructed. This observation confirms that the relief of obstruction seen immediately after stent insertion with an increase in peak flow rate from a mean of 7.9 to 22.3 ml/s detoriates with time.[22]

Complications

As for the Urospiral, the most common complications with the Prostakath are encrustations,[22,26] migration,[22,23]

considerably in both groups, to 2 and 3, respectively. Since 1987, the author has personally treated 318 patients with the Prostakath. Voiding symptoms are

Table 39.3. *Results of studies using the Prostakath*

Reference	No. of patients	Age (years) [median (range)]	Follow-up (months)	Success rate (%)	Complications (number)
Yachia et al.[20]	26	(59–86)	< 12	77	Incontinence retention
Harrison and de Souza[21]	30	80 (65–93)	?	55	Urethral stricture (1) Failure in patient with chronic retention
Nordling et al.[22]	150	76 (40–95)	8.2 (0–40)	66	Calcification (21) Incontinence (25) Migration (42)

Table 39.4. *Voiding symptoms in 318 patients after insertion of the Prostakath*

Symptom	Incidence (number)		
	None	Moderate	Severe
Stress incontinence	244	20	17
Urge	155	79	46 (incontinence)
Frequency	162	63	45
Nocturia	205 (0–1 times/night)	61 (2–3 times/night)	12 (> 3 times/night)
Emptying problems	259	15	8
Urethral bleeding	271	9	2
Local discomfort	262	13	7

Table 39.5. *Reason for removal of Prostakath stent in 150 of 318 patients*

Reason for removal	No. of patients
Planned prostatectomy	29
Incontinence	17
Retention	35
Local discomfort	9
Irritative voiding symptoms	17
No symptomatic improvement	12
Stent migration	16
Not stent related (e.g. stroke)	14
Urethral bleeding	1
Infection	0

incontinence[22] and urethral stricture. Although in 318 patients the author found chronic bacteriuria in 53 and intermittent bacteriuria in 27, this never represented a significant clinical problem. Patients with irritative symptoms due to bacteriuria were normally well treated on long-term, low-dose antibiotics. All patients received prophylactic antibiotics before stent insertion. One death due to sepsis after stent removal in an 89-year-old man has prompted the use of intravenous antibiotics before any stent manipulation.

This death is one of two major complications seen during the last 8 years. The other case is that of an 84-year-old man who had his stent removed after 2 years owing to recurrence of obstructive symptoms. The head of the stent was buried in mucosa, which is often seen and normally represents a mucosal hyperplasia. At removal (by grasping the neck with a hook), 2–3 cm of the urethra was stripped in the whole circumference. The patient at present has an indwelling catheter, but the final outcome remains to be seen.

Encrustations have not been a major problem, although they may sometimes be fairly severe and become more so after extended follow-up. The stones are very soft and fracture easily.

Intraurethral catheter

The IUC was introduced at the same time as the Prostakath.[3] The device is a double malecot 16 Fr polyurethane catheter available in 25–80 mm lengths at 5 mm intervals (Fig. 39.5). It is inserted under local anaesthesia with gel, either cystoscopically or using a special insertion tube. The IUC lies in the posterior urethra with one of the expansions in the bladder and the second just above the external sphincter (Fig. 39.6). A non-absorbable nylon suture is connected to the distal end of the catheter and remains within the urethra. This makes removal of the stent very easy if necessary.

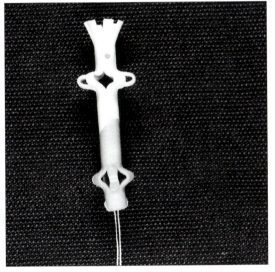

Figure 39.5. *Intraurethral catheter.*

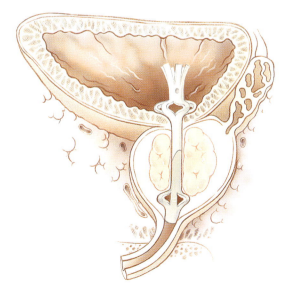

Figure 39.6. *Correct positioning of the IUC stent.*

Symptomatic outcome

'Success rate' is of the same order as with the coils (Table 39.6). Effects on symptom scores are not reported, mainly because the patients were mainly elderly, fragile men in urinary retention.

Effect on obstruction

Patients previously in retention are normally able to void freely with the device in the correct position.

Complications

Migration and encrustation are the main complications (Table 39.6).

Second-generation stents

The two available second-generation stents are both made of nickel–titanium, a metal increasingly used in medicine. The metal has an intrinsic memory, expands when heated (at a preselected temperature) and becomes flaccid and increasingly bendable when cooled.

Memokath

The Memokath is an intraprostatic coil with an outer diameter of 22 Fr and an inner diameter of 18 Fr. It is a coil of a nickel–titanium thread, 0.65 mm thick, which at a temperature of 45–50°C expands the lower five turns conically to a maximum diameter of 11 mm (Fig. 39.7). It is positioned in the prostatic urethra with the tip at the bladder neck and the expandable part at the apex above the external sphincter. The stent should not protrude into the bladder, thus minimizing the risk of encrustations (Fig. 39.8).

The stent is inserted and positioned endoscopically using a 14–16 Fr flexible cystoscope. The length of the prostatic urethra must be determined before implantation of the stent. The stent comes in lengths of 40, 50, 60 and 70 mm and a stent of appropriate length is chosen. A flexible cystoscope is passed through the insertion catheter and the stent, so that it projects 2–3 mm beyond the tip of the stent.

The urethra is lubricated with local anaesthetic gel and the stent is inserted under direct vision. The tip is positioned at the bladder neck and the distal part of the stent is flushed with 50 ml water at 50°C. This dilates the distal part of the stent, thereby releasing it from the

Table 39.6. *Results of studies using the Nissenkorn IUC*

Reference	No. of patients	Age (years) [median (range)]	Follow-up (months)	Success rate (%)	Complications (%)
Nissenkorn[27]	73	74 (54–100)	6–16	74	Migration (5) Obstruction (2) Stone (1)
Sassine and Schulman[28]	43	?	Up to 24	85	Migration (9) Stone (1)

(a)

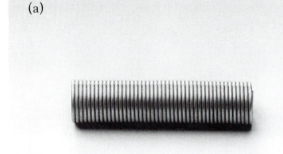

(b)

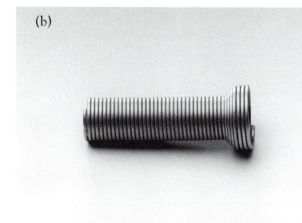

Figure 39.7. *Memokath: (a) during insertion; (b) after flushing with 50°C water.*

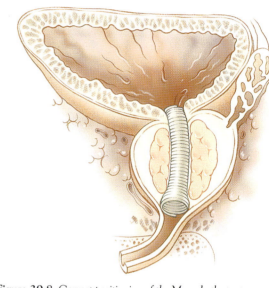

Figure 39.8. *Correct positioning of the Memokath stent.*

sheath. The sheath and the flexible cystoscope can then be gently retracted.

If the stent is to be removed, cold irrigation fluid is used. This makes the stent soft, bendable and easy to remove as a long thread.

Effect on symptoms

Poulsen et al.[29] reported a 'success rate' of 83% with a median follow-up of 3 months (range 0.2–9 months). Similarly, Booth et al.[30] reported a 'success rate' of 80%. The author has now treated 64 patients with the Memokath, with an observation time of up to 3 years. A total of 24 stents have been removed, but only ten because of stent problems: in five patients removal was because of urinary retention, in three because of urinary incontinence, in one because of local discomfort and in one because of migration. Patients' symptoms are outlined in Table 39.7. It must be remembered that the stent is mostly used in patients who are too old or frail for surgery, which is not comparable to a normal prostatectomy population. Seven patients received no further treatment after stent removal; seven had another

Table 39.7. *Voiding symptoms in 64 patients after insertion of the Memokath*

	Incidence (number)		
Symptom	None	Moderate	Severe
Stress incontinence	49	1	1
Urge	17	15	10 (incontinence)
Frequency	28	14	10
Nocturia	36 (0–1 times/night)	15 (2–3 times/night)	1 (>3 times/night)
Emptying problems	49	2	1
Urethral bleeding	49	2	1
Load discomfort	52	0	1

type of stent inserted, three received an indwelling catheter and only seven went on to prostatectomy.

Effect on obstruction

Peak flow rate increased from a mean of 8 to 16 ml/s immediately after insertion,[29] but tended to decrease after some months. No data are available on pressure–flow studies.

Complications

One distal and one proximal migration have been observed after 1 and 3 months, respectively. This is a much better migration rate than with the first-generation stents. Encrustations seem to be less, as well. Of 24 stents removed, 12 were without macroscopic encrustations, three had minor, three slight and three severe encrustations. Of 42 evaluable patients, 13 had persistent bacteriuria causing no clinical problems; in four, urinary infection was cured with antibiotics.

Prostacoil

This stent is also made of nickel–titanium and is wound on a delivery catheter. At insertion it has an outer calibre of 17 Fr, and after release it takes on a wavy form, with an alternating calibre of 24–30 Fr. The stent is, like the Urocoil and the Prostakath, composed of three sections (Fig. 39.9). The intraprostatic section is made in 40, 50, 60, 70 and 80 mm lengths, while the intrabulbar section has a length of 10 mm. The two parts are connected by a helical trans-sphincteric section.

The Prostacoil is provided on a delivery catheter and inserted under fluoroscopy (Fig. 39.10). The patient is

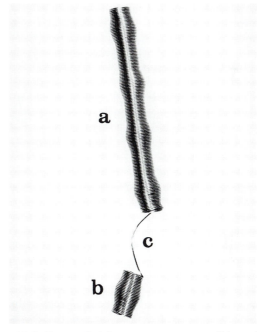

Figure 39.9. *Prostacoil: (a) intraprostatic section; (b) intrabulbar section; (c) helical trans-sphincteric section.*

catheterized at least 24 h previously with a 20 Fr Foley catheter. After removal of the catheter, a retrograde urethrogram is performed and the position of the external sphincter is marked with an external radio-opaque marker. The distance from the bladder neck to the external sphincter is measured using an open-tip measuring catheter. The tip of the stent is designed to protrude 5–10 mm into the bladder, so a stent of appropriate length is chosen. A guidewire is threaded through the measuring catheter, which is then removed,

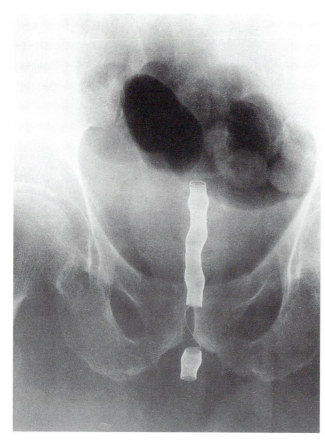

Figure 39.10. *Radiograph of the Prostacoil in situ.*

and the guidewire is used for insertion of the stent. When the stent is in place, the lock on the introducing catheter is released, first the distal and then the proximal part. A new endoscopic device for delivering the Prostacoil is currently being tested.

The Prostacoil may be removed either by using a 12 Fr Foley bag catheter inserted through the stent or by grasping the distal end of the stent and pulling it out through the endoscope.

Effect on symptoms

A 'success rate' of 88% is reported by Yachia et al.[31] in 65 patients with a mean follow-up of 16 months (range 3–28 months).

Effect on obstruction

Patients unable to void before stent insertion voided freely afterwards. No further data are available.

Complications

No incident of encrustation or migration has been reported. Patients with sterile urine remained sterile and, in 26 of 32 patients, a previous infection cleared within 2 months.

Discussion

Long-term indwelling catheters are simple to use, but are associated with significant complications,[32,33] besides the considerable embarrassment and bother associated with such a device.

Prostatectomy is by far the best treatment for a patient facing the need to carry an indwelling catheter because of infravesical prostatic obstruction. If the patient for some reason is unfit for surgery, several alternatives are possible, such as thermotherapy, clean intermittent self-catheterization or permanent and temporary stents. The temporary stents allow normal voiding for many months. They are easy to insert, even as an outpatient procedure, and are normally easy to remove, especially the second-generation nickel–titanium stents.

First-generation temporary stents carry a considerable risk of complications in the form of encrustation inside and outside the stent, and migration of the sent. Migration seems to be much less of a problem with the second-generation stents, but longer follow-up is needed before the encrustation issue can be evaluated.

Very few data exist on symptom scores, but it seems that these patients at longer follow-up are still fairly symptomatic.[17] In this context is must be remembered that a majority of these patients are very old and frail — a population often suffering from lower urinary tract symptoms that are due to causes other than infravesical obstruction. Furthermore, the effect on infravesical obstruction has been poorly described. Only with one type of temporary stent (Prostakath) have pressure–flow studies been performed, and those patients were clearly obstructed 4 months after stent insertion. Stent insertion initiates an oedemateous reaction in the urethral mucosa. Even in the large calibrated permanent stents this may become obstructive; in the temporary stents with their smaller diameter it is much more likely to happen. It seems that the ability to void freely immediately after insertion of a temporary stent is followed by increasing mucosal obstruction, leaving the patient able to void but with the problem of a moderate to severe infravesical obstruction.

First-generation temporary stents protruding into the bulbous urethra (Prostacoil, Prostakath) carry the risk of developing urethral strictures (Table 39.3) and many (30%) of these patients have some degree of urinary incontinence. This has not yet been described with the Urocoil, but it may become a consequence of having a metal thread running through the external sphincter. A bioabsorbable stent that desintegrates within a few weeks to months has been described.[34] This stent might be particularly useful after laser prostatectomy or in other conditions, where very short-term relief of infravesical obstruction is needed.

Conclusions

First-generation temporary stents are indicated only as an alternative for an indwelling catheter for short-term relief of prostatic obstruction, e.g. in patients waiting for surgery, or after laser prostatectomy, or as a treatment for a longer period in patients unfit for surgery. Effects on symptom scores and infravesical obstruction seem to be limited and poorly investigated.

Second-generation temporary stents seem to have less complications with the indications being the same as for the first-generation stents. Studies of their effect on lower urinary tract symptoms and on infravesical obstruction are needed.

References

1. Fabian K M. Der intraprostatische spirale 'Partielle Katheter' (Urologische spiral). Urologe A 1980; 19: 236–238
2. Fabian K M. Der intraprostatische 'Partielle Katheter' (Urologische spirale) II. Urologe A 1984; 23: 229–233
3. Nissenkorn I. Experience with a new self retaining intraurethral catheter in patients with urinary retention: a preliminary report. J Urol 1989; 142: 92–94
4. Nordling J, Holm H H, Klarskov P et al. The intraprostatic spiral: a new device for insertion with the patient under local anaesthesia and with ultrasonic guidance with 3 months follow up. J Urol 1989; 142: 756–758
5. Williams G, Jager R, McLoughlin L. Use of stents for treating obstruction of the urinary outflow in patients unfit for surgery. Br Med J 1989; 298: 1429–1431
6. Parker C J, Birch B R P, Connelly A et al. The porges urospiral: a reversible endoprostatic prosthetic stent. World J Urol 199; 9: 22–25
7. Guazzoni G, Montorsi F, Columbo R et al. Long term experience with the prostatic spiral for urinary retention due to benign prostatic hyperplasia. Scand J Urol Nephrol 1991; 25: 21–24
8. Billiet I, Mattelaer J, Van Brien P. Use of transrectal longitudinal sonography in the placement of a prostatic coil. Eur Urol 1990; 17: 76–78
9. Langkopf B, Oehlmann U, Geshe R, Rebmann U. Erste erfahrungen mit einer harnrohren endothese bein blasenhalsadenom. Z Urol Nephrol 1991; 74: 793–800
10. Fabricius P G, Matz M, Zefinich H. Die endourethral spirale — eine alternative zum Dauerkatheter? Z Arztl Fortbild (Jena) 1983; 77: 482–483
11. Rohl H F, Bauhe H P, Andersen O P. Den urologiske spiral. Et endoprostatisk kateter. Ugeskr Laeger 1987; 149: 2076–2077
12. Flier G, Seppelt U. Erfahrungen mit der urologischen spiral. Urologe (B) 1987; 27: 304–307
13. Schopes W, Kierfeld G. Die urologische spirale und ihr klinischer stellenwert. Urologe (B) 1987; 27: 308–309
14. Langemeyer T N M, Ferwerda W H H. De prostaat spiral als alternatief voor een verblijtscatheter. Ned Tijdschr Geneeskd 1987; 131: 2022–2025
15. Roth S T, Rathert P. La 'spirale urologique'. Une possibilité therapeutique dans le traitement du carcinoma prostatique. J Urol (Paris) 1988; 94: 261–263
16. Garbit J L, Blitz M, Bomel J et al. La prothese endo-prostatique spirale de Fabian. J Urol (Paris) 1988; 94: 265–267
17. Guazzoni G, Montorsi F, Bergamaschi F et al. Prostatic spiral versus prostatic urolume Wallstent for urinary retention due to benign prostatic hyperplasia. Eur Urol 1993; 24: 332–336
18. Conart P as cited in Smith P H. Other non-medical therapies (excluding lasers) in the treatment of BPH. In: Cockette A T K, Khoury S, Aso Y et al. (eds) Proceedings of the 2nd International Consultation on benign prostatic hyperplasia (BPH). Jersey: SCI 1993: 470–471
19. Holmes S A V, Miller P D, Crocker P R, Kirby R. Encrustation of intraprostatic stents — a comparative study. Br J Urol 1992; 69: 383–387
20. Yachia D, Lask D, Robinson S. Self retaining intraurethral stent: a alternative to long-term indwelling catheters or surgery in the treatment of prostatism. AJR 1990; 154: 111–113
21. Harrison N W, de Souza J V. Prostatic stenting for outflow obstruction. Br J Urol 1990; 65: 192–196
22. Nordling J, Ovesen H, Poulsen A L. The intraprostatic spiral: clinical results in 150 consecutive patients. J Urol 1992; 147: 645–647
23. Thomas P J, Britton J P, Harrison N W. The prostakath stent: four years experience. Br J Urol 1993; 71: 430–432
24. Nielsen K K, Kromann-Andersen B, Poulsen A L et al. Subjective and objective evaluation of patients with prostatism and infravesical obstruction treated with both intraprostatic spiral and transurethral prostatectomy. Neurourol Urodyn 1994; 13: 13–19
25. Nielsen K K, Kromann-Andersen B, Nordling J. Relationship between detrusor pressure and urinary flow rate in males with an intraurethral prostatic spiral. Br J Urol 1989; 64: 275–279
26. Rosenkilde P, Pedersen J F, Meyhoff H H. Late complications of prostakath treatment for benign prostatic hypertrophy. Br J Urol 1991; 68: 387–389
27. Neissenkorn I. Prostatic stents. J Endourol 1991; 5: 79–82
28. Sassine A M, Schulman C C. Intraurethral catheter in high-risk patients with urinary retention: 3 years experience. Eur Urol 1994; 25: 131–134
29. Poulsen A L, Schou J, Ovesen H, Nordling J. Memokath: a second generation of intraprostatic spirals. Br J Urol 1993; 72: 331–334
30. Booth C M, Al-Dabbagh M A, Lyth D R, Nordling J. The memokath: a second generation 'memory alloy' prostatic stent. Proc BAUS Ann Meet, Harrogate, 1993: 153

31. Yachia D, Beyar M, Aridogan I A. A new, large calibre, self-
     expanding and self-retaining temporary intraprostatic stent
     (ProstaCoil) in the treatment of prostatic obstruction. Br J Urol
     1994; 74: 47–49
32. Onslander J G, Greengold B, Chen S. Complications of chronic
     indwelling catheters among male nursing home patients: a
     prospective study. J Urol 1987; 138: 1119–1195

33. Brietenburger R B. Bacterial changes in the urine sample of patients
     with long-term indwelling catheters. Arch Ind Med 1984; 144:
     1585–1588
34. Kemppainen E, Talja M, Riihelä M et al. A bioabsorbable urethral
     stent. Urol Res 1993; 21: 235–238

Prostatic endoprosthetics

A. E. Te S. A. Kaplan

40

Introduction

The hallmark of therapy designed to alleviate the symptoms associated with prostatism is to decrease bladder outlet obstruction. The use of tubes or catheters to open or bypass this obstruction is a time-honoured concept in urological teaching. Thus, the concept of a prostatic stent to 'open' the prostatic urethra is a logical natural extension of these ideas.

The modern medical concept of a stent — the placement of a foreign body through a stenotic lumen to maintain patency — is only two decades old. Stents have been commonly utilized in other medical specialties such as vascular surgery (Table 40.1). Dotter et al. reported in 1969 on the use of a coilspring in the popliteal artery.[1] Recently, there have been reports of successful stenting of coronary arteries and Food and Drug Administration approval for its application within the coronary arteries.[2] Self-expandable stainless steel stents (Wallstent) were also used in 26 iliac and 15 femoropopliteal artery lesions of 31 patients to treat stenoses or occlusions. In the iliac artery group, 96% of the stented lesions were patent at a mean follow-up of 16 months while in the femoropopliteal artery group, six of 11 patients had patent stents at 7–26 months.[3] This is consistent with the work of others who have reported greater success in larger-diameter vessels.[4,5] Plastic biliary endoprosthetic stents have also been applied successfully to relieve malignant obstructive jaundice in 80–90% of patients.[6] Its use has been recommended because it is well tolerated and ideal in palliatively treated tumour patients.

Over the past decade, a number of investigators have reported on the use of prostatic urethral stents. In both Europe and Asia, urologists have reported clinical efficacy employing a variety of different stents. However, in the United States, urologists have only recently reported favourable experiences with prostatic stents. Given the explosion of alternative therapeutic devices for prostatism, the attention directed towards prostatic urethral stents has lagged behind that focused on other therapies. Owing to strict regulatory restrictions of use of the prostatic stent in the United States, other alternative therapeutic alternatives such as laser prostatectomy, which is widely available, have been accepted with more enthusiasm by the urological community. Currently, there is debate whether the indications for stents should be limited to frail elderly patients or expanded to younger men with prostatism.[6]

The purpose of this chapter is to review and update the current status of prostatic urethral stents both in the United States and worldwide (Table 40.2). Most of the literature to be reviewed concerns first-generation stents. Currently, there is a major research effort to develop more favourable and biocompatible stents. The ultimate role of prostatic urethral stents in the urological armamentarium for therapy of benign prostatic hyperplasia (BPH) therapy remains to be determined.

Table 40.1. *Role of endoprostheses*

Specialty	Location/indication for use of stent
Vascular surgery	Coronary artery Peripheral (iliac, femoral, popliteal) Renal artery
Gastrointestinal tract surgery	Biliary
Urology	Urethral stricture Detrusor–external sphincter dyssynergia Renal artery stenosis BPH

Prostatic endoprostheses

Prostate springs

Prostakath

The prostatic spring or spiral was first described by Fabian in 1980.[7] There have been many subsequent modifications including the Prostakath (Engineers

Table 40.2. *Types of prostatic urethral stent*

Type	Stent
Spiral	Prostakath
	Porges Urospiral
	Prostacoil
Self-expandable	Superalloy mesh
	(Urolume Wallstent)
	Stainless steel
	(Gianturco stent)
Balloon expandable	Intraprostatic
	stent (titanium)
(On the horizon)	Intraurethral
	catheter (IUC)
	Biodegradable (SR-PLLA)
	Thermoexpandable
	(Nitinol) SMA
	stent (Memotherm,
	Memokath, Chinese SMA)

& Doctors A/S, Copenhagen, Denmark). The stent, which is composed of stainless steel, is coated with 24 carat gold, which helps to prevent encrustation. The outer diameter is 21 Fr and the stent is supplied in four lengths — 4.5, 5.5, 6.5 and 7.5 cm. The straight portion, consisting of multiple spiral loops, remains in the prostatic urethra with the most proximal portion extending through the bladder neck into the bladder. The distal portion consists of a 2 cm straight wire segment traversing the membranous urethra and two spiral loops in the bulbar urethra. It is important to note that the spiral does not become epithelialized. The practical implications of this phenomenon are the lack of obstruction through the lumen of the stent.

The Prostakath can be placed either under direct vision or under ultrasound guidance. Vincente et al. reported on 49 patients (40 with BPH, seven with prostatic carcinoma and two patients with 'sclerosis' of the bladder neck) who were followed up for 22 months after cystoscopic insertion.[8] There was normal voiding in 74%, decreases in post-void residual in 88.5% and flow rates between 6 and 12 ml/s in 60% of cases.

In a multicentre study from Finland, 75 patients underwent placement of the Prostakath (80% under ultrasound guidance).[9] A good or excellent result was

noted in 58% of patients, while eight remained in urinary retention. Three patients required removal of the Prostakath because of urinary tract infection. Yachia et al. reported their experience in 26 men who were poor operative risks.[10] The treatment was successful in 20 (77%); all 20 were able to void satisfactorily, and four of the 20 resumed sexual activity, which previously had been prevented by indwelling catheters. Two patients who had delayed prostatic surgery because of fear of impotence were able to empty their bladders properly and to remain sexually active. Three patients subsequently had surgery, two after anticoagulant therapy had been withdrawn and one after renal function had improved: no difficulties caused by the stent were encountered during surgery. Four patients who had the stent in place for 12 months had no difficulties. In 16 of the 18 patients who had indwelling catheters and infected urine before insertion of the stent, sterilization of the urine was obtained after relatively short courses of antibiotic treatment. Short-term complications associated with the stent were incontinence or urinary retention. These were treated by repositioning the stent. Frequency of urination after insertion of the stent either disappeared spontaneously or was treated with anticholinergic drugs. In six patients, frequency was so severe that removal of the stent and insertion of an indwelling catheter were necessary. Slight to mild dysuria occurred immediately after surgery in all patients but eventually disappeared.

Thomas et al. reported the successful use of the Prostakath in 57 of 64 patients in urinary retention.[11] A stent-related problem that required further treatment occurred in 16 patients. Displacement was the most common side effect noted.

Nordling et al. reported the largest experience using the Prostakath in 150 men (age 40–95 years).[12] Of the 150 patients, 70 had severe prostatism, while the remaining 80 were in urinary retention. Peak flow rates increased from a mean of 7.9 to 22.3 ml/s. However, 75 patients required removal of the stent for various reasons, including proximal (42 patients) and distal (13 patients) migration.

Porges Urospiral

Miller reported that of 36 patients who underwent endoprostatic helicoplasty using a similar spiral — the

Porges Urospiral — 67% had a successful outcome.[13] A major predisposing factor for failure included patients with chronic retention; in addition, eight patients had incontinence. In a Turkish study, 18 patients in retention were all able to void after stent insertion.[14] However, 44% had persistent urinary tract infection, and upward migration of the stent occurred in 55% of cases.

In a study of 184 patients who underwent insertion of the Porges Urospiral (81 in urinary retention, 84 with severe outflow obstruction and 19 with severe detrusor instability complicating obstruction), a success rate of 72% was reported.[15] Although 51 patients were classified as technical failures, only 17 (9.3%) proceeded to prostatic surgery.

Prostacoil

The Prostacoil (Instent, Inc., Minnesota, USA) is a new self-expanding and self-retaining, large-calibre, temporary intraprostatic coil. The stent is supplied wound on a delivery catheter to reduce its calibre to 17 Fr, with a wavy form containing alternating calibres of 24/30 Fr in its expanded form. It is supplied in lengths of 40, 50, 60, 70 and 80 mm. The entire lumen is hollow and instruments up to 17 Fr can easily be passed through it. Yachia et al. reported their results in 65 patients with BPH (follow-up of 3–28 months). Of these 65 patients, 30 became eligible for surgery and had their stents removed within 3–12 months after insertion. Only one stent was removed because of urgency and incontinence. Repositioning was required in five patients; 14 complained of dysuria or perineal pain. Twenty-seven patients have their stent in place and voided without difficulty. Infected urine was reported in 32 patients. The major advantages of this stent are ease of insertion, ease of removal and the potential for subsequent instrumentation. Most importantly, it does need to be placed precisely within the confines of the prostatic urethra.[16]

Self-expandable stents

Wallstent

The Urolume Wallstent (American Medical Systems) is a biomedical superalloy prosthesis woven in a tubular mesh and produced in various diameters and lengths

(Fig. 40.1). It is stable when expanded and will not suffer elastic recoil. It is preloaded in a special delivery system that allows direct visualization of the prosthesis and the urethra throughout the entire insertion procedure. As the Urolume is deployed from the delivery system, it expands to a diameter of 14 mm. The elastic properties and radial force of the prosthesis allow it to remain in place and prevent migration.

The stent can be placed under spinal, caudal or local anaesthesia with a prostate block and i.v. sedation. In the authors' experience, a saddle block has been particularly effective with minimal patient discomfort or morbidity. The length of the prostatic urethra is calibrated using either a standard ureter stent or a calibration catheter. A deployment tool (Fig. 40.2) is

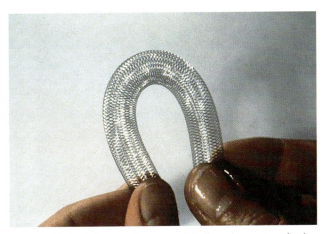

Figure 40.1. *Self-expanding stent (Wallstent), composed of a superalloy mesh.*

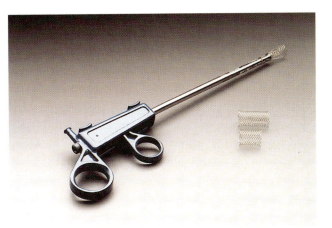

Figure 40.2. *Delivery tool. The stent is positioned at the bladder neck and distally to the verumontanum.*

used to place the stent (2 or 3 cm in length) under direct vision. In patients with longer prostatic urethras, two or even more overlapping stents may be used. The deployment tool contains the stent in a compressed state and is 21 Fr in diameter. As the stent is released, it expands to its full diameter and length. In the authors' experience, and that of others, it has been determined that one of the keys to successful placement is that no portion of the stent protrudes through the bladder neck into the bladder or distally beyond the verumontanum. Chapple et al. reported their preliminary experience using the Wallstent in 12 patients with prostatic outflow obstruction.[17] All were in a high-risk group for surgery and 11 were treated successfully, with a follow-up of 1–11 (median 9) months. The majority of patients (11 of 12) were satisfied with the procedure, which provided a quick, safe and effective alternative to conventional surgical treatment. In this series, the stent was delivered using combined ultrasound and endoscopic control under local anaesthesia. The procedure was well tolerated, the stent becoming covered with epithelium by 6–8 months following insertion, yet allowed easy removal within the first 4–6 weeks should the need arise. In that series, mean peak flow rate improved to 13.4 ± 4.7 ml/s. All patients had postoperative urgency, which usually resolved within 4–6 weeks; however, in one patient these symptoms persisted, consistent with de novo detrusor instability.

The same group has updated their experience in 54 patients, 46 (85%) of whom were in urinary retention. For the retention patients, mean peak flow rate was 16.6 ml/s and the mean post-void residual was 74 ml. At 1 year, total Madsen symptom score decreased to 6.5 in the non-retention men and to 6.0 in the patients originally in retention.[18] The majority demonstrated marked objective and subjective improvement, while five stents had to be removed. Harrison and DeSouza reported a similar experience in 30 patients with outflow obstruction:[19] most had urinary retention and were unfit for conventional surgery. The prostatic stent was readily inserted under local anaesthesia and successfully relieved obstruction in 80% of patients with acute retention.

McLoughlin et al. reported that all of 19 patients in urinary retention were able to void spontaneously after placement of the Wallstent.[20] Similarly, a high percentage of patients (79%) reported postoperative urgency, which resolved within 8 weeks. In a subsequent study, the same group reported that in 21 patients, endoprostheses were placed under fluoroscopic guidance. The procedure was technically successful in all patients, although in one case a second stent was required 2 months later.[21] One patient developed a urethral stricture in the 12–16-month follow-up period. One case of epididymo-orchitis and one case of septicaemia after stenting were treated successfully with antibiotics.

In the United States, Oesterling et al. in 1994 reported the use of the Wallstent in different populations, including those who had moderate symptoms yet were relatively health.[22] The group consisted of 126 men, 95 of whom had moderate to severe prostatism, and 31 were in urinary retention. For the non-retention cohort, mean symptom score decreased from 14.3 to 5.4 ($p<0.001$); at 24 months peak flow rate increased from a mean of 9.1 to 13.1 ml/s ($p<0.001$) and post-void residual decreased from 85 to 47 ml ($p=0.02$). For the retention group, mean symptom score, peak flow rate and post-void residual were 4.1, 11.4 ml/s and 46 ml, respectively. By 12 months, nearly all endoprostheses were 80–100% covered with urothelium; more than 50% had complete coverage. The explantation rate was 13% (n=17).

In a recent multicentre study in Europe, Guazzoni et al. examined a modified prostatic Urolume Wallstent which has a 'less shortening' feature compared with the commercially available Urolume Wallstent.[23] It was developed to counter placement problems associated with pronounced shortening after deployment in the commercially available stent. Although similar clinical efficacy is demonstrated in this study of 135 healthy patients, the high long-term complication rate (38%) of this modified stent has led to its abandonment. The standard Urolume stent has been shown to relieve bladder outlet obstruction successfully in healthy patients with BPH.

Gianturco stent

A self-expanding metal stent — the Gianturco stent — which differs from the Wallstent in that it is made of stainless steel, has greater spacing between each of the interstices, is inserted with a stent pusher and is 1.5 cm in diameter, was investigated recently in the prostatic urethras of dogs.[24] There was no epithelial overgrowth and marked infiltration of lymphoid cells.

Morgentaler and DeWolf reported their initial experience using the Gianturco-Z stent in 25 frail men, 21 in urinary retention, with bladder outlet obstruction. Spontaneous voiding occurred in 20/21 patients in retention, with 16/21 demonstrating long-term success. Symptom scores and flow rates were not reported. Complications included five cases of stent migration, calcifications on two stents, symptomatic urinary tract infection in two patients and treated asymptomatic bacteriuria in three patients. Approximately 50% of patients had transient increases in irritative voiding symptoms. At 3 months, eight of 13 patients evaluated had 90% epithelialization of the stent.[25]

Balloon expandable stents

Intra–prostatic stent (titanium)

Titanium possesses excellent biocompatibility, with a long history of safety as a biomaterial for both dental and orthopaedic implants. It is particularly useful where stresses are moderate to low and where the implant is intended for long-term use. The Intra-prostatic stent, when expanded, is 11 mm in diameter and is available in lengths ranging from 12 to 65 mm in 4 mm increments (Fig. 40.3). The stent is placed

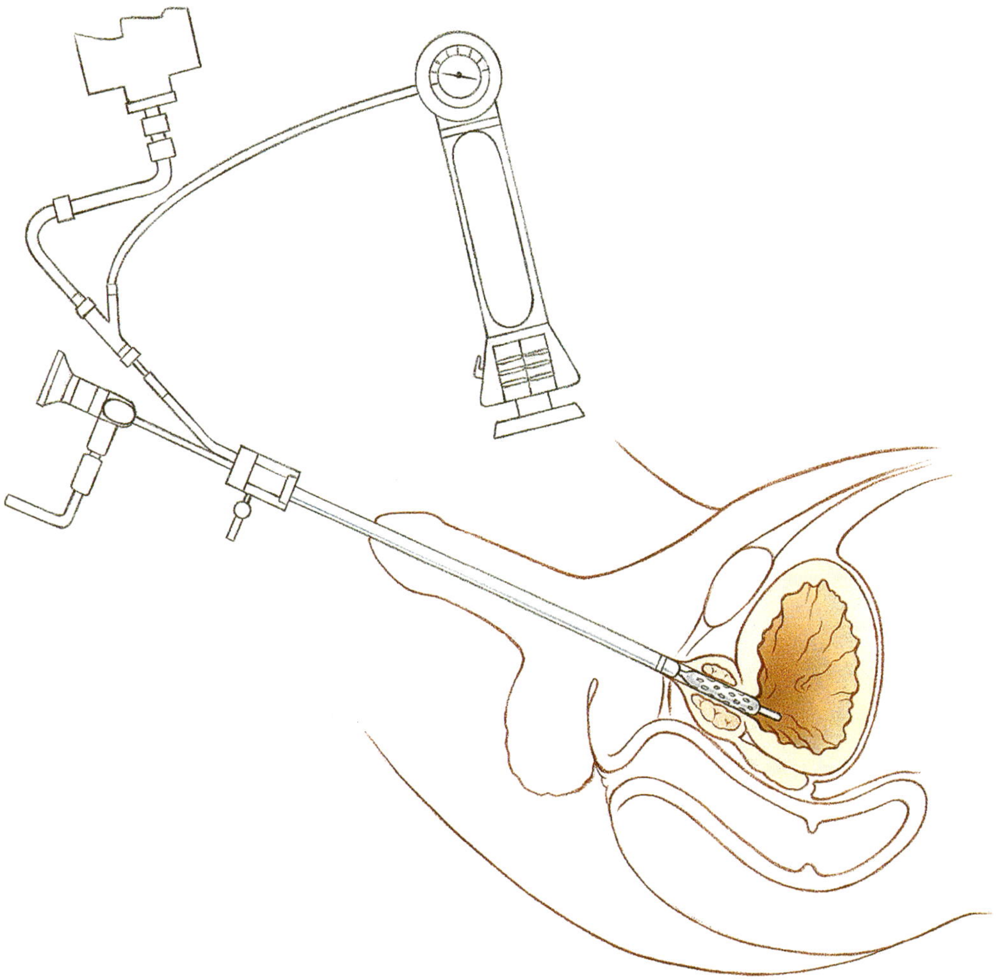

Figure 40.3. *The titanium stent in the correct position within the prostatic urethra.*

cystoscopically under local anaesthesia and sedation. As with the Wallstent, a calibration catheter is inserted cystoscopically and the length of the prostatic urethra from the bladder neck to the external urethral sphincter is measured under direct vision. The elongated stent is mounted on an insertion catheter that can be adapted to a special urethroscopic sheath. The expansion of the stent in the prostatic urethra is performed by inflating the balloon on the insertion catheter to 130 p.s.i. (approximately 9 atm or 900 kPa) for 30 s. The position of the stent can be confirmed either cystoscopically or by ultrasound (Figs 40.4, 40.5). The position of the stent can be adjusted by using grasping forceps through the cystoscope.

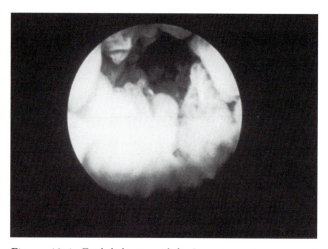

Figure 40.4. *Epithelialization of the Intra–prostatic stent at 12 months.*

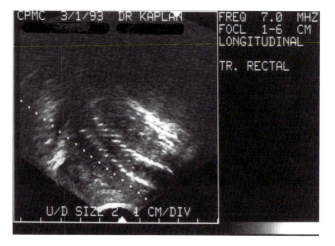

Figure 40.5. *Transrectal ultrasound examination and biopsy can be performed readily with the Intra-prostatic stent in place.*

In a series from England, Kirby et al. noted that 28/32 patients in acute urinary retention were able to void satisfactory after placement of the Intra-prostatic stent.[26] Asymptomatic urinary tract infections were noted in eight patients. In a more recent update of their data, 36/42 patients in retention were able to void spontaneously with a mean peak flow rate of 10.5 ml/s.

Recently, a multicentre cooperative study representing the initial United States experience using the Intra–prostatic stent was conducted in a total of 144 consecutive patients with moderate to severe prostatism.[27,28] Voiding symptoms were graded according to the Madsen–Iversen scale. The diagnostic work-up included history and physical examination with laboratory evaluation (urinalysis, urine culture, serum electrolytes, complete blood count and prostate-specific antigen). Patients with a known neurogenic bladder, cancer of the prostate or prior history of prostate surgery were excluded. Patients were seen at 1 week, as well as 1, 3, 6, 12, 18 and 24 months (as well as yearly thereafter) after completion of treatment to assess symptoms, peak flow rate (Q_{max}) with a minimum voided volume of 125 ml, urine culture and residual urine.

Participants ranged in age from 55 to 95 (mean 73.5) years. Before placement of the stent, two distinct groups could be identified: group 1 comprised 59 patients (41%) who presented in urinary retention and group 2 comprised 85 patients (59%) who presented with moderate to severe symptoms of bladder outlet obstruction.

The type of anaesthesia included 18 general, 47 spinal or epidural, 57 intravenous sedation and 22 with intraurethral xylocaine only. Of the 144 patients, 140 (97%) were able to void spontaneously within 36 h after stent insertion. However, four developed persistent urinary retention after initial stent placement, necessitating prolonged periods of suprapubic catheterization.

Symptom scores improved and were statistically significant at all follow-up intervals compared with pretreatment values ($p<0.001$). The mean symptom scores had improved by 53.4, 61.4 and 62% at 12, 18 and 24 months, respectively. Symptom scores decreased from 16.3 ± 0.3 to 7.8 ± 0.7, 6.5 ± 1.0 and 6.2 ± 0.5 at 12, 18 and 24 months, respectively.

The differences in Q_{max} for the entire group were significant at all follow-up intervals compared with pretreatment levels ($p<0.01$). Q_{max} increased from a mean of 5.0 ± 0.4 ml/s to 12.2 ± 0.8, 11.8 ± 0.7 and 12.0 ± 1.2 ml/s at 12, 18 and 24 months, respectively.

Post-void residual urine (PVR) was measured in obstructed patients prior to treatment, in all patients at 6 and 12 months after treatment (when measured by catheterization) or at all follow-up assessments (when measured by ultrasound). The PVR pretreatment measurement for the combined obstructed patients was 70 ± 12.9 ml and measured 70.7 ± 23 ml at 24 months. After 12 months, retention patients' measured volumes were 20.1 ± 5.7 ml. For group 2 patients, the PVR decreased from a mean of 117 ± 20 ml before stent placement to 99.3 ± 34.2 ml and 74.4 ± 36.2 ml at 12 and 24 months, respectively ($p<0.04$).

In 35 patients who underwent synchronous video–pressure–flow urodynamic studies, pretreatment maximum detrusor pressure (P_{det}) was 67.5 ± 13.5 cmH$_2$O. In those patients who had follow-up urodynamic studies at 1 year, P_{det} decreased to 49.4 ± 9.7 cmH$_2$O. In addition, six cases of de novo detrusor instability were noted.

Elective cystoscopy was performed at follow-up intervals between 1 and 12 months after treatment. The procedures revealed varying degrees of epithelial covering and no evidence of encrustation. Bladder stones (free-floating within the bladder and not adherent to the stent) and urethral strictures were noted in one and two patients, respectively. These findings, however, were not reported by the attending physician as attributable to stent placement. All other cystoscopies (n=64) revealed a well-healed and patent prostatic urethra. Multiple stent placement occurred when a stent was removed and replaced with another stent. Most of the second stent placements followed incorrect placement or incorrect sizing of the first stent.

Multiple stent placements were performed in eight patients, four (50%) of whom were in retention, the remaining four being in group 2. In these eight cases the device was, in the opinion of the investigator, dislodged because of external manipulation by a urethral catheter or, more probably, misplacement.

Adverse reactions (n=30) that occurred at the time of treatment or during the follow-up interval included haematuria requiring a transfusion (one), discomfort (five), tissue occlusion of the stent (two), postoperative retention (four), irritative voiding symptoms, either de novo or sustained (six), impotence (one), incontinence (four) and urinary tract infection (one). In most cases, this occurrence was transient and resolved within 4 weeks. Transient haematuria was associated with virtually all stent placements but usually resolved within days of placement. A total of 41 stents have remained in place for more than 3 years.

Stents were removed from 28 patients (19.4%), two of whom (7.1%) had been in the retention group. Ten of the stent removals (35.7%) were performed by one of the investigators because of 'migration'. Stent removal was secondary to either technical failure (15) or treatment failure (13). Of these patients, eight had a second stent placed, while the remaining patients underwent transurethral resection of the prostate (TURP). Although cystoscopy was not routinely part of the investigative protocol, patients who had persistent symptoms or lack of objective improvement underwent endoscopic evaluation at the discretion of the investigator. Technical failures were secondary to either inaccurate positioning or incorrect stent sizing and were categorized according to each investigator. Those patients who had persistent symptoms and upon cystoscopic evaluation were noted to have appropriate sizing and placement of the stent, were categorized as treatment failures. All treatment failures resulted primarily from either persistence or recurrence of symptoms.

On the horizon

Intraurethral catheter

Researchers in Israel have developed an intraurethral catheter (IUC) as an alternative to long-term indwelling catheters. Between 1988 and 1991, Nissenkorn and Lang placed 130 IUCs in 94 patients.[29] All insertions took place under local anaesthesia and in an outpatient setting. The IUC was left in place for from 1 to 19 months. All patients were able to void freely, were continent and had no residual urine. In three patients there was unresolved urinary tract infection, requiring removal of the IUC. In addition, patients who were sexually active prior to catheter placement continued to achieve normal ejaculations with the IUC in place.

These findings were confirmed by Sassine and Schulman, who inserted the IUC in 43 patients with poor life expectancy or high surgical risk over 3 years.[30] Of these, 84% were able to void without incontinence or significant PVR. There were four instances of early and five of late prothesis migration into the bladder. Six patients had symptomatic urinary tract infections while five had documented bacteriuria. The IUC remained in position without encrustations for up to 9 months.

Biodegradable stents

The advantage of a biodegradable stent is that there is no need for removal of the implanted material. Kemppainene et al. reported their experience using bioresorbable urethral stents.[31] Biodegradable self-reinforced poly-L-lactide (SR-PLLA) stents were used in 16 male rabbits after urethrotomy and seven stainless steel stents were used as controls. The SR-PLLA stent demonstrated favourable implantation properties and was completely implanted with minimal tissue reaction at 6 months. No calcifications were noted and the stent was completely degraded at 14 months. This early information suggests that this is a promising material for stents in the urinary tract.

Thermoexpandable stents

A stent made of an equi-atomic intermetallic compound, NiTinol (a titanium–nickel compound), has had early encouraging results. The stent has the ability to change from one configuration to another at different temperatures. Flushing the catheter with water at 45°C makes the coil expand to its maximum diameter. If the stent has to be removed, the coil can be irrigated with water at 15°C, which softens the metal, allowing the coil to be removed as a long thread. The titanium–nickel shape memory alloy (SMA) features of this stent have been studied and reported by Mori et al.[32]

Gottfried et al. reported their experience using the Memotherm stent.[33] This SMA stent is thermosensitive and comes in variable lengths of 2–8 cm. In 109 patients with BPH, the mean American Urological Association (AUA) symptom score decreased from 27.2 to 8.5 and mean peak flow rate increased from 4.1 to 15.6 ml/s. Stent correction was necessary in 11 patients. Complications included stress incontinence in nine patients and persistent urgency in 46. Complete epithelialization was seen in 60% of patients at 6 months and in 80% of patients at 1 year.

Poulsen et al. reported on the Memokath (Engineers & Doctors A/S, Hornbaek, Denmark), another SMA titanium–nickel alloy intraprostatic stent.[34] In 30 consecutive patients with a follow-up of up to 9 months, a success rate of 83% was reported. No migration was noted; however, encrustation appeared to be a persistent problem. (See also Chapter 39.)

Finally, Qiu et al. described the use of a Chinese SMA titanium alloy stent in 25 patients and reported a 92% success rate with no encrustation or migration in up to 20 months' follow-up.[35]

Conclusions

The use of stents to bridge the prostatic urethra has met with considerable enthusiasm. On the basis of initial results, it seems clear that this technology will have a lasting impact on how some patients with BPH are treated. In the authors' experience, the optimal patient has been the fail elderly patient in urinary retention. Others have advocated endoprostheses, particularly the prostatic spiral, as 'stress tests' to determine how patients will fare after definitive prostatectomy.[36] In fact, Nielsen et al. reported on a small series of patients who had a prostatic stent placed for 4 months followed by removal and a subsequent TURP.[37] A control group, who did not receive a stent, was observed and treated with prostatectomy later. All groups underwent evaluation with serial reporting of symptom scores and urodynamic studies at inclusion, 4 months after initial treatment (observation vs stent) and 4 months after TURP. Nielsen and colleagues concluded that the intraprostatic spiral decreased both symptoms and urethral resistance, but that a TURP was still more effective overall.

Future prospects, particularly the use of biodegradable materials, should make the prostatic stent more attractive to a greater segment of the BPH population. Appropriate clinical trials will help to direct the urologist in selecting the appropriate clinical setting for the use of prostate stents and the correct type of stent.

References

1. Dotter C T, Buschmann R W, McKinney M K et al. Transluminal expandable nitinol coil stent grafting: preliminary report. Radiology 1983; 147: 259–260

2. Bucx J J, DeCheerder I, Beatt K et al. The importance of adequate anticoagulation to prevent early thrombosis after stenting of stenosed venous bypass grafts. Am Heart J 1991; 121: 1389–1396

3. Zollikofer C L, Antonucci F, Pfyffer M et al. Arterial stent placement with use of the Wallstent: midterm results of clinical experience. Radiology 1991; 179: 449–456

4. Rousseau H, Puel J, Mirkovitch V et al. Self expanding endovascular prosthesis: an experimental study. Radiology 1987; 164: 709–714

5. Foerster E C, Hoepffner N, Domschke W. Bridging of benign choledochal stenoses by endoscopic retrograde implantation of mesh stents. Endoscopy 1991; 23: 133–135

6. Kaplan S A, Koo H P. Prostatic stents. Curr Tech Urol 1990; 3: 1–8

7. Fabian K W. Der intraprostatische 'Partielle Katheter' (urologische Spirale). Urologe A 1980; 19: 236–238

8. Vincente J, Salvador J, Izquierdo F et al. Long term follow up of patients with intraprostatic prostheses. Société Internationale d'Urologie, Seville 1991: abstr 617

9. Ala-Opas M, Talja M, Hellstrom P et al. Prostakath —Urospiral in urinary outflow obstruction. Société Internationale d'Urologie, Seville 1991: abstr 622

10. Yachia D, Lask D, Rabinson S. Self-retained intraurethral stent: an alternative to long-term indwelling catheters or surgery in the treatment of prostatism. AJR 1990; 154: 111–113

11. Thomas P J, Britton J P, Harrison N W. The Prostakath stent: 4 years experience. Br J Urol 1993; 71: 430–432

12. Nordling J, Oveson H, Poulson A L. The intraprostatic spiral: clinical results in 150 consecutive patients. J Urol 1992; 147: 645–647

13. Miller R A, Birch B R, Parker C J. Endoprostatic helicoplasty: the Porges Urospiral. J Urol 1991; 145: 397A

14. Karaoglan U, Alkibay T, Tokucoglu H et al. Urospiral in benign prostatic hyperplasia. Société Internationale d'Urologie, Seville 1991: abstr 621

15. Lewi H J, Des U, Krappel F. The role of the intraprostatic spiral in 184 patients — 15 month follow up. Xth Congr Eur Assoc Urol, July 1992: abstr 232

16. Yachia D, Beyar M, Aridogan I A. A new, large calibre, self-expanding and self-retaining temporary intraprostatic stent (ProstaCoil) in the treatment of prostatic obstruction. Br J Urol 1994; 74: 47–49

17. Chapple C R, Milroy E J, Rickards D. Permanently implanted urethral stent for prostatic obstruction in the unfit patient: preliminary report. Br J Urol 1990; 66: 58–65

18. Milroy E, Chapple C R. The UroLume stent in the management of benign prostatic hyperplasia. J Urol 1993; 150: 1630–1635

19. Harrison N W, DeSouza J V. Prostatic stenting for outflow obstruction. Br J Urol 1990; 65: 192–196

20. McLoughlin J, Jager R, Abel P D et al. The use of prostatic stents in patients with urinary retention who are unfit for surgery. An interim report. Br J Urol 1990; 66: 66–70

21. Adam A, Jager R, McLoughlin J et al. Wallstent endoprostheses for the relief of prostatic urethral obstruction in high risk patients. Radiology 1990; 42: 228–232

22. Oesterling J E, Kaplan S A, Epstein H B et al. The North American experience with the Urolume endoprosthesis as a treatment for benign prostatic hyperplasia: long term results. The UroLume Study Group. Urology 1994; 44: 353–362

23. Guazzoni G, Montorosi F, Coulange C et al. A modified prostatic Urolume Wallstent for healthy patients with symptomatic benign prostatic hyperplasia: a European multicenter study. Urology 1994; 44: 364–370

24. Dobben R L, Wright K C, Dolenz K et al. Prostatic urethra dilation with the Gianturco self-expanding metallic stent: a feasibility study in cadaver specimens and dogs. AJR 1991; 156: 757–761

25. Morgantaler A, DeWolf W C. A self expanding prostatic stent for bladder outlet obstruction in high risk patients. J Urol 1993; 150: 1636–1640

26. Kirby R, Lui S, Eardley I et al. The use of the ASI titanium intraprostatic stent in the treatment of bladder outlet obstruction due to benign prostatic hyperplasia. J Urol 1992; 148: 1195

27. Kaplan S A, Merrill D C, Mosely W G et al. The titanium intraprostatic stent: the United States experience. J Urol 1993; 150: 1624–1629

28. Kaplan S A, Chiou R K, Morton W J et al. Long–term experience utilizing a new balloon expandable prostatic endoprothesis: the Titan stent. North American Titan Stent Study Group. Urology 1995; 45: 234–240

29. Nissenkorn I, Lang R. The intraurethral catheter — 3 years of experience. Congr Eur Assoc Urol, July 1992: abstr 233

30. Sassine A M, Schulman C C. Intraurethral catheter in high-risk patients with urinary retention: 3 years of experience. Eur Urol 1994; 25: 131–134

31. Kemppainene E, Talja M, Riihela M et al. A bioresorbable urethral stent. Urol Res 1993; 21: 235–238

32. Mori K, Okamoto S, Akimoto M. A new self-expansive intraurethral stent using shape memory alloy: a preliminary report of its availability. Urology 1994; 45: 165–170

33. Gottfried H W, Hautmann R E, Sintermann E, Zechner O. Memotherm stent for BPH treatment in high risk patients — experience of more than 100 cases. J Urol 1994; 151: 397A

34. Poulsen A L, Schou J, Ovesen H, Nordling J. Memokath: a second generation of intraprostatic spiral. Br J Urol 1993; 72: 331–334

35. Qiu C Y, Wang J M, Zhang Z X et al. Stent of shape-memory alloy for urethral obstruction caused by benign prostatic hyperplasia. J Endourol 1994; 8: 65–67

36. McLoughlin J, Williams G. Prostatic stents and balloon dilatation. Br J Hosp Med 1990; 43: 422–426

37. Nielsen K K, Kromann-Andersen B, Poulsen A L et al. Subjective and objective evaluation of patients with prostatism and infravesical obstruction treated with both intraprostatic spiral and transurethral prostatectomy. Neurourol Urodyn 1994; 13: 13–19

41

Transurethral electrovaporization of the prostate

B. J. Miles L. Sirls

Introduction

Electrosurgery is the application of a high-frequency electric current to cut or coagulate tissue. In 1891 the French physicist d'Arsonval first applied electrosurgery by using an alternating current of specific frequency that would heat tissue without causing muscle and nerve stimulation.[1] The collaborative work of Bovie (a physicist) and Cushing (a surgeon) led to the development of the first specific machine for widespread surgical use.[2] Wappler's subsequent development of the complex oscillator allowed the use of both a cutting and a coagulation current from a single machine.[3]

The main interest of urologists in this context is the application of electrical energy to the prostate to achieve the mechanical debulking of obstructing prostatic tissue in a precise, controlled manner. However, the tissue response to electrical energy is dependent on many factors. A thorough understanding of these factors is important, as their modification allows the surgeon to cut, coagulate or vaporize prostatic tissue as needed. This chapter discusses the basic principles of electric currents, the basic electrosurgical wave-forms and their tissue applications, and the clinical results of transurethral electrovaporization of the prostate.

Basic electrosurgical principles

An electric current consists of electrons that flow freely through conducting substances but not through insulating substances. Voltage (V) is the force required to push the electrons through a wire, analogous to the pump required to push water through a pipe. Amperes measure the flow rate of electrons flowing down the wire, analogous to the volume of water flowing down the pipe. Electricity flowing down a wire, like water flowing down a pipe, has a certain force and rate of flow. This force (voltage) and rate of flow (amperage) can be used to do work. The power (joules) of the electric current flowing down the wire is the product of the force (voltage) and flow (amperes) and is measured in watts (W): Power (P) = current (I) × volts (V), or P = IV.

Unlike water that may flow out of a pipe, electrons must complete a circuit in order to flow. The complete electrosurgical circuit consists of the current flowing from the generator to the active electrode (the working element) through the patient and to a return electrode (the 'Bovie pad'). Tissue resistance to electrical flow, measured in ohms, is important conceptually since it is this tissue resistance, not the active electrode, that generates heat.

Various tissues have different resistances to electrical flow, ranging from blood with a low resistance of about 30 ohms to fat with a high resistance to current flow of 1000–2000 ohms. Muscle is intermediate at 300–400 ohms. The difficulty in coagulating in a bloody field is secondary to easy current dissipation through the blood. This easy vascular conduction is further illustrated by the rare reports of significant tissue damage and slough after paediatric circumcision.[4] The usual resistance of a tissue can change after being denatured by heat. For example, after desiccating the normal prostate there is an increase in the resistance to current flow; however, the increase in applied power usually allows for continued coagulation or vaporization.

The power density of the electrosurgical instrument is another important parameter that may be manipulated to the surgeon's advantage. Power density is the amount of power delivered, divided by the area over which the power is applied. For a complete circuit, the same amount of alternating current that enters the patient must leave the patient. As the active electrode applies the energy to a very small area (usually a needle tip), the high power density causes a controlled area of tissue coagulation or vaporization. However, because the energy leaving the patient does so over a much larger surface area (the 'Bovie pad'), the power density is significantly decreased and no heat or thermal injury

results. The practical application of this principle is that
a roller-ball electrode with a large surface area will
demand that the power settings be increased compared
with a standard wire loop (with a much smaller surface
area and thus greatly increased power density). In fact,
power settings for electrovaporization of the prostate
will be 25–75% higher than the settings for a standard
transurethral resection of the prostate (TURP) in order
to achieve the necessary high power densities.

Electrosurgical wave-forms

The electrosurgical unit generates a high-frequency
oscillating sine wave similar to that seen on an
oscilloscope. Understanding the characteristics of the
sine wave and its modification is critical to the correct
application of electrosurgical techniques. The height or
amplitude of the sine wave represents voltage, the
wavelength is the distance between the wave peaks, and
the frequency is the number of waves per second (Hz;
kHz=1000 waves/s).

All high-frequency electrosurgical units generate an
oscillating radio sine wave, which may be 'pure' or
'damped'. A pure sine wave (cutting current) is a
balanced, symmetrical wave in which the amplitude of
all oscillations is the same (Fig. 4.1). A pure sine wave
produces a highly localized effect on the tissue with very
focused molecular oscillations resulting in 'tissue
separation' with very little coagulation. The power
density of a continuous pure sine wave as applied
through a thin transurethral wire loop is so intense that
the water in the cells with which the loop makes
contact is immediately brought to over 100°C, thereby
causing the cells to vaporize (explode), leaving nothing
in their wake except a space. The result is a surgical cut.
Hence, the pure continuous sine wave is a cutting
current with no haemostasis.

The damped wave-form (coagulation current) is a sine
wave that occurs as clusters or bursts, with the first wave
the largest, and each successive wave smaller (Fig. 4.1). A
highly damped wave is one in which the first wave is
large and the subsequent waves rapidly approach zero.
The damped wave-form is not continuous, i.e. the
electrosurgical generator pauses between pulses. In fact,
the generator is usually off more than it is on, and
therefore less power passes through the instrument,

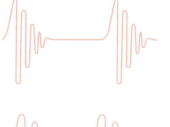

Highly damped

High haemostasis
less tissue damage
slower healing

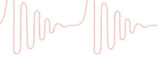

Moderately damped

Moderate haemostasis
less tissue damage
moderate wound healing

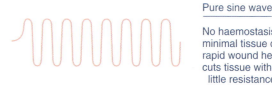

Blended current

Mild haemostasis
variable tissue damage
cuts tissue with
coagulation

Pure sine wave

No haemostasis
minimal tissue damage
rapid wound healing
cuts tissue with
little resistance

Figure 41.1. *All high-frequency electrosurgery is a variation of the
sine wave. Different tissue effects are created by altering the basic sine
wave. The pure sine wave is the 'cutting current'' and the highly
damped wave the 'coagulation current'. (From ref. 11 with
permission.)*

decreasing the power density. As much less overall energy
is applied, the tissue heats (coagulates or dessicates) but
does not vaporize. The more the wave-form is damped,
the more heating and tissue coagulation occurs. The non-
continuous damped wave-form is therefore used as a
coagulation current for haemostasis because it creates
significant heat and subsequent tissue destruction.

Pure sine waves offer no haemostasis and therefore
have no advantage over a scalpel. Hence, most 'cutting'
currents are really a blend of a pure sine wave and
damped sine wave (Fig. 4.1). These blended currents
allow simultaneous cutting and haemostasis. With the
correct blend, an instrument that cuts and that provides
satisfactory haemostasis and minimal tissue damage can
be achieved.

The alternating current used in electrosurgery is in
the radiofrequency band and must be within a certain

range to avoid adverse physiological effects within the patient and other complications in the operating room. Most electrosurgical generators operate at a frequency of 400–1000 kHz. Low-frequency waves of 100 kHz cannot be used because they will stimulate the neuromuscular system. These low-frequency waves in fact are responsible for the adductor muscle reflex (obturator reflex) triggered during standard transurethral surgery.[5] The obturator nerve is stimulated when arcing occurs at the active electrode and artefactual lower-frequency currents are generated. Higher-frequency currents (i.e. over 4000 kHz) are difficult to contain within the circuit and may flow out from the circuit and interfere with other electrical equipment in the operating room.

High-frequency electrosurgery

High-frequency electrosurgery is the most common form of electrosurgery. The 110V 60 Hz alternating current is boosted by an electrosurgical unit to a very high voltage and frequency level while decreasing the amperage. A high-frequency, high-voltage, low-amperage current has essentially no effect on the human body as it passes through, unless the entrance or exit point is very small (such as a needle electrode). If the entrance point is small, the high-frequency oscillations will generate intense heat at that highly focused point. Modification of this current–tissue interaction is the basis of modern electrosurgery.

Examples of applied electrosurgery

Electrocautery

Electrocautery technically is not electrosurgery since it does not transfer electric current to the patient. The electric current is used to heat a treatment filament, which is not an electrode. The filament tip becomes hot and transfers heat to the tissue, producing thermal damage. The current is direct and of low voltage, but the amperage is high to provide sufficient current flow through the wire to generate heat. No tissue conduction of the electric current is required. Since there is a large amount of coagulation, there is considerable heat damage to surrounding tissue and tissue healing may be slow. Electrocautery cannot be used in bloody fields

since the electrical energy is dissipated over the large surface area.

Electrosurgery

Electrosurgery may result in three distinct tissue responses that are dependent on the type of electric current applied and the manner in which it is applied. The tissue response to applied heat depends on the power density and the wave-form of the current.

Electrosurgical desiccation

Electrosurgical desiccation involves using heat to drive water slowly out of tissue, effectively drying it out (Fig. 41.2). This is technically simple, and may be performed by placing an electrode in contact with the tissue surface and using either the cut (at low power) or coagulation wave-form. Good contact is necessary for this heat transfer; a charred or dirty electrode desiccates poorly. When the electric current is applied the resistance of the tissue generates heat, which dries the tissue out. The tissue visibly turns brown when desiccated. Desiccation is important in electro-vaporization of the prostate, because desiccated tissue does not vaporize well. When the high-power vaporizing roller ball is applied to the surface of the prostate, a zone of vaporization occurs and a zone of desiccation occurs for approximately 2–3 mm below this vaporized trough. This zone of desiccation provides the improved haemostasis observed with electrovaporization. When the surgeon moves on to another area of the prostate,

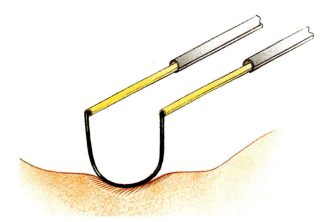

Figure 41.2. *Lower power settings or a damped wave-form combined with excellent tissue contact results in tissue desiccation. (From ref. 12 with permission.)*

the desiccated zone rehydrates from the continuous fluid flow (fluid diffuses into the desiccated tissue) and is able to be vaporized on a subsequent pass.

Electrosurgical fulguration

Fulguration is a product of both the electric current wave-form (coagulation current) and the power density. If insufficient energy is applied to the prostate, the tissue will coagulate and not vaporize. The coagulation current does not vaporize because the generator is in the pause mode more than it is pulsing current (which decreases the power density), and the wave is damped. Similarly, if a cutting current wave-form is used but the power is turned down, there will not be sufficient energy to vaporize and the tissue will coagulate. A power level that may be routinely used for cutting with a standard wire loop may, therefore, coagulate only when the larger surface area roller ball is used. Typically, because the electrode is continually moving over the prostatic surface, the coagulation current results in both fulguration (carbonized tissue) and desiccation (Fig. 41.3).

Electrosurgical vaporization

The object of electrosurgical vaporization is identical to that for a cutting current, i.e. to apply enough power to cause the cells to heat rapidly and explode, leaving nothing behind but a space (Fig. 41.4). Because the surface area of the rollerball is large, more power than usual is required from the electrosurgical generator. This

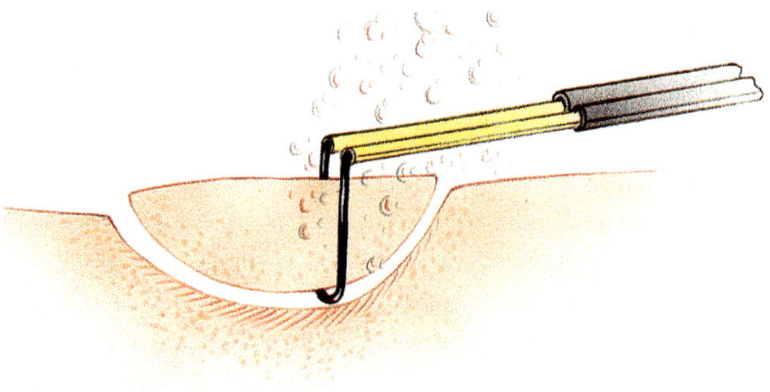

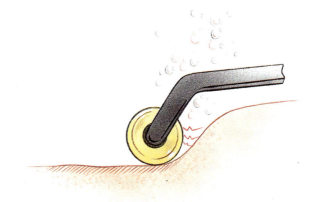

Figure 41.4. *Higher power settings and a pure sine wave ('cutting current') creates intense heat that vaporizes tissue on contact, leaving a surgical cut. (From ref. 12 with permission.)*

assures a high enough power density to vaporize tissue without excessive fulguration which would make the tissue more resistant to further attempts at vaporization.

Application to the prostate

The clinical application of electrovaporization of the prostate depends on a combination of tissue effects. First, the high power density applied through the larger surface area roller ball is used to vaporize a trough, effectively debulking the tissue. As the power density vaporizes 3–4 mm of tissue, 1–3 mm of underlying tissue is heated, but not sufficiently for vaporization (Fig. 41.5). This underlying tissue is desiccated, which accounts for the haemostasis observed. When the surgeon moves on to another area of the prostate, this small rim of desiccated prostate rehydrates from the continuous fluid flow and is able to be vaporized on a subsequent pass. This zone of desiccation also provides a barrier to fluid absorption.

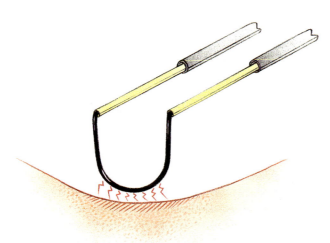

Figure 41.3. *Less tissue contact as the electrode moves over the tissue surface results in fulguration (carbonization) and desiccation. (From ref. 12 with permission.)*

Figure 41.5. *The combination of a 'cutting current' and high power density applied through a roller ball results in tissue vaporization with an underlying zone of desiccation, minimizing bleeding and fluid absorption. (From ref. 12 with permission.)*

Transurethral vaporization of the prostate: clinical application

Equipment

The equipment necessary to carry out transurethral vaporization of the prostate (TVP) is the same as that used for TURP — a standard Iglesias or continuous flow resectoscope — and in place of the cutting loop a modified roller ball is used. Numerous TVP roller balls are available and an early ACMI version is shown in Figure 41.6. All TVP electrodes share a common feature, of either ridges or some other projection (spikes) above the surface of the 'ball' that serve as points of extremely high power density. Vaporization occurs when these ridges/projections come into contact with tissue. In order to achieve the necessary power density for vaporization, the power generator settings must be increased by 25–75% over standard power settings for TURP. Power settings up to 230–250 W for pure cut may be used for vaporization and 60–80 W for coagulation. The standard electrical generator used for TURP should be able comfortably to generate 300 W; otherwise, it is possible to overburden the generator or to have less than optimal results, owing to inadequate power generation.

Technique

Because the technique of TVP is similar to that of TURP, the learning curve is short. The technique is familiar to urologists and can easily be learned and adapted to clinical practice. The vaporization electrode is rolled over the surface of the prostate with gentle to minimal pressure (Fig. 41.7). Firm pressure can lead to excessive desiccation and poor vaporization. The surgeon should not leave the roller ball in one place for too long, as this will create divots or pockets with large surrounding zones of desiccation. Subsequently, these pockets are difficult to vaporize and may result in an unsatisfactory prostatic channel and a frustrated surgeon.

The TVP procedure should be started in the same fashion as a standard TURP. The zone of prostate vaporization is extended in the routine fashion until capsular fibres are seen. It is possible to sculpt the prostate at the apex by gently rolling the electrode retrograde towards the bladder. When debris accumulates on the electrode, it is easily removed by switching to the coagulation mode and rolling the electrode over the prostate. This carbonized tissue should be removed at frequent intervals because it can diffuse and decrease power density on the roller-ball ridges. If tissue is required for permanent section, a standard transurethral resection loop can be used and tissue harvested for this purpose.

Medium-sized (30–40 g) or small prostate glands are ideal for TVP but large glands may be approached as well. Glands over 100 g have been managed successfully using TVP. Vaporization proceeds until a zone of desiccation prevents further vaporization. Standard resection (TURP) can be used to remove the zone of desiccation and vaporization continues until the capsule is evident or the surgeon is satisfied with the degree of tissue ablation.

Theoretical advantages

The risk of transurethral syndrome is minimized because blood vessels are electrodesiccated during the vaporization process. For similar reasons, the risk of significant blood loss is also decreased. High-risk patients, and patients on anticoagulants requiring surgery, may therefore be excellent candidates for TVP, just as visual laser ablation of the prostate (VLAP) has theoretical advantages. Potential advantages of TVP over VLAP are a more rapid clinical response (due to more immediate debulking) and less postoperative irritative voiding symptoms.

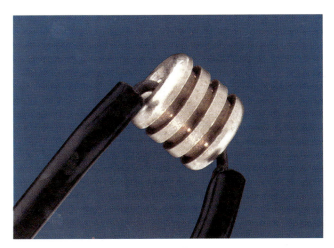

Figure 41.6. *An early Circon ACMI® roller ball.*

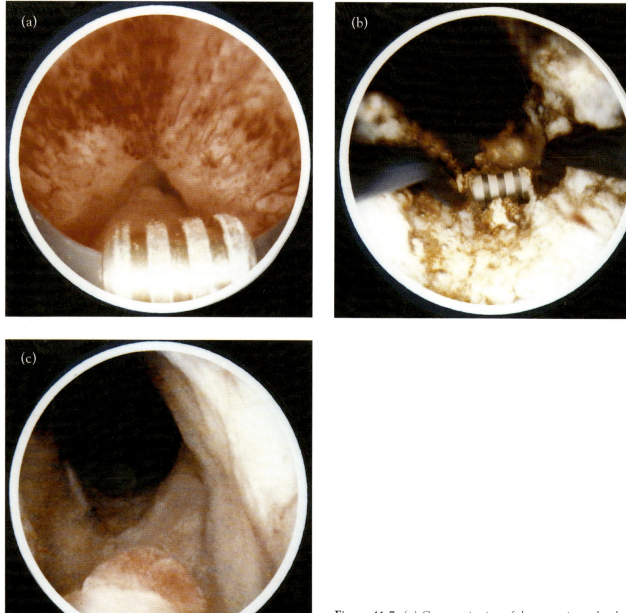

Figure 41.7. (a) Cystoscopic view of the prostatic urethra before TVP; (b) the same prostatic fossa during TVP; (c) postoperative result at 12 weeks, showing the TURP-like defect.

Clinical experience

Few published data exist on electrovaporization of the prostate. Canine studies have demonstrated that the zone of tissue necrosis extends 1–3 mm beyond the zone of vaporization.[6] By 7 weeks, tissue necrosis is resolved and re-epithelialization of the prostatic fossa is complete. Few controlled human studies have been carried out since 1993, and only one peer-reviewed article has been published at the time of this writing.[7]

Dr Irving Bush has the greatest surgical experience with electrovaporization of the prostate, dating back to 1966.[8] He reported on the successful use of this technique in over 500 men with bladder outlet obstructive symptoms due to benign prostatic hyperplasia (BPH), carcinoma of the prostate and bladder neck contractures, with 76% of the men voiding normally within 24 h. However, his reports do not include standardized subjective or objective measures of outcome.

Barua et al. reported on 12 patients, three of whom were in urinary retention.[9] Although all patients voided after TVP, neither the American Urological Association (AUA) Symptom Index nor objective urodynamic parameters were presented. No change in serum electrolytes and minimal changes in the serum haemoglobin (0.43 g/dl) were noted. Similarly, Stuart et al. reported on 34 patients, 11 of whom reported a mean AUA score decrease from 26 to 12; the mean postoperative peak urine flow rate was 13 ml/s .[6]

The only peer-reviewed published report on TVP is that on 25 men treated by Kaplan and Te.[7] The mean AUA score decreased from 17.8 to 5.9 at 1 month, and to 4.2 at 3 months postoperatively. The mean peak urine flow rate increased from 7.4 to 15.3 ml/s at 1 month and to 17.3 ml/s at 3 months; all these results were statistically significant. The serum haematocrit and sodium were not significantly changed. The reported complications included 'mild haematuria' in three and a urethral stricture in one. Operative time averaged 40 min for a 'moderate-sized' gland. No patient experienced irritative postoperative voiding symptoms. Of the 25 men, 14 were potent preoperatively and remained so postoperatively; however, all men developed retrograde ejaculation.

A team at Baylor College of Medicine reported on 12 men who were in urinary retention treated by TVP (B J Miles, personal communication). All voided on the first postoperative day and there were no significant changes in serum haemoglobin or electrolytes during the procedure. Three high-risk cardiac patients received full anticoagulant therapy, two with coumadin and one with heparin, and none had intraoperative or immediate postoperative bleeding. One patient experienced delayed bleeding 1 week postoperatively, requiring recatheterization.

Early reports of TVP suggest that the rate of intraoperative and postoperative complications is low.[6–9] The improved haemostasis and the resistance of desiccated prostate tissue to fluid absorption should, theoretically, minimize intraoperative complications. The major theoretical advantage, however, is that the TVP patient should have less blood loss than that associated with standard TURP. However, it is likely that, as experience increases, the postoperative complications, in particular, should approach those reported after TURP.[10] Retrograde ejaculation, reported in all of Kaplan's patients, is to be expected because the bladder neck is opened in a fashion similar to that with TURP. Although no bladder neck contractures have been reported, vaporization at the bladder neck may result in a contracture rate similar to that reported after TURP. The estimated impotence rate of approximately 4% after TURP may be observed after TVP. Rectal injury has not been reported.

Finally, another possible advantage of TVP over TURP and VLAP is the reduction in procedural and postoperative costs. The cost of the roller ball and disposable equipment required for TVP is significantly lower than that of the specialized equipment required for VLAP. In the Miles (Baylor) experience, TVP patients were discharged from the hospital 0.5–1 day sooner than those undergoing TURP. These cost differences, together with the improved intraoperative and postoperative complication profile, should make TVP an attractive alternative to TURP.

Conclusions

TVP is an easy technique for the endoscopic ablation of prostatic tissue. TVP is similar to traditional TURP, and uses the standard resectoscope equipment familiar and available to urologists. Preliminary data have demonstrated clinical efficacy with minimal intraoperative and postoperative morbidity. TVP has a potential advantage in its cost profile. Long-term follow-up is needed to confirm the durability of these encouraging results.

References

1. d'Arsonval A. Action physiologique des courants alternatifs. C R Soc Biol (Paris) 1891; 43: 283
2. McLean A J. The Bovie electrosurgical current generator: some underlying principles and results. Arch Surg 1929; 18: 1863
3. Kramolowski E V, Tucker R D. The urological application of electrosurgery. J Urol 1991; 146: 669–674
4. Laska S, Penis burned during circumcision–amputation — 2.75 million dollar award. Med Malpract Verdicts Settlements Experts 1986; 2: 8
5. Prentiss R J, Harvey G W, Bethard W F et al. Massive adductor muscle contraction in transurethral surgery: cause and prevention; development of new electrical circuitry. J Urol 1965; 93: 263
6. Stewart S, Benjamin D, Ruckle H et al. Transurethral vaporization of the prostate: a new technique for treatment of symptomatic BPH. 12th World Congr Endourol SWL, 6 Dec 1994; St Louis, Mo. J Endourol 1994; 8(suppl 1): 145 (abstr)

7.   Kaplan S A, Te A E. Transurethral electrovaporization of the prostate: a novel method for treating men with benign prostatic hyperplasia. Urology 1995; 45: 566–572

8.   Bush I, Maiters E, Bush J. Transurethral vaporization of the prostate (TVP): new horizons. Society for Minimally Invasive Therapy, 5 Nov 1994, Berlin (abstr)

9.   Barua J, Omer K, Mustafa T, Fowler C. Transurethral vaporization of the prostate (TVP). Society for Minimally Invasive Therapy, 5 Nov 1994, Berlin (abstr)

10.   Mebust W K, Holtgrewe H L, Cockett A T et al. Transurethral prostatectomy: immediate and postoperative complications. A cooperative study of 13 institutions evaluating 3,885 patients. J Urol 1989; 141: 243–247

11.   Sebben J E. Cutaneous electrosurgery. Chicago: Year Book Medical, 1989, p20

12.   Te A E, Kaplan S A. Curr Surg Techn Urol 1995; 8: 1–7

Future Directions

VI

42

Treatment outcomes and their interpretation in benign prostatic hyperplasia

C. G. Roehrborn

Introduction

The practice of clinical medicine is largely based on empirical data, which are used in a more or less formal way to guide physicians' decision-making. At the one end of the spectrum, a physician may recommend a certain treatment to a patient because he has just treated another patient in a similar situation successfully by the same method. At the other end of the spectrum, physicians' decision-making is often guided by opinions voiced in the form of review articles, which represent the combined experience of individual authors regarding a certain clinical problem.

This approach to clinical decision-making works sufficiently well in many situations where the choices are either limited or well known and time proven. A different situation arises when a new treatment alternative becomes available, for which no or insufficient clinical experience has been accumulated. In such cases it becomes important to find ways in which to compare the treatment with already existing therapies, so that physicians may make a rational choice between the different alternatives.

When comparing different treatment strategies a large array of parameters might be used, including such factors as safety, efficacy, cost, complications, time commitment and durability. These parameters used for comparison are outcomes of the treatment, in that they are the direct or indirect results of the therapeutic intervention.

Outcomes that are specific for the treatment intervention and the underlying disease are logically chosen for any such analysis. This is relatively easy in some disease processes, more difficult in others. For example, when comparing antihypertensive medications, it is self-evident that the ability of the drugs to lower blood pressure should be one of the most important outcomes to be considered. However, because of the multitude of drugs already on the market, it is also important to look at adverse events and side effects associated with a new drug, and the treatment cost in comparison with other alternatives. On a second look, from a patient's viewpoint, adverse events and side effects are actually more important as they are immediately felt by the patient, whereas the change in blood pressure might not be perceived at all. However, the gain in life years as a result of preventing cardiovascular mortality and morbidity associated with the lowering of blood pressure is an outcome in which the patient *is* very interested. The relative change in blood pressure thus is used only as a proxy parameter for the anticipated avoidance of morbidity and mortality. Once it is established that drug-induced normalization of blood pressure in fact results in avoidance of morbidity and mortality, not every new drug has to prove this fact in long-term studies, but rather the proxy — namely, the lowering of blood pressure — may be accepted as evidence instead.

Outcomes

As the above example indicates, there are basically two different kinds of outcomes — namely, direct or health outcomes and intermediate or biological outcomes.[1] Direct or health outcomes are those outcomes that patients can experience, feel and care about. They relate to the length and quality of life, including death, functional disability, appearance, pain, anxiety, reassurance and peace of mind. Some of the health outcomes are desirable (e.g. survival, improvement in function, improvement in appearance), whereas others are undesirable (e.g. pain, side effects, risks, cost, loss of time). Intermediate or biological outcomes thus are outcomes that patients cannot experience or feel directly. Although in some cases they may be unimportant, in other situations they are an important (or the only) proxy for an underlying important health outcome, which would be very difficult to measure otherwise.

For example, a patient with a myocardial infarction is admitted to the coronary care unit. All he cares about at that time is his pain, when it will get better, and whether he will survive this episode. Pain and survival are clearly the most important health outcomes to the patient. Physicians will be interested in the elevation of the creatine phosphokinase (CPK) isoenzymes or cardiac troponin-1 enzyme, which are specific for damage to cardiac muscle tissue. This value is of extremely limited interest to the patient. However, inasmuch as this value indicates the amount of cardiac muscle damaged, it carries some prognostic significance, and thus represents a proxy for the health outcome 'survival'.

Health outcomes are measured in a variety of ways:

1. Dichotomous (e.g. survival: yes or no);
2. Continuous (e.g. degree of pain);
3. Categorical (e.g. angina class); or
4. Counts (e.g. number of angina attacks per week).

The effect of a treatment intervention is measured by how it changes the probability (dichotomous outcome) or the magnitude (continuous, categorical or counts) of a health outcome.[1] An increase in the probability or the magnitude of a desirable health outcome, or a decrease in the probability or the magnitude of an undesirable outcome, may be called an intervention or treatment benefit. A harmful intervention or treatment is characterized by the opposite — namely, a decrease in the probability or magnitude of a desirable outcome or an increase in the probability or magnitude of an undesirable health outcome. Most treatments have both benefits and ill effects. For example, streptokinase treatment for a myocardial infarction increases survival probability and reduces pain, but it is associated with potentially harmful complications. Effects are measured as actual changes or differences, ratios, percentage changes, odds ratios, or effect sizes.

Table 42.1 lists the various types of outcomes and outcome measures, as well as the measures of effect. Outcome and effect measures should be chosen to be meaningful to a potential patient. This is usually best achieved by presenting both the outcomes with and without intervention, as well as the chosen effect measure. Reporting only the relative changes in outcomes without information about the absolute changes is often misleading. For example, the chance of a 55-year-old woman dying from breast cancer in the next 10 years is 1.2%. Annual screening will reduce the risk to 0.7%. This represents a relative decrease by 42% in the chance of dying of breast cancer, but an actual change in the probability of about 0.5%. If a physician advised a woman to be screened because she would

Table 42.1. *Outcomes and outcome and effect measures*

Outcome	Outcome measure	Effect measures	Symbol*
Dichotomous	Probability of outcome	Absolute differences in probabilities	$P_t - P_c$
		Ratio of probabilities	P_t/P_c
		Percentage difference in probabilities	$[(P_t - P_c)/P_c]$
		Odds ratio	$\{[P_t/(1-P_t)]/[P_c/(1-P_c)]\}$
Continuous	Mean	Difference in means	$\mu_t - \mu_c$
		Ratio of means	μ_t/μ_c
	Median	Difference of medians	$m_t - m_c$
		Ratio of medians	m_t/m_c
		Effect size	$(m_t - m_c)/\text{variance}$
Categorical	Probabilities of categories	Difference in probabilities of categories	$P_{t1} - P_{t2}$
Count	Number of occurrences in specified interval	Difference in number of occurrences	$C_t - C_c$
		Ratio of number of occurrences	C_t/C_c

* Subscript t indicates treatment group, c indicates control group. (From ref. 1 with permission.)

reduce her risk of dying by 42%, this information might be open to misinterpretation and misunderstanding and tends to provoke overly optimistic expectations on the part of the patient. The information that the annual screening would reduce her risk from 12 to 7 in 1000, however, would clarify both the baseline and the reduced risk and allow the patient to weight the benefit of the intervention against the disadvantages (such as the yearly mammography and physical examination with associated expenditure of time and money, and the possibility of a false-positive mammogram with the resulting anxiety and need for a biopsy).

Outcomes in BPH

When addressing the topic of outcomes in benign prostatic hyperplasia (BPH), it is implicitly understood that the discussion centres on outcomes of various treatment interventions. In this context, however, it is important to emphasize that watchful waiting, namely no active intervention apart from of regular follow-up (see Chapter 20) is considered as one of the possible

'treatment' interventions. Much can be learned from the natural history of the disease process (see Chapter 11) in relation to possible outcomes of a watchful waiting strategy, although important differences are introduced by a variety of parameters such as the 'clinic' or 'white coat' effect.

As in most disease processes, both direct health and indirect biological outcomes, desirable and undesirable, can be measured in BPH. In the process of the development of the Agency for Health Care Policy and Research (AHCPR) Guidelines for the diagnosis and treatment of BPH,[2] a panel of proxy judges and patients was asked to sort 15 different outcomes printed on cards and displayed before them in a random fashion. Without being given any information about expected or reported effect measured, their task was to sort the outcomes in the order of their importance in the process of choosing a treatment for BPH. Figure 42.1 lists the 15 outcomes in descending order of importance, as determined by dividing the sum total of all rankings by the number of respondents. By far the most important outcome for this panel was the probability of symptom

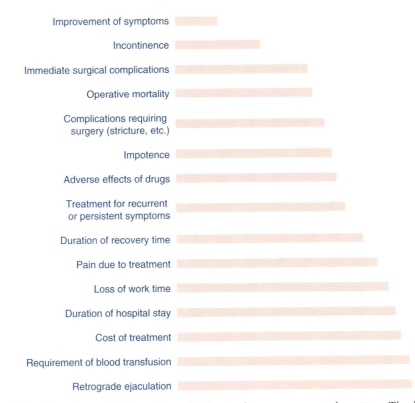

Figure 42.1. *Outcomes ranked in descending order of importance for choosing between treatment alternatives. The shorter the bar, the more important the outcome.*

improvement, followed by the probability of suffering urinary incontinence. All other outcomes were significantly less important in the process of deciding between treatment choices and, surprisingly, retrograde ejaculation ranked last among the members of the panel.

In Table 42.2 all outcomes commonly assessed in BPH treatments are listed and categorized regarding the type of parameter, outcome measure, the type of outcome, and the direction of the outcome. There are only a few direct benefits of treatment for BPH: these are symptom improvement, and also the magnitude of improvement in symptoms, bother and quality of life. All other benefits are indirect biological outcomes, which are not usually of particular interest to patients (flow rate, residual urine, prostate size, pressure–flow parameters). However, the latter are continuous outcomes and are measured as means/medians, with the effect being measured as difference or ratio of the means/medians. Obviously, all potential treatment benefits, direct and indirect, can also be undesirable if,

for example, during or after treatment the symptoms or the flow rate worsen. Most direct outcomes are dichotomous — that is, they either occur or do not occur (either the patient becomes impotent or he does not) and are measured in probabilities. A few outcomes, such as incontinence or pain, might be described in categorical terms or counts (i.e. grades or episodes of incontinence) and measured in terms of differences in probabilities of categories or number of occurrences. Most physicians are more comfortable, in evaluating different treatment strategies, when confronted with effect measures such as changes or differences in means or medians, rather than with probabilities and differences in probabilities. This is reflected in the relevant literature, where most authors report those continuous outcome data in great detail, with little attention being focused on the more important direct outcomes measured in terms of probabilities. A welcome and much-needed addition to the outcome parameters utilized was, therefore, the development of quantitative symptom, bother and quality-of-life assessment scores,

Table 42.2. *Direct and indirect, desirable and undesirable parameters used as outcomes of BPH treatments, and their outcome measures*

Outcome parameter	Outcome	Outcome measure	Type of outcome	Direction of outcome
Probability of symptom improvement	Dichotomous	Probability	Direct	Benefit
Magnitude of symptom improvement	Continuous	Mean/median		
Magnitude of bother improvement	Continuous	Mean/median		
Magnitude of quality-of-life improvement	Continuous	Mean/median		
Flow-rate improvement	Continuous	Mean/median	Indirect	
Pressure–flow improvement	Continuous	Mean/median		
Prostate size reduction	Continuous	Mean/median		
Residual urine volume reduction	Continuous	Mean/median		
Urinary incontinence	Categorical/count	Probabilities/number of occurrences	Direct	Harm
Surgical complications	Dichotomous	Probability		
Operative mortality	Dichotomous	Probability		
Pain and suffering from treatment	Categorical/count	Probabilities/number of occurrences		
Side effects of drugs	Categorical	Probabilities		
Requirement of blood transfusion	Dichotomous	Probability		
Retrograde ejaculation	Dichotomous	Probability		
Erectile dysfunction	Dichotomous	Probability		
Long-term complications	Dichotomous	Probability		
Re-treatment for recurrent/persistent BPH	Dichotomous	Probability		
Hospital stay	Continuous	Mean/median		
Loss of work time	Continuous	Mean/median		
Recovery time	Continuous	Mean/median		
Cost of treatment	Continuous	Mean/median		

which capture direct and relevant health outcomes, while at the same time they can be measured on a continuous scale, expressed in terms of means±standard deviation (variance), and allow comparison between treatments by comparing the changes and difference in these means, standard deviations or variances.

Benefits of treatment

Direct health outcomes

Symptom improvement (probability of symptom improvement)

The disease process of BPH is characterized by a constellation of lower urinary tract symptoms — often referred to as 'prostatism' — which are divided into obstructive and irritative symptoms. The former occur during the bladder-emptying phase and include hesitancy, decreased stream, feeling of incomplete emptying, straining to void, intermittency, post-void dribbling and urinary retention. The latter occur during the storing phase and include daytime frequency, nocturia, urgency and urge incontinence associated with involuntary detrusor contractions. These symptoms, however, are rather non-specific, and occur in a large percentage of men even in the absence of an enlarged prostate as the underlying cause.[3,4] Diokno et al.[5] provided estimates of the symptoms of prostatism in 802 non-institutionalized men 60 years or older and found a prevalence of 35% of one or more symptoms, with an annual incidence rate of 16.4 and 16.1% during 1 and 2 years of follow-up, respectively. Many men with such symptoms do not have a noticeably enlarged prostate; conversely, other men with an enlarged prostate do not have the same symptoms. Recently, it has even been shown that the frequency and severity of these symptoms in age-matched women is similar to that of men.[6,7] Because of this lack of specificity, it has been suggested that these symptoms should be referred to as 'lower urinary tract symptoms', thus leaving the underlying cause of the symptoms unspecified.

Nevertheless, patients usually seek consultation with a health-care provider because of these symptoms, and over 90% of all transurethral resection of the prostate (TURP) interventions in the USA are done either for symptoms alone or for a combination of symptoms and other indications (such as infections, residual urine or

bleeding).[8] As shown in Fig. 42.1, the probability of symptom improvement is the single most important outcome considered by patients when choosing a therapy for BPH.

The probability of symptom improvement is a dichotomous outcome with either an absolute difference in probabilities or a ratio of probabilities being the effect measure. The instrument used to determine whether symptom improvement has occurred is usually a global subjective question answered by either the patient himself or the physician. In most of the published literature this is done by asking a question such as 'Overall, are your symptoms better, unchanged or worse?' following the treatment or at a predetermined follow-up period.

The global subjective assessment of the treatment outcome by the patient himself is obviously of great importance, although there are many important biases that may affect the answers given. For example, patients may wish to please their treating physician and are likely to give a positive answer if asked directly by the physician, as opposed to questioning by a neutral person, such as a nurse who has not participated in the treatment. The global subjective assessment on the part of the treating physician is even more problematic. In most of the older literature dealing with surgical therapy, the assessing physician was also the treating physician, thus introducing a considerable bias in his judgement. In some of the newer publications, the physician who rendered the global subjective assessment was not involved in the treatment or (in the case of a randomized, double-blind study) did not know which treatment the patient received.

In this context, it is of interest to determine to what degree doctors and patients agree in their perception of health status and outcomes following therapeutic interventions. In one study of the effects of treatment for hypertension, 100% of doctors reported an improvement in the quality of life, whereas only 50% of the patients perceived such improvement.[9] In a similar study involving 385 men undergoing TURP, a relatively high rate of concordance was found between the patients' and the doctors' preoperative assessment and the outcomes after 12 months.[10,11] Preoperatively, agreement was high for obstructive symptoms (75%), but less good for irritative symptoms (59%). The greatest disagreement (41–46%) existed concerning the risk of urinary tract infections, renal damage and acute retention, in which cases the patients usually anticipated a higher degree of risk than did the physicians. Postoperatively, disagreement was found regarding incontinence (44% at 12 months), urgency (47% overall), and certain complications, namely urinary tract infections (20% overall) and sexual dysfunction (20% overall). In the vast majority of cases, patients reported symptoms and complications of which the physician was not aware. The level of concordance was unrelated to the experience of the individual surgeon, age, social class, education, employment or marital status of the patients, their expectations regarding the outcome of the surgery, or whether or not they felt that they had a choice about the operation.

For the purpose of the AHCPR BPH Guidelines, the reported global subjective symptom improvement rates were analysed as a categorical (improved, unchanged, worse) or a dichotomous (improved versus not improved) outcome, the latter using the Confidence Profile Method and a hierarchical Bayes model assuming a random effect[12–14] (Fig. 42.2). The probability of symptom improvement after a placebo treatment or during watchful waiting is slightly greater than 40%, while all other 'active' treatment interventions have a substantially (and significantly) greater probability of symptom improvement — with the exception of balloon dilatation, for which the confidence interval is large and overlaps with those for placebo and watchful waiting.

Tempting as it is to compare these treatment modalities with regard to the probability of symptom improvement, several caveats are in order. Little if anything is known about the severity and frequency of the patients' symptoms prior to treatment. It is reasonable to assume, that those patients treated by transurethral incision of the prostate (TUIP), TURP, or open surgery, were initially more symptomatic than those treated with placebo or by watchful waiting. The symptom severity level prior to treatment, however, undoubtedly affects the perception of symptomatic improvement on the part of the patient. Furthermore, patients who made a significant 'investment' (e.g. by undergoing a surgical procedure) are more likely to report improvement in their symptoms than are patients

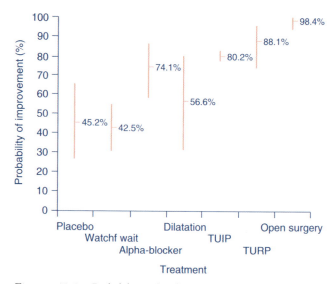

Figure 42.2. *Probability of achieving symptom improvement determined by global subjective assessment as a dichotomous outcome (improved versus not improved). Shown is the mean probability and the 90% confidence interval for improvement to occur following various interventions for which data were available (watchf wait, watchful waiting; TUIP, transurethral incision of the prostate; TURP, transurethral resection of the prostate). The number next to the horizontal dash indicates the mean probability. (Adapted from ref. 2 with permission).*

who only took a drug over a limited period of time — a phenomenon known as cognitive dissonance.

Thus, while it is of considerable value to learn patients' global assessment of treatment outcomes with regard to symptom improvement following different therapeutic strategies, a comparison of the effectiveness of these different strategies is significantly compromised by a limited understanding of the symptom severity level prior to therapy, and by the fact that patients tend to attribute greater improvements to more invasive therapies.

Magnitude of symptom, bother and quality-of-life improvement

The development of instruments to quantify symptoms has added a much-needed new dimension to the evaluation of men with lower urinary tract symptoms. In the past, two physician-administered symptom scoring instruments were available, both of which suffered from a series of shortcomings. The so-called Boyarsky or Ad Hoc Committee symptom score[15] was developed as part of an attempt to develop guidelines for the evaluation of

BPH, and the Madsen–Iversen symptom score[16] was published in 1983 as a point system to aid physicians in the proper selection of surgical candidates. Neither of these instruments was properly tested and validated. The following is a list of basic requirements for a symptom-severity assessment tool for BPH.

1. It should be easy to understand and, preferably, be self-administered by the patient.
2. It should avoid giving disproportionate weight to individual symptoms.
3. It should be internally consistent.
4. It should separate between patients with BPH and controls (criterion validity).
5. It should reflect the degree of bother the patient experiences.
6. It should not change in a test–retest situation (reliability).
7. It should change after effective treatment (sensitivity).
8. It should correlate with other scoring instruments (construct validity).

Many of these requirements are not fulfilled by the two above-mentioned instruments; their use should, therefore, be discouraged at present.

The American Urological Association (AUA) Measurement Committee recently developed an instrument[17–19] that has now gained widespread acceptance in the USA and worldwide (see Chapter 12). Through the 2nd International Consultation on BPH in 1993,[20] the AUA Symptom Index (AUA-SI) has been widely distributed as International Prostate Symptom Score (IPSS), and validation studies of its translation into many different languages have been conducted, making it undoubtedly the most useful and widely utilized assessment tool in BPH worldwide. The AUA-SI/IPSS is a seven-question self-administered questionnaire inquiring about the frequency or severity of lower urinary tract symptoms (Appendix 42.1a). The answer scheme for the first six questions ranges from the symptom being present 'not at all' (=0) to 'almost always' (=5 points). The seventh question regarding nocturia allows for a categorical answer ranging from 0 to 1, 2, 3, 4 times or 5 or more times per night. The total score thus ranges from 0 to 35 points, with the cutoff points being 0–7 (mild symptom frequency), 8–18 (moderate symptom frequency) and 19–35 points (severe symptom frequency). Although the presentations and publications that have utilized the AUA-SI are numerous, several investigators have criticized it as being not specific for BPH.[6,7,21] These authors have administered the AUA-SI to men and to age-matched women, and have demonstrated a similar symptom level within each age stratum in both sexes. To be useful as a measure of symptom severity in a given patient, however, an instrument does not have to be disease specific. For example, it is immediately evident that patients with severe arthritis would score poorly on the Karnofsky performance status scale or the Eastern Cooperative Oncology Group (ECOG) scale, commonly used to assess the impact of cancer on a patient's everyday activities. This does not mean that these patients suffer from cancer, but rather that their illness impacts on their everyday activities in a way similar to that of an advanced cancer disease. Despite these observations, improvements of performance following effective cancer treatment can still be measured by using the Karnofsky performance index, and different treatment regimens can be compared by comparing the resulting changes in the Karnofsky score. This is precisely the appropriate indication for the AUA-SI — to measure the baseline severity or frequency of symptoms and to allow monitoring of these symptoms during and/or after treatment in men who, on the basis of a comprehensive evaluation, have been diagnosed as having BPH. The lack of disease specificity has led some authorities to suggest that the term 'lower urinary tract symptoms' should be used, rather than 'BPH' until the diagnosis of BPH has been confirmed or established as the causative pathogenic mechanism responsible for the symptoms.

Symptom severity and frequency alone do not sufficiently explain the health-care-seeking behaviour of men. Whereas some men are bothered enough by mild symptoms to consult a physician, others tolerate much more severe symptom frequency and severity before seeking help. In general, a high degree of correlation has been found between symptom severity or frequency and bother. Jacobsen et al.[22] found, in a population-based study of men aged 40–79 years in Olmsted County, Minnesota, USA, a tight correspondence between the two measures (r^2=0.71). The AUA Measurement

Committee developed and validated an AUA Symptom Problem Index (SPI) as a companion to the AUA-SI[23] (Appendix 42.1b). Instead of inquiring about the frequency or severity of symptoms, the seven questions are aimed at the degree to which the present symptoms are a problem for the patient. The answer scheme ranges from 'no problem' (= 0) to 'big problem' (= 4 points), for a total score from 0 to 28 points. Baseline data from a medical treatment trial for BPH revealed a correlation of $r=0.74$ between the AUA-SI and the SPI in 1990 men with an AUA-SI of at least 13 points (unpublished data) (Fig. 42.3a). A comparison of populations in North America and Scotland demonstrated that similar symptom severity levels cause a similar impact and degree of bother for both American and Scottish men.[24] The degree to which patients are bothered by symptoms is more important in the decision about whether to seek help and undertake treatment and, in fact, men with a bother index greater than predicted from their symptom

index were more likely to have sought health care.[22] These men were older, poorer, more anxious, and had a lower general well-being score than those with a bother index closer to that predicted from their symptom index. Moreover, worry and embarrassment about urinary symptoms have also been shown to be important in determining health-care-seeking behaviour, beyond symptom frequency and severity alone.[25] In recognition of these facts, the AUA Measurement Committee has recently also developed and validated a BPH Impact Index (BII) that measures how much the urinary problems affect various domains of health[23] (Appendix 42.1c). Both have excellent test–retest ($r=0.88$ for both) reliabilities, correlate with the AUA-SI ($r=0.86$ and 0.77), and discriminate between men with BPH and controls [receiver operating characteristic (ROC) areas under the curve of 0.87 and 0.85].[23] In the aforementioned 1990 men with BPH, a correlation of $r=0.519$ was found between the AUA-SI and the BII (Fig. 42.3b).

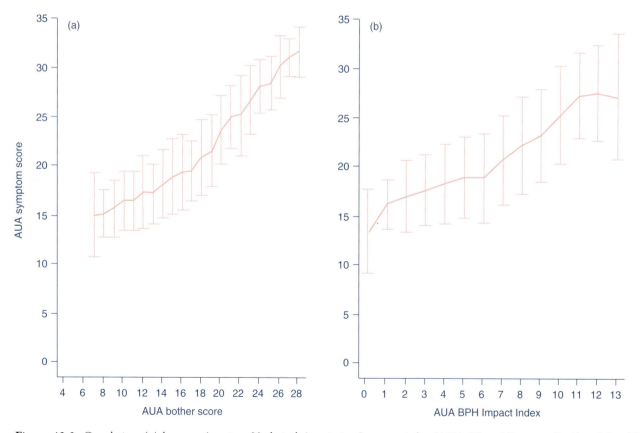

Figure 42.3. *Correlations (a) between American Urological Association Symptom index (AUA-SI) and Symptom Problem Index (SPI) (r=0.741), and (b) between AUA-SI and BPH Impact Index (BII) (r=0.519) in 1990 men with an AUA-SI greater than or equal to 13 points, an SPI greater than or equal to eight points, and clinical BPH.*

In recognition of the importance of the disease-specific quality of life, and the degree to which it is affected by the symptoms of the disease, a single quality-of-life question is currently recommended by the International Consultation on BPH.[20] The wording of this single question and the six possible answers are reproduced in Appendix 42.1d.

The AUA-SI, internationally known as the International Prostate Symptom Score or I-PSS, the SPI, the BII and the single disease-specific quality-of-life question, form a comprehensive set of tools to capture a patient's lower urinary tract symptom frequency and severity, the problems they cause him, and the degree to which they affect various domains of his health.

Other tools have been developed, parallel to those discussed above, by different groups of investigators, which might serve the same purpose in a similar fashion.[26–32]

A decided advantage of these quantitative scoring instruments is the fact that they represent a continuous outcome parameter. The effects of treatments can be measured and compared as absolute improvement (or worsening), percentage improvement (or worsening), and the difference or the ratio of means (or medians). Within each treatment group, comparisons can be made before versus after treatment, and the absolute and percentage changes in the mean±standard deviation (variance) from before to after treatment can be compared between treatment groups, provided that the two (or more) groups are similar enough at baseline to allow such comparison.

In the past, symptom index data have been reported using a variety of different approaches. Most investigators have reported the original data in the form of pre- and post-treatment mean±standard deviation (variance). Additionally, in many published BPH treatment studies the percentage improvements in symptom indices are also reported. The formula used to calculate the absolute decrease in symptom index (SI) from before treatment (SI_{pre}) to after treatment (SI_{post}) as a percentage of SI_{pre} is: $(SI_{pre} - SI_{post}) / SI_{pre} \times 100 = SI_{impr\%}$. A seven-point absolute improvement in SI, however, represents significantly different $SI_{impr\%}$ values depending on SI_{pre} (Fig. 42.4a). Indeed, the same seven point drop in SI, which equals 20% of the total 35-point

scale, represents a $SI_{impr\%}$ of 20% when SI_{pre} is 35, and a $SI_{impr\%}$ of 63.6% when SI_{pre} is 11 points. Similarly, a five-point drop (14.3% of the total scale) represents an $SI_{impr\%}$ ranging from 14.3 to 45.5%, and a ten-point drop (28.6% of the total scale), represents an $SI_{impr\%}$ ranging from 28.6 to 90.9%.

The discrepancy between the $SI_{impr\%}$ calculated as above, and the point drop expressed as a percentage of the 35-point scale is further illustrated in Fig. 42.4b. By fixing the SI_{pre} at 28 points, a $SI_{impr\%}$ of, for example, 50% represents a 40% drop of the 35-point scale. Conversely, to reach a SI_{post} of eight points requires a drop of two points (5.7% of the 35-point scale) or a 20% improvement when the SI_{pre} is ten points, but requires a drop of 20 points (57.1% of the 35-point scale) or 71.4% improvement from baseline, when the SI_{pre} is 28 points (Fig. 42.4c).

The reporting of either absolute ($SI_{pre} - SI_{post} = SI_{impr}$) improvements in SI expressed as a decrease in points from before to after treatment, or the reporting of $SI_{impr\%}$, thus can be misleading, depending on the pretreatment SI. A practical example makes this point clear. A cohort of men treated with drug A experiences an SI_{impr} of eight points (mean) with a reported $SI_{impr\%}$ of 28.6%, while another cohort treated with drug B experiences an SI_{impr} of eight points (mean) with a reported $SI_{impr\%}$ of 50%. Both drugs lower the SI by the same absolute amount of points, but drug A induces an improvement from 28 to 20 points, whereas that with drug B is from 16 to 8 points.

The question of which drug is the better treatment choice cannot be answered without answering one fundamental question: does the perception of therapeutic benefit from treatment depend more on the pretreatment SI, on the absolute or percentage drop in points, or on the post-treatment SI? This question cannot be answered with certainty at present. Barry et al.[33] recently made an important observation in this regard. They assessed the relationship between changes in the SI and BII with patients' global ratings of improvement, in over 1200 men with clinical BPH treated in a double-blind medical treatment trial. Those patients rating themselves at least slightly improved had a mean decrease in SI of 3.1 points and a mean decrease in BII of 0.4 points. However, the baseline SI scores strongly influenced this relationship. For men with a

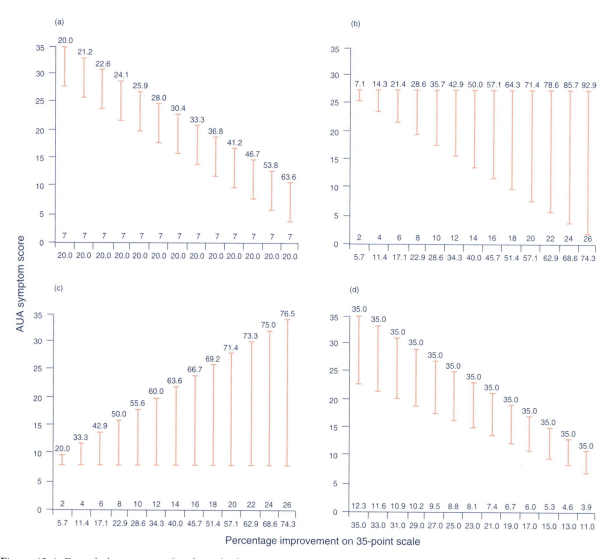

Figure 42.4. *Example demonstrating the relationship between pre- and post-treatment AUA-SI, the absolute drop in points (number at bottom of figure insert), the percentage drop from baseline (number above the vertical bars) and of the 35-point scale (number along x-axes): (a) inflation of the percentage drop with decreasing SI_{pre}; the impact of having either a fixed SI_{pre} (b) or a fixed SI_{post} (c). For example, a two- point drop from a baseline of 28 represents a 7.1% improvement, whereas the same absolute drop represents a 20% drop from ten to eight. In (d) the $SI_{impr\%}$ is fixed and the ever-decreasing corresponding absolute improvement (as well as the percentage improvement of the 35-point scale) with decreasing SI_{pre} is demonstrated. A 35% $SI_{impr\%}$ may represent a 12.3-point to a 3.9-point actual improvement.*

baseline SI of 10 points, a one-, three- and five-point decrease correlated with their perception of slight, moderate and marked improvement, respectively. For men with a baseline score of 20 and 30, the respective decreases were 3.5, 7.5 and 12 (20-point baseline score), and seven, 11 and 19 (30-point baseline score). Expressed as $SI_{impr\%}$, moderate improvement correlates with a 30% (ten-point baseline score), 37.5% (20-point baseline score) and 36.7% (30-point baseline score) improvement. These data indicate that both the baseline score and the

absolute or percentage drop in points are important in the perception of improvement, and that a constant $SI_{impr\%}$ across various strata of baseline severity is associated with a similar perception of improvement. Taking this into account, Fig. 42.4d illustrates the absolute drop in points associated with a $SI_{impr\%}$ of 35% (perceived as 'moderate' improvement), which ranges from 12.3 (baseline 35) to only 3.9 (baseline 11) points.

The importance of reporting *all* relevant outcome data associated with quantitative symptom scores becomes clear with an example (Fig. 42.5). There are five randomized trials comparing transurethral thermotherapy with sham treatment. All show superiority of the active treatment over the sham treatment. The absolute drop in SI ranges from 7.6 to 12.1 points for the active arms, and the percentage drop from 55 to 70%. However, the greatest drop in symptom score was achieved in a population of men with a baseline score of 19.2 points (trial 5), clearly more symptomatic than the patients in all four other trials. Whereas one might reasonably state that trials 1–4 yield a similar result in a similar patient population, the population in trial 5 is sufficiently different to make a direct comparison difficult or impossible.

A comparison of three alpha-1-receptor blocker trials makes this point even more strikingly. Eighty-two patients were treated with doxazosin versus placebo over 16 weeks,[34] 2064 patients with terazosin versus placebo over 52 weeks,[35] and 296 patients with tamsulosin

versus placebo over 12 weeks[36] (Fig. 42.6a). Although presumably in all three trials the patients treated with active drugs achieved a greater than 35% improvement in SI, which is perceived as at least a moderate improvement, the baseline symptom status is vastly different and precludes a direct comparison between the three drugs. Furthermore, in all three trials a different symptom score was used: the scale ranged from 0 to 30 points in the doxazosin trial, from 0 to 35 points (AUA-SI). in the terazosin trial, and from 0 to 27 (Boyarsky score) in the tamsulosin trial. In Fig. 42.6b all scores are rescaled to a 100% scale and the pre- and post-treatment mean scores are expressed as a percentage of the 100% scale. This manoeuvre allows a fairer comparison between the trials, eliminating at least the difference introduced by the different scales used. None the less, there is no overlap between the terazosin and the tamsulosin trial symptom scores; thus, it is impossible to determine whether the 21.7%

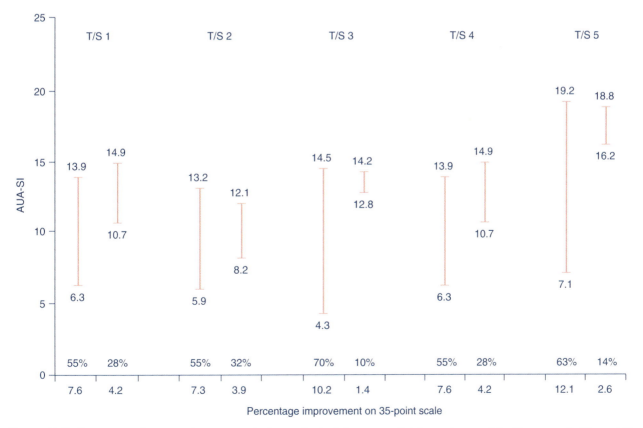

Figure 42.5. *Comparison of symptom improvement in five randomized sham-controlled thermotherapy trials. Shown are the SI_{pre} and SI_{post} (numbers above and below the vertical bars, respectively), the $SI_{impr\%}$ (numbers above the x-axis) and the absolute improvement for the active treatment and the sham arms (T, treatment; S, sham).*

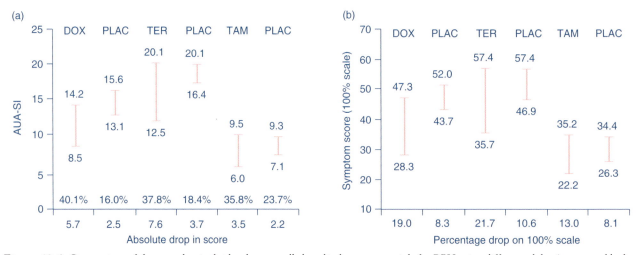

Figure 42.6. *Comparison of three randomized, placebo-controlled medical treatment trials for BPH using different alpha-1-receptor blockers (DOX, doxazosin; TER, terazosin; TAM, tamsulosin; PLAC, placebo). The three trials do not allow immediate comparison, as three different symptom scores were used, namely a 30-point scale instrument in the doxazosin trial, the AUA 35-point SI in the terazosin trial, and a 27-point instrument in the tamsulosin trial. While in (a) the absolute pre- and post-treatment scores are listed above and below the vertical bars, and the percentage and absolute drops are listed on the bottom of the figure and along the x-axis, (b) illustrates a better way to compare the data by rescaling all scores to 100%. Listed are the pre- and post-treatment scores expressed as a percentage figure, and the percentage drops on the 100% scale are listed along the x-axis. While this method illustrates that the 5.7-point drop in the doxazosin trial is comparable to the 7.6-point drop in the terazosin trial, it also demonstrates the limits of comparability. The tamsulosin-treated patients, even after rescaling of the score show no overlap with the terazosin-treated patients before or after treatment.*

improvement on the 100% scale (terazosin) is better than the 13.0% improvement on the 100% scale (tamsulosin).

Both thermotherapy trial 5 and the terazosin trial have similar entry criteria and baseline mean symptom indices. A comparison (Fig. 42.7) shows that the improvement in the device sham and the drug placebo arms are fairly similar, namely 2.6 and 3.3 points, or 13.8 and 18.4%. Although the alpha-blocker provides at least a moderate improvement, the thermotherapy treatment provides a 63% improvement, perceived by patients as a marked improvement. In such cases, direct comparison is possible and may be justifiable.

The above discussion should have demonstrated clearly that, at present, when investigators use different inclusion and exclusion criteria and different symptom scores, at least a unified style of reporting should be demanded. To facilitate comparison, the mean pre- and post-treatment indices should be made available [including standard deviation (variance) or preferably confidence intervals], the range of the scale that was used, and the percentage improvement from baseline as well as the percentage improvement on the scale. The lower limits of the symptom score allowing inclusion in

trials often differ; thus the pretreatment mean symptom scores will differ too: in a trial with a minimum SI of ten, the mean will be lower than in a trial where the minimum SI is 15. Although this effectively precludes comparison of the entire population as a whole, at least subsets might be comparable, namely those subsets that are common to both trials, for example patients with an SI from 15 to 20, from 20 to 25, from 25 to 30 etc. Authors should, therefore, give serious consideration to stratification of the study population by baseline symptom severity score, and to reporting all items listed above for each stratum. An example of such stratification is presented in Fig. 42.8. Using results from the HYCAT trial,[35] the effectiveness of treatment with terazosin can be assessed within each symptom severity stratum. This allows immediate comparison with other trials being analysed using similar stratifications. The findings reported by Barry et al.,[33] demonstrating a correlation between perceived improvement and baseline symptom score, further emphasize the usefulness of such a stratification system.

In an effort to utilize quantitative symptom improvement measures, all available symptom score data for the various treatment modalities discussed in the

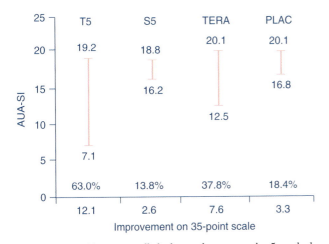

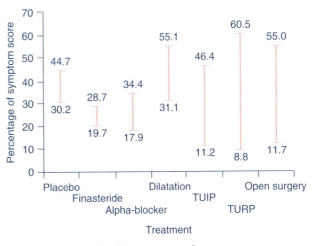

Figure 42.7. *Sham-controlled thermotherapy study 5 and the terazosin (TERA) trial have similar entry criteria and comparable patient populations. Active thermotherapy appears to be more effective in improving symptoms than alpha-blockade, while sham treatment appears to have the same efficacy as placebo (PLAC) treatment.*

Figure 42.9. *Combined mean pre- and post-treatment symptom scores (rescaled to 100% scale) for different treatments for BPH (Adapted from ref. 2 with permission.)*

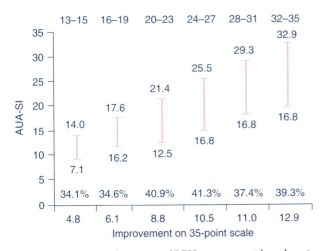

Figure 42.8. *Suggested reporting of BPH treatment trial results using the results from the HYCAT terazosin treatment trial.[35] As well as reporting the percentage improvement from baseline (numbers above the x-axis), the absolute improvement and the pre- and post-treatment scores with standard deviations (variance) or confidence intervals should be listed. To facilitate comparison between matched groups, a stratification by baseline symptom severity is suggested (numbers at top of figure), and pre- and post-treatment scores (above and below the vertical bars), and absolute and percentage improvement, should be reported for each stratum.*

perceived improvement on the baseline symptom level, illustrates why it currently is exceedingly difficult — if not impossible — to compare different treatments with regard to symptom improvement.

The considerations elaborated above for the symptom score, apply directly to other outcomes that are quantitative and continuous, specifically bother and quality-of-life scores. Although, hitherto, fewer reports using such instruments have been published, it can be expected that, with a deeper understanding of the factors that drive patients to seek help, a deeper appreciation of bother and quality of life will stimulate physicians to use these tools to an ever-increasing extent. Outcome reporting using these tools should follow the principles outlined above. Preference should be given to the reporting of raw scores before and after treatment, and consideration should be given to stratification by baseline score. These recommendations are in agreement with those made by the BPH Clinical Trials Subcommittee of the American Urological Association (Dr John D. McConnell, personal communication).

Indirect outcomes

Urinary flow rate

Although the direct benefits of treatment are clearly most important to patients, indirect outcomes such as changes in urinary flow rate, residual urine volume,

AHCPR BPH Guidelines[2] were rescaled to a percentage scale and the mean pre- and post-treatment symptom severities were plotted (Fig. 42.9). The tremendous variability of the pretreatment (baseline) symptom severities between the different treatments, and our increasing knowledge about the dependence of prostate size and urodynamic pressure–flow parameters are useful in reporting and comparing different treatment modalities. They are continuous outcomes and effect measures such as differences in means (medians)±standard deviation (variance) before and after treatment, both within and between treatment groups, can be calculated and reported.

Urinary flow rate recording is a non-invasive technique of assessing the strength of the urine stream (see Chapter 15). Of the various parameters obtained, the peak or maximum urinary flow rate — often indicated by the symbol Q_{max} — is the most useful. The voided volume is the total volume expelled during the voiding act, and the average flow rate — often indicated by the symbol Q_{avg} — is the voided volume divided by the flow time (time during which measurable flow occurs). In the case of intermittent flow patterns, the intervals between flow episodes are disregarded and the voiding time (entire duration of all voiding episodes) is reported instead.

There are some aspects of flow rate recording that are of immediate relevance to the outcome reporting of BPH treatments. The first is the concern that patients may improve their performance from measurement to measurement, owing to a learning effect. Both the actual effect and its magnitude have been debated. If, in fact, patients on average would have an improved maximum flow rate on second and any subsequent voidings compared with the first recording, then any possible treatment effect would be overestimated by that effect. Golomb et al.[37] studied the variability and circadian changes in 32 men with BPH by repeated home flow rate recording (total number of recordings 476, average per subject 15). In 87.5% of patients the maximum flow rate varied by at least one standard deviation (SD) and in 47% by two SD. Circadian changes were insignificant, and no comment was made on a systematic improvement of the flow rate from the first to the subsequent recordings. In a similar experiment, 164 men performed four consecutive flow rate recordings in a flow clinic.[38] The average peak flow rate increased from the first to the fourth voiding, from 9.0 to 11.3, 12.3 and finally 14.3 ml/s. An increase of more than 3 ml/s between the first and the second recording was noted in 27% of men, from the first to the third in 52%, and from the first to the fourth in 69% of

men. These findings illustrate the need for multiple (at least two) baseline flow rate recordings prior to enrolment of patients in BPH treatment trials. Preferably, all recordings should have peak flow rates under the selected cutoff inclusion criterion.

Grino et al.[39] analysed 23 857 flow rate recordings of 1645 patients enrolled in a finasteride versus placebo trial. On average, machine-interpreted maximum flow rates were 1.5 ml/s higher than manually read values, as a result of significant artefacts of more than 2 ml/s in 20% of tracings and of more than 3 ml/s in 9% of tracings. Although the differences between treatment groups were the same when assessed by both methods, confidence intervals were up to 25% larger with the machine-read values. Since confidence intervals have a significant impact on statistical power calculations, flow rate recordings should be manually read and interpreted to avoid this bias.

Many authors have addressed the dependency of maximum flow rate on the voided volume in cohorts of both male and female volunteers, as well as patients (for an overview see ref. 2). In general, it is accepted that over a wide range of voided volumes there is a direct positive correlation between voided volume and maximum flow rate. Many nomograms and formulae have been developed to correct for this problem, and to make maximum flow rates comparable, independent of the voided volume. However, other authors have suggested that this phenomenon may not occur — or may occur only to a lesser and perhaps insignificant degree — in men with clinical BPH. At present the International Continence Society (ICS) does not recommend a mathematical correction of the maximum flow rate based on the voided volume.

Urinary flow rate recordings were obtained from 2113 participants in the Olmsted County study, and normal reference ranges stratified by age and voided volume have been established.[40,41] The median maximum flow rate decreased from 20.3 in men 40–44 years old to 11.5 ml/s in men 75–79 years old. The decrease in maximum flow rate was 2 ml/s per decade of life. Between 24% (40–44 years) and 69% (75–79 years) of men between these age strata had a maximum flow rate of less than 15 ml/s, while between 6 and 35% of men had a maximum flow rate of less than 10 ml/s. Keeping this age-dependent decline of the maximum flow rate in mind, it is understandable that this parameter by itself is not specific for the diagnosis of BPH. Furthermore, it has been shown that there are poor correlations between the maximum flow rate and other assessment tools such as symptom severity (correlation coefficient $r=-0.07$; $p=0.27$), bother ($r=0.02$; $p=0.81$), residual urine ($r=-0.19$; $p=0.009$), and prostate size ($r=-0.14$; $p=0.06$) (analysis based on 198 patients).[42] In another cohort of 274 men with an AUA-SI of 13 points or more, similarly poor correlations between the maximum flow rate and AUA-SI and SPI were found (Fig. 42.10). The mean AUA-SI was 20.8 ± 5.5 in those men with a Q_{max} of less than 10 ml/s, and was 19.5 ± 5.1 in men with a Q_{max} of more than 10 ml/s (not significant). Although these observations limit the diagnostic usefulness of flow rate recordings, they do not affect their usefulness in following patients during and after treatment, reporting and comparing treatment outcomes.

Probability of flow rate improvement. Many older studies have reported the probability of the maximum flow rate, as with the probability of symptom improvement, of improving, staying the same or deteriorating. Whereas in the case of changes in symptom

perception this method provides some meaningful information, in the case of flow rate recordings it is a very poor way to describe the data. A minor change in the maximum flow rate in either direction (e.g. less than ±1.0 ml/s) is very likely unnoticed by the patient. Thus, it would be possible to report a seemingly impressive percentage of patients with 'an improvement', whereas in fact, the magnitude of that improvement could be clinically insignificant. The reporting of number and/or percentage of patients who experience a not further specified change in any of the parameters of the flow rate recording is, therefore, inadequate.

Magnitude of flow rate improvement. Like the continuous outcome parameter of magnitude of symptom changes, flow rate changes can be measured quantitatively. The effects of treatments can be measured and compared as absolute improvement (or worsening), percentage improvement (or worsening) and the difference or the ratio of means (or medians). Within-treatment-group comparisons can be made before versus after treatment, and the absolute and percentage changes in the mean±standard deviation (variance) from before to after treatment can be compared between treatment groups, provided that the

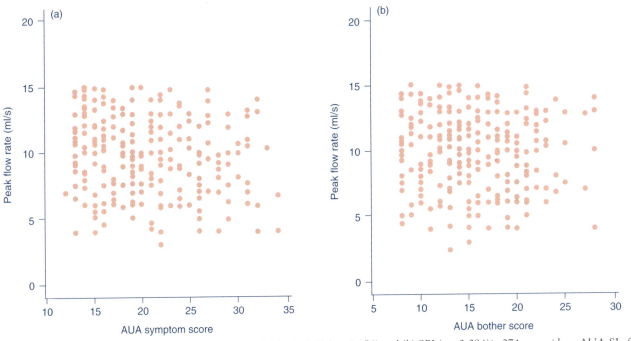

Figure 42.10. *Correlation between maximum flow rate and (a) AUA-SI (r=–0.156) and (b) SPI (r=–0.084) in 274 men with an AUA-SI of 13 or more.*

two (or more) groups are similar enough at baseline to allow such comparison.

Fundamentally, the discussion above regarding the magnitude of symptom improvement applies to the magnitude of flow rate improvement, but with a few important exceptions. For one, nothing is known about the relationship between numerical changes in maximum flow rate and the patients' perception of such changes. In other words, we cannot define the smallest improvement in flow rate that would be experienced as an improvement by most patients. Secondly, the desired direction of the change in flow rate is upward, whereas for almost all symptom assessment scales it is downward. For example, a mean improvement in the maximum flow rate from 5 to 10 ml/s represents a 100% improvement, a change from 10 to 15 ml/s a 50% improvement, and so on. An improvement in symptom score from ten to five points, however, represents a 50% improvement, and a change from 15 to ten points equals only a 33% improvement. Furthermore, the flow rate scale is open ended, and a maximum possible flow rate is not defined. Percentage changes cannot, therefore, be anchored to a scale as is possible for the symptom score. On the other hand, the scale is identical for each investigator and every patient. Data from different cohorts and trials can thus more readily be compared.

The AHCPR BPH Guideline panel compared mean pre- and post-treatment maximum flow rate data (Fig. 42.11). A striking difference from the symptom score data discussed earlier is the similarity of the mean pretreatment maximum flow rate in all combined treatment groups.

In the absence of a threshold flow rate change perceptible to patients, outcomes should be reported in terms of the baseline (based on two or more recordings) and post-treatment maximum flow rate (population mean). Changes may be expressed as absolute and as a percentage change from baseline, notwithstanding the limitation of the percentage improvement. Stratification of the data is strongly recommended. Data should be provided concerning the percentage of patients who experience a change in maximum flow rate in either direction (e.g. –4 to –2, –2 to 0, 0 to +2, +2 to +4 or +4 to +6 ml/s).

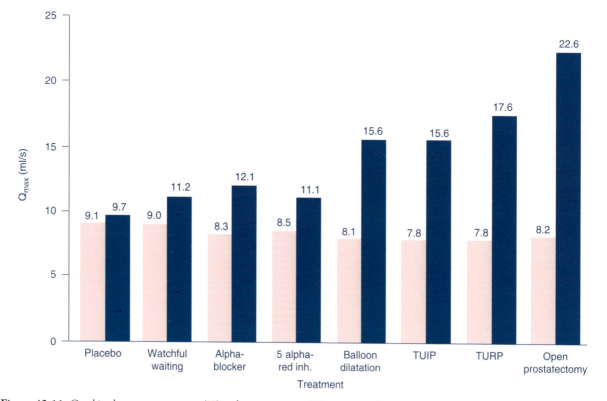

Figure 42.11. *Combined mean pretreatment ( ) and post-treatment (■) maximum flow rates (Q_{max}) for different treatments for BPH (5 alpha-red inh., 5 alpha-reductase inhibitor). (Adapted from ref. 2 with permission.)*

Residual urine

The measurement of post-void residual urine has been considered by some to be an integral part of the study of micturition.[43] Healthy volunteers have been found to have residual urine volumes ranging from 0.09 to 2.24 ml,[44] and Di Mare et al.[45] demonstrated that virtually all healthy men had less than 12 ml of residual urine. Thus, the presence of residual urine constitutes an abnormal finding, although it certainly is not specific for the diagnosis of BPH (see Chapter 15).

Residual urine can be measured by in-and-out catheterization and several non-invasive methods. Many investigators have demonstrated that transabdominal ultrasonography allows measurement of residual urine volume with sufficient accuracy (for a review see ref. 2); it should, therefore, be the preferred method of measuring residual urine.

A substantial problem in the interpretation of residual urine data is the wide intra-individual variability from measurement to measurement, even within a 24 h period.[46,47] Multiple measurements of residual urine using non-invasive techniques are therefore recommended. Whether the mean of two measurements provides a more reliable value than any single measurement has yet to be determined.

Reservations similar to those discussed above for flow rate recordings are in order for residual urine measurements. Increased amounts of residual urine are not specific for BPH, and no threshold has been described that would identify patients with BPH with sufficient accuracy. Furthermore, correlations between residual urine and AUA-SI ($r=0.01$; $p=0.84$), SPI ($r=-0.09$; $p=0.25$), maximum flow rate ($r=-0.19$; $p=0.009$) and prostate size ($r=0.07$; $p=0.35$) are non-existent or poor.[42]

Probability of decrease in residual urine volume.
Many older studies have reported the probability of the residual urine volume (like those of symptom improvement and of maximum flow rate) to decrease, to stay the same, or to increase. As discussed for the flow rate recording, this is a poor way of describing outcomes, as minor and most clinically insignificant changes in the residual urine volume would count as 'improvement' or 'deterioration'.

Magnitude of decrease in residual urine volume.
Changes in residual urine volume can be measured quantitatively. The effects of treatments can be measured and compared as absolute decrease (increase), percentage decrease (increase), and the difference or the ratio of means (medians). Within-treatment-group comparisons can be made before versus after treatment, and the absolute and percentage changes in the mean from before to after treatment can be compared between treatment groups, provided that the two (or more) groups are similar enough at baseline to allow such comparison.

As is the case with the changes in flow rates, it is unknown what change (if any) in residual urine volume can be perceived by the patient as an improvement, and what amount of change may affect the ultimate outcome in either a positive or negative direction.

The AHCPR Guideline Panel[2] analysed mean pre- and post-treatment residual urine volume data (Fig. 42.12). In striking contrast to the flow rate data, the baseline mean residual urine volume differs greatly between the different treatment modalities, and, as a result, both the absolute and the percentage changes in residual urine volume differ significantly between the treatments under consideration. Thus, it is exceedingly difficult to compare these treatments in relation to their ability to alter residual urine volume.

In the absence of a threshold residual urine volume change perceptible to patients, outcomes should be reported (like those for flow rates) in terms of the baseline (based on two or more measurements) and post-treatment residual urine volume (population mean). Changes may be expressed as absolute and percentage change from baseline, notwithstanding the limitation of the percentage improvement. Stratification of the data is strongly recommended. Data should be provided concerning the percentage of patients who experience a change in residual urine in either direction (e.g. −150 to −100, −100 to −50, -50 to 0, 0 to +50, +50 to +100 ml).

Urodynamic pressure–flow studies

Urodynamic pressure–flow studies represent the most sophisticated — but also the most invasive — method of assessing men with clinical BPH, and measuring their response to treatment (see Chapter 16). None of the

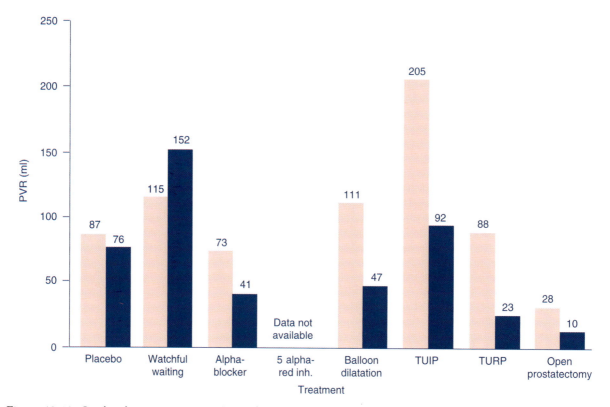

Figure 42.12. *Combined mean pretreatment (▢) and post-treatment (■) residual urine (PVR) volumes for different treatments for BPH (5 alpha-red inh., 5 alpha-reductase inhibitor). (Adapted from ref. 2 with permission.)*

assessment tools discussed thus far, including pressure–flow studies, are specific for the diagnosis of BPH. However, although lower urinary tract symptoms can be caused by a large variety of disorders, and a reduced maximum flow rate can be caused by either outlet obstruction or a weak detrusor muscle, pressure–flow studies can at least reliably differentiate the latter two.[48] It still can not be assumed that outlet obstruction is caused by BPH in all cases, but the post-test probability is substantially increased.

The proper techniques of performing and reporting pressure–flow studies are poorly documented, standardized, and adhered to. The ICS is currently conducting a large BPH study, with one of the declared goals being the comparison of properly conducted pressure–flow studies with other assessment tools.[49]

Pressure–flow studies record continuously the intravesical and intra-abdominal pressure, and the urinary flow rate. The difference between intra-abdominal and intravesical pressure (P_{abd}–P_{ves}) is calculated as the detrusor pressure (P_{det}). Because of the continuous recording of these parameters, pressure–flow

studies generate a tremendous amount of data that might be of diagnostic use. Among these parameters are the maximum flow rate (Q_{max}), detrusor pressure at the moment of maximum flow rate ($P_{det\ at\ Qmax}$), maximum detrusor pressure, the time from the beginning of the voiding contraction to the beginning of urine flow (opening time), the pressure at the beginning of urine flow (opening pressure), and various mathematical transformations and calculations performed with these variables. Although there is general agreement that the most useful of the parameters recorded is the $P_{det\ at\ Qmax}$, greater diagnostic accuracy can be achieved by relating $P_{det\ at\ Qmax}$ to the Q_{max} itself.[48]

Several ways of displaying the results of pressure–flow studies have been proposed, among them the linear passive urethral resistance relation (LPURR),[50,51] the group-specific urethral resistance (URA)[52] and a three-parameter model.[53] The most popular form of reporting the results of pressure–flow studies, however, is the use of the Abrams–Griffiths nomogram[48,54] (Fig. 42.13a). By plotting P_{det} and Q_{max} on an x–y graph, a categorical assignment of obstructed,

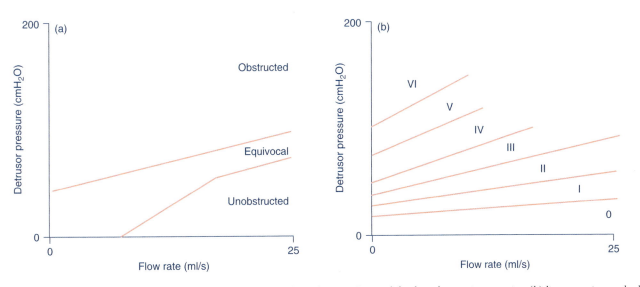

Figure 42.13. (a) Abrams–Griffiths plot of maximum flow rate (Q_{max}) versus P_{det} and the three diagnostic categories; (b) linear passive urethral resistance relation (LPURR) with the six diagnostic classes.

equivocal and unobstructed can be made. Various refinements allow a further segregation of the equivocal group into obstructed and unobstructed patients. The severity of obstruction can be graded by using the Abrams–Griffiths (AG) number.[55,56] The AG number is calculated as $P_{det\ at\ Qmax} - 2Q_{max}$, and a value of over 40 indicates obstruction. Both $P_{det\ at\ Qmax}$ and the AG number are continuous variables and thus allow comparison before and after treatment, and between treatment groups.

The LPURR line is constructed by drawing a line from the $P_{det\ at\ Qmax}$ to the point of $P_{det\ at\ Qmin}$ (Fig. 42.13b). This method allows a classification into six categories, labelled 0–VI, with patients in the 0 category being unobstructed and patients in category VI being severely obstructed. A continuous variable, the detrusor-adjusted mean PURR factor (DAMPF), has also been introduced.[57]

Probability of improvement in pressure–flow studies. Regardless of the parameter used, reporting of the number and/or percentage of patients who experience any improvement in these parameters following treatment is probably meaningless. Little, if anything, is known about threshold changes that would convey benefit to the patient regarding his ultimate outcome, and changes that are probably clinically insignificant might be reported as 'improvement'. Thus, the practice

of reporting the probability of improvement should be avoided.

Probability of change in category in pressure–flow studies. The Abrams–Griffiths nomogram allows categorical assignment of patients into three categories of obstructed, equivocal and unobstructed. Accordingly, it is possible to report the number and percentage of patients who change assignment before and after treatment, and to compare these numbers/percentages between treatments. Although this semiquantitative way of reporting has been used in the past, it has several shortcomings. A substantial number of patients fall in to the equivocal category, and thus make meaningful interpretation more difficult. The LPURR also permits categorical assignment into one of six groups, and the agreements between the assignments using different ways of displaying the pressure–flow studies is high.[48] However, as continuous variables can be extracted from pressure–flow studies, it is clearly advantageous to report outcomes in relation to one of the continuous variables available.

Magnitude of improvement in pressure–flow studies. Of the possible continuous variables ($P_{det\ at\ Qmax}$, AG number, DAMPF), $P_{det\ at\ Qmax}$ has enjoyed most widespread use, and is currently recommended by several international organizations.[20] Because of the previously mentioned difficulties in comparing the results of pressure–flow studies performed in different laboratories under different conditions and using different techniques, outcome reporting should include a brief description of the precise technique utilized, including information on the rate of filling the bladder, the position of the patient during voiding, the way in which the pressure in the bladder was recorded (suprapubic versus transurethral) and the size of the catheter (in the case of a transurethral catheter).

Mean±standard deviation (variance) values for $P_{det\ at\ Qmax}$ before and after treatment should be reported, as well as absolute and percentage decrease (increase) of the same parameter from baseline to after treatment. Provided that similar techniques have been used and that the populations are similar at baseline regarding their urodynamic evaluation, comparisons between the improvements in mean $P_{det\ at\ Qmax}$ from baseline to after treatment can be made between treatment groups. Stratification of the entire population should be considered. The mean absolute or percentage improvement in the chosen parameter from baseline to after treatment might be reported for patients stratified by baseline $P_{det\ at\ Qmax}$ (e.g. in increments of 20 cmH$_2$0), or stratified by categorical assignment according to the Abrams–Griffiths plot or the LPURR.

Prostate size

It is well established that prostate size does not correlate with patients' symptoms, perception of bother, or other commonly used measures.[42,58,59] Although there are many cross-sectional studies reporting average prostate size stratified by age,[60] there is a paucity of longitudinal data concerning the growth of BPH. From a community-based study conducted in Olmsted County,[61] a growth rate of 0.6 ml/year, or 6 ml per decade of life, has been estimated. However, the growth rate appears to be age dependent, with a rate of 0.4 ml/year for men 40–59 years of age versus 1.2 ml/year for men 60–79 years of age.

Changes in prostate size due to natural history or induced by treatments are the indirect outcomes least likely to be noticed by patients. However, changes in prostate size are commonly reported for several newer, minimally invasive treatment modalities, most notably treatments based on microwave- or radiofrequency-generated heat. Of the medical treatment modalities, those interfering with the normal hormonal milieu are all likely to alter prostate size by specifically shrinking the glandular epithelial component of the prostate. Although a variety of medications can effect such changes, the only drug classes of practical relevance are the 5-alpha-reductase inhibitors and the aromatase inhibitors.

Accurate and reproducible measurement of prostate size is very difficult if not impossible to achieve.[2] Digital rectal examination, cystoscopy, intravenous urography, transabdominal ultrasonography, transrectal ultrasonography (TRUS), computerized tomography scanning and magnetic resonance imaging (MRI) have all been utilized. Of these, TRUS and MRI have been most extensively used in the European and North American arms of the phase III trials of the 5-alpha-reductase inhibitor finasteride.[62] Despite standardization of techniques, considerable interexaminer and intra-individual variability in prostate size measurements remains with both of these modalities.

Probability of prostate volume reduction. In view of the considerable variability of prostate size, using even the most sophisticated assessment techniques, reporting of the probability of any changes in prostate volume is unacceptable. Small changes may be due to unrecognized physiological variables or may be of no clinical relevance.

Magnitude of prostate volume reduction. Most hormonal medical treatment modalities for BPH reduce the prostate size by between 20 and 30% after up to 6 months of therapy, independent of the baseline size of the prostate.[2] In the phase III finasteride trials, over 50% of patients receiving the active drug experienced a volume reduction of greater than 20%, while 20% of placebo-treated patients experienced the same magnitude of size reduction.[2] The magnitude of size reduction did not correlate with the magnitude of symptom or flow rate improvements in a TURP series.[58] A recently completed meta-analysis of the finasteride treatment database (P. Boyle, personal communication) indicated, however, that men with larger prostate glands at baseline experienced a greater improvement in their symptom score. Given these findings, reporting of prostate size as an outcome parameter should include the following parameters: methods of size assessment, baseline and post-treatment mean±standard deviation (variance), absolute and percentage change from baseline to treatment, and stratification by baseline size in large datasets.

Harms (ill effects) of treatment

Direct health outcomes

Probability and magnitude of symptom, bother and quality-of-life deterioration

Reporting of only the pre- and post-treatment mean±standard deviation (variance) score and the percentage change may give the false impression that, in fact, none of the patients treated experienced deterioration of any of these outcome assessment parameters. Considering the emotional and financial investments that patients make when undertaking treatment for BPH, they have a right to be fully informed about the probability of such a deterioration in symptoms, bother and quality of life, and the expected degree to which this may occur. Traditionally, authors have not given due consideration to the reporting of these outcomes in an unfavourable direction. It is simple and effective to report the number and percentage of total patients who experience *any* deterioration in these outcomes. However, changes occurring in a unfavourable direction are hidden in the global absolute and percentage changes, even when these changes are stratified by symptom severity. The ways of displaying and comparing treatment outcomes that currently exist and that have been discussed so far do not allow a detailed analysis of these changes. The less invasive a treatment modality (e.g. watchful waiting), the more likely that patients will, in fact, deteriorate. A possible model to display such information is shown in Fig. 42.14. For each baseline symptom severity stratum, the probability of actually deteriorating is indicated with an estimate of the magnitude of the effect. Thus, the two fundamental questions asked by patients (what is the probability that I will experience symptom improvement or worsening; how much symptom improvement or worsening will I experience?) can be answered.

Other harmful health outcomes

The health outcomes discussed in the following paragraphs are not usually employed as primary or secondary endpoints in BPH treatment trials. However,

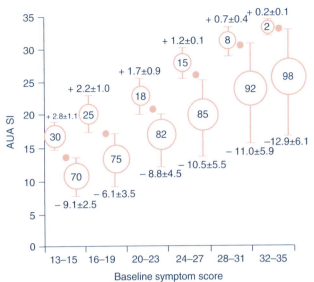

Figure 42.14. *Theoretical model to display symptom improvement or deteriotation following treatment. Patients are stratified by baseline symptom severity (AUA-SI). The number of stratifactions and the lowest and highest stratifaction depends on inclusion and exclusion criteria of the trial. In this example patients with > 13 points were included. The ● represent the mean baseline symptom score for each stratifaction. Within each stratification there exists a probability of improving or not improving/deteriorating. This probability is indicated by the size of the open circles and numerically by the percent of patients experiencing improvement or deterioration. The vertical bars indicate the standard deviation of the observed changes. The numbers below (improvement) and above (deterioration) indicate the mean changes ± standard deviation in each stratification. E.g, a patient with a baseline symptom score of 21 point (third stratification) has a 82% probability to improve, and a 18% probability to deteriorate. The mean improvement is −8.8±4.5 SD points, and the mean deterioration (if it occurs) is +1.7±0.9 SD points.*

as they all have a direct impact on patients' health, appropriate attention should, therefore, be devoted to their reporting.

Not all the outcomes discussed below can be expected to occur after every treatment modality; rather, some are unique to certain types of therapy. It is also conceivable that, in the future, therapies may be developed that have possible outcomes that are unforeseen and that have not been discussed here. Such outcomes should be reported in the most objective and accurate format possible.

The majority of outcomes described here are dichotomous — they either do or do not occur. Thus, they are reported as a probability of occurrence. Other outcomes allow categorization (e.g. by severity of incontinence), or the number of episodes of occurrence (e.g. urine leakage) may be counted and reported. Lastly, some outcomes — such as hospital stay, loss of work time and recovery time — are continuous, and mean (median)±standard deviation may be reported.

The goal in reporting should be to move more and more towards quantitative outcome reporting by replacing dichotomous outcomes with continuous measures. Examples of such improvements are scoring instruments for urinary incontinence or erectile dysfunction.

Adverse events and side effects of medical treatment

Every medical treatment is associated with a certain incidence of adverse events and side effects that may or may not be attributable to the drug itself. Adverse events are any health-related events that take place during the time of the treatment, whether causally related to the drug or not, while side effects are effects of a drug on a tissue or organ system other than the one thought to be benefited by the administration of the drug. Consequently, the list of adverse events taking place during a treatment is considerably longer than the list of side effects of a drug. Patients may not volunteer at every visit all adverse events that took place during the preceding interval. Thus, it should be indicated whether only those adverse events or side effects volunteered by the patient were reported, or whether the patient was prompted, for example by a printed list or a standardized questionnaire specifying possible adverse events or side

effects. A particular problem with tabulated adverse events and side effects is one of accounting. A patient may have one or more adverse events or side effects, and thus the total number of adverse events or side effects encountered may be greater than the number of patients affected by them. Furthermore, some adverse events or side effects may occur only at the beginning of the treatment and then disappear, while others may surface later in the therapy, adding a time dimension to the problem of reporting. Greatest informational value may be achieved by greatest clarity in reporting, and a possible way of reporting adverse events or side effects is shown in Table 42.3. Adverse events may occur equally in patients treated with placebo or active drug, and direct side-by-side comparison, as illustrated in this example, is needed to allow a tentative conclusion as to whether a certain event may be related to the drug itself.

Some adverse events or side effects lead to premature withdrawal from a trial. This subset of events should be reported separately in a similarly styled table.

Statistical comparisons can be made regarding the incidence of adverse events or side effects under drug and placebo treatment either during each follow-up period or over the entire trial, and reported separately for those events allowing continuation versus those leading to premature withdrawal from the trial.

If the adverse events or side effects are clearly defined (e.g. by using ICD-9 codes), different treatments can be compared.

Table 42.3. *Example for the reporting of adverse events (A to D) in a double-blind, placebo-controlled, 12-month drug trial for BPH*

Adverse event	3-month visit		6-month visit		12-month visit		Occurrences per patient months (PM)	
	Drug (n=100)	Placebo (n=100)	Drug (n=88)	Placebo (n=92)	Drug (n=76)	Placebo (n=85)	Drug PM=1020	Placebo PM=1086
A	12	11	9	7	8	6	29	24
B	8	2	7	1	6	1	21	4
C	2	0	5	1	10	1	17	2
D	1	1	1	0	0	1	2	2

Listed are the number (n) of patients available for follow-up, the episodes of occurrence for the four adverse events (A to D) within each period of follow-up, and the total number of occurrences during the treatment related to the total number of patient months (=sum of the number of months that each patient received treatment). 'A' might be a typical adverse event such as headache occurring equally commonly during drug and placebo treatment, 'B' might be a drug-related side effect occurring at similar frequency throughout treatment, 'C' a side effect occurring more commonly later in the treatment, and 'D' a rare adverse event.

Operative morbidity (complications)

The reporting of operative morbidity or complications, occurring either during or immediately after surgical or minimally invasive procedures, should adhere to the same standards as discussed for the reporting of adverse events. With the advent of more minimally invasive treatment modalities, sham-controlled trials become commonplace, and it seems logical to report complications that occurred in the sham controls as well as those encountered during active treatment. Complication reporting is particularly important in trials comparing two active modalities, such as TURP and microwave thermotherapy. As discussed above, the number of occurrences related to the total number of treatment episodes should be reported, and the complications should be defined as accurately as possible (use of ICD-9 codes) to allow comparisons between trials and treatments.

Operative mortality

Intra- or perioperative mortality reporting is of obvious interest to patients and providers. Separate values may be provided for the number of patients dying of any causes versus those dying (presumably) as a direct result of the intervention. The time interval considered for reporting (30 or 90 days) must be stated to allow comparison between treatment modalities and reported series.

Pain and suffering associated with treatment

Pain associated with treatment is notoriously under-reported in BPH treatment trials. As more minimally invasive treatment becomes available, every effort should be made to report these important outcomes in a quantitative form. Several approaches are feasible: patients may be asked to rate their pain daily (weekly during follow-up) following the intervention, using either a numerical pain scale (0=no pain and 10=worst possible pain), or a visual analogue scale by placing a cross or a checkmark along a line, the distance of which is then measured and transformed into a number between 0 and a chosen extreme, or by choosing one of several pain categories (e.g. no pain, mild, moderate, severe, unbearable pain) (Fig. 42.15). By using any one of these methods, a categorical or continuous outcome parameter can be derived, allowing for appropriate statistical assessment of postprocedural pain along a time axis of follow-up.

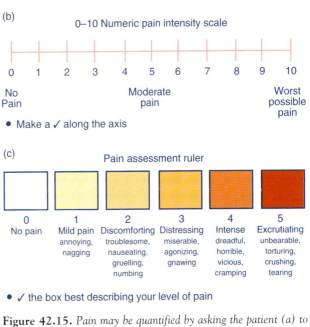

Figure 42.15. *Pain may be quantified by asking the patient (a) to place a checkmark along a visual analogue scale between two extremes ('no pain' and 'worst possible pain'), (b) to place a checkmark along a numerical scale between two extremes, and (c) to check one of several categories of pain severity.*

Another approach to quantitative pain assessment is the counting of the number and dosage of pain medications administered either parenterally, per rectum or orally in a predefined peri- and postoperative period. By converting the different pain medications used to a single equivalency measure (e.g. mg morphine sulfate equivalent), a continuous outcome parameter is again created, allowing for statistical assessment of need for pain medication following various treatment interventions.

Urinary incontinence

The prevalence of urinary incontinence in non-institutionalized persons over the age of 60 years has been estimated to range from 15 to 30%, with the prevalence being twice as high in women compared to men. Up to one-third of those identified as incontinent have frequent episodes, usually daily or weekly.[63] The prevalence of incontinence in nursing home residents is even higher and is estimated to be 50% or more.

Every reporting of incontinence as a result of treatment for BPH must be seen and interpreted against this background. Whereas traditionally, incontinence following surgery has been reported as either 'stress' or 'total' incontinence at an unspecified time interval,[2] every effort should be made in future to specify the type, onset and severity of incontinence, as well as the treatment necessary and given for it. This could, ideally, be accomplished by the administration of an incontinence questionnaire before and shortly after treatment, and at appropriate follow-up time points. A standardized, validated incontinence questionnaire for men should be developed, perhaps modelled on incontinence questionnaires already existing for women.[64,65]

Incontinence thus could be reported as a continuous variable, and appropriate statistical analyses before and after treatment, as well as comparisons between therapies, could be performed.

Erectile dysfunction and retrograde ejaculation

The prevalence of erectile dysfunction increases with advancing age.[66–70] The prevalence of impotence in men with BPH is similar to that in age-matched controls (Fig. 42.16).[70] Erectile dysfunction following treatment for BPH has to be interpreted in the context of these prevalence figures. In the past, reporting was limited to global statements regarding the percentage of patients rendered impotent after TURP, often regardless of their potency status prior to surgery. Even when the literature is limited to those series allowing for a separate analysis of preoperatively potent patients, a mean probability of impotence induced by TURP of 13.6% was calculated.[2] Newer studies have refuted this high estimate,[71] indicating that impotence induced by TURP is a very rare event (see Chapter 31).

Every effort should, therefore, be made to report erectile function and dysfunction following treatment for BPH, as accurately and quantitatively as possible. Thus, the method of assessment [such as unstructured interview, questionnaire, snap gauge or nocturnal penile tumescence (RigiScan™) testing] should be specified,

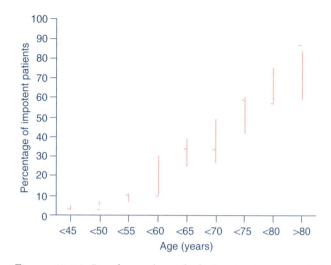

Figure 42.16. *Prevalence of erectile dysfunction in age-matched controls and patients with BPH. Shown is the range reported for normal controls stratified by age and the prevalence in men with BPH (horizontal dash). (Adapted from ref. 2 with permission.)*

and the degree of dysfunction quantified and converted to a continuous variable by the use of a standardized validated questionnaire[72] (Appendix 42.2). The use of such a tool allows for statistical analyses before and after treatment, and for comparisons between treatments.

Retrograde ejaculation is of concern mostly to young patients interested in maintaining fertility. Both surgical and minimally invasive treatments, as well as therapy with an alpha-blocker may affect antegrade ejaculation. Retrograde ejaculation may be present only temporarily after certain interventions; thus, the number of men suffering from this outcome in relation to the total number of men followed should be reported for the appropriate time points.

Hospital stay, loss of work time and recovery time

Although efforts should be made to measure and report accurately the recovery time and loss of work time, these are usually estimates at best. The only variable that can be measured and reported accurately is the number of days of hospital stay. Unfortunately, owing to changing economic factors, this number is quite meaningless when comparing hospital stay from one country to another, and from one health-care delivery system to another (e.g. Veterans Administration versus managed care versus private practice; rural versus urban environment). Even within a given health-care delivery system, hospital stay may vary significantly from year to year, and certainly from one decade to another, making comparisons between treatment modalities all but meaningless. However, recovery time and loss of work time are much less influenced by economic considerations, and improved ways to capture and report these outcomes should be sought.

Cost of treatment

Cost can be divided into the direct, the indirect and the intangible cost of treatment for BPH (see Chapter 44). Although there is a growing consensus that cost data should be collected and reported,[73] much additional work is needed to provide data on intangible and indirect costs, and cost–effectiveness analysis of individual treatment strategies. Indeed, a formal cost–effectiveness analysis has been conducted and reported only for the alpha-receptor-blocker terazosin in an all-cost analysis compared with placebo.[74] A formal discussion of the problems involved in the reporting of cost data is beyond the scope of this chapter.

Long-term complications

There are several well-recognized long-term complications of surgical treatment for BPH that in turn require health-care intervention in their own right. The classic complications are the development of a bladder neck contracture and/or of a urethral stricture following either TURP or open prostatectomy (see Chapter 31). Several of the minimally invasive treatment modalities may also have long-term complications, as yet unrecognized. When reporting treatment outcomes, it is important to specify the number of patients available at each of the long-term follow-up time points, and to relate the number of occurrences to the number of patients at each time point. To facilitate comparison between treatments, standardized definitions (ICD-9 codes) should be utilized. Whereas some of these complications do not require any interventions beyond a single dilatation, others require formal surgical repair. The outcomes should therefore be categorized in relation to their severity and requirements for subsequent treatment.

Treatment failure and need for re-treatment

Treatment failure and re-treatment rates are rather difficult to estimate from currently existing literature,[2]

for several reasons. Older surgical literature tended to report the perioperative outcomes without giving much considerations to subsequent treatments. Newer medical treatment trials enrol patients with the declared intent of following them for a defined period. Once the last follow-up visit is completed, patients are all but forgotten and the case-report books are closed. There is a considerable incentive for patients to stay in a trial until it is officially terminated: they receive free medication and some form of care. Even without appreciable improvements in symptoms, some patients might be content to continue until the end, and then to opt either for no further treatment, or for the purchase of medication to continue their treatment, or for surgical intervention — once they had learned whether they had been receiving a placebo or active drug. Thus, it is very difficult to extrapolate from the number of patients who withdraw from a trial to the number of actual treatment failures. This problem is often bypassed by defining a priori a certain symptom improvement margin as success as opposed to failure. The number of patients seeking alternative treatments at the end of a trial may also be misleading, because a significant number of participants wait patiently until the end of the study to choose from a variety of other therapeutic modalities. This situation is further complicated by the fact that treatment failure, by any definition, is not the same as the need for re-treatment. If definition and accounting of treatment failures are imprecise, the definition of 'need for re-treatment' is even less precise. It is very well understood that the threshold differs for each patient to undergo treatment by whatever modality, and surgical treatment for BPH is a notoriously poor study endpoint.

A review of the available literature was performed for the AHCPR BPH Guidelines and probabilities of re-treatment were calculated (Fig. 42.17). The only therapeutic modalities for which reliable data are available, are open surgery, TURP and TUIP. The confidence intervals around the mean estimates for all other modalities are unacceptably wide, and much additional information is needed to come to a better understanding of failure and re-treatment rates.

Very similar to the US Food and Drug Administration mandate, that every patient with a penile implant or artificial urinary sphincter should be 'captured' in a database and followed indefinitely by the manufacturing

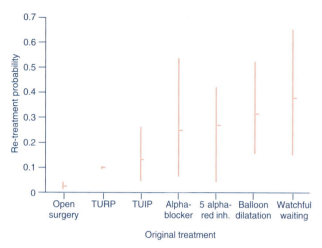

Figure 42.17. *Mean and 95% confidence interval for the probability of undergoing re-treatment within 5 years of the original treatment, based on a comprehensive meta-analysis of data from the literature. The large confidence intervals indicate the uncertainty involved in estimating re-treatment rates for all therapies with the exception of open surgery, TURP and TUIP. 5 alpha red inh., 5 alpha-reductase inhibitor.*

company, sponsors of medical or device treatment trials in BPH should contact patients following the end of the official trial at regular intervals to ascertain the behaviour of men in the years after the trial. It is very likely that the treatment choices in the years after the end of a trial, without the additional incentive of the participation in the trial, give a much more realistic estimate of the rates of treatment failure and of re-treatment.

Non-compliance with therapy and re-treatment with another form of therapy are powerful economic forces driving the cost of the original treatment modality upward, if one holds that the apparent failure of the original treatment to provide lasting symptomatic relief is responsible for the additional cost incurred by the subsequent treatment. Thus, there is a scientific and economic reason to quantify treatment failures and re-treatment rates as accurately as possible, and to report them stratified by years of follow-up, to allow comparison between treatment modalities.

Indirect health outcomes

Probability and magnitude of deterioration in flow rate, residual urine, pressure–flow parameters and prostate size

A certain number of patients will experience a deterioration or worsening in their maximum flow rate

and the pressure–flow parameters, and/or an increase in the residual urine. At present, no data are available to predict what magnitude of change in any of these parameters might be perceived by the patient as a worsening. Furthermore, little information is available to predict, from deterioration of these indirect outcomes, untoward long-term direct health outcomes. If, for example, one knew that an increase in the amount of residual urine by 100 ml predicts ultimate urinary retention within the next year, it would be important to report such data. However, at present almost all predictions of ultimate outcomes based on any of the indirect outcomes (flow rate, residual urine, pressure–flow parameters) are speculative and not substantiated by actual findings. In a study comparing TURP with watchful waiting, a higher rate of failures was noted in the watchful waiting cohort that was attributable to three outcomes — urinary retention (2.9 vs 0.4%), high residual urine volume (5.8 vs 1.1 %) and high symptom score (4.3 vs 0.4%).[71] It would, however, be an overinterpretation of such data to state that an increase in the amount of residual urine predicts ultimate failure of conservative treatment regimens. In a population-based study, Guess et al.[75] were unable to demonstrate a statistically significant relationship between amount of residual urine or peak flow rate and renal function. If one accepts an elevation of serum creatinine as a reasonable proxy for an 'ultimate' outcome, namely upper tract deterioration, one can conclude that, in fact, none of the indirect outcomes have ever been shown to be a useful predictor of such outcomes. Although pressure–flow parameters might be the best candidates for this purpose, long-term follow-up studies are not available to document that a deterioration in these parameters is followed by ultimate deterioration in upper urinary tract function.

Given the rather modest increases in prostate size reported in longitudinal studies,[61] it is unlikely that patients will ever perceive the growth of the prostate during watchful waiting or other treatments that do not affect the size of the gland. Although not scientifically established, it may be assumed that the regrowth of BPH following tissue ablative treatments follows similar rules. Consequently, the growth and/or regrowth of the prostate is of little relevance and no practical importance in the outcome reporting of BPH treatments.

The reporting of unfavourable changes in any of these parameters, therefore, is of less importance than that of unfavourable symptom score changes.

Combination of outcome parameters in reporting and categorization of outcomes

In the past, many investigators have attempted to overcome the lack of uniform reporting criteria by combining several outcome parameters into a single global assessment. Intuitively this approach has several advantages. Patients and physicians might like the concept of having to consider only one single assessment criterion, rather than a host of different parameters. Comparison between various treatments could be greatly facilitated by the availability of such a single criterion, both intuitively and statistically. However, several shortcomings of such approach have also to be considered. For one, there might be a disagreement as to which outcome parameter should contribute to a greater or lesser degree to the single criterion, and a treatment comparison based on individual parameters is impossible. In everyday life, most of us prefer to have the various parameters presented in separate columns. For example, when purchasing a car, we like to look at acquisition and maintenance cost, petrol (gas) consumption, passenger room, room for luggage, average time spent at the garage for repairs, and many other features. Rather than rolling all these parameters into a single criterion, such as a number from 1 to 100, we reserve the right to look at the individual components, since for some the luggage room is most important, for others the petrol consumption, and for yet others the reliability of the car. Even if a combined rating is offered, it usually reflects the value judgement of one single person regarding the importance of the various parameters or outcomes.

A particularly treacherous problem in reporting BPH treatment outcomes in such a fashion is the fact that, usually, a direct health outcome such as symptom improvement is combined with an indirect outcome such as flow rate recordings. A statement such as 'six months after [balloon] dilation 46% of the patients demonstrated at least a 25% improvement in subjective (symptom score) and objective (corrected peak flow rate) parameters, while 6 (21%) experienced excellent (greater than 50%) symptomatic improvement despite unchanged corrected peak flow rates and 3 (11%) showed significant (greater than 50%) improvement in corrected flow rate alone',[76] illustrates the problem that a reader (consumer) might encounter when trying to interpret and compare these data with other treatment options.

Reporting of raw baseline and post-treatment symptom score means±standard deviation (variance), however, also poses a problem for the consumer. Patients want to know what *their* chances are to *experience* symptom improvement, and not just what is the mean change in symptom index. This information cannot be learned from population statistics alone. Rather, every patient enrolled in a treatment trial has to be analysed individually and an assignment made regarding magnitude of improvement or deterioration. Using the data reported by Barry et al.,[33] a patient experiencing a drop in symptom index of three points could be assigned 'slight improvement', a patient with a drop of five points 'moderate improvement', and a patient with a drop of nine points 'marked improvement'. On the basis of the assignment of the individual patients, the probability of a new patient experiencing either improvement or worsening of his symptoms can be predicted. Using such a system, a treatment with few side effects might produce a large number of patients with slight to moderate improvement, whereas another treatment producing more marked improvements might have a higher incidence of more severe side effects.

Unfortunately, at present not enough is known about the subjective perception of changes in the various outcome parameters to facilitate such categorical assignment for other scoring systems and the indirect outcomes such as flow rate recording.

At the 3rd International Consultation on BPH in the summer of 1995 in Monaco, a system was proposed to categorize outcomes of treatment regarding symptoms, quality of life, flow rate and pressure–flow studies (Table 42.4).[77] Much additional work needs to be done before such a grid might become a useful tool in the reporting of trials in BPH for both physicians and consumers.

Table 42.4. *Response evaluation criteria proposed by the 3rd International Consultation on BPH*

Response*	I-PSS	Quality of life	Q_{max}	LPURR
Maximal				
Pretreatment	< 19	5 or 6	< 10 ml/s	> III
Post-treatment	< 8	0 or 1	> 15 ml/s	0 or I
Intermediate				
Poor	Change ≤3	No change	Change < 3 ml/s	Change in grade ≤ I

I-PSS = International Prostate Symptom Score (=AUA-SI) (range from 0 to 35 points in order of increasing symptom severity). Quality of life = assessment question for disease-specific quality of life (range from 0 to 6 points in order of decreasing quality of life). LPURR = linear passive urethral resistance relation, categorized from grade 0 to VI in increasing magnitude of obstruction. *All responses not classified as 'maximal' or 'poor' are 'intermediate' responses.
(From ref. 77 with permission.)

Reporting of follow-up of trial particpants

It is often difficult to follow the flow of patients throughout a trial, and the number of patients for whom outcomes are reported changes frequently. The Standards of Reporting Trials Group recently suggested the use of flow diagrams (Fig. 42.18) to illustrate the flow of participants through the stages of a trial, including withdrawals and timing of outcome assessments.[78] Such a diagram should accompany each reported trial, controlled or uncontrolled, to help the understanding and interpretation of the reported outcomes and the subpopulation in which they were noted.

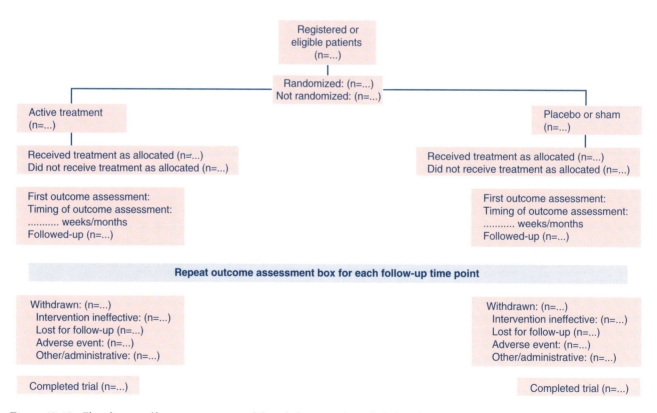

Figure 42.18. *Flow diagram of how participants passed through the stages of a trial. (Adapted from ref. 78 with permission.)*

Summary

To facilitate comparison between different treatments for BPH, certain uniform reporting criteria should be adopted by researchers in the field. Possible outcomes following treatment can be conveniently categorized as 'beneficial' or 'harmful'. Furthermore, they represent either direct health outcomes, which are felt and perceived by the patient, or indirect or proxy outcomes, which sometimes can be related to direct outcomes by way of modelling. The increased popularity of symptom, bother, quality-of-life, and sexual function scoring instruments has given us a set of continuous outcome parameters, thus facilitating quantitative reporting and comparison within and between treatment groups. Additionally there are numerous direct outcomes that are either dichotomous or categorical in nature, and for which only probabilities can be reported. It might, in future, be desirable and possible to convert some of these into quantitative outcome parameters.

A second problem in comparing different treatments for BPH is the fact that the populations differ with regard to such factors as baseline symptom severity, bother and flow rate data, as a result of different entry, inclusion and exclusion criteria. To facilitate the comparison of at least subsets of patients, reporting of outcome data stratified by baseline parameters should be encouraged.

By standardizing trial entry criteria and inclusion and exclusion parameters, and by making standardized reporting mandatory, we will in future be able to assess rapidly new treatment modalities for BPH. Furthermore, comparison of new treatments with already established older treatments can be expedited. Selection of a treatment modality may be based on many considerations and depends on the circumstances. Among two equally effective treatment modalities, a patient may select the one with fewer complications, whereas a managed-care organization may select the less expensive. Intelligent and rational choices should be based on intelligible presentation and comparison of data.

References

1. Eddy D M. A manual for assessing health practices and designing practice policies: the explicit approach. Philadelphia: American College of Physicians, 1992

2. McConnell J D, Barry M J, Bruskewitz R C et al. Benign prostatic hyperplasia: diagnosis and treatment. Clinical Practice Guideline, Number 8. Rockville, Md: Agency for Health Care Policy and Research, Public Health Service, US Department of Health and Human Services, 1994

3. Beier-Holgersen R, Bruun J. Voiding pattern of men 60 to 70 years old: population study in an urban population. J Urol 1990; 143: 531–532

4. Britton J P, Dowell A C, Whelan P. Prevalence of urinary symptoms in men aged over 60. Br J Urol 1990; 66: 175–176

5. Diokno A C, Brown M B, Goldstein N, Herzog AR. Epidemiology of bladder emptying symptoms in elderly men. J Urol 1992; 148: 1817–1821

6. Lepor H, Machi G. Comparison of AUA symptom index in unselected males and females between fifty-five and seventy-nine years of age. Urology 1993; 42: 36–41

7. Chai T C, Belville W D, McGuire E J, Nyquist L. Specificity of American Urological Association voiding symptom index: comparison of unselected and selected samples of both sexes. J Urol 1993; 150: 1710–1714

8. Mebust W K, Holtgrewe H L, Cockett A T K, Peters P C. Transurethral prostatectomy: immediate and postoperative complications. A cooperative study of 13 participating institutions evaluating 3885 patients. J Urol 1989; 141: 243–247

9. Jachuck S J, Brierley H, Jachuck S, Willcox PM. The effect of hypotensive drugs on the quality of life. J R Coll Gen Pract 1982; 32: 103-105

10. Black N, Petticrew M, Ginzler M et al. Do doctors and patients agree? Int J Technol Assess Health Care 1991; 7: 533–544

11. Doll H, McPherson K, Davies J et al. Reliability of questionnaire responses as compared with interview in the elderly: views of the outcome of transurethral resection of the prostate. Soc Sci Med 1991; 33: 1303–1308

12. Eddy D. The Confidence Profile Method: a Bayesian method for assessing health technologies. Oper Res 1989; 37: 210–238

13. Eddy D M, Hasselblad V, Shachter R. A Bayesian method for synthesizing evidence: the Confidence Profile Method. Int J Technol Assess Health Care 1990; 6: 31–56

14. Eddy D M, Hasselblad V. FAST*PRO. Software for meta-analysis by the Confidence Profile Method. San Diego: Academic Press/ Harcourt Brace Jovanovich, 1992

15. Boyarsky S, Jones G, Paulson D F, Prout G R Jr. A new look at bladder neck obstruction by the food and drug administration regulators: guide lines for investigation of benign prostatic hypertrophy. Trans Am Assoc Genitourin Surg 1976; 68: 29–32

16. Madsen P, Iversen P. A point system for selecting operative candidates. In: Hinman F (ed) Benign prostatic hypertrophy. New York: Springer-Verlag, 1983: 763–765

17. Barry M J, Fowler F J Jr, O'Leary M P et al. Correlation of the American Urological Association symptom index with self-administered versions of the Madsen–Iversen, Boyarsky and Maine Medical Assessment Program symptom indexes. Measurement Committee of the American Urological Association. J Urol 1992; 148: 1558–1563; discussion 1564

18. O'Leary M P, Barry M J, Fowler F J Jr. Hard measures of subjective outcomes: validating symptom indexes in urology. J Urol 1992; 148: 1546–1548; discussion 1564

19. Barry M J, Fowler F J Jr, O'Leary M P et al. The American Urological Association symptom index for benign prostatic hyperplasia. The Measurement Committee of the American Urological Association. J Urol 1992; 148: 1549–1557; discussion 1564

20. Cockett A T K, Aso Y, Denis L et al. Recommendations of the International Consensus Committee. In: Cockett A T K, Khoury S, Aso Y et al. (eds) The 2nd International Consultation on Benign Prostatic Hyperplasia (BPH). Jersey, Channel Islands: SCI, 1993: 553–564

21. Chancellor M B, Rivas D A. American Urological Association symptom index for women with voiding symptoms: lack of index specificity for benign prostatic hyperplasia. J Urol 1993; 150: 1706–1710

22. Jacobsen S J, Girman C J, Guess H A et al. Natural history of prostatism: factors associated with discordance between frequency and bother of urinary symptoms. Urology 1993; 42: 663–671

23. Barry M J, Fowler J F J, O'Leary M P et al. Measuring disease-specific health status in men with benign prostatic hyperplasia. Med Care 1995; 33: AS145–155

24. Guess H A, Chute C G, Garraway W M et al. Similar levels of urological symptoms have similar impact on Scottish and American men—although Scots report less symptoms. J Urol 1993; 150: 1701–1705

25. Roberts R O, Rhodes T, Panser L A et al. Natural history of prostatism: worry and embarrassment from urinary symptoms and health care-seeking behavior. Urology 1994; 43: 621–628

26. Hald T, Nordling J, Andersen J T et al. A patient weighted symptom score system in the evaluation of uncomplicated benign prostatic hyperplasia. Scand J Urol Nephrol Suppl 1991; 138: 59–62

27. Epstein R S, Deverka P A, Chute C G et al. Urinary symptom and quality of life questions indicative of obstructive benign prostatic hyperplasia. Results of a pilot study. Urology 1991; 38: 20–26

28. Bolognese J A, Kozloff R C, Kunitz S C et al. Validation of a symptoms questionnaire for benign prostatic hyperplasia. Prostate 1992; 21: 247–254

29. Eri L M, Tveter K J. Measuring the quality of life of patients with benign prostatic hyperplasia. Assessment of the usefulness of a new quality of life questionnaire specially adapted to benign prostatic hyperplasia patients. Eur Urol 1992; 21: 257–262

30. Epstein R S, Deverka P A, Chute C G et al. Validation of a new quality of life questionnaire for benign prostatic hyperplasia. J Clin Epidemiol 1992; 45: 1431–1445

31. Lukacs B, McCarthy C, Grange J C. Long-term quality of life in patients with benign prostatic hypertrophy: preliminary results of a cohort survey of 7,093 patients treated with an alpha-1-adrenergic blocker, alfuzosin. QOL BPH Study Group in General Practice. Eur Urol 1993; 24 (suppl 1): 34–40

32. Lukacs B, Leplege A, MacCarthy C, Comet D. Construction and validation of a BPH specific health related quality of life scale including evaluation of sexuality. J Urol 1995; 153: 320A

33. Barry M J, Williford W O, Chang Y C et al. BPH-specific health status measures in clinical research: how much change in AUA Symptom Index and the BPH Impact Index is perceptible to patients? J Urol 1995; 154: 1770–1774

34. Gillenwater J Y, Conn R L, Chrysant S G, et al. Doxazosin for the treatment of benign prostatic hyperplasia in patients with mild to moderate essential hypertension: a double-blind, placebo-controlled, dose-response multicenter study. J Urol 1995; 154: 110–115

35. Roehrborn C G, Oesterling J E, Auerbach S et al. Effectiveness and safety of terazosin versus placebo in the treatment of men with symptomatic benign prostatic hyperplasia in the HYCAT study. 1995;

36. Abrams P, Schulman C C, Vaage S. The efficacy and safety of 0.4 mg tamsulosin once daily in symptomatic BPH. J Urol 1995; 153: 274A

37. Golomb J, Lindner A, Siegel Y, Korczak D. Variability and circadian changes in home uroflowmetry in patients with benign prostatic hyperplasia compared to normal controls. J Urol 1992; 147: 1044–1047

38. Reynard J, Lim C-S, Abrams P. The value of multiple free-flow studies in men with lower urinary tract symptoms (LUTS). J Urol 1995; 153: 397A

39. Grino P B, Bruskewitz R, Blaivas JG et al. Maximum urinary flow rate by uroflowmetry: automatic or visual interpretation. J Urol 1992; 149: 339–341

40. Girman C J, Panser L A, Chute C G et al. Natural history of prostatism: urinary flow rates in a community-based study. J Urol 1993; 150: 887–892

41. Oesterling J E, Girman C J, Panser L A et al. Correlation between urinary flow rate, voided volume, and patient age in a community-based population. Prog Clin Biol Res 1994; 386: 125–139

42. Barry M J, Cockett A T, Holtgrewe H L et al. Relationship of symptoms of prostatism to commonly used physiological and anatomical measures of the severity of benign prostatic hyperplasia. J Urol 1993; 150: 351–358

43. Abrams P, Blaivas J G, Stanton S L, Andersen J T. Standardization of terminology of lower urinary tract function. Neurourol Urodyn 1988; 7: 403–427

44. Hinman F, Cox C E. Residual urine volume in normal male subjects. J Urol 1967; 107: 641–645

45. Di Mare J R, Fish S, Harper J M, Politano V A. Residual urine in normal male subjects. J Urol 1963; 96: 180–181

46. Birch N C, Hurst G, Doyle P T. Serial residual volumes in men with prostatic hypertrophy. Br J Urol 1988; 62: 571–575

47. Bruskewitz R C, Iversen P, Madsen P O. Value of postvoid residual urine determination in evaluation of prostatism. Urology 1982; 20: 602–604

48. Abrams P. Objective evaluation of bladder outlet obstruction. Br J Urol 1995; 76: 11–15

49. Schäfer W, de la Rosette J J M C H, Hofner K. The ICS BPH study: pressure–flow studies, quality control and initial analysis. Neurourol Urodyn 1994; 13: 491–492

50. Schaefer W, Ruebben H, Noppeney R, Deutz F-J. Obstructed and unobstructed prostatic obstruction. World J Urol 1989; 6: 198–203

51. Schaefer W, Noppeney R, Ruebben H, Lutzeyer W. The value of free flow rate and pressure/flow-studies in the routine investigation of BPH patients. Neurourol Urodyn 1989; 7: 219–221

52. Griffiths D, van Mastrigt R, Bosch R. Quantification of urethral resistance and bladder function during voiding, with special reference to the effects of prostate size reduction on urethral obstruction due to benign prostatic hyperplasia. Neurourol Urodyn 1989; 8: 17–27

53. Spangberg A, Terio H, Engberg A, Ask P. Quantification of urethral function based on Griffith's model of flow through elastic tubes. Neurourol Urodyn 1989; 8: 29–52

54. Abrams P H, Griffiths D J. The assessment of prostatic obstruction from urodynamic measurements and from residual urine. Br J Urol 1979; 51: 129–134

55. Lim C S, Abrams P H. The Abrams–Griffiths nomogram. World J Urol 1995; 13: 34–39

56. Lim C S, Reynard J, Cannon A, Abrams P H. The Abrams–Griffiths number: a simple way to quantify bladder outlet obstruction. Neurourol Urodyn 1994: 13: 475–476

57. Schäfer W. A new concept for simple but specific grading of bladder outflow conditions independent from detrusor functions. J Urol 1993; 149: 356A

58. Roehrborn C G, Chinn H K, Fulgham P F et al. The role of transabdominal ultrasound in the preoperative evaluation of patients with benign prostatic hypertrophy. J Urol 1986; 135: 1190–1193

59. Simonsen O, Möller-Madsen B, Dorflinger T et al. The significance of age on symptoms and urodynamic and cystoscopic findings in benign prostatic hypertrophy. Urol Res 1987; 15: 355–358

60. Berry S J, Coffey D S, Walsh P C, Ewing L L. The development of human benign prostatic hyperplasia with age. J Urol 1984; 132: 474–479

61. Rhodes T, Girman C J, Jacobsen S J et al. Longitudinal measures of prostate volume in a community-based sample: 3.5 year followup in the Olmsted County study of health status and urinary symptoms among men. J Urol 1995; 153: 301A

62. Gormley G J, Stoner E, Bruskewitz R C et al. The effect of finasteride in men with benign prostatic hyperplasia. The

Finasteride Study Group [see comments]. N Engl J Med 1992; 327: 1185–1191

63. Diokno A C, Brock B M, Brown M B, Herzog A R. Prevalence of urinary incontinence and other urological symptoms in the noninstitutionalized elderly. J Urol 1986; 136: 1022–1025

64. Uebersax J S, Wyman J F, Shumaker S A et al. Short forms to assess life quality and symptom distress for urinary incontinence in women: the incontinence impact questionnaire and the urogenital distress inventory. Neurol Urodyn 1995; 14: 131–139

65. Shumaker S A, Wyman J F, Uebersax J S et al. Health-related quality of life measures for women with urinary incontinence: the incontinence impact questionnaire and the urogenital distress inventory. Qual Life Res 1994; 3: 291–306

66. Kinsey A C. Sexual behavior in the human male. Philadelphia: Saunders, 1948

67. Finkle A L, Moyers T G, Tobenkin M I. Sexual potency in aging males. 1. Frequency of coitus among clinic patients. JAMA 1959; 170: 1391–1393

68. Newman G, Nichols C R. Sexual activities and attitudes in older persons. JAMA 1960; 173: 33–35

69. Bowers L M, Cross R R, Lloyd F A. Sexual function and urologic disease in the elderly male. J Am Geriatr Soc 1963; 11: 647–652

70. Pearlman C K, Kobashi L I. Frequency of intercourse in men. J Urol 1972; 107: 298–301

71. Wasson J H, Reda D J, Bruskewitz R C et al. A comparison of transurethral surgery with watchful waiting for moderate symptoms of benign prostatic hyperplasia. The Veterans Affairs Cooperative Study Group on Transurethral Resection of the Prostate. N Engl J Med 1995; 332: 75–79

72. O'Leary M P, Fowler F J, Lenderking W R et al. A brief male sexual function inventory. J Urol 1995;

73. Holtgrewe H L, Ackerman R, Bay-Nielsen H et al. Economics of BPH. In: Cockett A T K, Khoury S, Aso Y et al. (eds) The 2nd International Consultation on Benign Prostatic Hyperplasia (BPH). Jersey, Channel Islands: SCI, 1993: 37–44

74. Hillman A L, Schwartz J S, Willian M K et al. The cost-effectiveness of terazosin and placebo in the treatment of moderate-to-severe benign prostatic hyperplasia. 1995;

75. Guess H A, Girman C J, Jacobsen S J et al. What levels of peak urinary flow and residual urine volume are associated with impaired renal function? J Urol 1995; 153: 475A

76. Goldenberg S L, Perez-Marrero R A, Lee L M, Emerson L. Endoscopic balloon dilation of the prostate: early experience. J Urol 1990; 144: 83–89

77. Aso Y, Abbou C, Abrams P et al. Clinical research criteria. In: Cockett A T K, Khoury S, Aso Y et al. (eds) 3rd International Consultation on Benign Prostatic Hyperplasia (BPH). Jersey, Channel Islands: SCI, 1995

78. Standards of Reporting Trials Group. A proposal for structured reporting of randomized controlled trials. JAMA 1995; 272: 1926–1931.

Appendix 42.1

(a)   **AUA SYMPTOM INDEX (range from 0 to 35 points)**

	Not at all	Less than 1 time in 5	Less than half the time	About half the time	More than half the time	Almost always
1. Over the last month how often have you had a sensation of not emptying your bladder completely after you finished urinating?	0	1	2	3	4	5
2. Over the last month, how often have you had to urinate again less than two hours after you finished urinating?	0	1	2	3	4	5
3. Over the last month, how often have you found you stopped and started again several times while urinating?	0	1	2	3	4	5
4. Over the last month, how often have you found it difficult to postpone urination?	0	1	2	3	4	5
5. Over the last month, how often have you had a weak stream while urinating?	0	1	2	3	4	5
6. Over the last month, how often have you had to push or strain to begin urinating?	0	1	2	3	4	5
7. Over the last month, how many times did you most typically get up to urinate from the time you went to bed until the time you got up in the morning?	0 none	1 time	2 times	3 times	4 times	5 or more times

AUA-SI score [0–7 mild; 8–18 moderate; 19–35 points severe symptoms]: ....

(b)   **SYMPTOM PROBLEM INDEX (range from 0 to 28 points)**

	No problem	Very small problem	Small problem	Medium problem	Big problem
1. Over the past month, how much has a sensation of not emptying your bladder been a problem for you?	0	1	2	3	4
2. Over the past month, how much has frequent urination during the day been a problem for you?	0	1	2	3	4
3. Over the past month, how much has getting up at night to urinate been a problem for you?	0	1	2	3	4
4. Over the past month, how much has stopping and starting when you urinate been a problem for you?	0	1	2	3	4
5. Over the past month, how much has a need to urinate with little warning been a problem for you?	0	1	2	3	4
6. Over the past month, how much has impaired size and force of urinary stream been a problem for you?	0	1	2	3	4
7. Over the past month, how much has having to push or strain to begin urination been a problem for you?	0	1	2	3	4

AUA Symptom Problem Index: ....

(c)   **BPH IMPACT INDEX (range from 0 to 14 points)**

1. Over the past month, how much physical discomfort did any urinary problems cause you?	None 0	Only a little bit 1	Some 2	A lot 3
2. Over the past month, how much did you worry about your health because of any urinary problems?	None 0	Only a little 1	Some 2	A lot 3
3. Overall, how bothersome has any trouble with urination been during the past month?	Not at all bothersome 0	Bothers me a little 1	Bothers me some 2	Bothers me a lot 3

4. Over the past month, how much of the time has any urinary problem kept you from doing the kinds of things you would usually do?	None of the time 0	A little of the time 1	Some of the time 3	Most of the time 4	All of the time 5

BPH Impact Index: ....

(d)   **QUALITY OF LIFE QUESTION**

If you were to spend the rest of your life with your urinary condition just the way it is now, how would you feel about that?

Delighted	Pleased	Mostly satisfied	Mixed (about) equally satisfied and dissatisfied)	Mostly dissatisfied	Unhappy	Terrible
0	1	2	3	4	5	6

Quality-of-life score: ....

AUA SI	AUA SPI	AUA BII	QOL
0 to 35	0 to 28	0 to 14	0 to 6

Name	
First Name	
Date of Birth	
Date of Visit	

Appendix 42.2

BRIEF MALE SEXUAL FUNCTION INVENTORY

Let's define sexual drive as a feeling that may include wanting to have a sexual experience (masturbation or intercourse), thinking about having sex, or feeling frustrated due to lack of sex:

During the past 30 days, on how many days have you felt sexual drive?	No days 0	Only a few days 1	Some days 2	Most days 3	Almost every day 4
During the past 30 days, how would you rate your level of sexual drive?	None at all 0	Low 1	Medium 2	Medium high 3	High 4
During the past 30 days, how often have you had partial or full sexual erections when you were sexually stimulated in any way?	Not at all 0	A few times 1	Fairly often 2	Usually 3	Always 4
During the past 30 days, when you had erections, how often were they firm enough to have sexual intercourse?	Not at all 0	A few times 1	Fairly often 2	Usually 3	Always 4
How much difficulty did you have getting an erection during the past 30 days?	No erection at all 0	A lot of difficulty 1	Some difficulty 2	Little difficult 3	No difficulty 4
In the past 30 days, how much difficulty have you had ejaculating when you have been sexually stimulated?	No sexual stimulation 0	A lot of difficulty 1	Some difficulty 2	Little difficulty 3	No difficulty 4
In the past 30 days, how much did you consider the amount of semen you ejaculate to be a problem for you?	No climax 0	Big problem 1	Medium problem 2	Small problem 3	No problem 4
In the past 30 days, to what extent have you considered a lack of sex drive to be a problem?	Big problem 0	Medium problem 1	Small problem 2	Very small problem 3	No problem 4
In the past 30 days, to what extent have you considered your ability to get and keep erections to be a problem?	Big problem 0	Medium problem 1	Small problem 2	Very small problem 3	No problem 4
In the past 30 days, to what extent have you considered your ejaculation to be a problem?	Big problem 0	Medium problem 1	Small problem 2	Very small problem 3	No problem 4
Overall, during the last 30 days, how satisfied have you been with your sex life?	Very dissatisfied 0	Mostly dissatisfied 1	Neutral or mixed 2	Mostly satisfied 3	Very satisfied 4

Score of Brief Sexual Function Inventory (range from 0 to 44 points): ....

43

Guidelines for diagnosis and management of benign prostatic hyperplasia

J. D. McConnell

Introduction

Despite the high prevalence of benign prostatic hyperplasia (BPH) in the general population, management of the condition varies significantly, both internationally and regionally. For example, rates of prostatectomies performed per population unit vary greatly among different countries. These variations are unlikely to be due to purely geographic differences in disease prevalence or severity and may often be the result of variations in decision-making by individual practitioners.

The high prevalence of BPH in the ageing population, the unexplained geographic variations in practice patterns, the high cost of treatment and the ever-increasing number of alternative treatments entering the market-place, all make BPH an appropriate candidate for practice guidelines. Several groups have made an effort to generate BPH guidelines to assist the practitioner. The United States Government convened a panel of experts from the American Urological Association (AUA) and other specialities to develop BPH practice guidelines. This effort was funded by the Agency for Health Care Policy and Research (AHCPR), a division of the Department of Health and Human Services. The AHCPR BPH guideline panel worked for 3 years to develop practice recommendations based on 'explicit methodology'. The world's literature on BPH diagnosis and treatment was reviewed and critiqued by the panel before recommendations were made. Draft guidelines were then extensively peer-reviewed by experts and practitioners in the fields of urology, internal medicine and family practice. Further input was obtained from men affected by BPH before the final report was published.[1]

The International Consultation on Benign Prostatic Hyperplasia has met three times since 1991, most recently in June 1995, to develop practice recommendations. The International Consultation, patronized by the World Health Organization (WHO), is an international group of experts in prostatic disease who meet as individual committees to develop recommendations on the diagnosis and treatment of BPH, utilizing a 'consensus approach'.[2] However, the committee have relied heavily on published data during their review, even though explicit methodology was not utilized.

Despite the fact that these two groups have utilized different approaches for the development of practice guidelines, it is remarkable that they have come to very similar conclusions.[1,2] The 1995 report of the International Consultation was not published at the time this chapter went to press. Therefore, comparisons between the two recommendations focus on the AHCPR document and the 1993 International Consultation report. There are slight differences between the two documents, primarily concerning the appropriate role of diagnostic tests; however, the treatment recommendations are very similar. The author chaired the AHCPR panel and relied heavily on text from the previously published report[1] for the current review.

Initial evaluation

Medical history

In the AHCPR guidelines, a detailed medical history focusing on the urinary tract, previous surgical procedures, general health issues, and fitness for possible surgical procedures is recommended.[1] In the International Consultation recommendations, a history is highly recommended.[2]

Specific areas to discuss when taking the history of a man with BPH symptoms include a history of haematuria, urinary tract infection, diabetes, nervous stricture disease, urinary retention, and aggravation of symptoms by cold or sinus medication. Current prescription and over-the-counter medications should be examined to determine if the patient is taking drugs that impair bladder contractility (anticholinergics) or that increase outflow resistance (sympathomimetics).

Physical examination

In the AHCPR guidelines, a digital rectal examination (DRE) and a focused neurological examination are recommended.[1] In the International Consultation recommendations, these tests are highly recommended.[2]

The DRE and neurological examination are done to detect prostate or rectal malignancy, to evaluate anal sphincter tone and to rule out any neurological problems that may cause the presenting symptoms. The presence of induration is as important a finding as the presence of a nodule.

The outcomes of these tests are not entirely known, and the specificity of the rectal examination for the detection of prostate cancer is limited. Only 26–34% of men with suspicious findings on DRE have positive biopsies for cancer.[3–5] The sensitivity is equally low and in one study was found to be only 33%.[6] Nevertheless, given the minimal expense, discomfort and time involved, most patients would opt to have the DRE done. Although the Preventive Services Task Force[7] could not recommend for or against inclusion of the DRE in periodic health examinations, that recommendation applies to screening of asymptomatic men and not specifically to ageing men with symptoms of prostatism.

Furthermore, the rectal examination establishes the approximate size of the prostate gland. In patients who choose or require invasive therapy such as surgery, estimation of prostate size is important to select the most appropriate technical approach. DRE provides a sufficiently accurate measurement in most of these cases. However, the size of the prostate should not be considered in deciding whether active treatment is require. Prostate size does not correlate with symptom severity, degree of urodynamic obstruction or treatment outcomes.[8–12] If a more precise measurement of prostate size than can be obtained from a DRE is needed to determine whether to perform open prostatectomy rather than transurethral resection of the prostate (TURP), ultrasound (transabdominal or transrectal) is more accurate than intravenous urography or ureterocystoscopy.

Urinalysis

In the AHCPR guidelines, a urinalysis is recommended, either by using a dipstick test or by examining the spun sediment to rule out urinary tract infection and haematuria.[1] In the International Consultation recommendations, urinalysis is highly recommended.[2]

There is insufficient evidence that urinalysis is an effective screening procedure for asymptomatic men.[7] Because serious urinary tract disorders are relatively uncommon, the positive predictive value of screening for them is low, and the effectiveness of early detection and intervention is unproven. However, in older men with BPH and a higher prevalence of these disorders, the benefits of an innocuous test such as urinalysis clearly outweigh the harms (disadvantages) involved. The test permits the selective use of renal imaging and endoscopy for patients with the greatest chance of benefiting from them. More important, urinalysis assists in distinguishing urinary tract infections and bladder cancer from BPH. These conditions may produce urinary tract symptoms (such as frequency and urgency) that mimic BPH.

The positive predictive value of urinalysis for cancer or other urological diseases is 4–26% depending on the patients screened and the rigour of follow-up studies.[13–15] If a dipstick approach is used, a test that includes leucocyte esterase and nitrate tests for the detection of pyuria and bacteriuria should be utilized.[7]

Creatinine measurement (assessment of renal function)

In the AHCPR guidelines, measurement of serum creatinine is recommended in all patients with symptoms of prostatism.[1] In the International Consultation recommendations, creatinine is highly recommended.[2]

There are many reasons for recommending creatinine measurement. One is the percentage of BPH patients who may have renal insufficiency. An analysis of basic BPH treatments contained seven studies in which the percentage of patients with renal insufficiency is mentioned.[1] In these studies, the percentage of patients with renal insufficiency ranges from 0.3 to 30%; the mean is 13.6% This may be an overestimation because the reports contain information only on those patients eventually receiving treatment. Nevertheless, the number of patients with renal insufficiency, in a population of patients seeing a physician for symptomatic prostatism, may be as high as one in ten.

It is well established that BPH patients with renal insufficiency have increased risk for postoperative complications. The risk is 25% for patients with renal insufficiency, compared with 17% for patients without the condition.[16] Moreover, the mortality increases up to sixfold for BPH patients treated surgically if they have renal insufficiency.[17,18] Of 6102 patients evaluated in 25 studies by intravenous urography prior to prostate surgery, 7.6% had evidence of hydronephrosis. Of these patients, 33.6% had associated renal insufficiency.

Elevated serum creatinine in a patient is a reason for recommending appropriate imaging studies to evaluate the upper urinary tract. In a retrospective analysis of 345 patients who had undergone prostatectomy, 1.7% (n = 6) had occult and progressive renal damage.[19] These patients had minimal or no urinary symptoms and presumably fit the category of patients with 'silent prostatism'. Measurement of serum creatinine is one modality to identify such patients. Although renal insufficiency from minimally symptomatic BPH is probably rare, the probability has yet to be defined. Meanwhile, routine creatinine measurement is reasonable.

Prostate-specific antigen

In the AHCPR guidelines, measurement of serum prostate-specific antigen (PSA) is an optional test in men with prostatism.[1] In the International Consultation recommendations, serum PSA is optional, but recommended 'if the diagnosis of prostate cancer would change the patient's management'.[2] The 1995 recommendations highly recommend that the PSA test be offered to patients with an anticipated life expectancy over 10 years, and in whom the diagnosis of cancer once established would change the treatment plan.

Measurement of the serum PSA, in combination with a DRE, increases the detection rate of prostate cancer over DRE alone. However, a policy mandating the measurement of serum PSA in all men would be controversial because of (a) the significant overlap in PSA values between men with BPH and men with pathologically organ-confined cancer, (b) a lack of consensus concerning the optimal evaluation of minimally elevated PSA values and (c) a lack of

evidence showing that PSA testing reduces the morbidity or mortality of men with prostatic disease.

A summary of four major studies demonstrated that 28% of men with histologically proven BPH have a serum PSA greater than 4.0 ng/ml.[1] Other studies confirm the association between BPH and elevated serum PSA levels. Stamey et al.[20] used the Pros-Check PSA assay (Yang Laboratories, Bellevue, WA, USA) to evaluate 73 patients with BPH and found 86% to have an elevated serum PSA level. The preoperative values ranged from 0.3 to 37 ng/ml, with the mean level being 7.9 ng/ml. After TURP, the mean value decreased to 1.3 ng/ml, with the range being 0.1–6.7 ng/ml. On the basis of these findings, the investigators concluded that benign hyperplastic tissue elevates the serum PSA level at a rate of 0.3 ng/ml/g BPH tissue (0.2 ng/ml by the Tandem-R PSA assay). Daver et al.[21] found elevated PSA levels in 68 and 70%, respectively, of clinically and histologically confirmed BPH patients (n = 150). Another study,[22] using the Tandem-R PSA assay with an established upper limit of normal of 5 ng/ml, found that 21 of 45 patients (47%) with histologically proven BPH had an elevated serum PSA level. Filella et al.,[23] also utilizing the Tandem-R PSA assay, found that 87% of patients with BPH had PSA levels greater than 2 ng/ml; 13% had levels greater than 10 ng/ml.

To be a valuable detector of early prostate cancer in patients with symptoms of prostatism, a PSA test must be able to identify and distinguish curable cancer from purely benign conditions of the prostate. In other words, a PSA test must have high sensitivity and specificity, low false-negative and false-positive rates, and high negative and positive predictive values.

Because BPH tissue contributes to the serum PSA concentration and has a high prevalence among men aged 50 and over, one way to evaluate the serum PSA value as a reliable detector of early, curable prostate cancer is to compare serum PSA values in men with organ-confined prostate cancer (patients who have the greatest likelihood of cure from definitive therapy) with serum PSA values in men who have BPH only. Pooling data from three studies shows that, of patients with organ-confined prostate cancer, 43% (136 of 319) had a PSA value within the normal range (0.0–4.0 ng/ml);[24–26] of men with BPH, 25% (148 of 597) had a PSA value above 4.0 ng/ml. Further analysis of the data demonstrates mediocre sensitivity (57%) and specificity (75%) for PSA when the values are between 4 and 10 ng/ml. The false-positive rate is significant (25%). However, true positive and negative predictive values cannot be calculated from these data because the ratio here between cancer and BPH cases is artificially high.

Comparing the individual serum PSA values for men who have BPH with the values for patients who have organ-confined prostate cancer, Partin et al.[24] found no statistically significant difference between the two groups. The mean value (± standard error) for men with BPH was 5.98±1.0 ng/ml, whereas the mean level for the patients with organ-confined prostate cancer was 5.62±0.6 ng/ml. Similar results are obtained when clinical stage A and B prostate cancer patients are compared with men who have BPH.[27] These findings indicate that serum PSA concentration does not have either the sensitivity or the specificity of an ideal detector. On an individual basis, serum PSA is not a reliable test for distinguishing men with BPH from patients with early prostate cancer. New tests, such as the 'free' versus complexed PSA test, may improve PSA performance.

When the role of PSA in the diagnostic work-up of patients with BPH is evaluated, a key question is how many of the approximately 10–15% of patients found to have stage A1 or A2 prostate cancer at the time of TURP would be detected prior to surgery. The approach to some of these men might be different if a preoperative evaluation uncovered an impalpable prostate cancer.

Although most of this discussion has focused on the accuracy of PSA testing, a more important issue is that the value of early prostate cancer detection itself is controversial. Unfortunately, no data are available to establish that earlier diagnosis leads to decreased morbidity or mortality. The average age of patients undergoing surgical treatment of BPH is 67 years. A substantial number of men presenting with prostatism will, therefore, be over 70, when the value of aggressive treatment with radical prostatectomy or radiation therapy is subject to question even by advocates of early detection and treatment.

Several large-scale investigations are under way to address these issues. Until this information becomes available, it is reasonable that a serum PSA determination be considered an optional diagnostic test in evaluating men presenting with prostatism. PSA determination would presumably be of most value in those men for whom the diagnosis of non-palpable prostate cancer would change the BPH treatment recommendation.

Symptom assessment

In the AHCPR guidelines, the International Prostate Symptom Score (I-PSS), which is identical to the AUA Symptom Index, is recommended as the symptom scoring instrument to be used in the initial assessment of each patient presenting with symptoms of prostatism. When the I-PSS system is used, symptoms should be classified as mild (0–7), moderate (8–19) or severe (20–35). The symptom score should be the primary determinant of treatment response or disease progression in the follow-up period.[1] In the International Consultation recommendations, use of the I-PSS is highly recommended in the initial evaluation.[2] The 1995 International Consultation will also recommend routine use of a voiding diary, especially when nocturia is the predominant symptom.

Most patients seeking treatment for BPH do so because of bothersome symptoms that affect the quality of their lives. Tools to quantify those symptoms are important to determine the severity of the disease and to document the response to therapy, to assess the patient's symptoms, and to follow them over time to determine the progression of the disease and points of necessary intervention. Such assessment tools also allow comparison of the effectiveness of various interventions. To the patient, of course, relief of symptoms is the single most important outcome, not flow rate, detrusor pressure or urethral resistance factors.

The I-PSS was developed by the Measurement Committee of the AUA. A full questionnaire was administered to patients with a clinical diagnosis of BPH, who were drawn from urological practices, and to younger control subjects without urinary complaints, who were drawn from a general medical practice.[28] On the basis of how well the individual symptom questions correlated to two ratings of the overall 'bother' of each subject's urinary difficulties, a seven-question set was selected for further testing; it covered the symptoms of incomplete emptying, frequency, intermittency, urgency, a weak stream, hesitancy and nocturia. This seven-question set was internally consistent (Cronbach's alpha = 0.85). Moreover, the reliability of the index was high, with a test–retest correlation of 0.93.

The index correlated strongly with patients' global ratings of their urinary difficulties ($r = 0.78$), providing evidence of the construct validity of the instruments. The tentative AUA index was also correlated with the Madsen–Iversen and Boyarsky scores obtained on the same subjects. The correlations, 0.85 and 0.93, respectively, were high. This provided additional evidence of construct validity.[29]

Finally, as a test of criterion validity, the ability of the index to separate the BPH patients from the control subjects in the validation study was examined. The area under the receiver operating characteristic (ROC) curve for these indices, a measure of discrimination that uses each patient's score as a diagnostic test for BPH, was 0.87. This measure suggests that a randomly selected BPH patient and a randomly selected control subject from the study population would be correctly classified 87% of the time.

On the basis of the results of this initial validation study, several questions were modified (in response to subject feedback), and the seven-item index was re-validated using the same design (this time with 107 BPH patients and 49 control subjects). Each question on the AUA Symptom Index can yield 0–5 points, producing a total symptom score that can range from 0 to 35. On re-validation, the scores again demonstrated high internal consistency (Cronbach's alpha = 0.86) and high test–retest reliability ($r = 0.92$). Scores were again correlated with subjects' two global ratings of their urinary problem ($r = 0.65$ and 0.72) and again discriminated BPH patients from control subjects (ROC area = 0.85).

As a final validation step, the sensitivity of the AUA Symptom Index — its ability to capture clinically important changes in patients' conditions — was assessed. Twenty-seven men with symptomatic BPH answered the questionnaire before and 1 month after having a prostatectomy. Their scores dropped from a mean of 17.6 to 7.1 over this period (95% confidence interval 8.1–12.9%). This is statistically a highly significant result.

Data from the two validation studies were pooled to correlate subjects' symptom scores with the subjects' global ratings of how bothered they were by their condition. These data can be used to divide the range of the AUA score into 'mild', 'moderate' and 'severe' symptom categories. Only one of 120 men with scores from 0 to 7 was bothered more than a little by his symptoms; these men can be considered the mild symptom group. The majority of the 108 men with symptom scores from 8 to 19 were still bothered 'not at all' or 'a little', only four of the 108 being bothered 'a lot'; these men can be labelled as having moderate symptoms. Most men with scores from 20 to 35 were bothered by their condition, 'some' or 'a lot' and can be considered to have severe symptoms.

Clearly, symptom scores alone do not capture the morbidity of a prostate problem as perceived by the individual patient. Symptom impact on a patient's life style must be considered as well. An intervention may make more sense for a moderately symptomatic patient who finds his symptoms very bothersome than for a severely symptomatic patient who finds his symptoms quite tolerable.

In conclusion, the objective documentation of a patient's symptom level is the most essential part of current US and international recommendations for the diagnosis, evaluation, treatment planning and follow-up of patients with prostatism. The I-PSS (AUA Symptom Index), currently the best available instrument, is recommended. However, it should be emphasized that optimal treatment decisions in individual patients will also need to take into account how a given level of symptoms affects each patient's quality of life (bothersomeness).

Additional diagnostic tests

In the AHCRP guidelines, patients with a normal initial evaluation and only mild symptomatology on the I-PSS (scores of 0–7), do not need additional diagnostic evaluation (Fig. 43.1). These patients should be placed in a watchful waiting programme and followed. Urinary flow rate, post-void residual urine (PVR), and pressure–flow urodynamic studies are optional in the evaluation of men with moderate to severe symptoms (AUA symptom score ≥ 8). Ureterocystoscopy is optional during later evaluation if invasive treatment is being strongly considered.[1] In the International Consultation recommendations, urinary flow rate and PVR are recommended.[2] This International Consultation recommendation is maintained in the 1995 report.

The urinary symptoms commonly seen in men with BPH are not specific. Urinary tract infection, urethral stricture disease, bladder cancer and primary bladder disease may mimic the symptoms of BPH. In most cases, the differential diagnoses can be ruled out by the medical history or the basic evaluation. In some cases, further diagnostic evaluation is warranted.

After reviewing the available diagnostic tests, including ureterocystoscopy, urinary flow rate and pressure–flow studies, the panel concluded that

evidence was insufficient to mandate use of any of these tests in patients with moderate to severe symptoms before offering treatment alternatives. The decision to perform additional diagnostic testing should be left to clinical judgement.

It may be appropriate for the physician to offer treatment alternatives to the patient without performing any further diagnostic tests. In particular, if the patient chooses watchful waiting or non-invasive therapy, invasive diagnostic tests may not be necessary. Conversely, even if optional diagnostic tests were not performed initially and if the patient chooses an invasive treatment option, it may be appropriate for the physician to consider further evaluation.

Diagnostic tests in men who require BPH surgery

Both the AHCPR and International Consultation recommendations recommend surgery if the patient has refractory urinary retention (failing at least one attempt

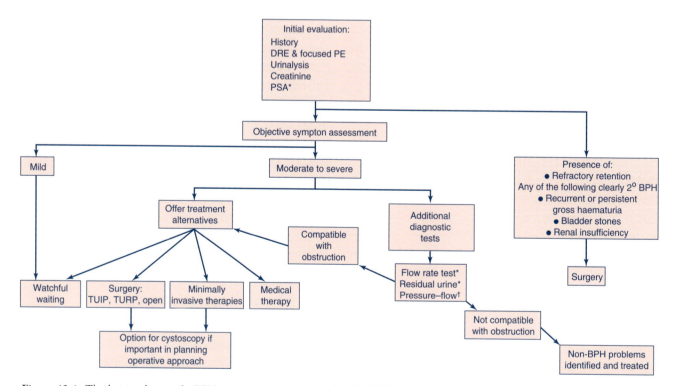

Figure 43.1. *The decision diagram for BPH management recommended by the AHCPR BPH Guideline Panel. *Optional in AHCPR guidelines; recommended by the International Consultation. †Optional in both AHCPR and International Consultation recommendations. PE, physical examination. (From ref. 1 with permission.)*

at catheter removal) or any of the following conditions, clearly secondary to BPH: recurrent urinary tract infection, recurrent gross haematuria, bladder stones, renal insufficiency or large bladder diverticula (Fig. 43.1).[1,2] In this situation, the performance of further diagnostic tests is not necessary unless there is reason to suspect that the patient's retention may be due to primary bladder disease. In that case, urodynamic studies (filling cystometry, for example) may be helpful. Pressure–flow urodynamic studies are not possible if the patient cannot urinate. Ureterocystoscopy is appropriate to consider prior to the operative procedure, to help plan the most prudent approach.

The presence of infection and haematuria in patients should prompt appropriate evaluations for these conditions prior to treatment of the BPH.

Uroflowmetry

In the AHCPR guidelines, urinary flow rate recording (uroflowmetry) is an optional test in the evaluation of men with prostatism.[1] In the International Consultation recommendations, flow rate is a recommended test.[2]

Uroflowmetry is the electronic recording of the urinary flow rate throughout the course of micturition. It is a common, non-invasive urodynamic test used in the diagnostic evaluation of patients presenting with symptoms of bladder outlet obstruction. The results of uroflowmetry are non-specific for causes of the symptoms. For example, an abnormally low flow rate may be caused by an obstruction (hyperplastic prostate, urethral stricture, meatal stenosis or other obstruction) or by weakness of the detrusor (bladder) muscle. The following statements can be made regarding uroflowmetry:

1. Flow-rate recording is the single best non-invasive urodynamic test to detect lower urinary tract obstruction. Current evidence, however, is insufficient to recommend a given 'cutoff' value to document the appropriateness of therapy.
2. The peak flow rate (Q_{max}) identifies patients with BPH more specifically than does the average flow rate (Q_{ave}).
3. Although Q_{max} decreases with advancing age and decreasing voided volume, no age or volume correction is currently recommended for clinical practice.

4. Although considerable uncertainty exists, patients with a Q_{max} greater than 15 ml/s appear to have somewhat poorer treatment outcomes after prostatectomy than patients with a Q_{max} of less than 15 ml/s.
5. A Q_{max} of less than 15 ml/s does not differentiate between obstruction and bladder decompensation.

The crucial issues for flow-rate recording in regard to patients with symptoms of prostatism are (a) the test's sensitivity in detecting patients with BPH, (b) the test's specificity in excluding those with symptoms due to some other cause than BPH, and (c) the test's ability to identify those patients most likely to have a positive outcome following treatment and those patients who probably will not have a positive outcome.

Despite its limitations, flow-rate recording has demonstrated some sensitivity in diagnosing BPH. Scott et al.[30] and Shoukry et al.[31] found that Q_{max} correlated better than symptoms with the presence or absence of obstruction as determined by pressure–flow studies. Siroky et al.[32,33] concluded that uroflowmetry was able to separate physiologically unobstructed and obstructed patients. Gleason et al.[34] found that Q_{max} distinguished between normal men and patients with BPH, urethral stricture or prostatitis. However, they also noted that a subgroup of patients with a decompensated detrusor muscle could not be separated from the obstructed men on the basis of Q_{max} alone. In a similar study, significant differences were noted in both Q_{max} and Q_{ave} between normal volunteers and 16 patients with BPH who were to undergo prostatectomy.[35] After prostatectomy, both parameters improved significantly in the 16 patients, and the postoperative values approximated those of the normal population.

Chancellor et al.[36] found that flow-rate recording cannot distinguish between bladder outlet obstruction and impaired detrusor contractility as the cause for a low Q_{max}. None of eight measured, non-invasive urodynamic parameters differed significantly in 31 patients with outlet obstruction compared with those in 14 patients with impaired detrusor contractility.

Abrams and colleagues[37,38] studied the value of uroflowmetry prior to prostatectomy. Failure rates for surgery were found to decrease with the addition of flow-rate measurement to symptom assessment in preoperative evaluation.

Q_{max} appears to predict surgical outcome in some studies. In one study,[39] 53 patients underwent prostatectomy on the basis of clinical indication alone. The study population was divided according to Q_{max} into three groups — Q_{max} less than 10 ml/s, or between 10 and 15 ml/s, or greater than 15 ml/s. Patients in all three groups experienced improvement in their symptom score after surgery, but the group with a Q_{max} less than 10 ml/s before treatment had a better overall subjective outcome, as assessed by global subjective judgement.

In a report that included men studied before and 6 months after prostatectomy,[40] patients were divided into three groups — Q_{max} greater than 15 ml/s, Q_{max} between 10 and 15 ml/s, and Q_{max} less than 10 ml/s. Subjective evaluation revealed an overall symptomatic improvement rate of 89% after surgery. The difference in success rates for men falling above or below the cutoff of Q_{max} = 10 ml/s was not significant (p <0.2). When a Q_{max} cutoff of 15 ml/s was used, success rates for men above or below the cutoff value differed significantly.

Unfortunately, not all investigators have utilized 15 ml/s as the cutoff. McLoughlin et al.,[41] using urodynamic testing and a cutoff of 12 ml/s, evaluated 108 men with prostatism before and 1 year after surgery and derived the following conclusions:

1. A Q_{max} less than 12 ml/s as indicator for obstruction would subject only 3% of patients unnecessarily to TURP.
2. Routine pressure–flow studies or cystometrograms are not indicated, but the screening of flow rates followed by further urodynamic testing in patients with a Q_{max} of greater than 12 ml/s is recommended. Studies to rule out uninhibited detrusor contractions are also indicated if symptoms persist after treatment.
3. The data confirm the independent predictive value of symptoms and flow rate.

Very low flow rates do not appear to portend poor treatment outcome. In one study[10] of 84 patients undergoing surgery for symptomatic BPH, patients with a low preoperative Q_{max} (less than 7 ml/s) improved

symptomatically as much as patients with a Q_{max} greater than 7 ml/s.

Neither subjectively assessed symptoms nor quantified symptom-score analysis correlate strongly with uroflowmetry measurements. Both are independent assessment tools. Patients with a Q_{max} greater than 15 ml/s have somewhat poorer outcomes than those with a Q_{max} less than 15 ml/s (although the majority of patients still improve). Other investigators report similar findings for different Q_{max} cutoff values (for example, 12 ml/s). Patients with very bothersome symptoms suggestive of prostatism, but with a Q_{max} greater than 15 ml/s, may benefit from further urodynamic testing (that is, pressure–flow studies) to reduce the number of surgical treatment failures. A Q_{max} less than 15 ml/s does not differentiate between outflow obstruction and detrusor impairment. Apparently, no minimal threshold of Q_{max} reliably diagnoses detrusor failure or predicts a poor surgical outcome. The wide range of Q_{max} 'cutoffs' used by individual government organizations is not surprising. Every flow-rate threshold used can be supported by at least one small study.

Post-void residual urine

In the AHCPR guidelines, measurement of PVR is an optional test in the evaluation of men with prostatism; a high PVR may suggest a slightly higher likelihood of failing watchful waiting.[1] The International Consultation recommendations recommend PVR measurement.[2]

PVR is the volume of fluid remaining in the bladder immediately following the completion of micturition. Studies indicate that residual urine normally ranges from 0.09 to 2.24 ml, with a mean of 0.53 ml;[42] 78% of normal men have residual urine volumes of less than 5 ml, and 100% have volumes of less than 12 ml.[43] The following points can be made regarding PVR:

1. Residual urine volume measurement has significant intra-individual variability that limits its clinical usefulness.
2. Residual urine volume does not correlate well with other signs or symptoms of prostatism.
3. Large residual urine volumes may predict a slightly higher rate with a strategy of watchful waiting.

However, the threshold volume defining a poorer outcome is uncertain.

4. It is uncertain whether residual urine volume predicts the outcome of surgical treatment.

5. It is uncertain whether residual urine volume indicates impending bladder or renal damage.

6. Residual urine volume can be measured with sufficient accuracy non-invasively by transabdominal ultrasonography. The measurement variation due to the method is less than the biological range of patient PVR variation.

PVR measurement can be performed by non-invasive (ultrasound) and by invasive (catheterization) methods. The most common method is urethral in-and-out catheterization. Invasive techniques are accurate if performed correctly, but carry a small risk of discomfort, urethral injury, urinary tract infection and transient bacteraemia (which has not been quantified in the literature). In addition to standard diagnostic ultrasound instruments for abdominal scanning, there is a much smaller, portable and less expensive device to measure PVR (BladderScan; Bard, Inc., Covington, GA, USA). Its reported accuracy is comparable to those of more expensive ultrasound units and of catheterization. With this device, the mean difference between estimated PVR and 'true' PVR (that is, by catheterization) was 6.9 ml in 39 measurements taken in 20 children with neurogenic bladders.[44] In 164 measurements in adult patients,[45] the correlation coefficient was $r = 0.79$.

Birch et al.[46] reported that, of 30 men with BPH, 66% had wide variations in PVR when three measurements were done on the same day using five different formulae to calculate the volume. In 34% of patients there was no difference between the three measurements. In 58%, at least two volumes were significantly different; in 8% of patients, all three were different. In most patients, two measurements were statistically similar while the third one yielded quite different results. This study proves that the intra-individual variation of the amount of residual urine is greater than the differences between the various formulae used.

Bruskewitz et al.[47] found similarly wide variations of the measured amount when they performed repetitive measurements of PVR (repeated 2–5 times) by in-and-out catheterization on 47 men prior to prostatectomy. They also found no correlation between the amount of residual urine and any ureterocystoscopic or urodynamic findings, symptoms, or the presence or absence of a history of urinary tract infections.

The intra-individual variation in PVR measurement is significant, regardless of the techniques used. Although repeated measurements may minimize the error, this is either costly (non-invasive techniques) or uncomfortable (invasive techniques) for the patient.

Shoukry et al.[31] found that 22% of 44 men with significant levels of residual urine on intravenous urography films had a 'normal' Q_{max}. These data indicate a poor correlation between the volume of residual urine and other urodynamic assessments of obstruction severity.

Griffiths and Castro[48] measured PVR by radiographic methods in 45 men with prostatism and found a reasonable correlation with the amount determined by catheterization, but no correlation with other clinical data such as prostatic size, Q_{max}, maximal bladder pressure, urethral resistance and symptom scores. Most investigators believe that large amounts of PVR urine indicate severe obstruction; however, Griffiths and Castro[48] found that 24% of the patients with severe obstruction had less than 50 ml of PVR urine.

PVR was found to be of little help in assessing 117 patients with BPH in a study by Abrams and Griffiths,[49] who considered PVR urine to be an indication of abnormal bladder function or detrusor decompensation rather than evidence of urethral obstruction.

Neal et al.[50] found a significant association in 253 men between PVR, age, 'below normal' (undefined) Q_{max} and high urethral resistance; weak voiding pressure, however, did not correlate well with PVR. The authors concluded that outflow obstruction is related to the development of increasing amounts of PVR urine.

Traditionally, urologists have assumed that increasing amounts of PVR denote BPH progression and are thus an 'indication' for surgery. This concept underlies the common inclusion of PVR in the appropriateness criteria of individual governments. Unfortunately, data are lacking to support the predictive value of PVR.

Andersen[51] studied 104 men with BPH and reported two patterns of BPH progression. The slow course was characterized by the development of high levels of PVR that resulted in decompensation of the detrusor muscle and eventually led to urinary retention. The fast course was associated with uninhibited detrusor contractions (UDCs). The amount of PVR, the presence of UDCs, and symptoms correlated poorly in the study. Nevertheless, Andersen recommended PVR as a safety parameter, when measured longitudinally throughout the clinical course of a patient with prostatism.

Jensen et al.[52] examined the prognostic value of PVR and 14 other clinical and urodynamic variables in relation to outcome of surgery in 120 men with prostatism. They found PVR the second-best predictor of outcome, after pressure–flow studies. However, the combination of these two predictors did not allow the authors to predict correctly the outcome in any of 14 patients who failed treatment. The authors did correctly predict all successfully treated patients.

Unpublished data from a randomized trial comparing TURP with watchful waiting (Veterans' Affairs Cooperative Study Group), demonstrate that PVR does not predict the outcome of surgery, and there appears to be little evidence to support criteria that require a certain amount of PVR before surgery is justified.[53] High PVR did predict, in this trial, a slightly higher failure rate for watchful waiting. However, the majority of men with large residual urine volume did not require surgery during the 3 year duration of the trial.

The volume of PVR correlates poorly with other signs and symptoms of prostatism. The common assumption — that the amount of residual urine predicts which men will or will not improve after surgery for prostatism — is not adequately supported by enough evidence to mandate use of the test. The test was, therefore, considered by the AHCPR panel to be optional in the evaluation of men presenting with prostatism.

The AHCPR panel believes that present review criteria requirements, for certain amounts of residual urine before a prostatectomy is considered appropriate, cannot be justified on the basis of current data. Requiring the presence of residual urine before offering treatment implies that at least partial bladder decompensation must occur before intervention is appropriate. Nevertheless, although poorly studied in the literature, monitoring of PVR is a reasonable option for men being followed with BPH or for those selecting non-surgical therapies. It is likely that high residual urines may lead to a slightly higher failure rate for watchful waiting, but repeat measurements should be considered before making treatment decisions based on PVR values.

Prospective evaluation of the predictive value of PVR is needed. Specifically, the risks associated with given volumes must be determined in order to ascertain what PVR values are associated with a risk of urinary retention, infection or poor treatment outcome.

Pressure–flow studies

In the AHCPR guidelines, pressure–flow studies are optional in the evaluation of men with prostatism.[1] The 1993 International Consultation recommendations state that 'if the analysis of the mandatory and recommended tests [flow rate and PVR] is not sufficiently suggestive of bladder outlet obstruction, further urodynamic assessment by pressure flow studies should be proposed to the patient especially if an invasive treatment is considered (i.e. surgical)'.[2] The value of pressure–flow studies is further stressed in the 1995 International Consultation recommendations, but its use is not mandated in all cases.

Pressure–flow studies differentiate between patients with a low Q_{max} secondary to obstruction and those whose low Q_{max} is caused by a decompensated or neurogenic bladder. Pressure–flow studies may also identify high-pressure obstruction in symptomatic men with normal flow rates.

Evidence for the usefulness of pressure–flow studies to predict surgical failure is equivocal. Some investigations have reported reduced failure rates, whereas others have reported that pressure–flow studies performed no better than Q_{max} measurements in this regard. Some patients who are excluded from surgery based on the pressure–flow test may still benefit from surgery.

Pressure–flow studies are most useful for distinguishing between urethral obstruction and impaired detrusor contractility. They should be performed when the distinction between the two will affect therapeutic decisions. Patients with a history of neurological diseases known to affect bladder or sphincteric function, as well as patients with normal flow rates (Q_{max} >15 ml/s) but bothersome symptoms, may also benefit from urodynamic evaluation, particularly if surgical therapy is contemplated.

Pressure–flow studies have been developed to fill a diagnostic gap. Flow-rate measurements, although useful to document the presence or absence of an impairment of the urinary stream, cannot differentiate between obstruction and decreased bladder contractility, neither can they differentiate between types of obstruction (for example, between BPH and urethral stricture). Urodynamic experts have, therefore, developed tests that differentiate between patients who have a low Q_{max} secondary to obstruction and those who have an impaired Q_{max} secondary to detrusor failure or other causes.

The value of pressure–flow plots is accepted by many urodynamic experts. However, there is little standardization in interpretation of these plots and few clear 'cutoff' values for defining obstruction as opposed to non-obstruction. Investigators have proposed various ways to present the same sets of data and claim superior differentiation between patient groups.[38,54–58] This variability in data presentation and definition has made it difficult to analyse the evidence that supports the use of such pressure–flow plots.

The most important issue to address is predictive value. To what extent can invasive pressure–flow studies identify patients who will not improve after surgical treatment of their urinary symptoms? To what extent does the addition of pressure–flow studies enable the clinician to separate the truly obstructed from the unobstructed patients? To what extent does this distinction predict the outcome of BPH therapy? Unfortunately, only a limited number of reports present outcome data addressing the value of pressure–flow studies in reducing the symptomatic failure rate of surgery.

Bruskewitz et al.[59] studied prospectively the outcome in 46 patients with prostatism. Patients were divided into two groups with urethral resistance either less than or greater than 0.6. The authors concluded that in patients with moderate prostatism, a cutoff value of $r =$ 0.6 does not predict either indirect health outcomes (Q_{max}, detrusor pressure, resistance) or direct health outcomes (symptom score assessment, global subjective symptom assessment) after surgery.

Abrams et al.[38] examined 190 men (age 47–85 years) who underwent prostatectomy. Follow-up data after surgery were available for 152 patients. The decision to perform surgery was based on urodynamic testing, but the report did not clarify which criteria were applied to the decision to operate and whether the surgeons were blinded concerning the preoperative urodynamic evaluation. The patients were considered objectively improved after surgery if their Q_{max} was greater than 15 ml/s at a pressure less than 100 cmH_2O. Subjectively, 88% of the patients had symptom improvement, 12% showed no change, and one worsened postoperatively. Objective assessment revealed partial or complete relief of obstruction in 86% of patients. In those patients who failed to improve symptomatically, 7.5% were relieved of their urodynamic obstruction.

In an earlier study by Abrams,[37] the inclusion of urodynamic data in the preoperative evaluation and indication for surgery reduced the subjective failure rate to 12%, down from 28% when patients were certified as candidates for surgery without the urodynamic data. However, a 28% failure rate is significantly higher than that reported in other TURP series.[1]

Another study[49] used pressure–flow plots in addition to flow-rate measurement. The study found that, in about half the cases, the patients with prostatism could be correctly classified as obstructed or non-obstructed by Q_{max} alone, but that the addition of the detrusor pressure at Q_{max} allowed correct classification in two-thirds of patients. Combining the two parameters into a single urethral resistance factor did not help in the two-thirds group. The remaining one-third of the patients were assessed by pressure–flow plot. In many of these patients, both pressure and Q_{max} were low, indicating a decompensating muscle as the source for the low Q_{max}.

Jensen and Andersen[60] recommended invasive urodynamic testing for patients with a Q_{max} >15 ml/s. For the population in their study, this results in an additional 9% of patients excluded from surgery and a decrease in failure rate to 8.3%. The support for this recommendation has to be questioned, however, in the light of an earlier study by Jensen et al,[55] which found that most unsatisfied patients are incorrectly classified preoperatively, even with urodynamic testing.

Schäfer et al.[56,57] used sophisticated, computerized analysis of pressure–flow data to define passive and dynamic urethral resistance measures. They documented that approximately 25% of patients undergoing TURP are not obstructed, on the basis of the investigators' criteria, although these patients may have a low Q_{max}. The improvement rate based on objective measures (Q_{max} and PVR) was 100% in patients categorized as severely obstructed, but was lower in the mildly obstructed and non-obstructed patients. Direct health outcome data were not reported by these investigators.

The Schäfer model has been used and expanded by other investigators,[58] but correlation of the objective results with direct health outcomes (subjective results) is again lacking. Others have employed computer programs to analyse pressure–flow plots, but also do not report outcome data.[61,62] The details of the analysis and the computer program are not discussed in an outcomes context. These computer-assisted urodynamic assessments need further evaluation before they can be recommended routinely.

Pressure–flow studies provide much more specific insight into detrusor function and the aetiology of voiding dysfunction than do flow-rate measurements. However, the limited number of outcome-based investigations performed demonstrate a modest additional value of pressure–flow studies over symptom and flow-rate evaluation. The benefit of pressure–flow studies is clearest in those patients who have a Q_{max} greater than 15 ml/s or in whom the initial evaluation suggests bladder dysfunction rather than BPH as the cause of patient symptoms. Although pressure–flow plots are generally recognized to be more informative than measurement of urethral resistance, interpretation of such plots has not been standardized.

Given the uncertainties that exist concerning the pressure–flow study, its use should not be mandatory in routine cases at present. It is, however, an appropriate test in patients for whom the distinction between urethral obstruction and impaired detrusor function would affect therapeutic decisions. In addition, pressure–flow studies are appropriate in patients with underlying neurological disease that may affect detrusor or sphincteric function.

Prospective trials to demonstrate the predictive value of pressure–flow studies are under way in several countries.

Filling cystometry (cystometrography)

In both the AHCPR and International Consultation recommendations, filling cystometry, which adds limited information to the evaluation of most men with prostatism, is not recommended in routine cases. The test may have value in the evaluation of patients with known or suspected neurological lesions and prostatism, but pressure–flow studies provide more specific information. In patients with suspected primary bladder or neurological lesions and who cannot urinate (retention), filling cystometry may be useful.[1,2]

Filling cystometry, an invasive urodynamic study, provides information on bladder capacity, the presence and threshold of UDCs and bladder compliance. UDCs are present in about 60% of men with prostatism and correlate strongly with irritative voiding symptoms. Compliance is a measure of the elasticity and distensibility of the bladder wall and is expressed as the ratio of volume to pressure (ml/cm).

Filling cystometry may demonstrate UDCs, which are more common in men evaluated for prostatism than in randomly selected, age-matched controls. This urodynamic finding correlates significantly with the presence of irritative systems. Filling cystometry does not add significant new information to the evaluation of men with prostatism. UDCs resolve in most patients after surgery. Only about one-quarter of patients who have UDCs before treatment retain them afterwards. Patients whose symptoms do not improve following surgery are more likely to have persistent UDCs.

Although filling cystometry may demonstrate a poorly contractile detrusor in men with primary bladder dysfunction, pressure–flow studies provide much more insight into the interaction between bladder contraction and urethral resistance. Filling cystometry may be considered for men in urinary retention who cannot urinate for a pressure–flow study.

Urethrocystoscopy

In the AHCPR guidelines, urethrocystoscopy is not recommended to determine the need for treatment. The test is recommended for men with prostatism who have a history of microscopic or gross haematuria, urethral stricture disease (or risk factors, such as history or urethritis or urethral injury), bladder cancer, or prior lower urinary tract surgery (especially prior TURP). To help the surgeon determine the most appropriate technical approach, urethrocystoscopy is an optional test in men with moderate to severe symptoms who have chosen (or require) surgical or other invasive therapy.[1] In the 1993 International Consultation recommendations, urethrocystoscopy is an optional test.[2] However, the 1995 International Consultation recommends classifying urethrocystoscopy in a manner identical to that in the AHCPR guidelines.

Endoscopy of the lower urinary tract (urethrocystoscopy) provides visual documentation of the appearance of the prostatic urethra and bladder in men with BPH. Historically, many urologists believed that the visual appearance of the lower urinary tract defines the severity of disease or predicts the outcome of treatment. However, this common urological procedure has been poorly studied. No data are available on the sensitivity, specificity or predictive value of the test.

Urethrocystoscopy is associated with certain potential benefits and harms (although they are not quantified in the literature). Potential benefits include the ability to demonstrate prostatic enlargement and visual obstruction of the urethra and the bladder neck; identification of specific anatomical abnormalities that alter clinical decision-making; identification of bladder stones, trabeculation, cellules and diverticular; measurement of PVR; and the ruling out of unrelated bladder and urethral pathology. Potential harms include patient discomfort, anaesthetic or sedative risk, urinary tract infection, bleeding and urinary retention.

The probability of any of these harms occurring is uncertain. Except for discomfort, their occurrence is likely to be infrequent. Nevertheless, potential harms must be balanced against potential benefits of this invasive procedure.

The endoscopic appearance of the bladder and prostate is often felt to be helpful in the decision to treat. Although the linkage between the endoscopic appearance of the lower urinary tract and treatment outcome is poorly documented in the literature, available information suggests that the relationship is minimal. Bladder trabeculation may predict a slightly higher failure rate in patients managed by watchful waiting, but does not predict the success or failure of surgery. Urethrocystoscopy may, nevertheless, be useful in determining the technical feasibility of specific

invasive therapies. For example, if urethrocystoscopy reveals a large middle lobe, balloon dilatation and transurethral incision of the prostate (TUIP) are unlikely to be successful. The decision to perform an open prostatectomy may be appropriately influenced by the shape of the gland, as well as its size. In all these cases, however, the patient and his physician have already selected invasive therapy. Urethrocystoscopy is therefore performed to select (or rule out) specific techniques, not to determine the need for treatment.

The remote probability of identifying, by urethrocystoscopy, lower urinary tract complications possibly attributable to BPH, in men without haematuria, urinary tract infection, or a history of risk factors, makes the routine use of this procedure for all men with prostatism questionable. Available data suggest that there is a minimal relationship between the endoscopic appearance of the lower urinary tract and treatment outcome. However, urethrocystoscopy may be useful in determining the technical feasibility of specific invasive therapies.

Imaging of the urinary tract

In the AHCPR guidelines, upper urinary tract imaging is not recommended in the routine evaluation of men with prostatism unless they also have one or more of the following: haematuria; urinary tract infection; renal insufficiency (ultrasound recommended); history of urolithiasis; history of urinary tract surgery.[1] In the 1993 International Consultation recommendations, upper tract (renal) imaging and transabdominal/transrectal ultrasound imaging of the prostate was classified as optional, but in the 1995 recommendations the classification is identical to that in the AHCPR guidelines.[2]

Intravenous urography (IVU), to image the urinary tract of men with BPH before treatment, is performed by 73.4% of urologists in the United States.[63] The number of urologists using ultrasonography to image the urinary tract is unknown. IVU is associated with a 0.1% incidence of significant adverse events; no direct adverse events are known to be associated with ultrasonography.

Of all-imaging studies performed in men with BPH, results in 70–75% are entirely normal.[1] Only a small fraction of the 25–30% of abnormal findings mandate changes in the management of the patient. The incidence of any significant findings is no higher in the urinary tract of men with BPH, compared with age- and sex-matched controls, except for bladder stones, diverticula, and trabeculation indicating the presence of bladder outlet obstruction.[1] A decision to restrict upper urinary tract imaging to patients with haematuria, urinary tract infection, renal insufficiency, a history of urolithiasis and a history of urinary tract surgery could result in an improved diagnostic yield and reduce cost without jeopardizing quality of care.

Bundrick and Katz[64] reported a change in management in 2.2% (four of 180) of patients, based on findings obtained on IVU in a population preselected by excluding men with haematuria, infections and a history of bladder tumours. Pinck et al.[65] deferred TURP in favour of a more urgent intervention in 2.5% (14 of 557). These data indicate that a change in management would occur in about 10% of the 25% of patients in whom the imaging study is 'abnormal'.

The presence or history of haematuria, renal insufficiency, urinary tract infection, and/or history of stones or prior urinary tract surgery increases the likelihood that IVU or ultrasonography will demonstrate clinically significant findings.[66–74] Donker and Kakiailatu[75] reported that, by screening those men with urinary tract infections, gross haematuria and renal insufficiency, they would have diagnosed almost all of the abnormal findings in their population of 307 men with BPH.[1] Although there are no conclusive data on the combined incidence of the important clinical predictors listed above, approximately one-third of all men with BPH have one or another indication for urinary tract imaging.

Assuming that an indication for renal imaging exists, a number of investigators strongly recommend, instead of IVU, ultrasonography combined with a KUB and a determination of the renal function by measurement of the serum creatinine.[76–82] This policy is sound if the level of renal insufficiency prohibits the performance of an IVU (which is rarely the case). Ultrasonography is more specific in determining the nature of a renal mass lesion, thus not requiring as many confirmatory studies as IVU. In a significant percentage (7.5%) of patients, however, the imaging will be inadequate. For the evaluation of haematuria, IVU has been found to be the more sensitive study.

BPH treatment guidelines

The AHCPR BPH Guideline Panel and the 2nd International Consultation committee collected and reviewed data for commonly utilized, as well as experimental, BPH treatments available at the time.[1,2] There was adequate evidence in the literature to estimate outcomes for the following treatments:

1. *Watchful waiting*: a strategy of management in which the patient is monitored by his physician, but receives no active intervention for BPH.
2. *Alpha-blocker therapy*: treatment using any of the class of alpha-1-adrenergic receptor blockers (including doxazosin, prazosin and terazosin) that inhibit alpha-adrenergic-mediated contraction of prostatic smooth muscle.
3. *Finasteride therapy*: treatment using the drug finasteride, an inhibitor of the enzyme 5-alpha-reductase, which lowers prostatic dihydrotestosterone levels and can result in some decrease in prostate size.
4. *Transurethral incision of the prostate (TUIP)*: an endoscopic surgical procedure limited to patients with smaller prostates (30 g or less of resected weight) in which an instrument is passed through the urethra to make one or two cuts in the prostate and prostate capsule, reducing constriction of the urethra. This procedure can be done on an outpatient basis.
5. *Transurethral resection of the prostate (TURP)*: surgical removal of the prostate's inner portion by an endoscopic approach through the urethra, with no external skin incision. This is the most common active treatment for symptomatic BPH and usually requires a hospital stay.
6. *Open prostatectomy*: surgical removal (enucleation) of the inner portion of the prostate via a suprapubic or retropubic incision in the lower abdominal area. Rarely, the procedure done through the perineum. Open prostatectomy requires a longer hospital stay than do the other surgical procedures.

Treatment modalities such as thermal therapy, laser prostatectomy, electrovaporization and prostatic stents have not been analysed as part of the guidelines recommendations. These approaches appear, in initial trials, to be promising, but further data are required before they can be recommended as worldwide treatment standards. Two new medical agents, tamsulosin (alpha-blocker) and episteride (5-alpha-reductase inhibitor), are in clinical trails. Phytotherapy is a widely used treatment option in Europe, but current data are insufficient to recommend this approach. The 1995 International Consultation recommendations view thermal therapy and phytotherapy as treatment options, but state that these therapies may not relieve obstruction.

Treatment recommendations

On the basis of the AHCPR BPH Guideline Panel's review of treatment options available in clinical practice, as well as the preferences of patients, the following practice recommendations were made (see Fig. 43.1).[1]

Patients with mild symptoms of BPH (I-PSS score ≤7) should be followed in a strategy of watchful waiting. The patient's symptoms and clinical course should be monitored, usually annually. He should be instructed on behavioural techniques to reduce symptoms, such as limiting fluid intake after dinner and avoiding decongestants. Probabilities of disease progression or the development of BPH complications are uncertain. Until research defines these probabilities, patients in a strategy of watchful waiting should be monitored periodically by reassessment of symptom level, physical findings, routine laboratory testing, and optional urological diagnostic procedures. If the patient's symptoms progress to moderate or severe levels, as defined by the I-PSS, it is appropriate to reassess the symptoms with the patient, to determine whether the condition is bothersome or is interfering with his health and to offer him other treatment options, if applicable. The International Consultation recommendation is to pursue watchful waiting if the symptoms are not bothersome.[2] The international group did not suggest a specific I-PSS 'cutoff' value (e.g. 7).

Patients with moderate and severe symptoms (I-PSS score ≥8) should be given information on the benefits and harms of watchful waiting, alpha-blocker therapy, finasteride therapy and surgery. The International Consultation

recommendations do not mention the use of specific I-PSS values;[2] rather, they recommend that 'the patient with "bothersome symptoms" must be informed of all available and acceptable treatment options applicable to his clinical condition and the related risks and benefits of each modality'.[2] The international group did not recognize balloon dilatation as an option, but did consider stents an option for high-risk patients in retention. Although balloon dilatation was considered in the AHCPR guidelines, it is no longer considered an appropriate option. This information should be presented to the patient in an unbiased format that expresses not only the probabilities of benefits and harms but also the range of uncertainty associated with those probabilities. The physician's opinion about optimal treatment should not be the only information communicated to the patient: actual outcome data should be presented to allow the patient to determine the best treatment for him. However, health care providers should be cautious of using educational materials developed by groups with a vested interest in a particular form of treatment.

If patients initially choose watchful waiting or treatments other than surgery, and later experience symptom progression or deterioration, it is appropriate to reassess surgery as a treatment option. However, failure to respond to medical or balloon dilatation therapy is not an absolute indication for surgery. Many patients who fail to benefit from medical therapy, for example, will elect to return to a strategy of watchful waiting rather than accept the risks of surgery.

On the other hand, surgery should not be 'reserved' for those men who fail medical or device therapy. If the patient has been fully informed, it is appropriate for him to have the option of electing surgery as his initial treatment. Choice of type of surgery (TUIP, TURP or open prostatectomy) is primarily a technical decision; this choice should be based on the surgeon's experience and judgement and should be discussed with the patient. The panel noted, however, that TUIP is an underutilized procedure that should be strongly considered for patients in whom the estimated resected tissue weight (if done by TURP) would be 30 g or less.

The following types of BPH patients should be treated surgically: (1) those with refractory urinary retention who have failed at least one attempt at catheter removal; (2)

those who have recurrent urinary tract infections, recurrent gross haematuria, bladder stones or renal insufficiency clearly due to BPH. The International Consultation recommendations add large bladder diverticular to this list.[2] There is little evidence to suggest that treatment options other than surgery benefit patients with any of these BPH complications. Nevertheless, if patients refuse surgery, or if they have sufficient medical co-morbidity to present an unacceptable risk for surgery, alternative therapies may be considered.

The foregoing treatment recommendations should not diminish the pivotal role of a caring physician in reaching an optimal treatment decision. Rather, they should expand the physician's counselling role by providing the patient with sufficient information to permit his participation in the decision-making process to the extent he desires. In those cases where the patient seeks the physician's opinion on the optional treatment strategy, or even 'surrenders' the decision completely to the physician, it is appropriate for the physician to recommend the optimal treatment and to act as the patient's proxy in the decision-making process, if necessary. The physician should take this prerogative, however, only at the patient's request.

Indirect treatment outcomes

Q_{max} and PVR are the indirect outcomes most commonly used to determine objectively the efficacy of BPH treatment in clinical research. All active treatments (alpha-blockers, finasteride, TUIP, TURP and open surgery) increase Q_{max} and decrease PVR; both Q_{max} and PVR respond very little to placebo treatment. The degree of improvement in Q_{max} and of reduction in PVR is superior with surgical treatment.

The AHCPR panel's review of indirect outcomes reported in the literature, specifically of flow rate and PVR, is intended to provide clinicians with useful information for judging the relative efficacies of treatment options.[1] Until better data are available on use of the parameters to predict the occurrence of BPH complications or response to treatment, these measurements should not be used to influence a patient's decision regarding the appropriateness of a given therapy, once a diagnosis has been established.

Direct treatment outcomes

In considering treatment, a patient may not be particularly interested in such indirect outcomes as possible improvement of his peak urinary flow rate or decrease of his residual urine, notwithstanding the importance of these parameters to many physicians. The patient is likely to be more interested in such direct outcomes as his degree of symptom improvement after treatment, the chances of complications or side effects of treatment, duration of any hospital stay, and time lost from work, as well as cost.

Patient preferences

In choosing treatments for a disease such as BPH, which principally affects the quality rather than the quantity of life and where the optimal decision may be dictated by personal values rather than scientific evidence, different patients may have different opinions concerning the benefits and harms of direct outcomes, depending on how bothered they are by their symptoms. One patient may find the risks of surgery or of other treatments acceptable, given the potential benefit; another patient may not find the risk of any therapy acceptable, because he is not bothered by his symptoms or because he is averse to any risk, or both. These differences in how individual patients weigh risks and benefits are clearly shown in studies of patient preferences.

Most patients with mild symptoms prefer watchful waiting, whereas there is a very wide range of preferences in patients with moderate symptoms.[1] Although surgery is the most commonly elected therapy for those patients with severe symptoms, a significant number of patients elected watchful waiting or another alternative therapy.

It is clear from these studies that the majority of BPH patients with mild symptoms are not sufficiently bothered by their symptoms to accept the risks of therapy, including non-invasive therapies. In patients with moderate and severe symptoms there is a wide range of preferences, probably due to varying levels of 'bothersomeness' and risk of aversion among individual patients.[1]

Given the variations in patient preferences, and because the physician's values (personal perceptions of benefits and harms) may differ from those of the patient, it is important that the patient's values take precedence in determining choice of treatment.

It is also apparent that the 'need' for therapy in patients with symptomatic BPH should, in most cases, be determined by the informed patient rather than by the physician. As made evident above, most patients with mild symptoms do not perceive a need for therapy, even with non-invasive approaches. Patients with severe symptoms may choose surgery, but many will have a preference for non-surgical intervention. However, an appreciable number of patients with moderate symptoms, after being fully informed, will also opt for surgical intervention. The concept that patients should only receive surgery if they have failed medical therapy is, therefore, not appropriate. Some patients with moderate symptoms, and who are significantly bothered by their symptoms, view the potential benefits of surgery as clearly superior to other forms of therapy, and the risks as acceptable.

References

1. McConnell J D, Barry M J, Bruskewitz R C et al. Benign prostatic hyperplasia: diagnosis and treatment. Clinical Practice Guideline No. 8, AHCPR Publication No. 94-0582. Rockville, Md: Agency for Health Care Policy and Research, Public Health Service, US Department of Health and Human Services, February 1994

2. Cockett A T K, Khoury S, Aso Y et al. (eds) Proceedings of the 2nd International Consultation on Benign Prostatic Hyperplasia (BPH). SCI Ltd, Jersey, Channel Islands, 1993

3. Thompson I M, Ernst J J, Gangai M P, Spence C R. Adenocarcinoma of the prostate: results of routine urological screening. J Urol 1984; 132: 690–692

4. Chodak G W, Keller P, Schoenberg H. Routine screening for prostate cancer using the digital rectal examination. Prog Clin Biol Res 1988; 269: 87–98

5. Lee F, Littrup P J, Torp-Pedersen S T et al. Prostate cancer: comparison of transrectal US and digital rectal examination for screening. Radiology 1988; 168: 389–394

6. Vihko P, Kontturi M, Lukkarinen D. Screening for carcinoma of the prostate: rectal examination, and enzymatic radioimmunologic measurements of serum acid phosphatase compared. Cancer 1985; 56: 173–177

7. Preventive Services Task Force (US). Guide to clinical preventive services; an assessment of the effectiveness of 169 interventions. Baltimore: Williams and Wilkins, 1989

8. Roehrborn C G, Chinn H K, Fulgham P F et al. The role of transabdominal ultrasound in the preoperative evaluation of patients with benign prostatic hypertrophy. J Urol 1986; 135: 1190–1193

9. Simonsen O, Møller-Madsen B, Dorflinger T et al. The significance of age on symptoms and urodynamic and cystoscopic findings in benign prostatic hypertrophy. Urol Res 1987; 15: 355–358

10. Donkervoort T, Zinner N R, Sterling A M et al. Megestrol acetate in treatment of benign prostatic hypertrophy. Urology 1975; 6: 580–587

11. Bissada N K, Finkbeiner A E, Radman J F. Accuracy of preoperative estimation of resection weight in transurethral prostatectomy. J Urol 1976; 116: 201–202

12. Meyhoff H H, Ingemann L, Nordling J, Hald T. Accuracy in preoperative estimation of prostatic size. A comparative evaluation of rectal palpation, intravenous pyelography, urethral closure pressure profile recording and cystourethroscopy. Scand J Urol Nephrol 1981; 15: 45–51

13. Mohr D N, Offord K P, Owen R A, Melton L J. Asymptomatic microhematuria and urologic disease. JAMA 1986; 256: 224–229

14. Mohr D N, Offord K P, Melton L J. Isolated asymptomatic microhematuria; a cross-sectional analysis of test-positive and test-negative patients. J Gen Intern Med 1987; 2: 318–324

15. Messing E M, Young T B, Hunt V B. The significance of asymptomatic microhematuria in men 50 or more years old: findings of a home screening study using urinary dipsticks. J Urol 1987; 137: 919–922

16. Mebust W K, Holtgrewe H L, Cockett A T K et al. Transurethral prostatectomy: immediate and postoperative complications. A cooperative study of 13 participating institutions evaluating 3,885 patients. J Urol 1989; 141: 243–247

17. Holtgrewe H L, Valk W L. Factors influencing the mortality and morbidity of transurethral prostatectomy: a study of 2,015 cases. J Urol 1962; 87: 450–459

18. Melchior J, Valk W L, Foret J D, Mebust W K. Transurethral prostatectomy in the azotemic patient. J Urol 1974b; 112: 643–646

19. Mukamel E, Nissenkorn I, Boner G, Servadio C. Occult progressive renal damage in the elderly male due to benign prostatic hypertrophy. J Am Geriatr Soc 1979; 27: 403–406

20. Stamey T A, Yang N, Hay A R et al. Prostate-specific antigen as a serum marker for adenocarcinoma of the prostate. N Engl J Med 1987; 317: 909

21. Daver A, Soret J Y, Coblentz Y et al. The usefulness of prostate-specific antigen and prostatic acid phosphatase in clinical practice. Am J Clin Oncol 1988; 11: 53–60

22. Buamah P K, Johnson P, Skillen A W. Comparative study of the clinical usefulness of prostate specific antigen and prostatic acid phosphatase in prostatic disease. Br J Urol 1988; 62: 581–583

23. Filella X, Molina R, Jo J et al. Clinical usefulness of prostate-specific antigen and prostatic acid phosphatase in patients with prostatic cancer. Tumor Biol 1990; 11: 289–294

24. Partin A W, Carter H B, Chan D W et al. Prostate specific antigen in the staging of localized prostate cancer: influence of tumor differentiation, tumor volume and benign hyperplasia. J Urol 1990; 143: 747–752

25. Lange P H, Ercole C J, Lightner D J et al. The value of serum prostate specific antigen determinations before and after radical prostatectomy. J Urol 1989; 141: 873–879

26. Hudson M A, Bahnson R R, Catalona W J. Clinical use of prostate specific antigen in patients with prostate cancer. J Urol 1989; 142: 1011–1017

27. Chan D W, Bruzek D J, Oesterling J E et al. Prostate-specific antigen as a marker for prostatic cancer: a monoclonal and a polyclonal immunoassay compared. Clin Chem 1987; 33: 1916–1929

28. Barry M J, Fowler F J Jr, O'Leary M P et al. The American Urological Association symptom index for benign prostatic hyperplasia. J Urol 1992; 148: 1549–1557

29. Barry M J, Fowler F J Jr, O'Leary M P et al. Correlation of the American Urological Association Symptom Index with self-administered versions of the Madsen–Iverson, Boyarsky and Maine Medical Assessment Program Symptom Indexes. J Urol 1992; 148: 1558–1563

30. Scott F B, Cardus D, Quesada E M, Riles T. Uroflowmetry before and after prostatectomy. South Med J 1967; 60(2): 948–952

31. Shoukry I, Susset J G, Elhilali M M, Dutartre D. Role of uroflowmetry in the assessment of lower urinary tract obstruction in adult males. Br J Urol 1975; 47(2): 559–566

32. Siroky M B, Olsson C A, Krane R J. The flow rate nomogram I: development. J Urol 1979; 122: 665–668

33. Siroky M B, Olsson C A, Krane R J. The flow rate nomogram II: clinical correlation. J Urol 1980; 123: 208–210

34. Gleason D M, Bottaccini M R, Drach G W, Layton T N. Urinary flow velocity as an index of male voiding function. J Urol 1982; 128: 1363–1367

35. Groshar D, Embon O M, Koritny E S et al. Radionuclide assessment of bladder-emptying function in normal male population and in patients before and after prostatectomy. Urology 1991; 37: 353–357

36. Chancellor M B, Blaivas J G, Kaplan S A, Axelrod S. Bladder outlet obstruction versus impaired detrusor contractility: the role of uroflow. J Urol 1991; 145: 810–812

37. Abrams P H. Prostatism and prostatectomy: the value of urine flow rate measurement in the preoperative assessment for operation. J Urol 1977; 117: 70–71

38. Abrams P H, Farrar D J, Turner-Warwick R T et al. The results of prostatectomy: a symptomatic and urodynamic analysis of 152 patients. J Urol 1979; 121: 640–642

39. Jensen K M-E, Bruskewitz R C, Iversen P, Madsen P O. Spontaneous uroflowmetry in prostatism. Urology 1984; 24: 403–409

40. Jensen K M-E, Jorgensen J B, Mogensen P. Urodynamics in prostatism I. Prognostic value of uroflowmetry. Scand J Urol Nephrol 1988; 22: 109–117

41. McLoughlin J, Gill K P, Abel P D, Williams G. Symptoms versus flow rates versus urodynamics in the selection of patients for prostatectomy. Br J Urol 1990; 66: 303–305

42. Hinman F, Cox C E. Residual urine volume in normal male subjects. J Urol 1967; 97: 641–645

43. Di Mare J R, Fish S R, Harper J M, Politano V A. Residual urine in normal male subjects. J Urol 1963; 96: 180–181

44. Massagli T L, Jaffe K M, Cardenas D D. Ultrasound measurement of urine volume of children with neurogenic bladder. Dev Med Child Neurol 1990; 32: 314–318

45. Ireton R C, Krieger J N, Cardenas D D et al. Bladder volume determination using a dedicated, portable ultrasound scanner. J Urol 1990; 143: 909–911

46. Birch N C, Hurst G, Doyle P T. Serial residual volumes in men with prostatic hypertrophy. Br J Urol 1988; 62: 571–575

47. Bruskewitz R C, Iversen P, Madsen P O. Value of postvoid residual urine determination in evaluation of prostatism. Urology 1982; 20: 602–604

48. Griffiths H J L, Castro J. An evaluation of the importance of residual urine. Br J Radiol 1970; 43: 409–413

49. Abrams P H, Griffiths D J. The assessment of prostatic obstruction from urodynamic measurements and from residual urine. Br J Urol 1979; 51: 129–134

50. Neal D E, Styles R A, Powell P H, Ramsden P D. Relationship between detrusor function and residual urine in men undergoing prostatectomy. Br J Urol 1987; 60: 560–565

51. Andersen J T. Prostatism III. Detrusor hyperreflexia and residual urine. Clinical and urodynamic aspects and the influence of surgery on the prostate. Scand J Urol Nephrol 1982; 16: 25–30

52. Jensen K M-E, Jørgensen J B, Mogensen P. Urodynamics in prostatism III. Prognostic value of medium-fill water cystometry. Scand J Urol Nephrol 1988; 114 (suppl): 78–83

53. Wasson J, Reda D, Bruskewitz R C et al.. Efficacy and cost of transurethral resection of the prostate for symptomatic benign prostatic hyperplasia. Forthcoming.

54. Jensen K M-E, Jørgensen J B, Mogensen P. Urodynamics in prostatism II. Prognostic value of pressure-flow study combined with stop-flow test. Scand J Urol Nephrol 1988; 114 (suppl): 72–77

55. Jensen K M-E, Jørgensen J B, Mogensen P. Urodynamics in prostatism IV. Search for prognostic patterns as evaluated by linear discriminant analysis. Scand J Urol Nephrol 1988; 114 (suppl): 84–86

56. Schäfer W, Noppeney R, Rübben H, Lutzeyer W. The value of free flow rate and pressure/flow-studies in the routine investigation of BPH patients. Neurourol Urodyn 1988; 7: 219–221

57. Schäfer W, Rübben H, Noppeney R, Deutz F-J. Obstructed and unobstructed prostatic obstruction. A plea for urodynamic objectivation of bladder outflow obstruction in benign prostatic hyperplasia. World J Urol 1989; 6: 198–203

58. Spångberg A, Teriö H, Ask P, Engberg A. Pressure/flow studies preoperatively and postoperatively in patients with benign prostatic hypertrophy: estimation of the urethral pressure/flow relation and urethral elasticity. Neurourol Urodyn 1991; 10: 139–167

59. Bruskewitz R C, Jensen K M-E, Iversen P, Madsen P O. The relevance of minimum urethral resistance in prostatism. J Urol 1983; 129: 769–771

60. Jensen K M-E, Andersen J T. Urodynamic implications of benign prostatic hyperplasia. Urologe [A] 1990; 29: 1–4

61. Rollema H J, van Mastrigt R, Janknegt R A. Urodynamic assessment and quantification of prostatic obstruction before and after transurethral resection of the prostate: standardization with the aid of the computer program CLIM. Urol Int 1991; 1 (suppl): 52–54

62. Rollema H J, van Mastrigt R. Objective analysis of prostatism: a clinical application of the computer program CLIM. Neurourol Urodyn 1991; 10: 71–76

63. Holtgrewe H L, Mebust W K, Dowd J B et al. Transurethral prostatectomy: practice aspects of the dominant operation in American urology. J Urol 1989; 141: 248–253

64. Bundrick T J, Katz P G. Excretory urography in patients with prostatism. AJR 1986; 147: 957–959

65. Pinck B D, Corrigan M J, Jasper P. Pre-prostatectomy excretory urography: does it merit the expense? J Urol 1980; 123: 390–391

66. Juul N, Torp-Pedersen S, Nielsen H. Abdominal ultrasound versus intravenous urography in the evaluation of infravesically obstructed males. Scand J Urol Nephrol 1989; 23: 89–92

67. Kreel L, Elton A, Habershon R et al. Use of intravenous urography. Br Med J 1974; 4: 31–33

68. Andersen J T, Jacobsen O, Strandgaard L. The diagnostic value of intravenous pyelography in intravesical obstruction in males. Scand J Urol Nephrol 1977; 11: 225–230

69. Christofferson I, Moller I. Excretory urography: a superfluous routine examination in patients with prostatic hypertrophy. Eur Urol 1981; 7(2): 65–67

70. Wasserman N F, Lapointe S, Eckmann D R, Rosel P R. Assessment of prostatism: role of intravenous urography. Radiology 1987; 165: 831–835

71. Wilcox R G, Mitchell J R A. Intravenous urography in the management of acute retention. Lancet 1977; 1: 1247–1249

72. Butler M R, Donnelly B, Komaranchat A. Intravenous urography in evaluation of acute retention. Urology 1978; 12: 464–466

73. Morrison J D. Help or habit? Excretion urography before prostatectomy. Br J Clin Pract 1980; 34: 239–241

74. Bauer D L, Garrison R W, McRoberts J W. The health and cost implications of routine excretory urography before transurethral prostatectomy. J Urol 1980; 123: 386–389

75. Donker P J, Kakiailatu F. Preoperative evaluation of patients with bladder outlet obstruction with particular regard to excretory urography. J Urol 1978; 120: 685–686

76. Matthews P N, Quayle J B, Joseph A E A et al. The use of ultrasound in the investigation of prostatism. Br J Urol 1982; 54: 536–538

77. Lilienfeld R M, Berman M, Khedkar M, Sporer A. Comparative evaluation of intravenous urogram and ultrasound in prostatism. Urology 1985; 26: 310–312

78. Cascione C J, Bartone F F, Hussain M B. Transabdominal ultrasound versus excretory urography in preoperative evaluation of patients with prostatism. J Urol 1987; 137: 883–885

79. Fidas A, Mackinlay J Y, Wild S R, Chisholm G D. Ultrasound as an alternative to intravenous urography in prostatism. Clin Radiol 1987; 38: 479–482

80. Hendrikx A J M, Doesburg W H, Reintjes A G M et al. Effectiveness of ultrasound in the preoperative evaluation of patients with prostatism. Prostate 1988; 13: 199–208

81. Solomon D J, Van Niekerk J P D V. Ultrasonography should replace intravenous urography in the pre-operative evaluation of prostatism. S Afr Med J 1988; 74: 407–408

82. Stavropoulos N, Christodoulou K, Chamilos E et al. Evaluation of patients with benign prostatic hypertrophy: IVU versus ultrasound. J R Coll Surg Edinb 1988; 33: 140–142

44

Economics of benign prostatic hyperplasia
H. L. Holtgrewe

Introduction

All nations of the world must confront the economic reality of the current highly competitive world economy. Health-care costs, like labour costs, constitute a significant component in the price of those goods and services that nations export into this global economy. Those nations with high health-care costs are placed in a position of relative disadvantage in relation to those nations with lesser costs — those who pay a lower health-care 'tax' on their exported products.

An example illustrates this fact. The aggregate health-care cost in a General Motors automobile manufactured in the United States in 1992 was US$1100;[1] health-care cost in a comparable imported Japanese automobile that same year was US$600.[1] The economic impact upon both foreign and domestic General Motors automobile sales created by this discrepancy is obvious.

Common diseases contribute most to total aggregate national health-care costs. Benign prostatic hyperplasia (BPH) is such a disease. In 1990, six nations of the developed world spent the equivalent of approximately three billion dollars simply for the surgical treatment of the disease (Table 44.1).[2]

This chapter assesses the economic aspects of BPH and the impact that the array of new emerging strategies of management — especially medical management — will have on future expenditure associated with this common disease of the male. Owing to the lack of accurate data from the nations of the developing world, attention is this chapter is focused on industrialized countries.

Background

There is a wide variation in the health-care delivery systems of the industrialized nations. Table 44.2 compares the ratio of public to private health-care funding in selected countries.[3] The past few years have witnessed a revolution within the United States health-care system, the world's largest. A consumer sovereignty fee-for-service system based upon indemnity insurance and out-of-pocket patient-to-physician payment, is rapidly being replaced by a private, for-profit, corporation system in which large managed-care organisations (MCOs) compete in providing US employers — the largest purchasers of health care — with total health-care packages for their employees. Within these MCOs, physicians — especially specialists such as urologists — are increasingly reimbursed for their services on a capitation basis where they are paid a prenegotiated annual sum. In return, the urologist

Table 44.1. *Estimates of direct costs of surgical treatment of BPH, 1990*

Nation	Direct costs (US$)	Population
United States	2 304 485 000	259 571 000
Japan	459 600 000	123 540 000
United Kingdom*	96 430 000	42 370 000
Belgium	55 670 000	9 993 000
France	37 800 000	56 735 000
Sweden	24 906 000	8 566 000

*England only. (From ref. 2 with permission.)

Table 44.2. *Health-care spending: public vs private funding, selected nations, 1992*

Nation	Percentage from public funds	Percentage from private funds
United States	42	58
Japan	72	28
Canada	73	27
Germany	73	27
France	74	26
United Kingdom	84	16

(From ref. 3 with permission.)

provides the urological care to the MCOs' enrollees, irrespective of those volumes of services required or provided. The capitated urologist thus shares financial risk. The fee-for-service incentive 'to do and to operate' is replaced by the capitation incentive of 'not to do and not to operate'. MCO executives and America's corporate leaders, who must purchase health insurance for their employees, view such a configuration as being intrinsically cost saving.

A poll commissioned by the American Urological Association (AUA) and conducted by the United States Gallup Organization of Princeton, New Jersey in February 1995 found, in seven select states (California, Florida, Illinois, Maryland, Massachusetts, Minnesota and New York), that 35.8% of urologists' incomes in those states were derived from MCO patient care.[4]

Even the US government-funded Medicare Program for citizens 65 years of age and over and the federal/state jointly funded Medicaid Program for the medically indigent are rapidly being privatized into these competing MCOs. Health policy planners view this as a means of containing the traditional severe annual inflation rates that have been experienced in these programmes over the past years and that have made these programmes the most rapidly expanding portion of the US federal government budget. These events have had, and will continue to have, inevitable impact upon the costs and the economics of the management of BPH in the United States.

Judged by any standard, the United States spends more on health care than any other nation. Table 44.3 depicts the per capita spending, spending as a percentage of gross domestic product (GDP) and annual health-care inflation rates among selected nations of the developed world.[5]

Urological manpower and its availability creates another variable in the management costs of BPH between nations. Table 44.4 reveals a dramatic variation in the numbers of urologists per capita within the community of nations.[6,7] Although there are no specific data that document a relationship between the numbers of urologists and numbers of prostatectomies for BPH, it is of interest to note that between 1976 and 1988 the number of urologists in Belgium increased from 153 to 210 (37%). During these same years the number of prostatectomies rose by 75% while the number of men

Table 44.3. *Health-care spending, 1992*

	Per capita (US$)*	Percentage of GDP	Growth rate in health spending, 1980–1992 (%)
Belgium	1485	8.2	8.3
Canada	1949	10.3	8.6
Denmark	1163	6.5	5.9
France	1745	9.4	7.9
Germany	1775	8.7	6.7
Italy	1497	8.5	8.4
Japan	1376	6.9	8.5
Netherlands	1449	8.6	6.3
Spain	895	7.0	8.8
Sweden	1317	7.9	3.7
United Kingdom	1151	7.1	8.0
United States	3094	13.6	9.3

*On basis of GDP purchasing power parities. (From ref. 5 with permission.)

Table 44.4. *World urological manpower, selected nations*

Nation	Ratio of urologists to population
Japan	1/16 000
Italy	1/23 000
United States	1/26 000
Germany	1/31 000
Ukraine	1/32 000
Czech Republic	1/34 000
Sweden	1/34 000
Belgium	1/37 500
Denmark	1/65 000
France	1/80 000
Venezuela	1/86 000
Chile	1/97 000
Ireland	1/211 000
United Kingdom*	1/250 000
South Africa	1/267 000
China	1/1 305 000
Zimbabwe	1/1 783 000
Pakistan	1/2 720 000

*England only. (From refs 6 and 7 with permission.)

65 years of age and over increased by an insignificant 1.3%.[8] Belgian urologists are not paid on a fee-for-service basis; this raises the question of whether the mere presence of urologists leads to more BPH therapy — including surgery.

Current costs of BPH management

Irrespective of its type — surgical, medical or device — the costs of BPH management must be divided into three components. *Direct costs* are those charges involved in patient evaluation and management — laboratory, imaging, medication and hospital/physician payment. These direct costs are the best chronicled and most visible, and receive the greatest attention. In a 1984 study from Sweden, Carlsson[9] reported that direct costs constituted 80% of total prostatectomy costs and indirect costs constituted the remaining 30%. *Indirect costs* are much more difficult to assess. They constitute the lost wages of the patient and his family, the costs of travel and other miscellaneous incidental expenses. The third component, *intangible costs*, is related to pain, suffering and mental anguish. In one of the few studies dealing with this issue, Standaert and Tarfs[10] measured the impact of these factors and reported that severe symptoms of BPH caused substantial adverse effect on the patient's quality of life and thus created significant intangible costs.

Direct costs (in 1995) of transurethral resection of the prostate (TURP) performed for BPH in selected nations, and the duration of hospitalization following surgery, are depicted in Table 44.5.[11] Whereas the duration of hospitalization following TURP is shortest in the United States, direct costs are highest. TURP constituted 95% of the operations performed for BPH in the United States in 1993.[12]

Ahlstrond et al.[13] report that 15% of total direct prostatectomy costs in Sweden are incurred prior to surgery, 70% are perioperative and the remaining 15% are incurred in the 5 years following surgery, owing to the management of complications and surgical failures.

From the first successful surgical enucleation of a prostatic adenoma a century ago,[14] surgery was the only effective means of BPH therapy. Prostatectomy to relieve the obstructive uropathy induced by BPH has, since that time, been central to urology. In 1962,

Table 44.5. *Total charges for TURP, 1995*

Nation	Direct costs (US$)	Duration of hospital stay (days; mean or range)
United States	6889	2.7
Japan	5000	10
Denmark	3218	5
Sweden	3045	5–7
United Kingdom	2217	7
Belgium	1842	4–7

(From ref. 11 with permission.)

Table 44.6. *Incidence of prostatectomy for BPH: selected nations, 1990 and 1993*

Nation	Prostatectomies per 1000 men	
	1990	1993
United States*	13	10.3
Sweden*	11	7.8
Japan*	9	8.7
United Kingdom[†]	5.9	6

*Men 55 years and over. [†]Men 45 years and over. (From refs 11 and 16 with permission.)

prostatectomy for BPH constituted over 50% of the American urologist's major surgery.[15] In 1987 the number of TURPs performed for BPH reached a peak of 253 000 within the US Medicare Program. Since then, the number has progressively fallen to 145 000 in 1994, a reduction of 43% (Fig. 44.1).[12] Reductions have occurred worldwide: the incidence of prostatectomy per 1000 men aged 55 years and older in selected countries is shown in Table 44.6.[11,16] Each of these nations experienced reductions between 1990 and 1993, apart from the United Kingdom which had a substantially lower rate than the other countries in 1990.

The era of medical treatment dawned with the early work of Caine et al.[17] and their description of the use of alpha-blockade in the treatment of BPH. The past half decade has witnessed an explosion in medical therapy. Table 44.7 documents the dramatic rise in the number of prescriptions written in the management of BPH in the United States from 1992 through 1994.[18] Table 44.8 documents the US dollar value of BPH prescriptions and their position among the top 20 medications prescribed by American urologists in 1994.[19]

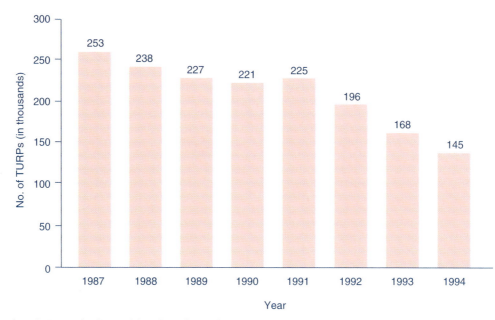

Figure 44.1. *Number of TURPS (in thousands) performed annually for BPH within the US Medicare Program.*

Table 44.7. *Medical therapy for BPH*

Drug	Prescriptions/year for BPH in US (thousands)		
	1992	1993	1994
Finasteride	317 000	1 345 000	2 040 000
Alpha-blockers	1 075 000	1 512 000	2 940 000

(From ref. 18 with permission.)

Table 44.8. *Prescriptions written by US urologists, 1994*

Product	Ranking*	Total sales (US$)
Cipro (ciprofloxin)	1	28 789 000
Proscar (finasteride)	2	27 917 000[†]
Hytrin (terozosin)	4	22 034 000[†]
Cardura (doxazosin)	17	2 508 000[†]

*Ranking within top 20 prescriptions written by US urologists. [†]Total of $52 459 000 for three BPH pharmaceutical products. (From ref. 19 with permission.)

The magnitude of the penetration of medical therapy into the treatment of BPH is further documented by another 1994 poll conducted by the Gallup Organization for the AUA:[20] 70% of American urologists reported that their first therapeutic recommendation for men with moderate symptoms [International Prostate Symptom Score (I-PSS) score of 8–9] was medical (Table 44.9). American urologists are even recommending initial medical management in one-third of their patients with severe symptoms (I-PSS 20 and higher).

Not only is BPH increasingly being treated medically but 1994 data revealed that 59% of terazosin prescriptions and 55% of finasteride prescriptions written for the treatment of BPH in the United States were written by primary care physicians.[18] Once the exclusive domain of the urologist, BPH patients are now being managed by their primary physicians — a further adverse economic reality for urologists whose reimbursement is based upon fee for service.

A recent random survey of the retail price of finasteride, terazosin and doxazosin — commonly used medical pharmaceutical agents in the treatment of BPH — reveals a substantial variation between selected countries (Table 44.10).[11]

Emergence of guidelines

The first government-endorsed guidelines for the evaluation and management of BPH were published in February 1994 by the Agency for Health Care Policy

Table 44.9. *First treatment recommendations for BPH patients not in retention (with no major complications)*

AUA score	First treatment	Percentage of US urologists
0–7 (mild)	Watchful waiting	77
	Alpha-blockers	17
	Other	4
	Finasteride	1
	No response	1
8–19 (moderate)	Alpha-blockers	65
	Other	15
	Watchful waiting	6
	Finasteride	6
	Transurethral resection	4
	Laser	2
	No response	2
20–35 (severe)	Transurethral resection	41
	Alpha-blockers	31
	Other	16
	Laser	6
	Finasteride	3
	No response	3

(From ref. 20 with permission.)

Table 44.10. *Retail price of medical BPH therapies, selected nations*

Nation	Retail price (US$)		
	Finasteride	Terazosin	Doxazosin
United States	2.04	1.30	0.97
Sweden	1.24	1.31	—
France	1.43	—	—
Belgium	1.82	1.92	—

(From ref. 11 with permission.)

and Research (AHCPR), an agency of the United States Department of Health and Human Services.[21] Motivation for the development of these guidelines was multifactorial but was largely due to the high cost of surgical BPH treatment and a scientifically unaccountable threefold variation in the incidence of prostatectomy in age-adjusted populations in different geographic regions of the United States.[22] The AHCPR guidelines were produced by a multidisciplinary panel with representation from urology, internal medicine, family medicine, radiology and nursing. Central to the guidelines is the seven-question self-administered AUA

Symptom Index.[23] Yielding a symptom sum ranging from between 0 and 35, symptom severity is divided into three groups — mild (0–7), moderate (8–19) and severe (20 and over).

The World Health Organization (WHO) 2nd International Consultation on BPH held in Paris, France in June 1993 adopted the AUA Symptom Index and added an eighth quality-of-life question, creating the I-PSS.[2] The degree of awareness of the I-PSS of urologists in selected nations and the degree of impact that the I-PSS has had in altering their practice patterns in the management of BPH is presented in Table 44.11.[11] International awareness has not, as yet, brought about alteration of patterns of practice.

Recommendations for the evaluation of the BPH patient contained within the AHCPR guidelines have the potential for achieving great cost savings. On the basis of the world's peer-reviewed literature, the guidelines recommend that imaging of the upper urinary tracts by radiographic or sonographic means should *not* be performed routinely and that these studies should be reserved for complicating factors such as haematuria or uraemia, or where there is a history of stone disease, flank pain, previous renal trauma or previous renal surgery — all of which, in their own right, constitute an indication for such investigations.[21] Similarly, a purely diagnostic routine cystoscopy is *not* recommended, as there is no literature-based evidence that the procedure provides any useful information in treatment decision-making. Complicating factors, such as a history suggesting the presence of a urethral stricture or haematuria, constitute an indication for cystoscopy. Once the decision for surgical treatment has been made,

Table 44.11. *Awareness and impact of I-PSS: selected nations, 1995*

Nation	Percentage of urologists aware of I-PSS	Percentage of urologists altering practice due to I-PSS
Denmark	100	0
United States	99	21
Sweden	66	32
Belgium	47	35

(From ref. 11 with permission.)

cystoscopy is often useful in planning the type of surgery to be undertaken and best suited to the patient (TURP, transurethral incision of the prostate, or open prostatectomy).

Despite the lack of utility of such studies, urologists worldwide continue to employ routine diagnostic upper tract imaging and cystoscopy, thus wasting enormous health-care resources, as depicted in Tables 44.12 and 44.13.[11]

The AHCPR guidelines contain comparisons of the first and second years' costs of surgical and medical strategies of management in the United States (Table 44.14).[21] These data are based upon 1988 and 1989 information and they are unique to the United States. They are dated but, nevertheless, provide some insight into the comparative costs during the interval of the first 2 years of medical and surgical treatments, as well as their comparison with the strategy of watchful waiting. Two years is, however, an inadequate interval of follow-

Table 44.14. *Average individual direct costs of treatment for BPH, United States, 1988–1989*

Primary modality	Cost* of primary treatment and 1 year follow-up[†] (US$)	Cost of 2nd year of treatment after primary treatment (US$)
Watchful waiting	1162	640
Finasteride	1326	778
Alpha-blocker	1395	845
TURP	8606	360
Open prostatectomy	12 788	69

*Calculated from Medicare data years 1988–1989 (Parts A and B), drug-cost estimates from pharmaceutical companies in seven states, and device-cost estimates from materials supplied by product manufacturers. [†]Included in cost estimates for first year after treatment are cost of failure (re-treatment with TURP) and cost of complications following surgical treatment (urinary incontinence, urethral stricture, bladder neck contracture). The estimates for watchful waiting, finasteride and alpha-blockers are probably higher than actually seen because not all patients who fail go on to TURP. (From ref. 21 with permission.)

Table 44.12. *BPH evaluation practices, selective nations: routine use of upper tract imaging*

Nation	Percentage of urologists*
Japan	60
United Kingdom	29
Belgium	25
United States	18
Sweden	5
Denmark	0

*Percentage of urologists routinely obtaining i.v. urogram or renal sonogram in the evaluation of the BPH patient. (From ref. 11 with permission.)

Table 44.13. *BPH evaluation practices, selected nations: routine use of cystoscopy*

Nation	Percentage of urologists*
Sweden	55
Belgium	52
Denmark	45
United States	41
Japan	10

*Percentage of urologists doing routine diagnostic cystoscopy in the evaluation of the BPH patient. (From ref. 11 with permission.)

up to allow for an accurate comparison of costs. Durability, the costs of retreatment and, thus, cost efficacy can be assessed only after a much longer duration of study. Furthermore, the data contained in Table 44.14 were derived from multiple published studies that were based on different cohorts of patients who could have presented with varying degrees of disease and with different severities of co-morbidity. Such variations could affect the reliability of the data and confound the comparisons.

It is still not clear what effect the AHCPR guidelines will have on physicians' compensation in the United States. From personal conversations with US government Health Care Financing Administration (HCFA) officials, it seems possible to this author that, after a reasonable interval to allow for adaptation, the future reimbursement for BPH therapy in the United States could well be linked to guidelines compliance. It is equally possible, if not probable, that US managed-care administrators may embrace these guidelines, demanding their use by urologists and primary physicians working within their organizations.

It is even more unclear what use, if any, government or health-insurance executives of other nations might find for the AHCPR guidelines. However, given the enormous costs incurred in the management of this common disease, and the uniqueness and the potential for cost savings contained within the guidelines, it may well be increasingly difficult for health-care planners of the world to ignore them completely.

Future BPH costs

Central to the economics and costs of BPH management worldwide will be the impact of the shift away from surgical treatment to strategies of medical management and the new less-invasive emerging device treatments, including laser and thermal therapies. Will these therapies reduce the total aggregate costs of BPH management compared with traditional prostatectomy? At the time of writing, within the world's peer-reviewed medical and urological literature there are insufficient data of adequate duration of follow-up to allow a meaningful evaluation of the new device therapies, their efficacy and their costs. Their ultimate role must await further study, evaluating their outcomes over time.

Clearly, the most costly aspect of any strategy of BPH management is its failure rate. Ineffective treatments, even marginally effective treatments, although initially less costly than prostatectomy become very expensive when the costs of definitive therapies such as surgery must be added to costs incurred during the course of the ineffective or unsuccessful treatment. A 'cascade' of treatments inevitably increases the costs over that which would have been incurred had the initial therapy been definitive. The failure rates of various BPH treatments derived from the AHCPR guidelines are shown in Table 44.15.[21]

Proven clinical effectiveness and cost effectiveness documented in properly performed, prospective, randomized clinical trials are essential before any new emerging treatment is allowed to achieve common public use. Costs of the new therapy should be documented and compared with those of existing established treatments and with other new competing emerging strategies of management. The Committee on the Economics of BPH of the 3rd World Health Organization Consultation on BPH, held in Monte Carlo in June 1995, admonished the editors of the world's peer-reviewed medical and urological journals to reject those manuscripts dealing with new BPH

Table 44.15. *Five-year projected treatment failure rates*

Treatment modality	Failure rate (%)*	
	High estimate	Low estimate
Watchful waiting		38 (15–65)[†]
Alpha-blocker	39 (23–70)[‡]	13 (4–31)[†]
Finasteride	27 (25–29)[‡]	10 (9–12)[†]
TUIP[††]	9 (1–28)[§]	
TURP	10 (9–11)[§]	
Open surgery	2 (1–4)[§]	

*90% confidence intervals (%) in parentheses. [†]Reported initial failure rate with subsequent period up to 5 years assumed to have 20% of the initial failure rate, modelled after the study by Craigen et al.[24] [‡]Reported initial failure rate assumed to be linear up to 5 years. [§]Single point estimates and confidence intervals devised from large clinical series up to and past 5 years. [††]Transurethral incision of the prostate. (From ref. 21 with permission.)

treatments lacking such economic data, just as they would reject manuscripts lacking important clinical data.[11]

The era when a pharmacological or device treatment could be advocated for public use simply because 'it works' is over. The current medical economic climate demands to know how well it works, what are its comparative costs, and whether it provides a durable, validated and favourable impact upon the patient's quality of life. Only when these issues are documented should new therapies become part of the contemporary armamentarium of world urologists and paid for by the public purse. In the absence of these cost data it should be asked whose interests are being served by the premature adoption of (and the public payment for) new therapies, the costs of which remain undocumented. The answer would appear to be as follows: the interests of industries and those of physicians administering the therapy — not those of society.

Conclusions

Certainly, prostatectomy incurs much greater cost than does medical therapy. Those monies saved by the avoidance of surgery can be retained within the nation's health-care system, invested at interest or directed into other areas of need. However, these initial savings do *not* constitute the entire scenario.

During the area when surgery was the only therapy for the obstructive uropathy induced by BPH, many men avoided or postponed medical evaluation, realizing that a surgical operation would be the ultimate outcome. Fear of surgery, with its pain and potential complications, induced many men to reject prostatectomy even after an evaluation resulted in a recommendation for surgery. The dread of an operation outweighed their desire for symptom relief.

The advent of effective medical therapy provides the former 'silent sufferer' with new options. Not only will men previously adverse to surgical treatment accept daily oral medication, they will actively seek such treatment. Even if that medical therapy provides a lesser degree of symptom relief than would surgery, they willingly accept a lesser outcome in exchange for lesser risk.

Coupled with this increasing demand for medical therapy is increased public awareness of the disease, its symptoms and its treatment options. The pharmaceutical industry and the medical device industry, seeking return on their investments in research and development, will ensure that men of an age when BPH is likely — and their families — are made aware of their products. Their advertising is currently appearing not only in medical journals but also in the public media, both print and electronic.

The improved management of cardiovascular and other diseases has been attended with greater longevity. Men are living longer and more are living into the BPH age range. Table 44.16 depicts the population demographics of the United States.[25] The population over 65 years of age is the most rapidly growing segment within the nation. These United States trends are replicated in other nations of the developed world.

The multiple forces of an ageing male population, enhanced public awareness and increasing patient demand for the new less-invasive treatments, will combine to create a huge increase in the total number of men undergoing evaluation for — and receiving — treatment of BPH. The total aggregate cost of the foregoing will overwhelm and greatly exceed any savings derived from the reduction in the number of surgical operations currently being experienced worldwide. The

Table 44.16. *United States population trends*

Year	US population (millions)	
	Age ≥ 65 years	Age ≥ 85 years
1890	3	0.13
1930	6	0.27
1960	18	0.9
1990	33	3
2000*	37	4
2020*	65	6
2050*	80	18

*Estimates. (From ref. 25 with permission.)

final result will be a dramatic increase in BPH expenditures which will have to be borne by the health-delivery systems of the developed nations owing to the vast increase in the numbers of men under treatment. Adherence to BPH management and treatment guidelines can offer some cost savings, but nothing short of actual rationing of care will control these inevitable cost escalations. The opposing forces of BPH management costs are depicted in Figure 44.2.

To what extent health-care policy planners, health budget bureaucrats, insurance company executives and MCO controllers will impose economics-based rationing upon BPH patients for whom they are responsible, remains unclear. Budget capping, lack of ready access to urologists, waiting lists and denial of certain pharmaceuticals or therapies are all possibilities and, to some extent, are currently being imposed in some nations. Urologists' reimbursement by capitation or salary and the incentives to limit services that these forms of physician reimbursement may create, represent another cost-containment strategy.

As economic competition exists between nations, so, too, competition exists within the health-delivery systems of a single nation — competition between diseases and competition between the various specialties of medicine. Each vies for its proper allocation of those finite resources at the disposal of the nation's health-care system. In view of this reality, it must be asked what obligation the public purse has, through its tax revenues or collective insurance premiums, to improve the

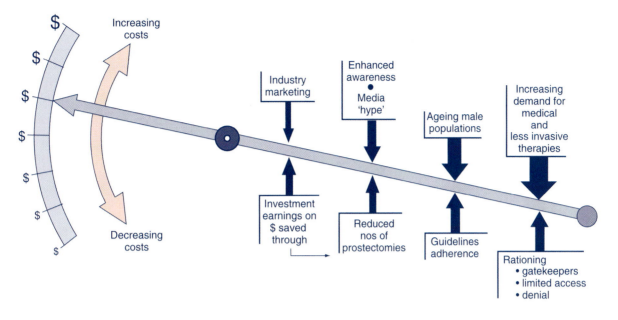

Figure 44.2. *Model depicting the opposing forces which will contribute to the increasing total future costs of the management of BPH in developed nations.*

symptoms of an older man suffering from a disease which, if properly evaluated and managed, is non-lethal. What obligation does the public purse have to reduce an older man's urinary frequency, nocturia and urgency, thus improving — to whatever extent — his quality of life? Could the same resources be better transferred to prenatal care, infant immunization programmes, cancer screening for younger adults, or for any one of an array of other worthy health needs? Only when BPH therapies document their durability and beneficial impact on quality of life can their payment be expected to come from the communal public purse.

The evaluation and management of BPH is an expensive growth industry destined to become ever more expensive. Its costs can be moderated only by practice guideline adherence and by government or managed-care rationing. These sobering facts make it mandatory that any new emerging treatment proves its cost efficacy and its long-term durability.

References

1. McAlinden S. Competitive survival: private initiatives, public policy and the North American automotive industry. Transportation Research Institute, Report 92-3. Ann Arbor: University of Michigan, 1992

2. Holtgrewe H L, Ackermann R, Bay-Nielsen H et al. The economics of BPH. In: Cockett A T K, Khoury S, Aso Y et al. (eds) The 2nd International Consultation on Benign Prostatic Hyperplasia (BPH). Paris, June 27–30, 1993. Jersey, Channel Islands: SCI, 1993; 37–44

3. Organization for Economic Cooperation and Development. OECD Health Data File, 1992

4. Gallup Organization. Managed care study for the American Urological Association. Columbia, Md: Gallup Organization Health Care Group, 1995

5. Schieber J, Poullier P, Greenwald L. Health system performance in OECD countries: 1980–1992. Health Aff (Millwood) 1994; 13(4)

6. Committee of the Société Internationale d'Urologie. Strategic issues in world urology. Data Report 3. Lille: SIU, 1995

7. World Population Statistics. In: 1994 Information Please Almanac, 47th ed. New York: Houghton Mifflin, 1994: 143–294

8. Holtgrewe H L, Ackermann R, Bay-Nielsen H et al. The economics of BPH. In: Cockett A T K, Aso Y, Chatelain C et al. (eds) The International Consultation on Benign Prostatic Hyperplasia (BPH). Paris, June 26–27, 1991. Jersey, Channel Islands: SCI, 1991: 261–267

9. Carlsson P. Diffusion and economic effects of medical technology in treatment of peptic ulcer, prostatic hyperplasia and gall bladder diseases. Likoping Studies in Art and Science No. 12 dissertation, 1987

10. Standaert B, Tarfs K. Economics of BPH: measuring the intangible costs. In: Kurth K, Newling D (eds) Benign prostatic hyperplasia. EORTC Genitourinary Monograph 12. New York: Wiley-Liss, 1994: 409–418

11. Holtgrewe H L, Ackermann R, Bay-Nielsen H et al. The economics of BPH. In: Cockett A T K, Aso Y, Chatelain C et al. (eds) The 3rd International Consultation on Benign Prostatic Hyperplasia (BPH) Paris, June 26–28, 1995. Jersey, Channel Islands: SCI, 1995, in press

12. Health Care Financing Administration, BESS Data, Washington, DC: 1994

13. Ahlstrond C, Carlsson P, Jonsson B. An estimate of the life-time cost of surgical treatment of benign prostatic hyperplasia. Scand J Urol Nephrol 1995, in press

14. Freyer P. A new method of performing prostatectomy. Lancet 1900; 1: 774

15. Holtgrewe H L, Mebust W, Dowd J et al. Transurethral prostatectomy: practice aspects of the dominant operation in American urology. J Urol 1989; 141: 248

16. National Inpatient Profile, October 1992–1993. Baltimore, Md: Health Care Investors Associated, 1994

17. Caine M, Pfau A, Perlberg S. The use of alpha adrenergic blockers in benign prostatic obstruction. Br J Urol 1976; 48: 255

18. Abbott methodology applied to NPA Plus™ and NDTT™ data, IMS America, Ltd, 1995; methodology on file at Abbott

19. Medical Economics Research Group. Urologists' facts about their practices. Walsh America/PMSI Alpha Data. Jan–Oct 1994. Montvale, NJ: 1995

20. Gee W, Holtgrewe H L, Albertsen P et al. Practice trends in the diagnosis and management of benign prostatic hyperplasia in the United States. J Urol 1995; 154: 205

21. McConnell J, Barry M, Bruskewitz R et al. Benign prostatic hyperplasia: diagnosis and treatment. Clinical Practice Guidelines No 8. AHCPR Publication No. 95-0582. Rockville, Md: Agency for Health Care Policy and Research, Public Health Service, US Department of Health and Human Services, 1994

22. Wennberg J, Gittelsohn A. Variations in medical care among small areas. Sci Am 1982; 246: 120

23. Barry M, Fowler F, O'Leary M et al. The American Urological Association's Symptom Index for benign prostatic hyperplasia. J Urol 1992; 148: 1549

24. Craigen A, Hickling J, Saunders C et al. Natural history of prostatic obstruction. J R Coll Gen Pract 1969; 18: 226

25. US Decennial Life Tables, State Life Tables; V. 1 ALMO 2MT-WY. Life expectancy; mortality (US) PHS 90-1151. Hyattsville, Md: US Department of Health and Human Services, Public Health Service, National Center for Health Statistics, 1990

45

Shared care for benign prostatic hyperplasia
R. S. Kirby J. M. Fitzpatrick M. G. Kirby A. Fitzpatrick

Introduction

To move forward in any walk of life one needs to manage change constructively. Internationally, the means of provision of medical care is now changing dramatically and urologists cannot ignore these changes (any more than a secretary could ignore the advent of the word processor). Governments and insurers, who hold the health-care purse strings, are demanding a shift of resources away from secondary and tertiary specialist care towards primary care, which is perceived as more cost-effective. This chapter examines the case for (and the drawbacks of) 'shared care' between specialists and family practitioners specifically for the management of benign prostatic hyperplasia (BPH).

What is shared care?

Shared care involves the constructive collaboration between specialists (in this case urologists) and family practitioners.[1] For it to work, it is necessary for an algorithm to be developed so that locally agreed protocols can be followed for the investigation of patients and clear guidelines can be issued, documenting which patients should be referred and which may be managed — by either watchful waiting or medical therapy — by the family practitioner. Moreover, the follow-up intervals to monitor disease progress and treatment effects and the criteria for subsequent referral have to be agreed.

In what other disease areas does 'shared care' work?

Shared care is widely employed in the UK in diabetes, asthma and hypertension. The large number of individuals affected by these prevalent diseases make it impracticable that each and every individual sufferer should be seen by a specialist; instead, therapy can be administered and its effects monitored by the family practitioner. Hypertension, asthma and diabetes are all within the remit of internal medicine, rather than surgically based as is the case with BPH, so there has been little resistance from family practitioners to picking up gradually the extra burden of management of these conditions. In an interesting parallel to prostatic disease, hypertension is generally considered to be appropriately managed at the family practitioner level; angina, by contrast, is usually regarded as an indication for specialist referral — presumably because of the invasive testing and therapy by angiography and angioplasty, as well as the unpredictable risk of sudden death from myocardial infarction. Similarly, it seems likely that, in the future, whereas uncomplicated mild to moderate BPH may become, in the first instance, the province of the family practitioner, prostate cancer (or suspicions thereof) will always prompt referral for evaluation (usually by transrectal ultrasound-guided biopsy) by a urologist.

The shared care initiative for BPH

In order to harmonize thoughts on these matters a committee was formed under the chairmanship of the late Professor Geoffrey Chisholm, CBE. The issues surrounding the presentation, evaluation and guidelines for referral were discussed and a nomogram devised (Fig. 45.1).[2] The feasibility and overall acceptance of the precepts and assumptions contained within that monogram were then field-tested by means of a questionnaire, which was sent to 2020 urologists, general surgeons with an interest in urology, geriatricians, family health service advisors (FHSA) and general practitioners. The absolute numbers and percentage of responders for each group are shown in Table 45.1.

Results of the survey
Scores for each question were compiled numerically (1 = I strongly agree; 2 = I agree; 3 = I disagree; 4 = I strongly disagree). There was consensus that *screening*

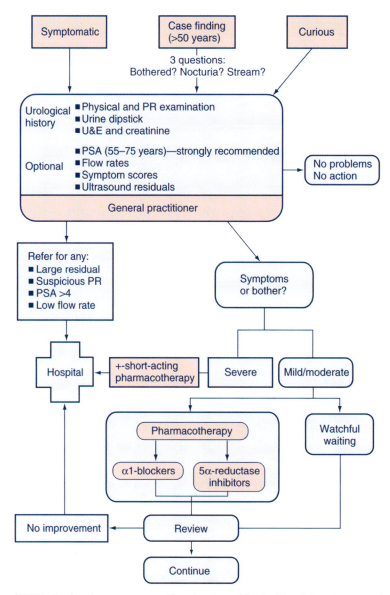

Figure 45.1. *Managing clinical BPH: the shared care initiative. Algorithm devised by the Shared Care Initiative Committee. (From ref. 2 with permission.)*

for BPH (i.e. inviting men aged between 50 and 70 years to attend for a prostate health check) was not generally practicable, although pilot screening studies in the UK have confirmed a 2% pick-up rate of apparently significant prostate cancer.[3] By contrast, the prospect of *case finding* was greeted with more enthusiasm. In this setting the American Urological Association (AUA) symptom scores or International Prostate Symptom Score (I-PSS) with their seven questions and possible cumulative score of 35 were regarded as rather too cumbersome. Instead, it was proposed that the family

practitioner could more readily ask all male patients of more than 50 years of age, presenting for whatever reason, three key questions: (1) do you get up at night to pass urine; (2) is your urinary stream reduced; (3) are you 'bothered' by your bladder function? Individuals responding positively to any of these questions might then be administered a targeted AUA/I-PSS symptom score and undergo a physical examination.

Physical examination for the symptomatic patient in whom BPH is suspected should include a focused neurological examination, as well as a palpation of the

Table 45.1. *Responders to the questionnaire sent out by the Shared Care Initiative Committee*

		Response	
Group	No. sent	n	%
Urologists	320	159	49.7
General surgeons	373	85	22.8
Geriatricians	712	160	22.5
Family practitioners	500	118	23.6
FHSA advisors	115	58	50.4
Total	2020	580	28.7

lower abdomen to exclude a chronically distended bladder. The cornerstone of the physical assessment is the digital rectal examination (DRE). Most respondents agreed that DRE was mandatory in the evaluation of BPH patients and that any induration or palpable nodule present should be regarded as an indication for referral to a urologist to exclude a diagnosis of prostate cancer. More work is necessary, however, to educate family practitioners in the skills of DRE, as a recent survey in the UK suggested that the majority were performing less than five of these examinations per month.[4]

The issue of prostate cancer raises the question of the necessity for prostate-specific antigen (PSA) testing in this context. In this respect, the respondents to the questionnaire were almost equally divided in their opinions. Although PSA testing will undoubtedly diagnose cases of early prostate cancer, there was concern that many patients, especially those in the mildly elevated PSA ranges, would be unnecessarily alarmed, perhaps undergo transrectal ultrasound-guided biopsy and, in fact, be found to have BPH. For this reason, PSA was included as an optional (but recommended) test for men aged between 50 and 70 years with prostatic symptoms, rather than a formal guideline requirement [the American Healthcare Policy Review (AHCPR) guideline committee came to similar conclusions].[5]

Who to refer?

The respondents generally agreed with the following guidelines for recommended patient referral to a urologist:

1. Severe symptoms (I-PSS > 18).
2. History of haematuria.
3. Palpably distended bladder or chronic retention on ultrasound.
4. Abnormal DRE (especially palpable nodule or prostatic induration).
5. Raised serum creatinine.
6. Raised PSA (> 4 ng/ml).
7. Any patient about whose diagnosis or treatment the GP has concern.

Who to treat?

Excluding the above categories of patient, it now seems legitimate for family practitioners to consider starting medical therapy either with an alpha-blocker or a 5 alpha-reductase inhibitor and to monitor the response to therapy in uncomplicated BPH. However, those patients with mild symptoms (I-PSS < 8) and who have little 'bother' from their BPH will usually be more appropriately managed by watchful waiting and annual review.

Follow-up for those managed medically

Patients with moderate symptoms of BPH and a normal DRE, as well as normal PSA and creatinine values, and who are managed medically will need to be reviewed regularly to monitor treatment response and evaluate side effects. The frequency of these visits will depend on the particular agent selected for therapy.

In general, alpha-blockers have a rapid onset of action in terms of symptom alleviation and flow rate improvement,[6] but most require careful dose titration to minimize side effects of dizziness and postural hypotension. Doxazosin and terazosin, for example, should be started at 1 mg/day and gradually increased to a maintenance dosage of 4 or 5 mg/day respectively (some patients may benefit from a further dose increment to 8 or 10 mg respectively). Patients treated thus should be reviewed in a timely fashion for these dose adjustments. Longer-term follow-up is also necessary because, although alpha-blockers relieve symptoms and improve peak flow rates, they do not reverse the underlying pathophysiology and prostate growth is, therefore, likely to continue.

5 alpha-reductase inhibitors, such as finasteride and epristeride, have a slower onset of action but achieve, eventually, a level of symptom reduction and peak flow rate enhancement which is very beneficial to patients.[7,8] Moreover, as they shrink the prostate and reverse the underlying pathophysiology of BPH, they may prevent longer-term complications, such as acute retention, and reduce the need for eventual surgery.[9] Finasteride also suppresses serum PSA levels (because PSA secretion is an androgen-dependent process) to around 50% of their pretreatment values within 6–12 months of therapy.[10] Patients treated medically for BPH should ideally be reviewed at 3, 6 and 12 months. Failure of PSA reduction and, in particular, evidence of an increase in PSA in spite of finasteride therapy, or failure to control symptoms, should prompt referral to a urologist.

Potential benefits of shared care

The algorithm featured in Figure 45.1 provides a framework for urologists and family practitioners to work together to optimize therapy for the many millions of sufferers from this most prevalent disease. Although some will argue that each and every man with symptomatic BPH should, ideally, be seen and evaluated by a urologist, logistics alone suggest that this will not be possible. To take the United Kingdom as an example, where there are an estimated 2.5 million men who constitute the 'iceberg' of BPH, to care for all these people there are only 350 urologists; by contrast, there are around 33 000 family practitioners.

In order for shared care of BPH to work effectively there are learning steps to be climbed by family practitioners. These are depicted in Figure 45.2. Urologists will need to involve themselves in this process of educating their colleagues in primary care in such skills as DRE and PSA interpretation.

Shared care for BPH in practice should permit more rapid access for patients to appropriate investigation and treatment. Family practitioners should benefit by being able to offer a more comprehensive range of therapies for their patients, as they gain experience in the management of BPH. Urologists should also gain, by building bridges between themselves and the family practitioners who refer to them. This will ensure that they see an increasing number of properly selected and

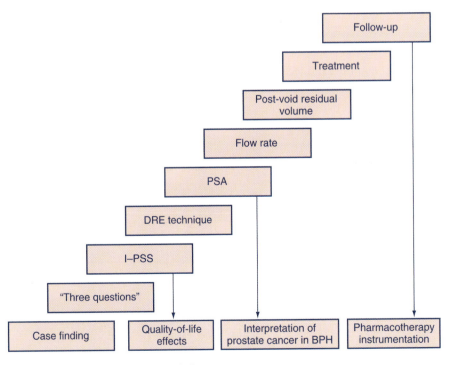

Figure 45.2. *Education of family practitioners by urologists: the learning steps.*

carefully assessed patients who more particularly require their special operative and interventional skills.

References

1. Orton P. Shared care. Lancet 1994; 344: 1413–1415
2. Kirby R S, Chisholm G, Chapple C R et al. Shared care between general practitioners and urologists in the management of benign prostatic hyperplasia: a survey of attitudes among clinicians. J R Soc Med 1995; 88: 284–288
3. Kirby R S, Kirby M G, Feneley M R et al. Screening for carcinoma of the prostate: a GP based study. Br J Urol 1994; 74: 64–71
4. Hennigan T W, Franks P J, Hocken D B, Allen-Mersh T G. Rectal examination in general practice. Br Med J 1990; 301: 478–480
5. McConnell J D, Barry M J, Bruskewitz R C et al. Benign prostatic hyperplasia: diagnosis and treatment. Clinical Practice Guideline No. 8. Rockville, Md: US Department of Health and Human Resources, 1994; 1–225
6. Eri L M, Tveter K J. Alpha-blockade in the treatment of symptomatic benign prostatic hyperplasia. J Urol 1995; 154: 923–934
7. Gormley G J, Stoner E, Bruskewitz R C et al. The effect of finasteride in men with benign prostatic hyperplasia. N Engl J Med 1992; 327: 1185–1191
8. Stoner E, Members of the Finasteride Study Group. Three-year safety and efficacy data on the use of finasteride in the treatment of benign prostatic hyperplasia. Urology 1994; 43: 284–294
9. Andersen J T, Ekman P, Wolf M et al. Can finasteride reverse the progress of benign prostatic hyperplasia? A two–year placebo–controlled study. Urology 1995; 46: 631–637
10. Guess H A, Heyse J F, Gormley G J. The effect of finasteride on prostate-specific antigen in men with benign prostatic hyperplasia. Prostate 1993; 22: 31–37

46

Prostate diseases beyond the year 2000: present and future burden of prostate diseases

P. Boyle P. Maisonneuve P. Napalkov

Introduction

The prostate gland is the site of the two most common urological diseases in elderly men: prostate cancer poses approximately a one-in-ten lifetime risk[1] and benign prostatic hyperplasia (BPH) can be found in 88% of autopsies in men aged 80 years and over with compatible symptomatology reported in nearly one-half of men aged over 50 years in the general population.[2,3] In the United States, BPH accounts for some two million physician office visits each year and over 400 000 prostatectomies are performed annually, making this the most common form of major surgery in men over 55 years of age. It has been estimated that a 40-year-old man who lives to the age of 80 would have around one chance in three of having a prostatectomy for BPH if current operation rates prevail,[4] although this has almost certainly increased.

Despite such a common occurrence, little is known with any certainty about the epidemiology of BPH.[5] The incidence, even the population prevalence, is difficult to determine, for a variety of reasons associated with difficulties surrounding the diagnosis of BPH and the identification of a source population to provide a denominator to calculate rates.[6] Knowledge of risk factors are sparse: analytical epidemiological studies of BPH are difficult to conduct. It is essential to establish an epidemiological definition of BPH for these reasons. Case–control studies, the most commonly employed design in epidemiology, are problematic in that a control group may be difficult to define in view of the likelihood that a large proportion of these may have undiagnosed BPH.

Furthermore, prostate cancer is now frequently the first or second most common form of cancer in men in many populations.[7,8] In many countries around the world the risk of incident prostate cancer is rising quite markedly although there is no evidence that the risk of fatal prostate cancer is changing to any great extent.[9] It is widely accepted that the risk of prostate cancer has environmental determinants, defining 'environment' in its broadest sense to include a wide range of lifestyle factors including dietary, social and cultural practices. Although a large number of risk factors have been investigated, the natural history and risk factors for prostate cancer are far from being clearly understood.[10]

Relationship between BPH and prostate cancer

The frequency of incidental prostate cancer during transurethral resection of the prostate (TURP) for BPH was reported to range from 13 to 22%.[11] The incidence of prostate cancer and BPH increases with age and both diseases are androgen-associated conditions.[12] BPH arises exclusively in the transition zone: by contrast, this is the site of origin of about 10–20% of prostatic adenocarcinomas.[13] Using prospective and retrospective approaches, Armenian et al.[14] demonstrated a 3.7 times higher death rate from prostate cancer in men with BPH than in controls and a 5 to 1 relative risk for prostate cancer for BPH patients.

However, it is generally accepted that BPH and prostate cancer are separate diseases with distinct aetiologies. In the prospective study of 838 men with BPH and 802 age-matched controls, Greenwald et al.[15] did not find any significant difference in the occurrence of prostate cancer. After 10.7–11.2 years of follow-up, prostate cancer risk of the BPH group was estimated to be 0.9.

A study from Rhode Island,[16] of 4853 men who had either TURP or a prostatectomy for BPH, demonstrated a non-significant risk for prostate cancer of 1.01 [95% confidence interval (CI) 0.77, 1.31] for those who underwent suprapubic prostatectomy compared with the expected rate determined from local cancer incidence statistics. For men who had undergone a TURP the risk was 1.18 (95% CI 0.94, 1.47) and was also statistically non-significant.

A recent follow-up study from Sweden[17] suggested that neither BPH nor TURP increased the risk of developing clinical prostate cancer in patients who underwent transurethral resection of a clinically benign prostate gland. The clinical incidence of prostate cancer was reported as 0.30% in the TURP group and 0.25% in the control group. In a retrospective case–control study of 198 patients who had TURP and 203 age-matched controls, investigators did not observe any significant difference in the incidence of prostate adenocarcinoma. Contrary to other studies, all patients with stage T1 prostate cancer found by TURP were included in the comparison between two groups. The reported odds ratio for development of clinically evident prostate cancer was 0.8 (95% CI 0.2, 3.1), and for death from prostate cancer was 1.3 (95% CI 0.24, 7.45). The authors concluded that neither TURP itself, nor BPH, increases the risk of clinical prostate cancer.

In contrast, Kearse et al.[18] in the long-term follow-up study of 269 patients who underwent TURP, found that a significant number (7.8%) subsequently developed clinical prostate cancer. Comparing these data with reports on disease progression in incidentally discovered prostate cancer, the authors suggested that the risk of progression and death from prostate cancer is similar in patients who underwent transrectal ultrasonography (TRUS) for BPH and for those who had incidentally discovered prostate cancer at TRUS. The authors suggested that this finding may be a result of both a combination of increasing patient age and the common hormonal basis for the development of BPH and prostate cancer.

Although most of the studies failed to demonstrate any significant relationship between the history of BPH and the development of prostatic adenocarcinoma, some common features in the natural history of these diseases and the frequent incidental findings of prostate cancer in TURP specimens may be considered as a sufficient reason for further studies.[19]

Impact of the ageing of the population on the prostate gland diseases

Life expectancy at birth has increased dramatically throughout this century. In many westernized countries, life expectancy of a boy or girl born today can be expected to approach 80 years. Furthermore, those born in the post-World War II 'baby boom' are approaching the age of 50 and early next century will attain an age when both cancer and prostatism become an important health concern. Unfortunately, little work has been undertaken to quantify the impact of this ageing process in years to come. However, the effect of the ageing that has already occurred is evident in the increasing burden of urological cancers around the world.

The ageing of the United States population has been well described by Brody.[20] In Europe less work has been done, although some data are available from United Nations publications in recent years. In qualitative terms it is clear where the major changes will take place in the elderly population in Europe:

1. In *Northern Europe*, the all ages population will increase between 1975 and 2000 by 3% in men and 2% in women. The population of Northern Europe for those over 60 will increase by 4% in men and 1% in women.
2. In *Western Europe*, the overall changes will be 3% in men and 1% in women. However, in those over 60 years there will be major changes, with a 20% increase in men and an 11% increase in women.
3. In *Eastern Europe*, the all ages population will increase by 15% in men and 13% in women. Lower life expectancy will limit the increases in the over 60 years population to 12% in both sexes.
4. In *Southern Europe*, the all ages population will increase by 15% in men and 14% in women. The over 60 population will increase by 24% in men and 27% in women.

With diseases so strongly linked to age, as is the case with BPH and prostate cancer, the greatest qualitative increase in the absolute numbers of cases of prostatic diseases will be experienced in Southern Europe, with substantial increases taking place also in Eastern and Western Europe, the latter related to the loss of life in generations affected by the two major wars that Europe experienced this century.

Descriptive epidemiology of BPH

Despite the high prevalence and public health impact, it is only recently that there has been any significant degree of interest in BPH epidemiology or in the natural history of the untreated disease. Although being a major cause of urinary problems in elderly men, BPH was not identified as a disease entity until the 19th century and it was only during the present (20th) century that effective treatment became available.[21] It has taken even longer for reliable and meaningful epidemiological information to become available about this condition.

BPH is one of the pathological conditions whose presenting symptoms are prostatism.[22] Several recent studies provide some indication of the distribution of symptoms of prostatism in the general population, and these are described below.

Descriptive epidemiology of prostatism

An important consideration to bear in mind when interpreting the prevalence/incidence figures for BPH derived from autopsy and clinical series is that not all BPH is symptomatic and not every case of prostatism is BPH. Thus some of the clinic-based material will be based on only symptomatic men. It is not clear what aspects of the disease relate to symptom development: it has, on the other hand, been shown consistently that symptomatology correlates poorly with prostatic size.[23]

A diagnosis of BPH is generally made in the clinic, based on clinical diagnosis and diagnostic criteria, or at surgery for clinically diagnosed BPH or at autopsy. A great deal of current knowledge regarding the prevalence of BPH comes from autopsy series. However, these are very selective in terms of who gets autopsied, and to make statements about population prevalence from such data is problematic.[6]

Each source of the diagnosis contains differing problems of potential errors and biases and all suffer, to a greater or lesser degree, from the potential problem of not having a clear definition of a source population (population at risk) to allow calculation of incidence or population-prevalence rates. Such considerations must always be borne in mind when evaluating the available data.

Berry et al.[2] summarized the information relating to BPH at autopsy and age from five studies. No prostate removed from men younger than 30 was found to contain BPH, and the prevalence of BPH rose with each age group, attaining a peak of 88% in men aged over 80.

Analysis of data from 6975 male patients who underwent life insurance examinations revealed that 20% of men in the sixth decade of life and 43% in the eighth decade had palpable enlargement of the prostate (a limitation to the reliability of this finding revolves around the findings being based on rectal palpation and performed by a substantial number of physicians). Lytton et al.[24] presented these data (first published in 1940) in such a way as to allow calculation of the prevalence of palpable prostatic enlargement by age. These findings show the rise in the prevalence of enlargement with age, although the levels attained are less than those found in the autopsy material.[2]

Despite some limitations to these studies, it can be concluded that BPH is a very common condition in males aged over 50 years and, in those over 80 the histological criteria for BPH can be fulfilled in up to 88% of subjects (see Chapter 10). Rotkin[25] observed that the frequency of symptomatic BPH in American men aged over 50 ranged between 50 and 70% in most series.

These striking estimates are complemented from the publication of the Veterans Administration Normative Aging Study, which followed 2036 volunteers and applied standards of clinical and surgical diagnosis of BPH. Using life-table methods, it was estimated from these data that the lifetime probability of surgical treatment for BPH was 29%.[4] In other words, three men in ten can currently expect to have surgical treatment for BPH in the absence of effective alternative therapy. This figure is higher than that calculated in the 1960s, when Lytton et al.[24] estimated that a 40-year-old man had a 10% chance of requiring surgery for BPH before he was 80.

The incidence of surgically treated BPH was recently investigated in a follow-up of 14 897 men (2175 Blacks and 12 722 Whites) receiving multiphasic health checks in the Kaiser Permanente Medical Care Program.[26] As expected, the incidence of prostate cancer was found to be higher among Blacks [the age-adjusted relative risk was 1.8 (1.4, 2.3)]. The incidence rate of surgically treated BPH was found to be somewhat higher in Blacks until the age of 65, after which it was higher among Whites. However, the age-adjusted risk of surgically treated BPH was the same for Blacks relative to Whites [odds ratio (OR) = 1.0; 95% CI 0.8, 1.2].

An important population survey has been conducted among men in Scotland.[27] Briefly, all men aged between 40 and 79 years in one community, and who were registered with a group general practice, were invited to complete a urinary symptom score and to undergo uroflowmetry. A total of 705 men (77% of those eligible) participated in the study and 214 (84% of those invited) of them were found to have signs and symptoms of prostatic dysfunction; they subsequently underwent TRUS for assessment of their prostate volume and, by inference, its weight. The prevalence rate of benign prostatic hypertrophy (sic) (defined as an enlargement of the prostate gland equivalent to a weight of more than 20 g in the presence of symptoms of urinary dysfunction and/or a urinary peak flow rate of less than 15 ml/s and without evidence of malignancy) was found to be 253 (95% CI 221, 285) per 1000 men in the community, rising from 138 per 1000 men aged 40–49 years to 430 per 1000 men aged 60–60 years. It could be concluded that apparently well men have a much higher frequency of BPH than previously shown by necropsy studies and other survey methods.

A similar study was conducted in Olmsted County, Minnesota among men aged 40–79 years and with no history of prostate or other urological surgery and who were also free from conditions associated with symptoms of neurogenic bladder.[28] Non-response-corrected scores for a composite of obstructive symptoms showed moderate to severe symptomatology among 13% of men aged 40–49 and 28% of men aged over 70 years. These figures were very similar to those obtained in a recent analysis of the Baltimore Longitudinal Study of Aging.[29] The similarity of these findings, and the large difference between these and the Scottish figures,[27] suggested that the difference between Scottish and American men could be cultural in origin.[28]

A large-scale survey of over 2000 men in the French population[30] also revealed quite different results from those obtained from Scotland.[27] The age-specific prevalence rates of prostatism in France and Scotland were respectively 80 and 237 per 1000 at age 50–59: 140 and 430 per 1000 at age 60–69; and 270 and 430 per 1000 at age 70–79 years. The French survey differed from the others in that it attempted to recruit a representative national sample and employed trained interviewers working throughout France to obtain the data.

At the present time, prostatism clearly represents an important disease for men and a major public health problem in many parts of the world. The focus of

attention in the contemporary management of BPH revolves around patient choices and quality of life. Surgery is effective and very safe, even in the elderly group of men affected by the condition, although there is still some discussion about increased post-surgical mortality rates in men receiving TURP compared with open prostatectomy.[31] The current era of BPH management, characterized by the focus on quality-of-life issues, is in sharp contrast to the situation of only 30 years ago when death from this condition was an important consideration.[32] A systematic analysis of all data available in the World Health Organization (WHO) Mortality Database between 1950 and 1990 revealed the mortality rates from BPH (i.e. deaths where it was decided that the underlying cause of death was BPH) have fallen in developed countries by an order of magnitude between the early 1950s and the late 1980s. The declines seen in western countries such as the United States, where 13 500 men fewer die each year now than would be expected if the mortality rates from the early 1950s still prevailed, indicate that this decline represents a considerable achievement for modern medicine. Unfortunately, such declines have not been observed to the same extent in countries of Central and Eastern Europe and South America.[32]

Temporal trends in BPH

In 1950–1954, the highest mortality rate from BPH was 22.9 per 100 000, in Denmark. In 24 countries with data available for this time period, 17 had a mortality rate that was greater than 10 per 100 000. In 1985–1989, data were available from 61 countries and in only one (Saint Vincent and Grenadines) was the mortality rate greater than 10 per 100 000.

The mortality rate from BPH has been declining noticeably in most developed countries. The decline is most notable in developed western countries such as the United States, Canada, Australia, New Zealand and the countries of Western Europe. The death rate has been decreasing much more slowly in countries of Central and Eastern Europe and is even stable in recent time periods. Rates in the former USSR, Byelorussian SSR and Ukrainian SSR are still very high but the only data available are the recent time periods excluding the examination of secular trends. High death rates are still observed from countries of South America.

Currently, there is still a cluster of countries around the Caribbean with high mortality rates. Although the number of cases in many of these countries is small, the rates appear to exhibit a tendency to stability over a period of time. For example, the death rates are still high in Trinidad, at 6.8 per 100 000 based on an average of 29 deaths per annum. In Saint Vincent and Grenadines the mortality rates appear to be consistently high, although based on very small numbers of deaths.

In the United States, the age-adjusted rate fell from 7.5 per 100 000 in 1950–1954 to reach 0.3 per 100 000 in 1985–1989. The (age-adjusted) relative risk of death in 1987 was only 6% of that in 1957. The largest declines have taken place in the oldest age groups. In absolute terms, this represents a decline from an average of 6261 deaths per annum in the period 1950–1954 to a total of 470 deaths per annum in 1985–1989. This is a saving of 5791 lives each year at least, since there are more men currently in these older age groups.

In the United Kingdom, the age-adjusted rate fell from 16.5 per 100 000 in 1950–1954 to reach 1.2 per 100 000 in 1985–1989. The (age-adjusted) relative risk of death in 1987 was only 9% of that in 1957. The largest declines have taken place in the oldest age groups. In absolute terms, this represents a decline from an average of 5027 deaths per annum in the period 1950–1954 to a total of 591 deaths per annum in 1985–1989. This is a saving of at least 4436 lives each year.

This estimate makes no allowance for the increased number of men in the oldest age groups in 1990, which would serve to increase further the magnitude of the decline seen. A better indication of the number of deaths prevented can be obtained by calculating expected numbers of deaths based on 1950s age-specific rates applied to 1990 populations. The age-specific rates for countries were calculated using the earliest 5 years of data available: this was generally 1950–1954. These rates were applied to the population of 1990; the expected number of deaths was calculated for each country and compared with the number of deaths observed (Table 46.1). In the United States, 449 deaths were observed in 1990 compared with 14 130 expected had the mortality rates of 1950–1954 applied: thus, an estimated 13 681 deaths were prevented in that single year. Similar figures are seen for the United Kingdom

(8706 deaths prevented), Federal Republic of Germany (9617), Italy (4700), France (2884) and Japan (875) (Table 46.1).

In Japan, the age-adjusted rate was initially lower at 1.2 per 100 000 per annum. This increased to 1.9 in 1965–1969 before falling to 0.4 per 100 000 in 1985–1989. In absolute terms this represents a slight increase from 260 deaths per annum in 1950–1954 to 269 deaths per annum in 1985–1989.

During the period examined (1957–1987) there was no country in which the age-adjusted mortality rate

Table 46.1. *Deaths from BPH observed in 1990 compared with those expected based on the application of age-specific rates for the first 5 years of data availability (usually 1950–1954) to the population of 1990 in selected countries*

Country	Deaths		
	Expected	Observed	Prevented
Canada	1750	65	1685
United States	14 130	449	13 681
Chile	360	153	207
Uruguay	185	23	162
Venezuela	208	80	128
Australia	1656	74	1582
New Zealand	279	27	252
Belgium	730	50	680
Denmark	1134	66	1069
France	3181	297	2884
Germany	9944	327	9617
Ireland	280	22	258
Italy	5203	503	4700
Netherlands	1802	142	1660
Portugal	416	36	380
Spain	1598	234	1364
United Kingdom	9171	465	8706
Austria	846	40	806
Finland	454	32	422
Norway	776	66	710
Sweden	1248	66	1182
Switzerland	1062	46	1016
Czechoslovakia	913	347	566
Hungary	718	161	557
Japan	1076	201	875

increased: in Mexico it remained virtually unchanged. In Central and Eastern Europe, rates have changed slowly but remain high, as do mortality rates in South America. However, countries in North America, Western and Northern Europe and the Caucasian populations of Australasia have experienced falls in the mortality rate from BPH over this 30-year period that have been greater than an order of magnitude.

Descriptive epidemiology of prostate cancer

Prostate cancer is an important public health problem, with over one-quarter of a million new cases diagnosed worldwide in the single year 1985.[33] It was predicted that, in the United States alone, 38 000 men would die of prostate cancer in 1994,[7] while in the countries of the European Community it accounts for more than 35 000 deaths each year.[8]

The incidence of the disease is increasing steadily in many countries around the world[9] and will pass half a million cases worldwide by the end of the 20th century if risk remains fixed at 1980 levels, or could reach 700 000 or more if the observed trends to increase continue.[5] Whereas major increases in the incidence of prostate cancer are apparent throughout the world, the mortality rate has remained constant in generations of men born since the early years of this century.[9]

In the 12 Member States of the European Community, it is estimated that in 1980 there were 85 000 new cases of prostate cancer, making this the second commonest form of cancer (after lung cancer) in men.[8] In the United States, prostate cancer has overtaken lung cancer in terms of absolute incidence, although it remains second to lung cancer as a cause of cancer death. Most importantly, given that in several countries the increased number of children born after World War II will be in their mid-fifties in the early part of the 21st century (at an age when cancer risk is becoming an important consideration) and coupled with the trends in increasing life expectancy (see ref. 20, for example), the consequence will be an increase in absolute terms in the number of cases of prostate cancer diagnosed[1]. In the absence of treatment improvements and with prospects for prevention by modification of lifestyle remote within current knowledge, there will

also be an increase in the number of deaths from prostate cancer worldwide. The situation would be further augmented by the presence of a temporal trend in risk that is widely reported from many countries and unlikely to be entirely artefactual.[1]

Higher rates in Black men than in White men, increases in overall trends in incidence and mortality rates and large geographical variations in occurrence are distinctive and recognized features of the descriptive epidemiology of prostate cancer.[34] The leading 23 rates of prostate cancer are reported from North America and the Black population of Bermuda. The highest rates of prostate cancer have been recorded in the Black population of the United States and are now at over 100 per 100 000; the lowest incidence rates (Asia and northern Africa) are around 1, indicating a 100-fold difference in the incidence of prostate cancer worldwide. In the United States, incidence rates of prostate cancer are higher in Afro-Americans than in Caucasians. The relative risk for prostate cancer in Afro-Americans is generally reported as around a factor of 1.7 when compared with Caucasians.

In contrast to the distribution pattern of overt prostatic cancers, the frequency of the smaller non-invasive lesions denoted 'latent' carcinoma does not appear to show much international variation.[35] This observation itself presents further difficulties in interpreting the international prostate cancer incidence pattern. The lifetime cumulative risk of prostate cancer (until age 75) approaches 10% in some population groups at present, compared with the 40% incidence of latent prostate carcinoma found in men over the age of 80 years.[11,36] This makes prostate cancer a unique malignancy with a very high prevalence of histologically identified tumours and relatively low clinical manifestation. Adenocarcinoma of the prostate, although exhibiting the histological signs of malignancy, may never have been life-threatening or have caused any clinical symptom in the lifetime of the individual. Obviously, any medical procedures or 'tests' that can detect such prostate cancers will have the effect of increasing reported incidence in the absence of any real increase in underlying risk.[37,38] TURP for BPH is normally accompanied by histological examination of all fragments removed and in 8–22% of all TURPs an incidental diagnosis of prostate cancer is made.[11,39]

Again, it is obvious that the increases in TURP rates since the 1970s will have led to corresponding increases in prostate cancer cases reported to the cancer registry: in fact, in Scotland this phenomenon appears to account for all the increase seen in the reported incidence rate of prostate cancer between 1977 and 1988.[9]

Japanese migrants to the United States have experienced a marked increase in prostatic cancer, although the rates of the Japanese in the San Francisco Bay area and in Los Angeles are still less than one-half of those of Whites.[40] Contrasts between United States Chinese and those elsewhere are even greater. In Singapore, the risk in foreign-born Chinese was 70% of that in the Singapore-born Chinese over 1968–1982. Polish migrants to the States also acquired higher mortality rates on migration,[41] again emphasizing the influence of environmental factors on the risk of this form of cancer. Recent studies suggests that several weak oestrogenic components of the predominantly vegetarian diet in Asian countries may have a protective role in the development of latent adenocarcinoma to clinical prostate cancer.[42]

Another feature of prostate cancer is the association between incidence (and mortality) rates and age, which is more striking than that for most other cancers. From an incidence rate of the order of 1–2 per 100 000 per annum in men in their 40s, the incidence rises dramatically to peak at 1200 per 100 000 in White men and 1600 per 100 000 in Afro-American men in their 80s. This association with age has enormous consequences for the future. Assuming that age-specific incidence rates remain fixed at 1980 levels, the number of cases of prostate cancer in men aged over 65 in the European Community will rise through 80 000 in 1990 to 92 000 in the year 2000. This increase in numbers of cases will be seen in every one of the 12 Member States, being most pronounced in France, Germany and Spain[1] because in these countries, life expectancy is increasing: boys at birth can now expect to live to 80 years of age.[20] More and more men, living to older ages, will result in increases in the absolute number of cases of prostate cancer diagnosed, even if the risk to an individual man remains fixed at 1980 levels. This increase is programmed to continue into the 21st century and to be exacerbated in many countries because, as mentioned earlier, those born in the post-World War II 'baby boom'

will be in their early 50s in the year 2000 and as they age will be prone to increasing numbers of cancers. This is the first group of men expected to go through life without the twin hazards of high infant mortality rates and a devastating war.

Temporal trends in prostate cancer incidence

Prostate cancer incidence data are currently available for over 160 cancer registries throughout the world.[43] However, few of them have long temporal series available covering uninterrupted time spans. Table 46.2 presents data covering over 25 years regarding prostate cancer incidence in selected cancer registries internationally. It is clear that there has been an increasing incidence of prostate cancer throughout the time period. Overall in Europe,[44] the incidence is increasing in the Nordic countries and Switzerland at between 5 and 10% every 5 years. In Hungary (Szabolcs and Vas), Spain (Navarra) and Italy (Varese) the incidence rates are lower but the rate of increase observed is greater, being over 20% every 5 years. The rate of increase is slightly less in France (Bas-Rhin) and the United Kingdom. The exception to this general increase is the significant and steady decline in Warsaw City (Poland), which is interesting but may reflect a local departure from the national pattern in Poland, where mortality is still increasing.[44] Taken together, the data from Southern Europe suggest that prostate cancer is increasing more rapidly than elsewhere in Europe, at more than 25% every 5 years.

In North America, there have also been considerable increases in the age-standardized incidence rate of prostate cancer. In Connecticut, generally considered the gold standard of United States cancer registries, the incidence rate has increased from 33.8 per 100 000 person-years to 42.7 over the 25-year period (Table 46.2). Large increases have taken place in other United States registries and they are also apparent in Canada. Overall, the increases in North American populations are substantial, being in the order of 15–25% every 5 years.[44] The incidence is generally rising more rapidly in Afro-American men than among Caucasian men.[44] Such are the underlying trends in the risk of prostate cancer that the lifetime risk for an Afro-American born around 1915 is 10% whereas the lifetime risk for an Afro-American born around 1940 appears to be closer to 15%.

Table 46.2. *Incidence of prostate cancer in selected cancer registries, 1960–1985*

Cancer registry	Incidence of prostate cancer (cases per 100 000 person-years)					
	1966 (ref. 57)	1970 (ref. 58)	1976 (ref. 59)	1982 (ref. 60)	1987 (ref. 62)	1992 (ref. 43)
Canada, Manitoba	30.59	31.06	37.62	43.22	44.36	54.71
Canada, Saskatchewan	33.43	39.04	39.01	46.13	57.58	52.99
US, Alameda: White	*	38.03	40.38	44.46	49.56	55.24
US, Alameda: Black	*	65.26	75.02	100.20	87.85	93.47
US, Connecticut	33.84	33.03	37.73	42.66	*	*
US, Connecticut: White	*	*	*	*	46.76	47.22
US, Connecticut: Black	*	*	*	*	72.28	65.00
India, Bombay	*	6.54	7.97	6.85	8.20	6.90
Japan, Miyagi	3.83	3.23	2.74	4.88	6.28	7.81
Denmark	17.71	19.45	21.76	23.02	27.74	29.88
Finland	17.56	17.43	22.67	27.17	34.23	36.11
Norway	25.04	29.80	33.07	38.89	42.04	43.83
Sweden	26.51	33.47	38.80	44.36	45.89	50.20
UK, Birmingham	17.30	18.39	17.70	18.57	18.90	24.97
New Zealand: non-Maori	*	39.95	25.91	30.66	33.32	35.38

*No data available for this period.

Increases have also taken place outside these developed countries with western cultures. In Japan, the overall incidence rate increased in Miyagi and Osaka Prefectures and there were increases in Singapore also, although the rates remain less than one-tenth those found in the United States. There was no increase in non-Maoris in New Zealand and in the population of Bombay in India (Table 46.2). In Shanghai (PR China) the incidence rate is low and unchanging and, although the rates in Chinese in Hong Kong and Singapore are approximately four times higher, the increases are small, being of the order of 6% every 5 years.[44]

Interpretation of these increases in incidence is not entirely straightforward. As discussed earlier, the entity recorded at a cancer registry ('prostate cancer') is the combination of three separate forms. Between registries, and within each registry as time advances, changes may take place in the incidence of prostate cancer recorded, owing to the influences of changes in either of the component entities. Thus, if there is a large increase in 'latent prostate cancer' due to an increased rate of TURP or widespread use of the prostate-specific antigen (PSA) test, this will influence the registration of prostate cancer and, hence, the overall incidence rate of prostate cancer recorded. Unfortunately, the data required to simplify interpretation of such changes are not available from the registries.

Another way to assess the magnitude of the problem of prostate cancer is by considering the cumulative lifetime (up to age 75) risk. Based on 1985 incidence and mortality rates remaining unchanged throughout their lifetime, White men in the United States have an 8.7% lifetime risk of developing prostate cancer and Afro-American men a lifetime risk of 9.4%.[45] With regard to mortality from prostate cancer, the lifetime risks among Whites and Afro-Americans in the United States are currently 2.6 and 4.3%, respectively.

Looking around the world, the age-adjusted incidence of prostate cancer is increasing at an average annual rate of around 3% per annum. Some of this increase is undoubtedly associated with diagnostic artefact, but the combined effect of this increase in incidence and the changing age structure of the population will be more pronounced for prostate cancer than for any other site in the majority of populations of the world. Again, assuming that the age-specific rates throughout the world remain fixed at their 1980 levels, the number of prostate cancers diagnosed throughout the world will increase from 235 000 in 1980 to 352 000 in 2000 if ageing is the only contribution considered. If, however, the temporal trend of increases in age-specific rate continues, the result will be to increase the total burden to 492 000 new cases in the year 2000. It is clear that, even though the incidence rate may increase noticeably, the ageing population will be the strongest determinant of the international prostate cancer burden in coming years.

Trends in mortality from prostate cancer

In view of the problems with 'latent carcinoma' of the prostate varying between countries for a variety of reasons, compounded recently by the increasing use of TURP as a treatment for BPH, which is associated with a 16% yield of unexpected focal carcinoma upon microscopical inspection,[11] and the increasing use of the PSA test for prostate cancer,[9] examination of mortality data may give a clearer picture of changes in life-threatening prostate cancer through time, particularly as there has been little change in survival after treatment.

There are two interesting features of trends in mortality from prostate cancer. First, the overall age-adjusted mortality rate is higher than the truncated rates (calculated on ages 35–64) and, secondly, the overall age-adjusted mortality rate increases much more rapidly than the truncated rates, if both are increasing.

In an attempt to investigate the nature of any changes in risk pattern for prostate cancer and to quantify any effect found, all available data in the WHO Mortality Database were employed in an age–period–cohort analysis of the changes in rates, conducted employing the method of DeCarli and La Vecchia.[46] In analysing and interpreting temporal changes in prostate cancer rates it is necessary to have mortality data available for a sufficiently long period and to be based upon large enough numbers of prostate cancer deaths to result in reasonably stable rates. Of more than 100 countries included in the WHO Mortality Database, 24 met the above criteria and have been included in the analysis of prostate cancer mortality rates.[47]

For each country, data have been analysed for ten 5-year age groups from 35–39 to 80–84 years and for

between six and eight 5-year time periods. Correspondingly, there are between 15 (1880–1950) and 17 (1870–1950) birth cohorts. For the first and last time periods, where data are not available for the whole of the 5-year period, rates have been based on years for which data are available. Results for time periods are expressed as relative risks, relative to the first available 5-year time period and for cohorts as risks relative to the birth cohort born during a period centred on 1915 — this was chosen as the earliest cohort that had data available in all the time periods considered. Cohort effects have been calculated for birth cohorts until 1940, because estimates for later cohorts are based on, at most, two observations.

The findings from statistical modelling indicate a clear pattern. First, the relative risks found in birth cohorts (relative to the 1910 cohort) are small. There is a clear pattern of increasing risk in cohorts until those born around 1910. Subsequently, in most countries the relative risk has either increased slowly or has remained fairly constant. In Scotland, England and Wales, Northern Ireland and the Irish Republic (Eire), there have been steady increases in risk among birth cohorts until those born in approximately 1900, and subsequent birth cohorts have experienced very little change in risk. There have been small and steady increases in risk in the grouping of Central and Eastern European countries [Austria, Hungary, Czechoslovakia and (the former Federal Republic of) Germany], which seem to have stabilized among cohorts born since approximately 1930. Similarly, small increases in risk have been experienced in Italy, Spain, Portugal, the Netherlands and Switzerland, which have also stabilized since around 1930. The patterns observed in the Nordic countries seem to be a little different, with more noticeable increases in risk taking place among recent birth cohorts. Despite a tenfold increase in risk between cohorts born around 1870 and 1910 in Japan, there has been a much smaller increase taking place in subsequent birth cohorts. There have been very few changes throughout the entire period of observation in cohort-specific prostate cancer risks in the populations of Australia, New Zealand, Canada and the United States.[47]

It appears that the risk of dying from prostate cancer has remained unchanged in many countries throughout this century. The increasing availability of TURP and the extensive use of currently available diagnostic modalities (PSA, TRUS and needle biopsies) may have resulted in a considerable increase in detection of clinically otherwise asymptomatic prostate cancers. The type of cancer found in such circumstances, generally T1a–c, is not commonly lethal and in many instances does not interfere with the normal lifespan of the man.[48] The small latent prostate cancers are considered to have lower potential for malignant behaviour.[49] Both 5- and 10-year survival rates for stage T1a–c prostatic adenocarcinomas are reported in many studies as around 75–87%,[50,51] and average local and/or distant progression rates are rarely reported as more than 10%.[18] This may explain the differences observed in the temporal trends in incidence and mortality from prostate cancer. The detection of 'latent' prostate cancers may expose a large number of patients with this usually non-fatal disease to the risks of surgical treatment, probably with little — if any — improvement in clinical outcome.[38,52]

Discussion and conclusions

The data currently available from descriptive epidemiological studies of BPH and prostate cancer indicate that these diseases constitute an important public health problem in many countries. Furthermore, they are both problems that seem set to increase in absolute terms and, in the case of prostate cancer incidence, in risk as well. Given the strong association between age and the occurrence rate of these conditions and the ageing of the population in those developed countries where these diseases are commonest, the number of men who develop either BPH or cancer will increase rapidly in the coming decade and beyond.

BPH is a very common condition (88% of autopsy specimens in men aged over 80 have histological BPH) and the cause of the commonest surgical procedure in elder men. Epidemiological data suggest that a 40-year-old man who survives to age 80 has a 10% chance of undergoing a TURP for BPH.[53] However, little is known with any certainty about the epidemiology of BPH. The incidence, even the population prevalence, is difficult to determine, for a variety of reasons associated with difficulties surrounding the diagnosis of BPH and

the identification of a source population to provide a denominator to calculate rates.

Lack of information on the natural history of untreated BPH has been identified as one of the major reasons underlying current controversies regarding indications for therapy. The standard treatments for BPH have traditionally been surgical, initially open prostatectomy but more recently TURP has dominated, and alternative therapies are more recent developments: these include medical therapy with alpha-blockers, 5-alpha-reductase inhibitors, antibiotics and plant extracts and innovative treatment approaches using hyperthermia and lasers.[54] The move from surgery has been driven to a large extent by quality-of-life issues and this is a major factor in the introduction of modern approaches to the treatment of BPH.

Surgery of BPH is effective and generally safe, even in this elderly group of men, although there is still considerable discussion about increased post-surgical mortality rates in men given TURP as compared with open prostatectomy.[31] Although this aspect of BPH was a common cause of death in elderly men just 20–30 years ago, improved medical care has seen dramatic reductions in mortality rates and, today, treatment choices in BPH are largely determined by considerations of quality of life.[5]

There is always the possibility of bias when comparing causes of death between countries and between time periods. It is credible that a physician may be less likely to think of BPH as a cause of death today then 30 years ago; however, that cannot begin to explain the order of magnitude of the declines observed in western countries with good-quality death certification schemes. These declines had generally taken place by the beginning of the end of the 1970s and the downward changes in the 1980s were not very marked.

It could be proposed that the greatest contribution to these declines has come from improvements in surgery and anaesthesia. Undoubtedly, the improved ability to visualize the operation and the ability to train surgeons in TURP by video monitoring has contributed to the improving safety of the procedure. With the tendency towards more and safer TURPs being accompanied by improvements in anaesthesia and improved medical management of the postoperative period, the resultant improvement in medical care has contributed in major part to the declining mortality rate. Such declines have taken place more rapidly and effectively in the major developed countries and there remains significant room for improvements in the outcome of care in Central and Eastern Europe and South America. This could be done with education programmes and by introducing state-of-the-art treatment schedules and materials in a widespread manner. Whatever their aetiology, these declines constitute an important contribution to the health of men and represent a considerable achievement for modern medicine.[32]

Like BPH, prostate cancer is a remarkably common disease in elderly men. Descriptive epidemiology has highlighted the wide geographical variation in prostate cancer occurrence and the large increases taking place in the reported incidence of the disease worldwide.[47] Even if age-specific incidence rates remain stable, the problem of prostate cancer seems sure to increase in absolute terms, simply because of the ageing of the population. Life expectancy at birth in many western countries is still increasing and 50% of boys today can expect to reach the age of 80 years. This has major implications for the future burden of prostate cancer.

Estimates of the population projections for many countries are available from United Nations publications. By simply taking these data and applying the 1985 age-specific estimated rates, it is clear that the absolute numbers of prostate cancers will increase consistently throughout the coming decades. There were an estimated 198 000 cases diagnosed in 1975,[55] which rose to 235 000 in 1980,[56] and to 290 000 in 1985.[33] Application of these 1980 rates to future populations reveals that the number of new cases of prostate cancer will be approximately 352 000 in the year 2000. However, given that the incidence of prostate cancer is increasing at around 3% per annum globally, the superimposition of this effect will see the estimated prostate cancer burden rise to 500 000. These figures were based on the incidence rates for 1980 and probably have been overtaken by events such as increasing TURP in many countries and increasing use of PSA testing. The net result could be closer to 700 000 if the international trends in the use of these tests continues.[5]

It is apparent that BPH and prostate cancer have important implications for the provision of health care in the next century. However, many aspects of the epidemiology of these diseases are poorly understood. The distribution of prostatism, which may indicate the prevalence of BPH, is unknown in many parts of the world. It was the great variation demonstrated in the incidence of prostate cancer that provided the first clues as to where to look for factors involved in the aetiology of the disease. However, for a disease that currently presents a near 10% lifetime risk in North Americans, knowledge of risk factors is extremely limited. Given the ageing population and the attainment early next century, by those born in the post-World War II baby-boom, of ages where BPH and prostate cancer begin to assume public health significance, the need for a better understanding of descriptive epidemiology and risk factors is obvious and it is clear that a major effort is required to reduce the impact of these diseases.

Acknowledgements

It is a pleasure to acknowledge the support of the Associazione Italiana per la Ricerca sul Cancro (Italian Association for Cancer Research). Dr Napalkov is supported by a Pfizer Fellowship in Urological Epidemiology.

References

1. Boyle P. Prostate cancer 2000: evolution of an epidemic of unknown origin. In: Denis L (ed) Prostate cancer 2000. Heidelberg: Springer-Verlag, 1994, 5–11
2. Berry S J, Coffey D S, Walsh P C, Ewing L L. The development of human benign prostatic hyperplasia with age. J Urol 1984; 132: 474–479
3. Isaacs J T. Epidemiology and natural history of benign prostatic hyperplasia. In: Prostate et Alpha-Bloquants. Amsterdam: Elsevier Science/Excerpta Medica, 1989: 219–227
4. Glynn R J, Campion E W, Bouchard G R, Silbert J E. The development of benign prostatic hyperplasia among volunteers in the Normative Ageing Study. Am J Epidemiol 1985; 121: 78–90
5. Boyle P. New insights into the epidemiology and natural history of benign prostatic hyperplasia. In: Kurth K, Newling D W W (eds) Benign prostatic hyperplasia. Recent progress in clinical research and practice. New York: Wiley-Liss, 1994, 3–18
6. Boyle P, McGinn R, Maisonneuve P, La Vecchia C. Epidemiology of benign prostatic hyperplasia: present knowledge and studies needed. Eur Urol 1991; 20: 3–10
7. Boring C C, Squires T S, Tong T. Cancer statistics. CA 1994; 44: 7–26
8. Jensen O M, Esteve J, Moller H, Renard H. Cancer in the European Community and its Member States. Eur J Cancer 1990; 26: 1167–1256
9. Alexander F E, Boyle P. The rise in prostate cancer: myth or reality? In: Garraway M J (ed) The epidemiology of prostate diseases. Edinburgh: Churchill Livingstone, 1995

10. Boyle P, Alexander F E, Luchini L, Bishop T. Aetiology of prostate cancer. In: Garraway M J (ed) The epidemiology of prostate diseases. Edinburgh: Churchill Livingstone, 1995

11. Epstein J I, Walsh P C, Brendler C B. Radical prostatectomy for impalpable prostate cancer: the Johns Hopkins experience with tumours found on transurethral resection (stages T1a and T1b) and on needle biopsy (stage T1c). J Urol 1994; 152: 1721–1729

12. Bostwick D G, Balcells S F, Cooner W H et al. Benign prostatic hyperplasia (BPH) and cancer of the prostate. In: Cockett A T K, Aso Y, Chatelain C et al. (eds) The International Consultation on benign prostatic hyperplasia (BPH). Jersey, Channel Islands: SCI 1992: 139–159

13. McNeal J E. Normal anatomy of the prostate and changes in benign prostatic hypertrophy and carcinoma. Semin Ultrasound CT MR 1988; 9: 329–334

14. Armenian H K, Lilienfeld A M, Diamond E L, Bross I D J. Relation between benign prostatic hyperplasia and cancer of the prostate: a prospective and retrospective study. Lancet 1974; ii: 115–117

15. Greenwald P, Kirmss V, Polan A K, Dick V S. Cancer of the prostate among men with benign prostatic hyperplasia. J Natl Cancer Inst 1974; 53: 335–340

16. Simons B D, Morrison A S, Young R H, Verhoek-Oftedahl W. The relation of surgery for prostatic hypertrophy to carcinoma of the prostate. Am J Epidemiol 1993; 138: 294–300

17. Hammarsten J, Andersson S, Holmen A et al. Does transurethral resection of a clinically benign prostate gland increase the risk of developing clinical prostate cancer? A 10-year follow-up study. Cancer 1994; 74: 2347–2351

18. Kearse W S Jr, Seay T M, Thompson I M. The long-term risk of development of prostate cancer in patients with benign prostatic hyperplasia: correlation with stage A1 disease. J Urol 1993; 150: 1746–1748

19. Griffiths K, Harper M E, Eaton C L et al. Endocrine aspects of prostate cancer. In: Denis L (ed) Prostate cancer 2000. Heidelberg: Springer-Verlag, 1994: 21–39

20. Brody J. Prospects for an aging population. Nature 1985; 315: 463–466

21. Steg A. Chronicle of achievements in the history of benign prostatic hyperplasia. Oxford: Oxford Clinical Communications, 1992

22. Schroder F H, Blom J H M. Natural history of benign prostatic hyperplasia (BPH). Prostate 1989; (suppl 2): 17–22

23. Isaacs J T, Coffey D S. Etiology and disease process of benign prostatic hyperplasia. Prostate 1989; (suppl 2): 35–50

24. Lytton B, Emery J M, Harvard B M. The incidence of benign prostatic hyperplasia. J Urol 1968; 99: 639–645

25. Rotkin I D. Epidemiology of benign prostatic hypertrophy: review and speculations. In: Grayhack J T et al. (eds) Benign prostatic hyperplasia. DHEW Publ. No. (NIH) 76-1113. Washington DC: US Government Printing Office, 1976: 105–117

26. Sydney S, Quesenberry C P, Sadler M C et al. Risk factors for surgically treated benign prostatic hyperplasia in a pre-paid health care plan. Urology 1991; 38: 13–19

27. Garraway W M, Collins G N, Lee R J. High prevalence of benign prostatic hypertrophy in the community. Lancet 1991; 338: 469–471

28. Chute C G, Panser L, Girman C J et al. The prevalence of prostatism: a population-based survey of urinary symptoms. J Urol 1993; 150: 85–89

29. Arrighi H M, Guess H A, Metter E J, Fozzard J L. Symptoms and signs of prostatism as risk factors for prostatectomy. Prostate 1990; 16: 253–261

30. Sagnier P P, Macfarlane C J, Richard F et al. Results of an epidemiological survey employing a modified American Urological Association symptom index for benign prostatic hyperplasia in France. J Urol 1994; 151: 1266–1270

31. Brendler C, Schlegel P, Dowd J et al. Surgical treatment for benign prostatic hyperplasia. Cancer 1992; 70(suppl): 371–373

32. Boyle P, Maisonneuve P, Steg A. Reduction in mortality from benign prostatic hyperplasia: a major unheralded health triumph. J Urol 1995

33. Parkin D M, Pisani P, Ferlay J. Estimates of the world wide incidence of eighteen major cancers in 1985. Int J Cancer 1993; 54: 594–606

34. Boyle P, Zaridze D G. Risk factors for prostate and testicular cancer. Eur J Cancer 1993; 29A-7: 1048–1055

35. Breslow N, Chan C W, Dhom G. Latent carcinoma of prostate at autopsy in seven areas. Int J Cancer 1977; 20: 680–688

36. McNeal J E. The prostate gland: morphology and pathobiology. Monogr Urol 1988; 9: 36–54

37. Severson R K. Have transurethral resection contributed to the increasing incidence of prostatic cancer? J Natl Cancer Inst 1990; 82: 1597–1598

38. Woolf H S. Public health perspective: the health policy implications of screening for prostate cancer. J Urol 1994; 152: 1685–1688

39. Murphy W M, Dean P J, Brasfield J A, Tatum L. Incidental carcinoma of the prostate. Am J Surg Pathol 1986; 10: 170–174

40. Haenszel W, Kurihara M. Studies of Japanese migrants: I. Mortality from cancer and other diseases among Japanese in the United States. J Natl Cancer Inst 1968; 40: 43–68

41. Staszewski J, Haenszel W. Cancer mortality among the Polish-born in the United States. J Natl Cancer Inst 1965; 35: 291–297

42. Griffiths K, Khoury S (eds) Primer on molecular control of prostate growth. Whitehouse Station, N J: Merck, 1994

43. Parkin D M, Muir C S, Whelan S et al. (eds) Cancer incidence in five continents, Vol 6. IARC Scientific Publication No. 120. Lyon: International Agency for Research on Cancer, 1992

44. Coleman M, Esteve J, Damiecki P et al. Trends in cancer incidence and morality. IARC Scientific Publication No. 121. Lyon: International Agency for Research on Cancer, 1993

45. Seidman H, Mushinski M H, Gelb S, Silverberg E. Probabilities of eventually developing or dying of cancer —United States 1985. CA 1985; 35: 36–60

46. DeCarli A, La Vecchia C. Age, period and cohort models: a review of knowledge and implementation in GLIM. Riv Stat Appl 1987; 20: 397–410

47. Boyle P, Evstifeeva T, Maisonneuve P et al. Temporal trends in prostate cancer mortality: is the risk rising? In: Cockett A B, Denis L, Aso Y et al. (eds) Proceedings of the Second International Consensus on Urological Disease. Oxford: Oxford University Press, 1995

48. Handley M R, Stuart M E. The use of prostate specific antigen for prostate cancer screening: a managed care perspective. J Urol 1994; 152: 1689–1692

49. McNeal J E, Viller A A, Redwine E A et al. Histologic differentiation, cancer volume, and pelvic lymph node metastasis in adenocarcinoma of the prostate. Cancer 1990; 66: 1225

50. Maeda O, Saiki S, Kinouchi T et al. Clinical study for incidental prostatic carcinoma. Hinyokika Kiyo 1991; 37: 135–139

51. Chodak G W, Thisted R A, Gerber G S et al. Results of conservative management of clinically localized prostate cancer. N Engl J Med 1994; 330: 242

52. Schwab L. Experts sharply divided on prostate cancer screening. J Natl Cancer Inst 1991; 83: 535–536

53. Barry M J. Epidemiology and natural history of benign prostatic hyperplasia. Urol Clin North Am 1990; 17: 495–507

54. Khoury S, Denis L. International consultation on benign prostatic hyperplasia. In: Kurth K, Newling D W W (eds) Benign prostatic hyperplasia. Recent progress in clinical research and practice. New York: Wiley-Liss, 1994: 617–624

55. Parkin D M, Dermaret E, Crosignani P C. The use of the computer in the cancer registry. Methods Inf Med 1983; 22: 151–155

56. Parkin D M, Laara E, Muir C S. Estimates of the worldwide frequency of sixteen major cancers in 1980. Int J Cancer 1988; 41: 184–197

57. Doll R, Payne P, Waterhouse J (eds) Cancer incidence in five continents, Vol 1. Lyon: International Agency for Research on Cancer, 1966

58. Doll R, Muir C S, Waterhouse J (eds) Cancer incidence in five continents, Vol 2. Lyon: International Agency for Research on Cancer, 1970

59. Waterhouse J, Muir C S, Correa P, Powell J (eds) Cancer incidence in five continents, Vol 3. IARC Scientific Publication No. 15. Lyon: International Agency for Research on Cancer, 1976

60. Waterhouse J, Muir C S, Shanmugaratnam K, Powell J (eds) Cancer incidence in five continents, Vol 4. IARC Scientific Publication No. 42. Lyon: International Agency for Research on Cancer, 1982

61. Muir C S, Waterhouse J A H, Mack T et al. (eds) Caner incidence in five continents, Vol 5. IARC Scientific Publication No. 88. Lyon: International Agency for Research on Cancer, 1987

Index